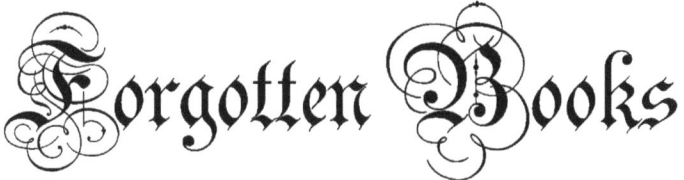
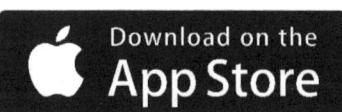
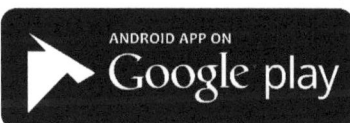

ISBN 978-1-332-09863-7
PIBN 10284380

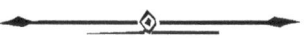

English
Français
Deutsche
Italiano
Español
Português

www.forgottenbooks.com

Mythology Photography **Fiction**
Fishing Christianity **Art** Cooking
Essays Buddhism Freemasonry
Medicine **Biology** Music **Ancient
Egypt** Evolution Carpentry Physics
Dance Geology **Mathematics** Fitness
Shakespeare **Folklore** Yoga Marketing
Confidence Immortality Biographies
Poetry **Psychology** Witchcraft
Electronics Chemistry History **Law**
Accounting **Philosophy** Anthropology
Alchemy Drama Quantum Mechanics
Atheism Sexual Health **Ancient History**
Entrepreneurship Languages Sport
Paleontology Needlework Islam
Metaphysics Investment Archaeology
Parenting Statistics Criminology
Motivational

THE
AMERICAN
ENCYCLOPEDIA AND DICTIONARY
OF
OPHTHALMOLOGY

EDITED BY
CASEY A. WOOD, M. D., C. M., D. C. L.

Professor of Ophthalmology and Head of the Department, College of Medicine, University of Illinois;
Late Professor of Ophthalmology and Head of the Department, Northwestern University
Medical School; Ex-President of the American Academy of Medicine, of the American
Academy of Ophthalmology. and of the Chicago Ophthalmological Society;
Ex-Chairman of the Ophthalmic Section of the American Medical
Association; Editor of a "System of Ophthalmic Therapeutics" and
a "System of Ophthalmic Operations"; Mitglied der Oph-
thalmologischen Gesellschaft, etc.; Ophthalmic
Surgeon to St. Luke's Hospital; Consulting
Ophthalmologist to Cook County
Hospital, Chicago, Ill.

ASSISTED BY A LARGE STAFF OF COLLABORATORS

FULLY ILLUSTRATED

Volume VIII—H. to Institutions for the Blind

CHICAGO
CLEVELAND PRESS
1916

INITIALS USED IN THIS ENCYCLOPEDIA TO IDENTIFY INDIVIDUAL CONTRIBUTORS

A. A.—ADOLF ALT, M. D., M. C. P. AND S. O., ST. LOUIS, MO.
Clinical Professor of Ophthalmology, Washington University, St. Louis, Mo.; Author of *Lectures on The Human Eye; Treatise on Ophthalmology for the General Practitioner; Original Contributions Concerning the Glandular Structures Appertaining to the Human Eye and its Appendages.* Editor of the *American Journal of Ophthalmology.*

.A. C. C. —ALFRED C. CROFTAN, PH. D., M. D., CHICAGO, ILL.
Author of *Clinical Urinology* and of *Clinical Therapeutics.* Member of the General Staff of the Michael Reese Hospital, Chicago. Formerly Physician-in-chief at St. Mary's Hospital; Physician to St. Elizabeth's Hospital; Physician to the Chicago Post-Graduate Hospital; Pathologist to St. Luke's Hospital. Late Professor of Medicine at the Chicago Post-Graduate College and the Chicago Polyclinic; Assistant Professor of Clinical Medicine, College of Physicians and Surgeons (University of Illinois); Member of the American Therapeutic Society.

A. E. B.—ALBERT EUGENE BULSON, JR., B. S., M. D., FORT WAYNE, IND.
Professor of Ophthalmology, Indiana University School of Medicine; Chairman of the Section on Ophthalmology of the American Medical Association; Ophthalmologist to St. Joseph Hospital, Allen County Orphans' Home, and the United States Pension Department; Editor of the *Journal of the Indiana State Medical Association,* etc.

A. E. H.—ALBERT E. HALSTEAD, M. D., CHICAGO, ILL.
Professor of Clinical Surgery, Northwestern University Medical School; Attending Surgeon, St. Luke's and Cook County Hospitals, Chicago; Consulting Surgeon, Illinois Charitable Eye and Ear Infirmary; Fellow American Surgical Association.

A. N. M.—ALFRED NICHOLAS MURRAY, M. D., CHICAGO, ILL.
Ophthalmologist, New Lake View Hospital. Formerly Clinical Assistant in Ophthalmology, and Assistant Secretary of the Faculty, Rush Medical College. Once Voluntary Assistant in the Universitaetes Augenklinik, Breslau. Author of *Minor Ophthalmic and Aural Technique.* Secretary, Physicians' Club of Chicago. Mitglied der Ophthalmologischen Gesellschaft, Heidelberg.

A. S. R.—ALEXANDER SANDS ROCHESTER, M. D., CHICAGO, ILL.
M. D. Jefferson Medical College; Ex-Chief, San Lazaro Contagious Hospital, Manila, P. I.; Adjunct Ophthalmologist to St. Luke's Hospital, Chicago.

B. C.—BURTON CHANCE, M. D., PHILADELPHIA, PA.
Assistant Surgeon, Wills Hospital, Philadelphia.

C. A. O.—CHARLES A. OLIVER (DECEASED).
Joint Editor of *A System of Diseases of the Eye;* Writer of numerous monographs on ophthalmic subjects.

iii

624255

C. E. W.—Lieut.-Col. Charles E. Woodruff, M. D., U. S. Army, Retired.

C. F. P.—Charles F. Prentice, M. E., New York City, N. Y.
President, New York State Board of Examiners in Optometry; Special Lecturer
on Theoretic Optometry, Columbia University, New York. Author of *A Treatise
on Ophthalmic Lenses* (1886); *Dioptric Formulæ for Combined Cylindrical
Lenses* (1888); *A Metric System of Numbering and Measuring Prisms (the
Prism-dioptry)* (1890); *The Iris as Diaphragm and Photostat* (1858), and
other optical papers.

C. H. B.—Charles Heady Beard (Deceased).
Surgeon to the Illinois Charitable Eye and Ear Infirmary (Eye Department);
Oculist to the Passavant Memorial Hospital and the North Star Dispensary
(Chicago); Member and Ex-president of the Chicago Ophthalmological Society;
Member of the American Ophthalmological Society, Etc. Author of *Ophthal-
mic Surgery* (1910); and of *Ophthalmic Semiology and Diagnosis* (1913).

C. P. S.—Charles P. Small, A. M., M. D., Chicago, Ill.
Late Clinical Assistant, Department of Ophthalmology, Rush Medical College.
Author of *A Probable Metastatic Hypernephroma of the Choroid.*

D. C. Mc.—Douglas C. McMurtrie, New York City.
Editor *American Journal of Care for Cripples;* former Secretary, American
Association for the Conservation of Vision; Author of *Education of and Occu-
pations for the Blind* in the *Reference Handbook of the Medical Sciences.*

D. H.—D'Orsay Hecht (Deceased).
Assistant Professor of Nervous and Mental Diseases, Northwestern University
Medical School; Consulting Neurologist to the Cook County Institutions for
the Insane at Dunning, Illinois; Attending Neurologist to the Michael Reese
and St. Elizabeth's Hospitals, Chicago.

D. W. G.—Duff Warren Greene (Deceased).
Formerly Oculist to the National Military Home, St. Elizabeth's Hospital, and
Ohio Soldiers' and Sailors' Orphans' Home, Xenia, Ohio.

E. C. B.—Edward C. Bull, Pasadena, Calif.

E. C. E.—Edward Coleman Ellett, B. A., M. D., Memphis, Tenn.
Professor of Ophthalmology, University of Tennessee, College of Medicine.

E. E. I.—Ernest E. Irons, M. D., Ph. D., Chicago, Ill.
Assistant Professor of Medicine, Rush Medical College; Assistant Attending
Physician, Presbyterian Hospital; Attending Physician, Cook County Hospital;
Consulting Physician, Durand Hospital of the Memorial Institute for Infec-
tious Diseases, Chicago.

E. H.—Emory Hill, A. B., M. D., Chicago, Ill.
Late House Surgeon, Wills Eye Hospital, Philadelphia; Assistant in Ophthal-
mology, Rush Medical College (in affiliation with the University of Chicago);
Assistant Ophthalmologist to the out-patient department of the Children's
Memorial Hospital, Chicago; Assistant Instructor in Ophthalmology, Chicago
Polyclinic. Member of American Academy of Ophthalmology and Oto-
Laryngology.

INDIVIDUAL CONTRIBUTORS

E. J.—EDWARD JACKSON, C. E., M. A., M. D., DENVER, COLO.
Professor of Ophthalmology in the University of Colorado; Former Chairman of the Section on Ophthalmology of the American Medical Association; Former President of the American Academy of Ophthalmology and Oto-Laryngology; The American Ophthalmological Society, and The American Academy of Medicine. Author of *Skiascopy and its Practical Application; Manual of Diseases of the Eye;* Editor of *Ophthalmic Year-Book* (nine volumes); *Ophthalmic Review; Ophthalmic Record;* and *Ophthalmic Literature.*

E. K. F.—EPHRAIM KIRKPATRICK FINDLAY, M. D., C. M., CHICAGO, ILL.
Assistant Clinical Professor of Ophthalmology, Medical Department, University of Illinois; Assistant Surgeon of the Illinois Charitable Eye and Ear Infirmary; Assistant Oculist at the University Hospital.

E. S. T.—EDGAR STEINER THOMSON, M. D., NEW YORK CITY, N. Y.
Surgeon and Pathologist, Manhattan Eye, Ear and Throat Hospital; Professor of Ophthalmology, New York Polyclinic Medical School and Hospital; Consulting Ophthalmologist to Perth Amboy and Ossining Hospitals; Member of the New York Academy of Medicine, New York Ophthalmological, and American Ophthalmological Societies. Author of *Electric Appliances and Their Use in Ophthalmic Surgery,* in Wood's *System of Ophthalmic Operations,* and various monographs.

F. A.—FRANK ALLPORT, M. D., LL. D., CHICAGO, ILL.
Ex-Professor, Ophthalmology and Otology, Minnesota State University; Ex-President, Minnesota State Medical Society; Ex-Chairman and Secretary, Ophthalmic Section, American Medical Association; Ex-Professor, Ophthalmology and Otology, Northwestern University Medical School; Ex-President, Chicago Ophthalmological Society. Author of *The Eye and Its Care;* Co-Author of *An American Text-Book of Diseases of the Eye, Ear, Nose and Throat; A System of Ophthalmic Therapeutics,* and *A System of Ophthalmic Operations.* Eye and Ear Surgeon to the Chicago Board of Education and to St. Luke's Hospital, Chicago.

F. C. T.—FRANK C. TODD, D. D. S., M. D., F. A. C. S., MINNEAPOLIS, MINN.
Professor of Ophthalmology and Chief of the Division of Eye, Ear, Nose and Throat, University of Minnesota, Medical Department; Chief of Eye, Ear, Nose and Throat Staff, University of Minnesota Hospitals; Eye, Ear, Nose and Throat Surgeon to Hill Crest Hospital; Eye Surgeon to the C. M. & St. P. R. R. Co., etc.; Chairman of the Section of Ophthalmology, A. M. A.; President of the Minnesota Academy of Ophthalmology and Oto-Laryngology; Vice-President of the A. M. A., etc. Monographs: *An Exact and Secure Tucking Operation for Advancing an Ocular Muscle; A Method of Performing Tenotomy which Enables the Operator to Limit the Effect as Required; Mules' Operation; Keratectasia; Report of a Case with Transparent Cornea; The Implantation of an Artificial Vitreous as a Substitute for Enucleation of the Eyeball; Simple Method of Suturing the Tendons in Enucleation; Malingering (Pretended Blindness); The Physiological and Pathological Pupil.*

F. E. B.—FRANK E. BRAWLEY, PH. G., M. D., CHICAGO, ILL.
Co-Author of *Commoner Diseases of the Eye, A System of Ophthalmic Therapeutics* and *A System of Ophthalmic Operations;* formerly voluntary assistant in the Universitaetes Augenklinik, Breslau, and the Royal London Ophthalmic Hospital (Moorfields); Oculist and Aurist to St. Luke's Hospital, Chicago. Editorial Secretary of *The Ophthalmic Record.*

F. P. L.—FRANCIS PARK LEWIS, M. D., BUFFALO, N. Y.
President American Association for the Conservation of Vision; President Board of Trustees N. Y. State School for the Blind; President N. Y. State Commissions for the Blind (1903 and 1906); Chairman Committee on Prevention of Blindness, American Medical Association; Ophthalmologist Buffalo State Hospital and Buffalo Homeopathic Hospital; Consulting Ophthalmologist J. N. Adam Memorial Hospital; Fellow Academy Ophthalmology and Oto-Laryngology.

G. C. C.—SEE *G. C. S.*

G. C. S.—G. C. SAVAGE, M. D., NASHVILLE, TENN.
Professor of Ophthalmology in the Medical Department of Vanderbilt University; Ex-President of the Nashville Academy of Medicine; Ex-President of the Tennessee State Medical Society. Author of *New Truths in Ophthalmology* and *Ophthalmic Myology*.

H. B. C.—H. BECKLES CHANDLER, C. M., M. D., BOSTON, MASS.
Professor Ophthalmology, Tufts Medical School, Boston; Senior Surgeon Massachusetts Charitable Eye and Ear Infirmary.

H. B. W.—HENRY BALDWIN WARD, A. B., A. M., PH. D., CHAMPAIGN, ILL.
Professor of Zoology, University of Illinois; Ex-Dean of the College of Medicine, University of Nebraska. Author of *Parasitic Worms of Man and the Domestic Animals; Data for the Determination of Human Entozoa; Iconographia Parasitorum Hominis; Human Parasites in North America.*

H. F. H.—HOWARD F. HANSELL, A. M., M. D., PHILADELPHIA, PA.
Professor of Ophthalmology, Jefferson Medical College; Emeritus Professor Diseases of the Eye, Philadelphia Polyclinic Hospital; Ophthalmologist to Jefferson Medical College Hospital; Ophthalmologist to Philadelphia Hospital.

H. G. L.—HENRY GLOVER LANGWORTHY, M. D., DUBUQUE, IOWA.
Surgeon to the Langworthy Eye, Ear, Nose and Throat Infirmary, Dubuque, Iowa; Member American Academy of Ophthalmology and Oto-Laryngology; of the Chicago Ophthalmological Society; of the American Medical Association, etc. Writer of numerous monographs on the special subjects of eye, ear, nose and throat.

H. S. G.—HARRY SEARLS GRADLE, A. B., M. D., CHICAGO, ILL.
Professor of Ophthalmology, Chicago Eye and Ear College; Director of Ophthalmic Clinic, West Side Free Dispensary; Member of the Ophthalmologische Gesellschaft, American Medical Association, American Academy of Ophthalmology and Oto-Laryngology.

H. V. W.—HARRY VANDERBILT WÜRDEMANN, M. D., SEATTLE, WASH.
Managing Editor, *Ophthalmology*, since 1904; Editorial Staff of the *Ophthalmic Record* since 1897; Managing Editor, *Annals of Ophthalmology*, 1897-1904. Member American Medical Association; Ex-Chairman Section on Ophthalmology, American Medical Association; Hon. Member, Sociedad Cientifica, Mexico; N. W. Wisconsin Medical Society and Philosophical Society. Fellow American Academy of Ophthalmology and Oto-Laryngology. Author of *Visual Economics* (1901); *Injuries to the Eye* (1912); *Bright's Disease and the Eye* (1912); and numerous monographs on the eye and its diseases. Collaborator on many other scientific books.

G. F. L.—GEORGE FRANKLIN LIBBY, M. D., OPH. D., DENVER, COLORADO.
Ex-Assistant Surgeon to the Maine Eye and Ear Infirmary; Ophthalmologist
to National Jewish Hospital for Consumptives, Mercy Hospital, and Children's
Hospital, Denver; and Denver, Laramie and North Western Railroad; Member
of the American Ophthalmological Society, Academy of Ophthalmology and
Oto-Laryngology, and Colorado Ophthalmological Society (its Secretary for six
years); Author of *Monocular Blindness of Fifty Years' Duration: Restoration
of Vision Following Hemiplegia; Polyps in the Lower Canaliculus; Silver Salts
in Ocular Therapeutics; Ocular Disease in Relation to Nasal Obstruction and
Empyema of the Accessory Sinuses (Bibl.); A Case of Complete Albinism:
Observations on the Changes in the Diameters of the Lens as Seen through the
Iris; Consanguinity in Relation to Ocular Disease; Heredity in Relation to the
Eye (doctorate thesis, Univ. of Colo., 1910); Acquired Symmetrical Opacities
of the Cornea of Unusual Type; Tuberculosis of the Bulbar Conjunctiva*, etc.

J. D. L.—JOSEPH D. LEWIS, A. M., M. D., MINNEAPOLIS, MINN.
Ophthalmic and Aural Surgeon to the Minneapolis City Hospital; Consulting Ophthalmic and Aural Surgeon to Hopewell Hospital and Visiting Nurses' Association; Member Minnesota Academy of Ophthalmology and Oto-Laryngology; Fellow American College of Surgeons.

J. G., JR.—JOHN GREEN, JR., A. B., M. D., ST. LOUIS, MO.
Assistant in Ophthalmology, Washington University Medical School; Ophthalmic Surgeon to St. Louis Children's Hospital; Ophthalmic Surgeon to St. Louis Eye, Ear, Nose and Throat Infirmary; Consulting Ophthalmic Surgeon to St. Louis Maternity Hospital; Consulting Ophthalmic Surgeon to St. John's Hospital, St. Louis.

J. L. M.—JOHN L. MOFFAT, B. S., M. D., O. ET A. CHIR., ITHACA, N. Y.
Editor *Journal of Ophthalmology, Otology and Laryngology*. Consulting Ophthalmic Surgeon, Cumberland Street Hospital, New York; Member (v.-p. 1905, 1908) American Homœopathic Ophthalmological, Otological and Laryngological Society; Member American Medical Editors' Association; Member (Senior) American Institute of Homœopathy; Senior Member (ex-pres.) New York State Homœopathic Medical Society; Senior Member (ex-pres.) Kings County (N. Y.) Homœopathic Medical Society; Honorary Member N. Y. County Homœopathic Medical Society.

J. M. B.—JAMES MOORES BALL, M. D., LL. D., ST. LOUIS, MO.
Dean and Professor of Ophthalmology, American Medical College of St. Louis, Medical Department of National University of Arts and Sciences. Author of *Modern Ophthalmology; Andreas Vesalius the Reformer of Anatomy.*

J. R. C.—JAMES RALEY CRAVATH, B. S., CHICAGO, ILL.
Electrical and Illuminating Engineer, Chicago; Vice-President, Illuminating Engineering Society; formerly associate editor *Electrical World;* joint-author *Practical Illumination* by CraVath and Lansingh; joint author *Light—Its Use and Misuse*, prepared by committee of the Illuminating Engineering Society; author of *Illumination and Vision; Tests of the Lighting of a Small Room;* and numerous other monographs.

L. H.—LUCIEN HOWE, M. A., M. D., SC. D., BUFFALO, N. Y.
Professor of Ophthalmology, University of Buffalo; Member of the Royal College of Surgeons of England; Fellow of the Royal Society of Medicine; Member of the *Ophthalmologische Gesellschaft* and of the *Société Française d'Ophthalmologie.* Author of *The Muscles of the Eye.*

M. S.—MYLES STANDISH, A. M., M. D., S. D., BOSTON, MASS.
Williams Professor of Ophthalmology, Harvard University; Consulting Ophthalmic Surgeon, Massachusetts Charitable Eye and Ear Infirmary and Carney Hospital, Boston, Mass.

N. M. B.—NELSON M. BLACK, PH. G., M. D., MILWAUKEE, WIS.
Author of *The Development of the Fusion Center in the Treatment of Strabismus; Examination of the Eyes of Transportation Employes; Artificial Illumination a Factor in Ocular Discomfort,* and other scientific papers.

P. A. C.—PETER A. CALLAN, M. D., NEW YORK CITY, N. Y.
Surgeon, New York Eye and Ear Infirmary; Ophthalmologist to St. Vincent's Hospital; Columbus Hospital and St. Joseph's Hospital, New York.

P. G.—PAUL GUILFORD, M. D., CHICAGO, ILL.
Ex-Resident Surgeon, Wills Eye Hospital, Philadelphia; Attending Oculist and Aurist, St. Luke's Hospital; Attending Oculist and Aurist, Chicago Orphan Asylum; Consulting Oculist and Aurist, South Side Free Dispensary. Co-Author of *A System of Ophthalmic Operations.*

R. D. P.—ROBERT D. PETTET, CHICAGO, ILL.
Author of *The Mechanics of Fitting Glasses.*

S. H. McK.—SAMUEL HANFORD McKEE, B. A., M. D., MONTREAL, QUE.
Lecturer in Pathology and Bacteriology, McGill University; Demonstrator in
Ophthalmology, McGill University; Assistant Oculist and Aurist to the Mont-·
real General Hospital; Oculist to the Montreal Maternity Hospital; Oculist to
the Alexandra Hospital; Member of The American Association of Pathologists
and Bacteriologists. Author of *The Bacteriology of Conjunctivitis; An Analysis of Three Hundred Cases of Morax-Axenfeld Conjunctivitis; Demonstration
of the Spirocheta Pallida from a Mucous Patch of the Conjunctiva; The Pathological Histology of Trachoma,* and numerous other monographs.

T. H. S.—THOMAS HALL SHASTID, A. B., A. M., M. D., LL. B., SUPERIOR,
WIS.
Professor of the History of Medicine in the American Medical College, St.
Louis, Mo.; Editorial Secretary of *The Ophthalmic Record.* Author of *A
Country Doctor; Practising in Pike; Forensic Relations of Ophthalmic Sur-
gery* (in Wood's *System of Ophthalmic Operations); Legal Relations of
Ophthalmology* (in Ball's *Modern Ophthalmology); A History of Medical Juris-
prudence in America* (in Kelly's *Cyclopedia of American Medical Biography).*

W. C. P.—WM. CAMPBELL POSEY, B. A., M. D., PHILADELPHIA, PA.
Professor of Ophthalmology in the Philadelphia Polyclinic Hospital and
Graduate Medical School; Ophthalmic Surgeon to the Wills, Howard and
Children's Hospitals; Chairman .of the Pennsylvania Commission for the
Conservation of Vision; Chairman of Section on Ophthalmology, College of
Physicians, Philadelphia. Editor of American Edition of Nettleship's *Text-
book of Ophthalmology;* Co-Editor, with Jonathan Wright, of *System of Dis-
eases of the Eye, Ear, Nose and Throat;* Co-Editor, with Wm. G. Spiller, of
The Eye and the Nervous System.

W. F. C.—W. FRANKLIN COLEMAN, M. D., M. R. C. S. ENG., CHICAGO, ILL.
Professor of Ophthalmology Post-Graduate Medical School; Professor of Ophthalmology Illinois School Electro-Therapeutics; Member Chicago Ophthalmological Society.

W. F. H.—WILLIAM FREDERIC HARDY, M. D:, ST. LOUIS, MO.
Assistant in Ophthalmology, Washington University Medical School.

W. H. W.—WILLIAM HAMLIN WILDER, A. M., M. D., CHICAGO, ILL.
Professor and Head of Department of Ophthalmology, Rush Medical College
(in affiliation with University of Chicago); Professor of Ophthalmology, Chicago Polyclinic; Surgeon, Illinois Charitable Eye and Ear Infirmary; Ophthalmic Surgeon, Presbyterian Hospital; .Member American Ophthalmological Society.

W. O. N.—WILLIS ORVILLE NANCE, M. D., CHICAGO, ILL.
Ophthalmic Surgeon, Illinois Charitable Eye and Ear Infirmary; Late Oculist
and Aurist to Cook County Hospital; President, Chicago Ophthalmological
Society.

W. R.—WENDELL REBER, M. D., PHILADELPHIA, PA.
Professor of Diseases of the Eye in the Medical Department of Temple University; Professor of Diseases of the Eye in the Philadelphia Polyclinic and
College for Graduates in Medicine; Ophthalmic Surgeon to the Samaritan
Hospital, to the Philadelphia General Hospital, to the Garretson Hospital; Consulting Ophthalmologist to the Friends' Asylum for the Insane; Member of the
Council of the Oxford Ophthalmological Congress; Past President of the American Academy of Ophthalmology and Oto-Laryngology; joint author of a *Handbook on the Muscular Anomalies of the Eye.*

LIST OF LEADING SUBJECTS IN THIS VOLUME

H

H. Abbreviation of hypermetropia. In chemistry, the symbol of hydrogen. In pharmacy, the symbol of *haustus,* a draught.

Haab's magnet. See **Electromagnet.**

Haab's reflex. See **Cerebral cortex reflex of pupil,** on p. 1971, Vol. III, of this *Encyclopedia.*

Haab's scales. This term has been applied to certain fundus lesions that Haab regards as pathognomonic of syphilitic degeneration of the retinal arteries. The changes consist of tiny white patches, suggestive of scales, scattered here and there over the walls of the arterioles. They may be so small that only close scrutiny, by the direct ophthalmoscopic method, will disclose them. Haab considers them to be the beginning of opacification of the vessel.

Haab's sign. See p. 1971, Vol. III, of this *Encyclopedia.*

Haaf, Gerhard ten. A well-known Dutch surgeon, of considerable reputation as an ophthalmologist. Born in 1720, he served for a time in the army, then settled in Rotterdam. Here in 1788 he was appointed Professor of Surgery in the College of Surgery. He was a brilliant teacher and a writer of some ability. He died in 1791.

His chief ophthalmologic writing was, "Korte Verhandeling Nopens de Nieuwe Wyze om de Cataracta te Genezen."—(T. H. S.)

Habenula. A ribbon-like structure. The superficial gray nucleus of the optic thalamus in front, and above the posterior commissure.

Habershon, S. H. A well-known general physician of London, who paid considerable attention to ophthalmology. Born in 1858, son of the celebrated Dr. Samuel Osborne Habershon (author of *"Diseases of the Stomach,"* etc.) he became secretary of the Ophthalmological Society of the United Kingdom (from 1894-1897) and a member of the Council of the same body (1897-1900). He was for years the physician of William E. Gladstone, and, at the time of his death (Feb. 26, 1915) was senior physician to the Hospital for Consumption and Diseases of the Chest, at Brompton.—(T. H. S.)

Habit-chorea. A form of muscle spasm that not infrequently invades the eyes. Oliver (*System of Diseases of the Eye,* Vol. IV, p. 471) has well described that form of it due to ametropia. It has a tendency to become increasingly uncontrollable and to invade other muscular groupings besides those of the eyelids and upper part of the face. Such cases, though controlled in a measure by constant mental effort, which frequently means undue vigilance and at times painful strain, are bettered by corrections of ametropia and heterophoria, which may set the mimicking clonic spasms of the affected muscles temporarily at rest. The condition, if at all times pronounced, can be cured only by additional therapy that is directed to the welfare of the system as a whole. In many cases the transfer of the patient from a sedentary life to an active, out-of-door occupation will be of the greatest benefit. Weak solutions of eserine or of any drug of like nature, with the employment of over-correcting convex lenses, may at times be of therapeutic advantage. Study of the nasal mucous surfaces should always be made, and attention should also be directed towards the possibility of osseous deformities in the upper portions of the nose. Antral disorder arising, as a rule, from carious teeth should be thought of. The possibility of the existence of more distant causes, such as uterine and pelvic disorders, particularly in young adults and even the more mature, must never be forgotten; and, lastly, the great army of so-called neurasthenics, gathered from every locality and social condition in this too-fast-running age of ours, should not be lost sight of. If to the results of these studies is combined carefully graded internal medication with arsenic, or, better, hypodermatic doses of the same drug, a cure can nearly always be secured.

Habit-spasm. A form of accommodative contracture usually associated with hypermetropia.

Habituation. The condition of having become accustomed to a particular environment or physical or mental state—generally abnormal. Thus, the strabismic individual may be said to be habituated to certain anomalous muscle and cerebral conditions. See, for example, the essay of Ammann (*Klin. Monatsbl. f. Augenheilk.*, p. 573, 1915) on stereoscopic vision and habituation; or that of Perlmann (*Zeitschr. f. Augenheilk.*, p. 244, 1915) on the habituation of one-eyed people.

Habitus glaucomatosus. The ocular condition established after one or more attacks of glaucoma, in which most of the typical signs and symptoms are present.

Habrahym. A Jewish Saracen of Spain who flourished about the middle of the 13th century. He is specially remembered for having cured Alphonse de Poitiers, Count of Toulouse (1220-1271), of a serious ocular affection, the exact nature of which is not known. On the recommendation of Raymond Gaucelm, Seigneur de Lunel, the count sent to Aragon for Habrahym, enclosing a safe conduct. Habrahym was immensely wealthy, and received large fees.—(T. II. S.)

Hachure. (F.) Massage.

Hæm- (in composition). For captions beginning with **Hæm-** see **Hem-**.

Hafer. (G.) Oats.

Hagelkorn. (G.) Chalazion.

Hager, Michael. A distinguished Austrian surgeon, who devoted considerable attention to ophthalmology. Born at Hermannstadt in Siebenbürgen, February (or March), 1795, he received his medical degree at Vienna in 1822, and, settling in Vienna, became Professor of Surgery at the Josephs Academy. He died Nov. 24, 1866.

Hager's only ophthalmologic writing was *"Ueber die Erhaltung der Augen und den Zweckmässigen Gebrauch der Brillen"* (Wien, 1823). —(T. H. S.)

Haguenot, Henry. A celebrated Monspellensian physician, who paid considerable attention to diseases of the eye. Born at Montpellier, Jan. 26, 1687, son of Jean Henri, grandson of Jean, and grandnephew of Thierry, Haguenot, all celebrated surgeons, he studied his profession at Montpellier, where his father was teaching surgery. In 1711, at the very early age of 24, he was elected a Fellow of the Royal Society of Sciences at Montpellier. Almost immediately afterward, he was made professor of surgery in the University, in succession to his father, who had just resigned.

Haguenot practised and taught at Montpellier for more than 50 years, and with great success. When 80 years of age, i. e., in 1767, he relinquished his professorship and also retired from practice. Four years later—Dec. 11, 1775—he died, aged 84.

He had no children, and therefore left to the Hôtel Dieu St. Eloi his entire fortune, including his very large library. This became the nucleus for the present most excellent library of the Medical College at Montpellier.

Haguenot's writings were almost all concerned with general medicine. In one of his works, however, *Tractatus de Morbis Externis Capitis* (12 mo., Avignon, 1751), he gives a bare, uninteresting and highly unoriginal treatise on the diseases of the eye.—(T. H. S.)

Hahnemann, Christian Friedrich Samuel (1755-1843), the founder of the homeopathic method of treatment. See **Homeopathy in ophthalmology.**

Haidinger, Brushes of. See **Brushes of Haidinger.**

Hailstone. A vulgar synonym of chalazion or Meibomian cyst.

Hair dyes. See p. 4100, Vol. VI, of this *Encyclopedia.*

Hairion, Frédéric. A celebrated French hygienist, syphilographer and ophthalmologist, one of the institutors of the International Congress for Ophthalmology at Brussels (1857) and for some years, beginning with 1837, one of the editors of the *Annales d'Oculistique.* Born at Beaumont, Hennegan, May 6, 1809, he received the medical degree at Lyons in 1832, pursued further studies at Paris, Brussels, and again at Paris, became for a number of years a military surgeon, and in 1835 settled permanently in Lyons. Here he at first taught syphilis, diseases of the skin, and hygiene; later, ophthalmology was added to his subjects. In 1840 or 1841 he founded the "Institut Ophtalmique Militaire," of which he was shortly afterwards made director.

The date of his death is not at present procurable, because of the European war.

Hairion's most important ophthalmologic writings are as follows: 1. Considérations Pratiques et Recherches sur l'Ophtalmie qui Règne dans l'Armée Belge. (Lyons, 1839.)   2. De l'Ophtalmie Gonor-rhoïque. (*Ibid.*, 1846.)   3. Des Granulations Palpébrales. (*Annales Belges d'Oculistique*, 1870.)   4. De l'Emploi du Collodion en Ophtal-mologie. (*Bull. de l'Académie Royale de Médecine*, 1848-49.)—(T. H. S.)

Hair-optometer. A device, commonly used in England, for measuring the range of accommodation and for ascertaining the near point. It resembles (see the cut) a miniature harp, in which the strings are

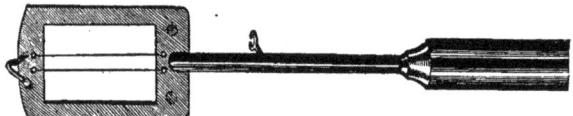

The Hair-optometer.

replaced by hairs. It is provided with a handle and a hook, to which a dioptre steel tape can be attached. The steel tape is marked in dioptres on one side and fractions of a metre on the other. In testing the accommodation the surgeon is to proceed as follows: A trial-frame is placed on the patient and one eye is covered with a metal disc. In front of the other eye the glass needed to make vision 6/6, in the test for far, is to be placed. The patient holds the hair-optometer in front of a white background and brings the instrument to the nearest point at which the hairs can still be distinguished. The distance from this point to the outer canthus of the eye is to be read off on the steel tape. This gives the amount of accommodation in dioptres.

Suppose, for example, the nearest point at which the hairs can be clearly seen is 12 centimetres. The amount of accommodation is then $100/12 = 8D$. The other eye is then to be tested in a similar manner and the result is recorded. The amplitude of accommodation is determined by using the formula: $A = P - R$, in which P and R are expressed in dioptres. To measure A in emmetropes, we find the nearest point (in centimetres) at which the patient can read small print, and divide this into 100 centimetres. In hypermetropes we add to the lens whose focal distance equals the distance of his near point that convex lens which enables him to see distant objects clearly without accommodative effort. In myopes we subtract the glass used for far vision.—(J. M. B.)

Hairs, Caterpillar. See **Conjunctivitis nodosa;** also p. 1781, Vol. III, of this *Encyclopedia*.

Hair, The. Woman's hair, burnt with litharge, was highly esteemed by Pliny (XXVIII, 20) as a remedy for *scabritia oculorum*.—(T. H. S.)

Haitz' campimeter. This is one of the modifications of the original blackboard perimeter. The author of the device says that all the campimeters should be printed on dull-gray carton, free from all reflections. The eight-sided figures should have strongly marked contours of clear gray. They are especially intended to excite fusion. At the same time it is not necessary that the two campimeters be viewed in toto; when portions of each are fused they fulfill their mission. On both sketches are two diagonals that should appear in relief and, therefore, should be printed white. These spur the eyes to maintain the normal position as they cross at the fixation point, where they double by vertical or horizontal deviation. There is a break in the center of each diagonal of 1 2/3 mm., or ½°, in order that the eye may not be blinded by any white at the fixation point, and so be able to distinguish saturation differences. The campimeter that has divisions into degrees is always placed in front of the eye to be examined. Two control signs, disks, are placed at the ends of one of the diagonals in each figure, and if binocular vision is present four disks will be seen, one at each corner of the stereoscopic picture. The divisions on the campimeter are in degrees from 0° to 10°, so that two adjoining lines are seen under an angle of 1°. The size of the intervals is determined empirically by finding the nasal border of the blind spot in the horizontal meridian. Its distance from the fixation point is first measured in the case of a number of emmetropes in angle degrees on the perimeter, and then in linear units in the stereoscope. Neither the different interpupillary distances nor the distance of the eyes from the stereoscope lenses has any appreciable influence on the test. Tests are performed as in perimetry in general, but one should be careful to avoid holding the test-square over one of a common contour. If one is testing the meridian 45° the square should be drawn alongside, not

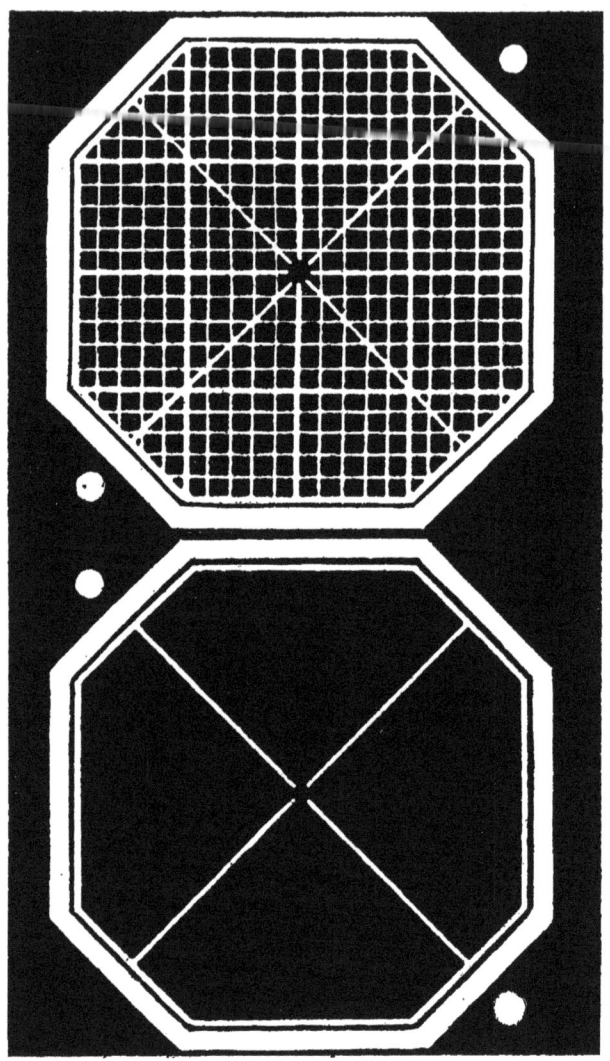

The Campimeters of Haitz to be used with a Stereoscope. (Davis.)

over the diagonal. In going from the nasal side toward the middle of the field the carrier should be held upright. The holders should be of the size of a needle and the test objects of two sizes, one $1\frac{1}{4}$ mm. square and one 2 mm. square. The smaller one is to be used in testing the zone between 0 and 5, the larger the zone between 5 and 10. The Heidelberg color papers make the best test objects. Ametropes should wear their correction. See, also, p. 4767, Vol. VI, of this *Encyclopedia*.

Haken. (G.) Hook or tenaculum.

Hakenpincette. (G.) Toothed forceps.

Halaf at-Tuluni. Once a slave, this gifted Arabian became a celebrated physician and skilful operator on the eye. His one known writing, *"Book of the Final Aim and Sufficiency concerning the Structure of the Two Eyes and Their Condition and Their Treatment and Their Medicines,"* though of great importance in its day, is not now extant.—(T. H. S.)

Halation. The photographic action of light reflected within the camera.

Halbbild. (G.) The image seen by each eye in binocular vision.

Halberstaedter-Prowazek bodies. See **Bacteriology of the eye**; also **Trachoma.**

Halbmesser. (G.) Radius.

Halbsehen. (G.) Hemiopia.

Haldat du Lys, Charles Nicolas Alexander de. A famous French surgeon and ophthalmologist. Born at Bourmont, Dec. 24, 1770, he was for a time a surgeon in the French army, but, having retired into civil practice at Nancy, he there became Instructor in Physics at the Ecole Centrale de la Meurthe. In 1803 he received the degree of Doctor in Medicine at Strassburg. Returning to Nancy, he became in 1824 Inspector of the University, a position which he held for eight years. He also became a Fellow and Secretary of the Academy of Science, Letters and Arts at Nancy. He died Nov. 26, 1852.

His ophthalmologic writings are as follows: 1.. Expériences sur la Vision Double. (Laméthrie, *Jour. de Physique,* 1806.) 2. Recherches sur les Limites de la Vision Simple et les Points de Correspondance de la Rétine, etc. (*Ibid.,* 1807.) 3. Optique Oculaire, Suivi d'Un Essai sur l'Achromatisme de l'Oeil. (Paris, 1849.)—(T. H. S.)

Hâlé. (F.) Sun-burnt; tanned.

Half-blindness. Hemianopia.

Half-prism spectroscope. A form of spectroscope in which the rays enter the prism at right angles to one of its faces, and are only dispersed on emerging from the opposite side.

Half-shadow apparatus. A modification of the ordinary polaristrobometer, in which the sensitive part is so constructed that the field of view is divided into two or more surfaces which, the analyser being in a certain position, show a uniform degree of partial shadow.

Half-sight. Hemiopia or hemiopsia. See **Hemiopia.**

Half-vision centre. A centre situated in the apex of the occipital lobe; so called because it receives impressions from corresponding halves of the two retinæ.

Halifa b Abil-Mahasan. A distinguished ophthalmologist of Aleppo, who flourished in the latter half of the 10th century. Concerning the man himself we know almost nothing; his one writing, however, entitled *"The Book of Sufficiency in Ophthalmology,"* is still extant, and for many reasons is worthy of note.

Of great importance is the list of Arabian ophthalmologists and ophthalmologies with which the book begins. As Halifa was one of the latest of the Arabian writers on the eye, the list, of course, is about complete, so far, at all events, as concerns the more important writers and books. The following is a translation of the highly interesting passage in question: "Generally recognized is the advantage of visual power, and the profit which one is in a position to create out of that power for his spiritual completeness. After I had studied in detail the works concerned especially with eye diseases and their treatment— as, for example, (1) the ten books of Hunain on the eye, and (2) his three books on the same subject, in the form of question and answer; (3) the book of his sister's son, Hubais, which he calls 'The Book of the Explanation of Eye-Diseases,' and in which he has provided the eye and a few diseases, as for example the large pterygium and the pannus, with illustrations; (4) The Memorandum-Book of the Oculist, Ali ben Isa; (5) The Commentary thereto by Daniel, the son of Saja; (6) The Tables of Rhazes; (7) The Final Aim of Ophthalmology; (8) The Memorandum-Book of Mansur; (9) The Book of Akbari; (10) The Book of the Oculist of Amid; (11) the work of Ibn Abi as-Sajjar; (12) The Work on Cataract, its Treatment and its Operation, by the Egyptian Ibn Dubail; (13) the book of the oculist Abdan; (14) the book of the oculist ad-Dan of Tiberias; (15) the work composed by the double-minister Abul Mutariff, of the Magrib, on the visual spirit, wherein he writes with excellent ideas concerning the treatment of the visual power; (16) The Book of the Correction of the Seer and of the Sight; (17) The Book for the Examination of the Oculist; (18) the iambic poem of al-Misri concerning the eye, its pathology and its treatment—as indeed still many others; for there is no book on the art of healing, whether short or long, that does not contain the anatomy of the eye and the description of a few of its diseases, and their treatment;—then I found in all these works the ordinary rules of the art, but still a neglect of a few subordinate subjects out of the chapters relating to this special branch."

The contents of Halifa's important book can best be given in his own words: "The Book comprises two main divisions. The first treats of the anatomy of the eye and of its various conditions. The second, of everything connected with its treatment.

"The first section of the first division treats of the definition of the eye, of its mingling, and of its color, and of the causes of the latter. The second, of the anatomy of the membranes of the eye and of their origin. The third, of the humors of the eye. The fourth, of the visual spirit" [see, herein, **Ali ben Isa** and **History of ophthalmology**] "and its nerves and of the condition of vision. The fifth, of the nerve of motion of the eye and of its origin. The sixth, of the anatomy of the muscles of the eye, and of the lids and the lashes and their roots and their nourishment. After that, I give the figure of the brain and of the two eyes and the nerves of both of them, as availably to the understanding as is for me possible." This figure is reproduced and discussed later in this section.

"The second main division comprises six sections. The first treats of the general rules concerning the scientific specialty, of the preservation of health and of the times of disease. The second contains an explanation of the preservation of the health of the eye, and also an explanation of such things as assist and injure the eye and of those which preserve its health and strength. The third section of this treats of this, how one opens the eye and introduces medicine into it. The fourth, of the best kind of sound and its employment. The fifth mentions the apparatus by means of which each kind of collyrium is fortified. The sixth mentions the most appropriate kind of clothing for the eye-doctor.

"Hereupon follow tables, which contain the number of the diseases of the lids as well as of the eyes themselves, and how such diseases arise, and at what seasons of the year and in what periods of life their occurrence is most frequent; and their causes and their symptoms and the treatment of such of them as man can treat. To eye-diseases belong those perceptible to the senses, as well as those not so perceptible.

"I add to each table the simple remedies, according to the expression of the learned as to what is specific for each affection—in order that thou mayest find occasionally indemnification for the compounded remedies. Thereupon follows the enumeration of several anesthetic [benumbing] remedies, which, by their mingling, benumb sensation, also specific means for the same purpose—according to the best knowledge and as briefly as possible.

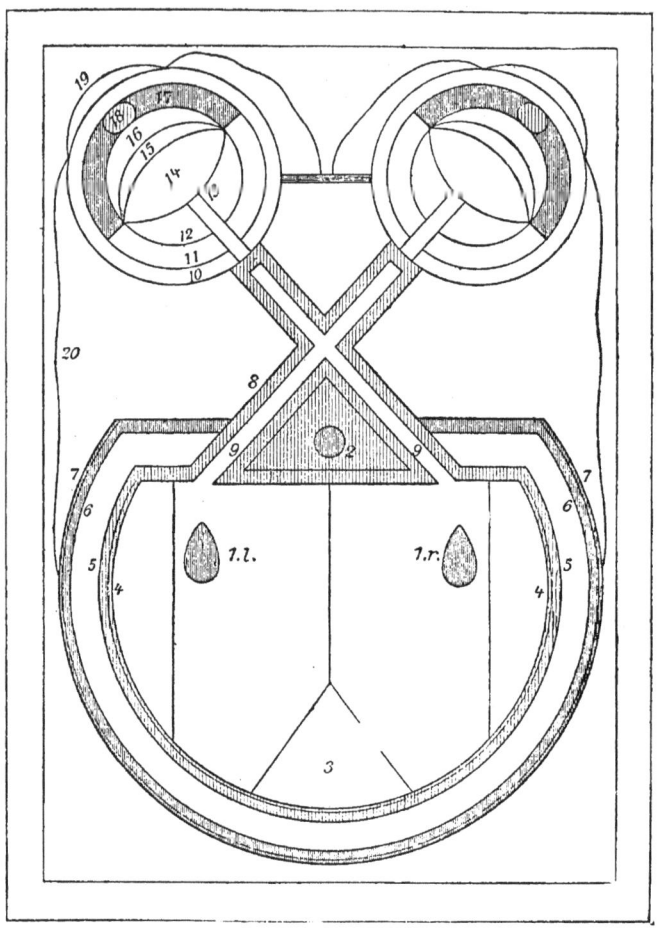

Halifa's Figure of the Brain, with both Eyes and the Optic Nerves.

The legend which should properly, but does not, appear beneath the cut is as follows: "This is the picture of the brain and of its three ventricles. These represent the place for the five powers: namely, common sense and the faculty of perception and the sense of locality sit in the anterior chamber (1); the imagination, together with the power of judgment, in the middle (2); the power of memory and proof in the posterior (3). Then there is shown in this figure a picture of the soft membrane (4) of the brain, which encloses the substance of the brain, and the hard membrane (5) over that. Then also a picture of the bones (6) of the skull and of the membrane (7) which lies thereupon and is known by the name of pericranium. Next, a representation showing how the Visual spirit passes forward in the hollow nerves (8) out of the substance of the brain, and how the hollow space (9) separates itself from the marrow substance of the brain. Then the forward prolongations of the membranes of the eye out of the substance of the nerves and out of that of its two membranes, the shapes of the former and those of the humors of the eye and their situation—so far as possible to show this on one plane and not upon a sphere. To what thou needest to know belongs this: The brain is the place of origin of each sensation and of each guiding and leading movement and also the place of the return. And specially for the eye is the place of origin thereof, and the limit of its function. Therefore must thou understand the construction of the brain and its singularity, and its working, if thou wishes to grasp the knowledge of the eye.'' The other numbered parts of this schematic eye are: 10, sclera, 11, choroid, 12, retina, 13, vitreous, 14, crystalline lens, 15, arachnoid membrane (anterior capsule of the lens), 16, egg-white fluid, 17, uvea, 18, pupil, 19, cornea, 20, conjunctiva.

''Finally follow tables on the treatment of those diseases which demand surgical intervention. . . . Then I add tables of the hidden diseases of the eyes and close the book with an index of remedies. I will keep short the table on compounded remedies, particularly as these have been already referred to. Thus is this appendix sufficient for the practitioner. May he, in my work, improve what is bad and complete what he finds to be defective. God is our trust.''

Much of the contents of his *''Book of Sufficiency''* Halifa undoubtedly borrowed from the earlier Arabians. Nevertheless, he has given us some new matter also, and even what he borrows he clarifies.

Probably most important, and at all events most interesting, of all the contents of this highly interesting book, is ''the figure of the brain and of the two eyes and of the nerves of both of them'' referred to above in Halifa's own analysis of the contents of his book. This illustration (which is here reproduced) is one of the earliest, possibly the very earliest, scientific illustration of the eye which has come down to our day.

Almost as interesting as this earliest illustration of the eye are the pictures given by Halifa, in the same work, of the various instruments which, in his time, were employed in ocular surgery.

Halifa's explanations are as follows: ''1· Shears, with broad blades. The length is always in proportion to that which is to be taken from the lid. 2. Shears, thinner than the preceding. For the cutting away of the skin from the conjunctiva. 3. Shears, thinner than the first pair and thicker than the second. For the removal of skin from the corneal circumference. [Peritomy?] 4. Opener. The best kind is of gold or silver; after these, copper. 5. The scalpel. Its iron is hidden in its copper, with two hooks. In many operations on the eye it is indispensable. [Hirschberg, with his usual insight, has suggested that this was a tiny knife concealed in a copper tube, or cylinder.] 6. Hooks. Pannus and pterygium are lifted with the large one and with the small one, to facilitate removal. Each renders the other indispensable. 7. Rose-blade. For the removal of excrescences from the lid; also for the cutting away of encysted tumors and for certain

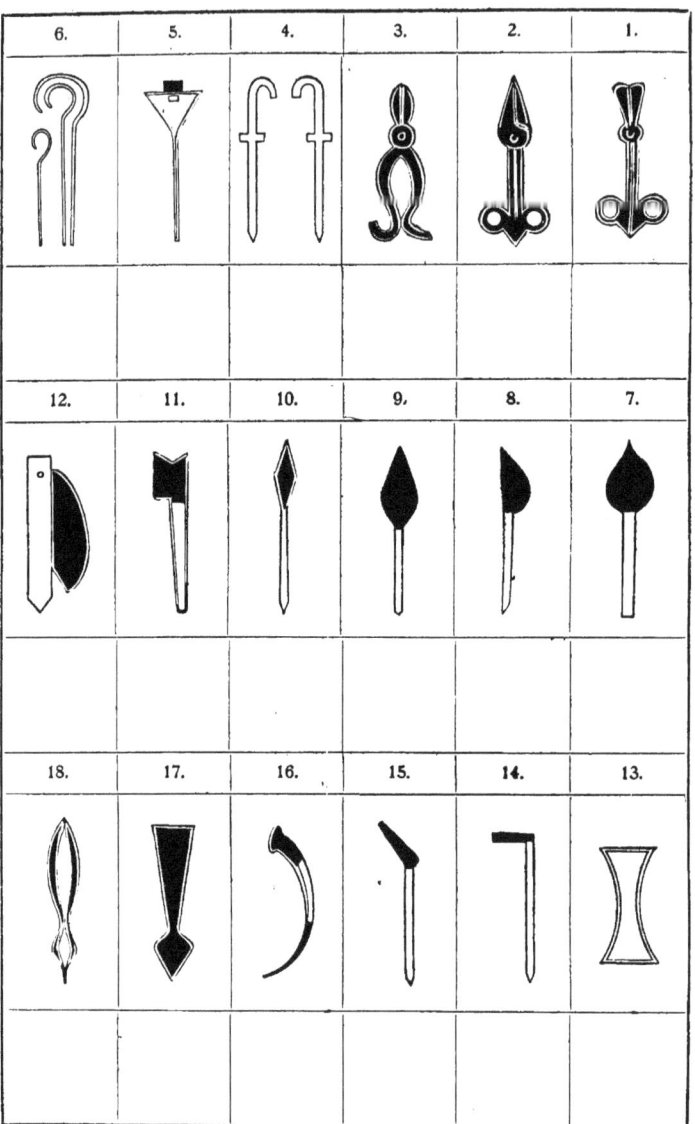

Ophthalmic Instruments. Described by Halifa.
Latter half of the thirteenth century.

other operations. 8. The half-rose. For the ablation of excrescences from the conjunctiva, in so far as it is finer than the foregoing; it can also be employed for that. 9. The spear. This splits the encysted tumor and passes in under it and cuts it off. It is rendered superfluous by the myrtle-blade. 10. The myrtle-blade. With this a pterygium is raised and peeled off, while, for the cutting away of the growth, the shears are employed. 11. The axe. For the opening of the frontal vein: according to the length, it is laid upon the vessel, and with the middle-finger of the right hand the division is accomplished. 12. The scissors-knife. Light of blade. With this is split the cystic tumor, carefully. 13. The cleaver. Against concealed pus. It is employed for opening chemosis, and is interchangeable with the lance. 14. The scraper. For rubbing the itch and for digging out the calcification. For this purpose can also be employed the half-rose. 15. The lancet. With round-headed point, for the eradication of a cyst. Also, chalazia and similar things are split with it. 16. The sickel. For splitting a union between the two lids. It is also used in cases of lagophthalmos. 17. The tensor. With this a wart is put upon the stretch; then the excrescence is removed with some other instrument. 18. The collector. With this is gathered superfluous hairs. With it one also takes from the eye the various things that may have fallen therein. 19. Burning-iron for the suture of the head and for the sides of the head. Therewith is burnt the head-suture and the two veins of the two sides of the head. 20. Burning-iron for both the temples. For burning both the veins in both the temples, and both the veins behind both the ears. 21. Burning-iron for lachrymal fistula. With this is burnt the lachrymal fistula after it has opened [begun to discharge]. 22. Burning-iron for the place of the hair. For burning the places of the superfluous hairs after these have been plucked out. 23. Purifier for a lachrymal fistula. With this the whole corner of the eye is purified—for him who does not like the burning of a fistula. 24. Raven's beak. For the taking out of that which clings fast to the eye or to the inner surface of the lid, as I have described this matter in the 14th chapter, on the diseases of the conjunctiva. 25. Little barleycorn-knife. A lancet. The length of its incision is that of a barleycorn—for opening the conjunctiva before a cataract operation. 26. Thorn-knife. With this are cut the frontal veins, of which I shall speak again. 27. Round cataract-needle. Thou knowest the procedure therewith. It and the three-cornered variety can be mutually interchanged. 28. Hollow cataract-needle. For sucking of cataract. Thou art acquainted with the operation. God knows best. 29. The tube for the ant [i. e., a swelling so called]. For pressing into the ant-swelling. The latter

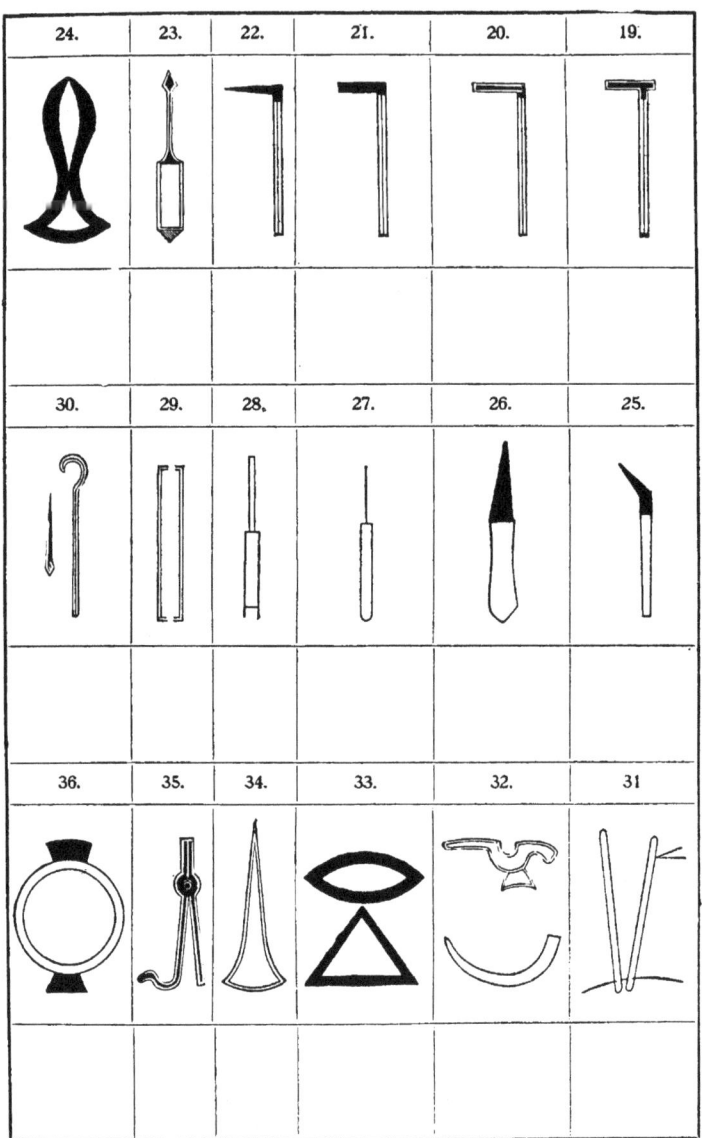

Ophthalmic Instruments. Described by Halifa.
Latter half of the thirteenth century.

is radically cured by this, as thou knowest. 30. Hook and needle. For threading-in a hair. When the superfluous lashes are few, they are removed in this way. 31. Bits of wood for tying-off [i. e., as a wart]. For him who cannot bear the iron. 32. Insufflator and horn for blowing-in. By means of the latter, powder is blown into the nose. The prophylactic medicine with the insufflator. 33. Leaden plate. It is round or triangular or longish, according to the given case. 34. A light cleanser. It is used in the treatment of lachrymal fistula. It renders the stronger cleanser superfluous. 35. Granule forceps. This is used when a grain or anything of the sort has fallen into the eye, as explained in The Diseases of the Conjunctiva. 36. A ring with handles. The management of this should be in proportion to the strength . . . according to my experience.'' Pictures of ocu-listic instruments occur in other works of Arabian writers—notably in the books of Abulkasim, Alcoati, Salah ad-din, and as-Sadili—but those in *"The Book of Sufficiency"* of Halifa are by far more numer-ous, and, feature by feature considered, more interesting and instruc-tive than those of all the other Arabian authors combined.—(T. H. S.)

Halikakabon. An unidentifiable plant, which, in Greco-Roman antiq-uity, was, on the authority of Archigenes, employed in "hot" dis-charges from the eyes.—(T. H. S.)

Hallauer glass. The invention, in 1905, of a smoky-green glass by Otto Hallauer of Basel, Switzerland. It is said by some to be more effective than Fieuzel's so-called chlorophyl, or greenish-yellow, glass in protecting the eye from injury by glaring. See, also, **Glare**; as well as **Colored glasses**; **Eyes of soldiers, sailors**, etc., and **Light**.

Haller's campanula. Since fishes have no ciliary muscles, in many of them accommodation occurs by means of a process of the choroid called the *processus falciformis,* which extends through the embry-onic choroid fissure into the vitreous humor towards the lens, around which it expands to form the so-called campanula Halleri. See, also, **Comparative ophthalmology**.

Haller's layer. One of the principal layers of the choroid, containing the larger vessels. See **Anatomy of the eye**; as well as **Histology of the eye**.

Haller's vascular circle. The circlet of arteries around the optic nerve.

Hall, John Charles. A celebrated English physician, especially re-nowned as an ophthalmologist and for his writings on occupational diseases. Born at Nottingham, England, in Dec., 1816, he studied at St. George's Hospital, as well as in Paris. Returning to England, he settled at first in Redford. In 1848 he became a Fellow of the Royal College of Physicians (Edinburgh) and in the same year settled in

Sheffield. A few years later he was made professor at the Sheffield School of Medicine.

His only ophthalmologic writing was entitled *"Clinical Remarks on the Eye."*—(T. H. S.)

Hallotype. HELLENOTYPE. A translucent photographic picture superposed on one similar in outline but stronger or opaque.

Hallucination. The highest degree of subjective sensation, dependent alone upon morbid stimulation of the sensory cortical centers. There is the perception of non-existent objects or impressions, creations of the imagination. Hallucinations may be of all the senses, and may be of every degree of variety and complication, from (eye) flashes of light to seeing armies of men, from (ear) hummings in the head to strains of "celestial music." Hallucinations were much more common among primitive peoples and in the early ages of the world than they are now.

As Swanzy (*System of Diseases of the Eye,* Vol. IV, p. 565 and 566) points out, visual hallucinations sometimes occur in cases of homonymous hemianopsia in the blind side of the field only, or may precede the hemianopsia. Some of these observed by patients were: a military officer in uniform, a boy, a pig eating oats, chairs and tables, a sheet of water, smoke, etc. Henschen is of opinion that hemiopic hallucinations occurring in focal brain-disease indicate the position of the lesion to be in the occipital lobe, and holds that they result from irritation of the center for visual memory. They would not occur if that center were destroyed; but the lesion, he believes, is likely to be situated not far from it, either in the cortical center for vision or in the subcortical fibres. De Schweinitz, however, has published a case in which there were homonymous hemiopic hallucinations in those sides of the fields which later on became hemianopic, and the lesion was found to be a gumma at the base pressing on the right optic tract. The author implies that there was no disease of the occipital lobe, but the latter does not seem to have been carefully examined.

Hallucinations of vision occur in connection with certain forms of insanity, in delirium tremens, and in acute fever; and the writer has seen a case of chronic simple glaucoma, without any brain-disease, in which there were marked, but not hemiopic, hallucinations,—brilliant flower-gardens for the most part; and a few other cases of glaucoma with this symptom are recorded. There may, therefore, occasionally be some danger of an error in diagnosis when the symptom appears in focal brain disease; yet the presence of other signs of focal brain disease, and the fact that the hallucinations are always in one or the other side of the binocular field, and are either accompanied or followed by blindness of the same side of the field, should prevent any serious difficulty of diagnosis from arising. But in this connection it must be mentioned that homonymous hemiopic hallucinations persisting for years without hemianopsia have been observed by Peterson in a case of chronic delusional insanity. Uniocular hallucinations— referred to one eye only, and not seen when that eye is closed, and to be well distinguished from the hemiopic form—have been described by several authors as occurring in the insane.

Hallucinations dédoublées. (F.) A term used by Michéa to designate hallucinations of both sight and hearing.

Halo. A circle of light around a luminous body due to the refraction of light through vapour; also the luminous or colored circles seen by the patient about lights in glaucoma.

Halos in the astronomic sense are circles of light surrounding the sun or moon and are due to the presence of ice-crystals in the air. The commonest and usually the brightest has a radius of about 22 degrees, i. e., this is the angular distance from the sun to its inner edge. As blue light is slightly more refrangible than red it is thrown farther out and the halo appears colored red inside and blue outside. Some of the crystals may, however, be lying so that the light enters at a side and leaves at one end, or *vice versa,* in which case the angle of minimum deviation is about 46 degrees, at which distance a second fainter halo is frequently seen with colors in the same order as in the first. In addition to the above a third, still larger, halo has been seen.

Another phenomenon sometimes seen with halos is the parhelic circle, which is a white circle passing through the sun and parallel with the horizon. It is caused by a light reflected from the surfaces of ice-crystals falling vertically through the air. When the sun is near the horizon this circle is intensified at distances of 22 degrees and 46 degrees from the sun, and forms parhelia or mock-suns, and another mock-sun is sometimes seen on this circle directly opposite the sun. Several other more complex forms of halo have been seen in the arctic regions.

Halos must not be confused with coronæ, which are smaller, colored circles that appear around the sun or moon when they shine through a thin cloud or mist. They are due to the diffraction the light undergoes in passing among the drops of which the cloud is composed.

When the sun shines on a bank of fog a large bow of about 40 degrees radius, resembling a rainbow, but not so brightly colored, is seen. It is often double, like the rainbow. Owing to the smaller size of the water-drops in a fog than in falling rain, the fogbow is wider and fainter than the rainbow. *(Standard Encyclopedia.)* See **Halo, Glaucomatous.**

Halo, Glaucomatous. In connection with this disease two entirely different meanings are attached to the term halo. It means, first of all, the peculiar circlet of light that certain patients with increased intraocular tension see about lights and, second, the circumpapillary ring described on p. 5411, Vol. VII, of this *Encyclopedia.*

Halo, Macular. HALO OF THE MACULA. HALO ABOUT THE MACULA. A glittering ring, or halo, around the macula lutea, seen with the ophthalmoscope.

This phenomenon is best seen by the direct method in young subjects, when with the pupil dilated and a good light the play of color can be observed about the rim of the fovea. It is almost identical with the brilliant reflexes that are observed about the course of the retinal vessels in children and probably in both instances are produced by the slight elevation of the semi-transparent retina in the neighborhood.

Haloscope. An experimental appliance by means of which the phenomena of halos can be exhibited.

Halo signatus. (L.) The ring of depressions in the vitreous made by the ciliary processes.

Haltenhoff, Georg. A prominent oculist of Geneva, Switzerland. Born at Geneva, June 8, 1843, he studied at Geneva, Würzburg, Zürich, Paris, Berlin, and Heidelberg, returning to Zürich to receive the medical degree in 1866. Concerning his life from 1866 to 1872, the present writer has not been able to secure the slightest information. In 1872, however, Haltenhoff settled as an ophthalmologist in Geneva, and, before the year was over, had qualified as privat docent in ophthalmology. In 1891 he became extraordinary, in 1903, ordinary, professor. Not till seven years later, however, was he placed in charge of the eye-division of a town clinic. He died April 24, 1915, after a long illness.

Some of Haltenhoff's ophthalmic writings are as follows: Mémoire sur la création d'une division ophthalmique à l'hôpital cantonal de Genève. *(Gen.,* 1872, p. 23.) Retinitis haemorrh. bei Diabetes mellitus. *(Klin. Mon.-Bl.,* pp. 291-298 and *Ann. d'Ocul.,* LXII, pp. 20-31.) Cataracte traumatique luxée, resorption spontanée. *(Bull, de la Soc. méd. de la Suisse Romande,* No. 12, 1873.) Fragment de bois dans la cavité orbitaire. *(Ibid.,* No. 10, 1873.) C. R. de quelques travaux récents sur les cavités lymphatiques de l'appareil visuel. *(Ann. d'Ocul.,* LXXI, pp. 208-212, 1874.) Apparat zu optischen Demonstrationen. *(Klin. Mon.-Bl.,* pp. 198-200, 1874.) Prolapsus traum. de la glande lacrim. orb. *(Ann. d'Oculist,* CXIII, p. 319,

1895.) Opération de la cataracte chez le chien. (*Ibid.*, CXXI, p. 129, 1898.) Un cas de tétanos céphalique avec paralysie faciale et oculaire. Guérison —. (*Ann. d'Ocul.*, CXXVIII, p. 467, 1902.) Cas de lépre avec localis. oc. (*Ibid.*, 1902.) Die Berger'sche Binokular-Lupe. (*Ophth. Klinik*, No. 22, and *Clinique opht.*, p. 281, 1905.) Hérédosyph. à la troisième génération. (*R. m. Suisse Rom.*, XXXVI, No. 6, 1906.) Double conj. diphtheroïde. (*Ibid.*, 1906.) Ophtalmoplégie externe double nucléaire (*Ann. d'Oc.*, CXXXIX, p. 290, 1908.) Mercure à prendre pour combattre l'ophtalmie des nouveau-nés. (*Ibid.*, CXL, p. 394, 1908.) Welches sind die gesetzlichen Massnahmen, die in der Schweiz zur Bekämpfung der Augen-Entzündung der Neugeborenen zu ergreifen sind? (St. Gallen, 1908.) Lésions ocul. tabétiques. *Revue gén. d'Ophtalm.*, p. 426, 1910.)—(T. H. S.)

Haly Abbas. A distinguished Persian physician of the Arabic period. See **Ali Abbas.**

Hamamelis. WITCH HAZEL. WINTER BLOOM. STRIPED ALDER. The medicinal parts are the dried leaves and bark, collected in the autumn, of *Hamamelis virginiana*. They contain tannic and gallic acids and are sedative and astringent. A decoction of the watery as well as of the alcoholic extract and the tincture are the best known preparations.

Whether there are distinct virtues in any of the preparations of "witch hazel" apart from the alcohol and other adjuvants that are commonly prescribed with it is difficult to say, but that a number of experienced surgeons prescribe it in collyria, washes and fomentations to the eye in hyperemia and simple infections of the conjunctiva is well known. For instance, J. L. Dickey has had much satisfaction from the following formula: Cocain. hydrochlor., gr. v; acid. boric., gr. x; tinct. hamamelidis; aquæ dest., āā. fl. ℥ss.

To be instilled every three or four hours.

The above would be a safer prescription if the cocaine were omitted, its dose reduced to half a grain, or alypin or beta eucaine substituted for it.

T. W. Moore often prescribes the following formula in inflammatory conditions of the conjunctiva, whether the increased secretion be purulent or not: Aqua hamamelidis, 10.00; cocain hydrochlor., 0.20; sodii chlor., 0.65; aqua rosæ ad. 30.00.

Three drops in each eye three times daily. To this he sometimes adds solution (1:1000) adrenalin chlor. 4.00 c.c.

Hamilton, Robert. An Edinburgh surgeon of the early 19th century, who seems to have devoted a considerable portion of his time to eye diseases. His life-dates are unknown. He was, however, for a time, surgeon at the Edinburgh Eye Infirmary, and, in 1843, published in the *Edinburgh Medical Journal* an article entitled "Substance of an Introductory Lecture to a Course upon the Structure, Functions and Diseases of the Eye; Comprising a Comparison of the State of Ophthalmic Science in Germany and England; and a Recommendation to Introduce the German Method of Instruction into the British Schools."—(T. H. S.)

Hamilton, Sir William Rowan. (1805-65), mathematician, was born in Dublin, Ireland. His earlier essays connected with caustics and contact of curves grew by degrees into an elaborate treatise on the *Theory of Systems of Rays.* To this he added various supplements, in the last of which, published in 1833, he predicted the existence of the two kinds of conical refraction, the experimental verification of which by Lloyd still forms one of the most convincing proofs of the truth of the undulatory theory of light. His next great work was *A General Method in Dynamics.* For these researches Hamilton was elected an honorary member of the Academy of St. Petersburg, a rare and coveted distinction.

While an undergraduate at Trinity College, Dublin, he was appointed in 1827 successor to Dr. Brinkley in the Andrews chair of Astronomy in the University of Dublin, to which is attached the astronomer-royalship of Ireland. This post he held until his death. In 1835 he was knighted on his delivering the address as secretary to the British Association for its Dublin meeting.—*(Standard Encyclopedia.)*

Hammer-head. HAMMER-HEADED SHARK. This animal belongs to a genus of fishes having the general form and characters of the family, but distinguished from all others by the unusual shape of the head, which, resembling a double-headed hammer laid flat, extends on both sides to a considerable length, carrying the eyes at the ends of the lateral expansions. The crescent-shaped mouth is below the center of the head, the nostrils are on the front edge of the head, and the eyes are covered by a nictitating membrane.

Hammock flap. Skin transplanted from a neighboring locality to fill in a defect due to disease or operative removal, as in the repair of the ravages of cancer of the *lower* lid by transplantation from the upper lid. See, for example, a reference to this method, devised by C. H. Mayo (*Jour. Am. Med. Assoc'n,* p. 752, Aug. 29, 1914).

Hammurabi, The Code of. An ancient Assyrio-Babylonian code, the oldest book on law in all the world, and, incidentally, the oldest document of any kind to mention matters medical or ophthalmic. The Egyptian *"Papyrus Ebers"* is, in fact, almost modern by comparison, for the date of its composition is about B. C. 1500, while that of the Hammurabic Code is actually B. C. 2250.

The parts of the Code in question which relate to ophthalmic matters are as follows (according to the translation of Robert Francis Harper, Ph. D.) :* 196.—If a man destroy the eye of another man, they shall destroy his eye. 198.—If one destroy the eye of a freeman or brake the bone of a freeman, he shall pay one mana of silver. 199.—If one destroy the eye of a man's slave or brake a bone of a man's slave, he shall pay one-half this price. 215.—If a physician .... open an abscess (in the eye) of a man with a bronze lancet and save that man's eye, he shall receive ten shekels of silver (as his fee). 216.—If he be a freeman, he shall receive five shekels. 218.—If a physician .... open an abscess (in the eye) of a man with a bronze lancet and destroy the man's eye, they shall cut off his fingers. 220.—If he open an abscess (in his eye) with a bronze lancet, and destroy his eye, he shall pay silver to the extent of one-half of his price.''—(T. H. S.)

Hampe. (F.) Stem or handle.

Hamulus lacrimalis. (L.) The name occasionally given to a small hook-like process at the lower end of the crest of the lachrymal bone.

Hamulus trochlearis. (L.) The tubercle on the orbital plate of the frontal bone for the attachment of the fibro-cartilaginous pulley of the superior oblique muscle.

Hancock, Henry. A famous London surgeon who devoted the most of his time to ophthalmology, and who invented the procedure of division of the ciliary muscle for glaucoma. Born at London, Aug. 6, 1809, he studied at first pharmacy, but appears never to have practised that profession. In 1830 he began the pursuit of medicine at the Royal Westminster Ophthalmic Hospital, later at King's College and at Westminster Hospital. For a time he was a pupil of Guthrie. In 1832 he was appointed house-surgeon at the Royal Westminster Ophthalmic Hospital, in 1834 prosector of anatomy in the Westminster School, and in 1837 lecturer on anatomy and physiology at the Charing Cross Medical Hospital. Two years later he was made assistant surgeon at the Charing Cross Hospital. For many years he was surgeon to the Westminster Ophthalmic Hospital, where his lectures were well attended. In 1846 he became president of the Westminster Medical Society, and, two years later, of the London Medical Society. In 1863 he became a Fellow of the Council of the Royal College of Surgeons.

Hancock's sclerocyclotomy, or division of the ciliary muscle for glaucoma, seems to have found little favor in his day, and, at the present time, is recommended only for the alleviation of pain in glaucoma absolutum. (See Wood's *System of Ophthalmic Operations* II, p. 1122,

---

* For the rest of this remarkable code, see *The Code of Hammurabi, King of Babylon*, by Robert Francis Harper, Ph. D., 2d ed., 1904, Chicago, Callaghan & Co.

article by William Campbell Posey on "The Operative Treatment of Glaucoma.") Ball is an ardent advocate of Hancock's operation for this one purpose.

Hancock died Jan. 1, 1880, at his country place, Standen House, Chute, Wiltshire.

Aside from numerous works on general surgery (the most important of which is entitled "On the Operative Surgery of the Foot and Ankle-Joint") he wrote "On the Division of the Ciliary Muscle in Glaucoma." (*Westminster Oph. Hosp. Reports,* No. 12, July, 1860, pp. 13-20.)—(T. H. S.)

Hancock, William Ilbert. A brilliant London ophthalmologist, who died very young. Born in 1874, he studied at Guy's Hospital, became, in 1896, a member of the Royal College of Surgeons, and in 1898 a

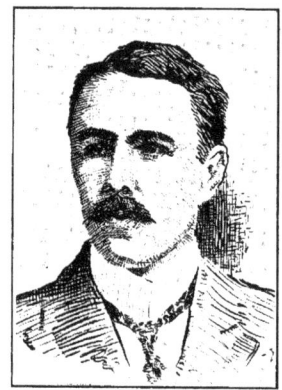

William Ilbert Hancock, F. R. C. S.

fellow of the same institution. The following year he became a member of the British Ophthalmological Society. He was assistant surgeon to the Royal London Ophthalmic Hospital (Moorfields), ophthalmic surgeon to the East London Hospital for Children (Shadwell's) and to the Bolingbroke Hospital. He contributed a number of excellent articles to the Transactions of the British Ophthalmological Society.

He was a gentle, modest man, with an enormous capacity for hard work. His only diversion was athletics, in which he greatly excelled.

He died Jan. 26, 1910, being only 36 years of age.—(T. H. S.)

Hand camera. A small portable camera.

Handführer. (G.) Cheiragon, or device to guide the hands of the blind in writing.

Hand-glass. A small magnifying glass for increasing the power of sight, especially for those whose near vision is unusually defective. Various forms are depicted herewith.

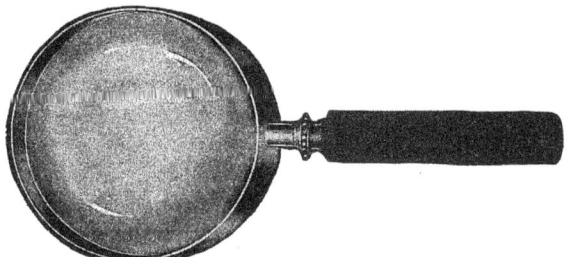

Hand Reading Glass.

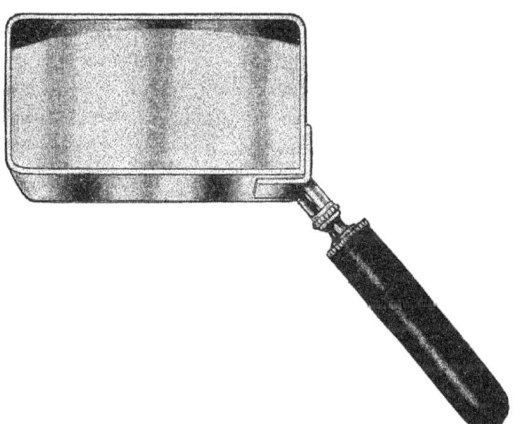

Hand Reading Glass.

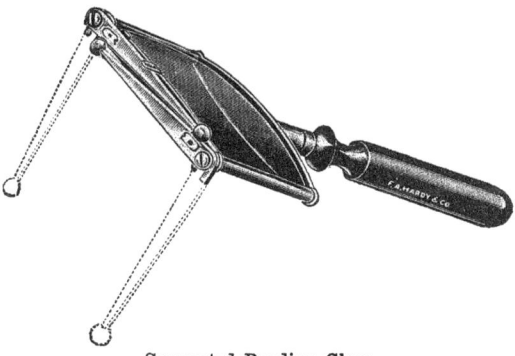

Supported Reading Glass.

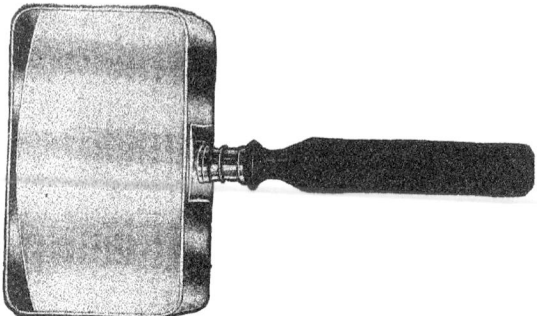

Cross Cylinder Hand Glass.

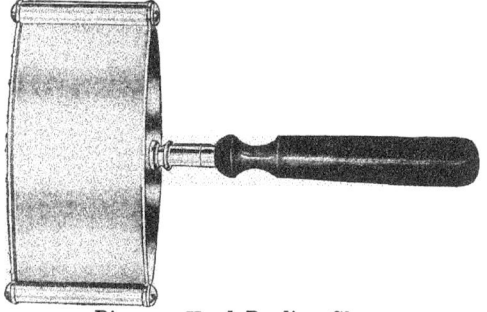

Biconvex Hand Reading Glass.

Hand-lamp. This useful apparatus has already been described on page 4602, Vol. VI, of this *Encyclopedia*.

Hand magnet. See **Electromagnet** and **Electricity.**

Hand perimeter. See **Examination of the eye;** as well as **Perimetry;** also, **Hird's hand-perimeter.**

Handschrift. (G.) Manuscript.

Hanging, Ocular indications of. See **Legal relations of ophthalmology,** about the middle third of the section.

Hannover, Adolf. A celebrated Danish anatomist, physician and ophthalmologist. Born at Copenhagen, Nov. 24, 1814, he was there admitted to medical practice in 1838. Later he studied for a number of years in Paris and Berlin. He then became a military surgeon; also assistant physician at the Royal Friedrich's Hospital, and for a time was privat docent in pathologic anatomy. In 1856, and again in 1878, he received the Monthyon Prize of the Institute of France for his investigations in ocular anatomy and pathology.

Hannover's chief ophthalmologic writings are: 1. Ueber der Netzhaut

u. s. w. (Müller's *Archiv* 1840.) 2. Die Linse. (*Ibid.*, 1845.) 3. Der Glaskörper. (*Ibid.*, 1845.) 4. Das Auge, Beiträge sur Anatomie, Physiologie und Pathologie dieses Organs. (Danish, 1850; German, Leipsic, 1852.) 5· La Rétine de l'Homme et des Vertébrés, Mém. Histologique, Historico-Critique et Physiologique. (Danish, 1875; French, Copenhagen and Paris, 1876.)—(T. H. S.)

Haplancyloblepharon. (Obsolete.) Simple ankyloblepharon.

Haploblepharocleisis. An old name for ankyloblepharon.

Haploscope. This term is sometimes applied to an instrument for measuring the visual axes, but Hering employed it to designate an apparatus that offers a special field of vision to each eye while the contents of

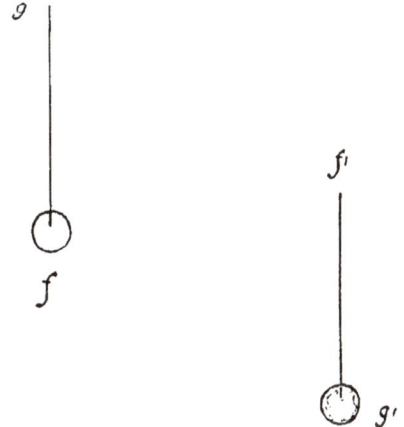

The Figures of the Haploscope. (Hering.)

these two fields are united in consciousness. In illustration of this device Cattell (Norris and Oliver's *System,* Vol. I, p. 553) describes it as consisting of a vertical screen upon which, at a horizontal distance apart, that is equal to the distance between the eyes, two points are marked, as, for example, f and f' in the figure. One is to look at this screen with both body and head held upright (the primary position) and with the visual lines (the lines which connect the nodal points of the eyes with their visual centers) placed horizontal and parallel. The left eye is to be directed upon the left mark f, and the right eye is to be fixed upon the right mark f'. If now at f a vertical line be drawn upward and one at f' drawn downward, the experimenter will see (since f and f' throw their images upon corresponding points) a continuous line gg'. This line, however, is not in general, as one might expect, a straight line, but the two lines form an obtuse angle with each other. The inclination of the two lines can be measured if one of the two lines—say f'g'—is made movable about an axis, and if the amount of its rotation can be read off upon the arc of a circle. This line can then be turned until it appears to be the exact continuation of the other. If in this new position of f'g' both lines should be produced beyond f and f' respectively, only a single straight line would be visible.

Hard cataract. An opacity of the lens, varying in color from gray to yellowish gray, involving the entire lens, and of hard, resistent consistence. It usually occurs in persons above 60 years of age, and by some authors is regarded as synonymous with senile cataract. See **Cataract.**

Harderian gland. HARDER'S GLAND. A small gland found in many animals, especially in birds, at the inner canthus of the eye. See page 2689, Vol. IV, of this *Encyclopedia;* also **Birds, Eyes of.**

Hard soap. See **Soap.**

Hare-eye. See **Lagophthalmos.**

Hare, The. The lung and the marrow of the hare were considered to be ophthalmic remedies in Greco-Roman antiquity. The dung of the hare, mixed with honey, was also a popular remedy.—(T. H. S.)

Hareus. A powerful arc light (rich in ultra violet rays) which Birch-Hirschfeld believes to be particularly injurious to the eyes.

Harlan, George Cuvier. A distinguished ophthalmologist of Philadelphia, inventor of Harlan's tests for malingering and Harlan's operation for symblepharon. He was born in Philadelphia, Pa., Jan. 28, 1835, the son of Dr. Richard Harlan. In 1855 he received the degree of Bachelor of Arts from Delaware College, and the Master's degree from the same institution in 1858—the year in which he received his medical degree from the University of Pennsylvania. His graduation thesis at the last named institution was entitled *The Iris.*

As early as April 6, 1857 (even before he had received his medical degree) he was appointed resident physician at the Wills Eye Hospital. From 1861 till 1864 he was surgeon at the same institution, although, for a time, in 1861, he was assistant surgeon in the U. S. Navy. In 1868 he again became full surgeon at the Wills Eye Hospital, and remained in that position till May, 1901—more than twenty-three years. On Oct. 29th of the same year he was made consulting surgeon. He was also connected at various times with numerous other hospitals in his capacity as ophthalmologist.

He was the first incumbent of the chair of ophthalmology at the Philadelphia Polyclinic and School for Graduates in Medicine. As a teacher he was clear, concise and practical.

He was also a very skilful operator, never quick and brilliant, but conservative and conscientious. His manner in the midst of an operation was, in fact, so placid and composed that the patient himself would often be considerably influenced by it. He used to tell his

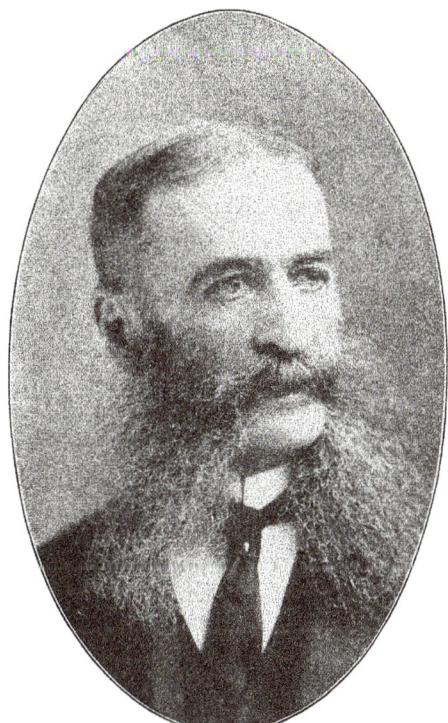

George Cuvier Harlan.

students that operation-fright was, at least in greater part, the offspring of too much haste.

He was a member of the College of Physicians of Philadelphia, the Philadelphia County Medical Society, the Medical Society of the State of Pennsylvania, the American Medical Association, the Wills Hospital Ophthalmic Society, the American Ophthalmological Society, and the International Congress of Ophthalmologists in 1876.

Aside from numerous journal articles, he wrote "Diseases of the Eyelids," and "Operations Performed upon the Eyelids," both for Vol. III of Norris and Oliver's *"System of Diseases of the Eye,"* and "Eyesight and How to Care for It" (1879). The latter composition was a popular manual, clear, practical and thorough, and of very great value to the laity. It had a large sale.

His operation for symblepharon, described in another portion of this volume, is widely employed, and the same may be said of his various tests for ocular malingering.

He was a very gentlemanly, unassuming man, courteous to all and especially helpful to the younger brothers in ophthalmology. He had but few amusements, or recreations. An occasional chat with a friend, the perusal of a good book, a ride on horseback; these were the "sum and circle" of all his diversions.

In the course of one of his horseback rides the accident occurred which resulted in his death. On the evening of Sept. 22, 1909, as he ambled along the Wissahickon bridle path, his horse slipped on a pebble and threw him against the side of a gully, fracturing his spine. For three hours he lay undiscovered. Found by a groom, he was taken to the Chestnut Hill Hospital, where he lingered for a few days, dying Sept. 25, 1909.—(T. H. S.)

Harlan's test. This test for pretended blindness (q. v.) is practically the same as Dujardin's test (q. v.).

Harley, George. A celebrated British physician, who devoted some attention to ophthalmology, and who was himself, for a time, almost blind. Born at Haddington, East Lothian, Feb. 12, 1829, he received his medical degree in 1850 at Edinburgh. He is said to have performed, before his graduation, a Cæsarean section, whereby, after the death of the mother, he delivered a living child who grew up and became a father of a family. After his graduation, Harley studied at Paris, Würzburg, Giessen, Berlin, Vienna and Heidelberg, and, returning to England in 1855, he settled as general practitioner in London. Here he became, in 1856, Instructor in Physiology and Histology at University College, three years later Professor of Legal Medicine, and in 1860 Physician at the University College Hospital. In 1854 he became a Fellow of the Royal College of Physicians, and in 1865 of the Royal Society. An ardent devotee of the microscope, he acquired, from excessive employment of the eyes in microscopic work, a retinitis which rendered him well nigh blind for nine or ten months. For all of this time he remained in a darkened room, and, after his recovery, wrote an account of his experiences, entitled "Autoclinical Remarks on Injury of the Retina from Overwork with the Microscope (*Lancet*, 1868). Harley died Oct. 27, 1896.—(T. H. S.)

Harman's aqueous needle. The attempt to catch the aqueous as it escapes through a corneal opening, by means of a scoop or pipette, is both wasteful and unreliable. Coming in contact with the conjunctiva its purity is questionable. Hence, Harman has devised a hypodermic needle, with a sharp, spear-shaped head which attaches to a lachrymal syringe. It can be introduced through the cornea, after thorough cleansing with saline solution, or even superficial

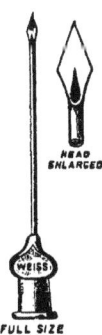

Harman's Hollow Spear-Headed Needle for Obtaining Aqueous for Bacteriologic Examination; to be used with a lachrymal syringe.

cauterization of the point through which it is introduced. It can be kept sterile and free from rust in absolute alcohol. (See the figure.)

Harman's lengthening operation. See **Muscles, Ocular.**

Harmonic colors. Complementary colors.

Harnstoff. (G.) Urea.

Harper, John. An early American surgeon, of some importance in ophthalmology. The date of his birth is not known. He was, however, a native of Ireland, received his degree at Glasgow, and, emigrating to America, settled in Baltimore. Here he was widely known as a cataract operator, performing, however, merely dislaceration of the capsule. He died in Baltimore in 1831.—(T. H. S.)

Harpoon needle. This is one of numerous devices for making an open-

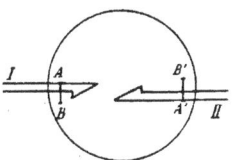

Weill's Method of Introducing the Harpoon Needles to Tear Secondary Membranous Cataract.

ing in the secondary membranes following extraction of cataract, or its partial absorption. This subject is fully described under **After-**

cataract. It may be added that Weill's method of accomplishing this and the instruments—harpoon needles—are worthy of special mention here. (See the figure.) Stilling's needles are practically the same and introduced and used in a similar fashion.

Harte Augenhaut. (G.) Sclerotic.

Hart, Ernest. A well known medical editor, hygienist, and oto oph thalmologist, inventor of gelatine discs for the medication of the eye. Born at London, in June, 1835, the son of a dentist, he studied at St. George's and St. Mary's Hospitals. In 1856 he became a member of the Royal College of Surgeons of England. He was for a time prosector at St. George's, and, later, instructor in diseases of the eye and ear at St. Mary's. In 1866 he was elected editor of the *"British Medical Journal"*—a position which he held until his death. He was also for a long time editor of *"The London Medical Record"* and of *"The Sanitary Record."* In addition to numerous journal articles, he wrote *"A Manual of Public Health"* (London, 1874). In 1893 he received the honorary degree of D.C.L. from the University of Durham, and died Jan. 7, 1898.—(T. H. S.)

Harter Staar. (G.) Hard cataract.

Hartley-Krause operation. Removal of the entire Gasserian ganglion.

Hartnack's loupe. This magnifying glass closely resembles a Coddington lens (see p. 2313, Vol. IV, of this *Encyclopedia*) and consists of a short, metallic tube twenty millimetres long, containing a series of lenses. They are equal to a convex lens of 60 D. The aperture is sixteen millimetres, the focal distance is very short (sixteen and sixtenths millimetres), and the linear enlargement is about five-fold. The field is quite as large as in the instruments previously mentioned.

Hartshorne, Edward. An American physician, famous, but of slight importance in ophthalmology. Born at Philadelphia in 1818, the second son of Dr. Joseph Hartshorne, he received the degree of A.B. at Princeton in 1837, that of A.M. at the same institution in 1840, and that of M.D. at the University of Pennsylvania in the same year. In 1844 he went to Europe, where he studied for several years. Returning to America, he settled in Philadelphia, and soon was widely known. His contributions to medical literature were numerous, extensive and valuable. In his practice he paid considerable attention to diseases of the eye, and in 1856 he edited the second American issue of T. Wharton Jones's *Principles and Practice of Ophthalmic Surgery* (Philadelphia, 1856).

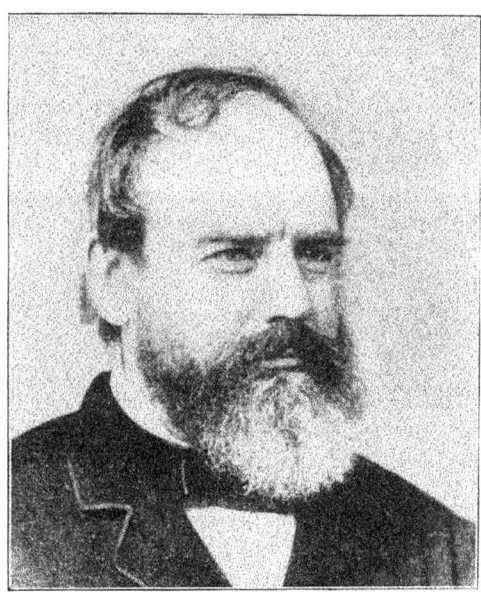

Edward Hartshorne.

Hartshorne married, in 1850, Mrs. Adelia C. Pearse, of Boston, by whom he had five children. He died in 1885, aged sixty-seven.— (T. H. S.)

Hartsoeker, Nicolas. A famous Dutch naturalist, of some ophthalmologic importance because of his *"Essai de Dioptrique"* (Paris, 1694; 1696; Dutch trans., Amsterdam, 1699). Born at Gouda, Holland, Mar. 26, 1656, he studied chiefly mathematics, physics, and astronomy at Leyden and Paris. From 1704 till 1716 he was Professor of Mathematics and Philosophy at Düsseldorf. Later he lived at Utrecht, where he died Dec. 10, 1725.—(T. H. S.)

Hart-trefoil. *Melilotus albus et officinalis.* The same as lote and melilot-clover. In ancient Greco-Roman times, melilot-clover was often employed in the form of a poultice for acute affections of the eye accompanied by swelling and discharge. It was also sometimes used for wounds of the eye.—(T. H. S.)

Harz. (G.) Resin.

Hasenauge. (G.) Lagophthalmus.

Hasner, Joseph, Ritter von Artha. A celebrated Austrian ophthalmologist, discoverer of "the valve of Hasner." He was born at Prague, Aug. 13, 1819, and there, in 1840, received his medical degree. For the next two years he was "secundärarzt" in the General Hospital at Prague, where he succeeded Arlt as first assistant in Fischer's eye clinic. In 1852 he was made extraordinary, and, in 1856, on Arlt's removal to Vienna, ordinary, professor. This full professorship, in 1884, he resigned, though he had not quite reached the age limit, because, owing to the foundation of the Czech University, his clinic was divided, and half of it assigned to the newly established institution. The division of his clinic gave him, in fact, a deep offense, from which he never fully recovered.

His more important publications are: 1. Entwurf einer Anatomischen Begründung der Augenheilkunde (Prague, 1847). 2. Physiologie und Pathologie des Thränenableitungsapparats (Prague, 1850). 3. Klinische Vorträge über Augenheilkunde (Prague, 1860-66). 4. Beiträge zur Physiologie und Pathologie des Auges (Prague, 1873). 5. Die Grenzen der Accomodation (Prague, 1875). 6. Phakologische studien (Prague, 1870). 7. Das Mittlere Auge in seinen Physiologischen und Pathologischen Beziehungen (Prague, 1879). 8. Die Verletzungen des Auges in Forensischer Hinsicht (1880). He also published a very large number of journal articles, and was for a long time one of the associate editors of the *"Prager Medicinischen Vierteljahrsschrift."* He died, after a long illness, Feb. 22, 1892.— (T. H. S.)

Hatpin, The, in ophthalmology. As an instrument capable of injuring the eye this article of woman's dress has occupied a prominent position, and a considerable literature has grown up about it. So frequently have serious penetrating wounds been intentionally and unintentionally caused by it that many municipalities have adopted laws regulating its use. See **Injuries of the eye.**

Hatton, George. A well known ophthalmologist of Portland, Me., whose life dates are unprocurable. His medical degree was received at Harvard in 1869. After a period of study abroad, he settled in Portland, Me., where he was winning an excellent reputation and a large practice, when he suddenly died.

He was a tall, thin man, red-haired, apparently tubercular; a man of clean life, and very religious. He is said to have carried his entire fortune ($25,000.00 in U. S. Government bonds) about on his person. These bonds he left to a Sunday school, or church, in Dedham, Mass.—(T. H. S.)

Hauptachse. (G.) Principal axis.

Hauptaugen. (G.) Principal eyes. A term applied to the pair of organs in four-eyed animals, usually insects and crustaceans, that chiefly functionate during the visual act.

Hauptblickpunkt. (G.) Principal point of fixation or regard.

Hauptbrennpunkt. (G.) Principal focus.

Hauptebene. (G.) Principal focal plane.

Hauptstrahl. (G.) Principal ray.

Haut. (F.) High; tall; upper.

Haut. (G.) Skin, derma.

Hauteur. (F.) Height; altitude.

Häutige Bindehaut. (G.) The conjunctiva changed to a skin-like membrane.

Häutiger Staar. (G.) Membranous cataract.

Hautkrankheiten. (G.) Diseases of the skin.

Hautleiden. (G.) Dermal affections.

Haut mal. (F.) Epilepsy.

Hautpfropfung. (G.) Skin grafting.

Hautreize. (G.) Irritation of the skin.

Hautverbrennunge. (G.) Burns of the skin.

Häuy, Valentin. (1745-1822.) A French philanthropist who, about 1782, first made tangible letters practically available for the blind and, later, established schools for teaching and training the sightless. He devoted his life to the education of the blind, and in 1786 wrote *Essai sur L'Education des Aveugles* (1786). See p. 250, Vol. I of this *Encyclopedia.*

Havers, Clopton. An English anatomist of the late 17th and early 18th centuries, of some slight ophthalmologic importance because of his "Extraordinary Bleeding at the Glandula Lacrymalis" (*Philos. Trans.,* 1694, Vol. III).—(T. H. S.)

Haw. A name given to the caruncle or remains of the third eyelid or winker of a horse; also a diseased or disordered condition of the same organ.

Hawk. The dung of the hawk, in ancient Greco-Roman times, was mixed with honey and employed externally for various diseases of the eye, probably because of the keen sight of the bird (Pliny, XXIX, 38).—(T. H. S.)

Hawksbee, or Hauksbee, Francis. An English physicist who was already a well-known experimentalist when in 1705 he was admitted a Fellow of the Royal Society. (He should not be confused with Francis Hawksbee the younger, 1687-1763, apparently his son, who was also an electrician and skilled instrument maker, and who, in 1723, was appointed clerk and housekeeper to the Royal Society.) Hawksbee the elder contributed forty-three memoirs to the *Philosoph-*

ical Transactions, chiefly on chemistry and electricity, between 1704 and 1713. His chief independent work, published in 1709, was entitled *Physico-Mechanical Experiments on Various Subjects; touching Light and Electricity producible on the Attrition of Bodies.* He is also well known as the improver of the earlier air-pumps of Boyle, Papin, and Hooke, and as the first who used glass in the electrical machine. He died soon after 1713.—*(Standard Encyclopedia).*

Hawkweed. *Hieracium pilocella.* According to the elder Pliny, an excellent poultice for epiphora is made by saturating with the juice of the hawkweed. The juice of the same weed, mixed with mother's milk, he believed to be good for ulcers of the cornea. Mixed with the juice of the poppy, the juice of the hawkweed was also well rubbed into the scalp "to clarify the vision."

The ancient Greeks and Romans believed that hawkweed juice was used by the hawks themselves to bring about an extraordinary clarification of the sight; hence the name of the plant.—(T. H. S.)

Haya poison. A powerful toxic agent from tropical Africa. It is said to be derived from some species of *Erythrophleum,* but this claim has been disputed. A solution of its impure alkaloid (1 to 2 per cent.) is a powerful local anesthetic, more persistent than cocain.

Hayden, Thomas. An Irish physician, of some ophthalmologic importance because of his "Function of the Yellow Spot of Soemmering in Circular Vision" (1858). He was born in Tipperary, became, in 1850, Licentiate of the Royal College of Surgeons of Ireland, and very shortly afterward Instructor in Anatomy at the Ledwich School of Medicine in Dublin. In 1855 he was appointed Assistant Professor of Anatomy and Physiology at the Dublin (Catholic) University. He died Nov. 30, 1881.—(T. H. S.)

Hay-fever. HAY-ASTHMA. SUMMER-CATARRH. This well-known disease is, as its name indicates, mostly met with in late summer. Its symptoms are usually those of the ordinary rhinitis, viz, redness and swelling of the nasal mucous membrane, a copious, watery discharge and repeated paroxysms of sneezing. The eyes exhibit intense itching, burning, lachrymation, scleral redness (sometimes definite catarrhal conjunctivitis); headache more or less marked; often general malaise, loss of appetite, some rise of temperature and difficulty of breathing when the bronchial mucous membrane is affected. Hay fever is most commonly a disease of adult life, but it may occur at all ages. It usually returns annually on a definite date, which varies with the locality in which the patient is subjected to the exciting cause, which is oftenest floating pollen of different grasses, most likely the ragweeds, goldenrods and timothy hay. Other causes of infection, or irritation, as dust or bright sunlight, may set up an attack. Three factors essential to the production of hay-fever are a nervous constitution or idiosyncrasy, a local irritability and an external exciting cause. The treatment, which is generally unsatisfactory, should be directed to improving the health by quinine, arsenic or other tonics and to soothing the nervous state by bromid of potassium or antipyrin. Local inhalations, as of iodine, adrenaline, etc., are also recommended but the best palliative remedy is to remove the patient from the probable source of his disease by sending him to the seaside or on a sea voyage. In the United States the region of the White Mountains in New Hampshire or the Lake Superior country also seems specially favorable for relief.

This is not the place to discuss the numerous other remedies that are constantly being lauded as cures (pollen extracts, vaccines, etc.) for this troublesome affection; suffice it to say, however, that apart from soothing collyria (containing holocain, chloretone, adrenaline) and protective glasses the indications are to relieve or cure the hay fever upon whose presence the ocular symptoms depend.

Hay, Gustavus. A well known ophthalmologist of Boston, Mass. He was born in Boston, May 11, 1830, received the degree of Bachelor of Arts at Harvard in 1850, graduated from the Lawrence Scientific School in 1853, and then, for a year, was connected with the work of the U. S. Coast Survey in the South.

Deciding to study medicine, he entered the Harvard Medical School in 1854, and there received his professional degree in 1857.

At first he settled in Boston as a general practitioner. Soon, however, he decided to become an ophthalmologist, and, in order to prepare himself as thoroughly as possible for the work of his new vocation, he studied for a time in Vienna. Here the teachers who chiefly influenced him were Jaeger and Arlt.

Returning to Boston, he practised ophthalmology and was very successful. From 1861-1873 he was one of the attending surgeons of the Massachusetts Charitable Eye and Ear Infirmary, and from 1873-1900 he was one of the consulting staff of the same institution.

His favorite recreation was mathematics, and, as Dr. Chas. H. Williams, of Boston, has related, "was never so happy as when working out some problem or when explaining some difficult proposition in optics or the higher mathematics, and his natural inclination would have led him to become a teacher of this science." Dr. James A.

Spalding, of Portland, Me., declares "Optic formulas were fun for him: he understood them as no one I ever before or since have met." He was very fond of etchings, and had an immense collection of them. Etchings, in fact, were hanging all over his house. He was slender, slim-faced, smoothly-shaven, and had a predilection for very large lenses in his own spectacles. He was always very dignified and deliberate, and, as a correspondent writes, "reminded one of a philosopher rather than a physician."

He married, in 1863, Maria Crehore, who died in 1875. In 1881 he married Miriam Parsons, who, with a son, survived him.

He died at his home in Jamaica Plain, April 26, 1908.—(T. H. S.)

Hays, Isaac. A famous American ophthalmologist, medico-economist, author and editor. Born at Philadelphia, Penna., July 5, 1796, the son of Samuel and Richea Gratz Hays, he received his general education at the University of Pennsylvania, obtaining the degree of A.B. in 1816. For a time, owing chiefly to the influence of his father, a prominent merchant, he devoted himself to commercial pursuits. His natural tendencies, however, soon asserting themselves, he began the study of medicine under the private instruction of Dr. Nathaniel Chapman.

Later he entered the Medical Department of the University of Pennsylvania, from which institution he received his degree in 1820. His thesis, on that occasion, was characteristically entitled "Sympathy." He then, for a time, devoted himself especially to the study of ophthalmology.

In 1822 he became surgeon to the Pennsylvania Infirmary for Diseases of the Eye and Ear, and, beginning in 1834, he was surgeon to the Wills Eye Hospital for twenty years. He reported the first case of astigmatism observed in America, and the fifth in all the world. He was also the first to report a case (that of Mary Bishop) of pathologic (not congenital) color-blindness. In February, 1826, he became one of the editors of the *"Philadelphia Journal of the Medical and Physical Sciences,"* which had been established six years before. A few months later, Dr. Hays was made sole editor of this journal, and then it was that he exchanged its title for one much better known, *"The American Journal of the Medical Sciences."* In 1869 he began to be assisted in his work as editor by his son, Dr. I. Minis Hays, but continued to act as editor-in-chief until his death—over fifty-two years.

Dr. Hays was never a teacher of medicine—a fact, no doubt, in some part due to his natural timidity before an audience.

Among the articles he wrote and the books which he either wrote or edited, are these:

1. The Forces by which the Blood is Circulated. (A leading article in *The Philadelphia Jour. of the Med. and Phys. Sciences,* 1826.)

2. Purulent Ophthalmia. (*Phila. Jour. of the Med. and Phys. Sciences,* 1827.)

3. Wilson's *"American Ornithology."* (Edited by Dr. Hays, 3 vols., 1828.)

4. Broussais' *"Chronic Phlegmasia."* (Trans. by Hays and Griffith; 2 vols., 1831.)

5. Diseases of the Eye. (A chapter in Dewees' *"Practice of Medicine,"* 1833.)

6. *The American Cyclopedia of Practical Medicine and Surgery:* A digest of Medical Literature. (Only 2 vols. issued—from A to Axilla —Phila., 1834-36.)

7. Laurence's *"Treatise on Diseases of the Eye."* (New ed. by Dr. Isaac Hays, 1843.)

When 38 years of age, Dr. Hays married Miss Sarah Minis, of Savannah, Ga. To them were born four children.

Dr. Hays died April 12, 1879, aged 83.—(T. H. S.)

Hazeline. This proprietary remedy is an extract of hamamelis (q. v.). Lawson (*Text-book,* p. 538) advises it as a soothing collyrium in the following formula: "Hazeline" gr. 15-20; aqua dest. fl.ʒi.

Headache, Blind. A popular name for migraine (q. v.); referring to the (often scintillating) scotoma that as a hemiopia or total obscuration of the visual field is seen in many cases.

Headache, Ocular. There are fewer symptoms for which the ophthalmic surgeon will be more frequently consulted, and hardly any of greater importance, than headache. Moreover, there is no affection that will more largely tax his diagnostic and remedial resources. Before he can properly decide to what class a particular headache belongs, he must have a practical knowledge of all of them. Ocular headache may be defined as that acute discomfort in and about the head that directly or indirectly results from organic or functional disorder of the visual apparatus.

The ocular element in all forms of headache is larger than is generally suspected. It is probably not less than 40 per cent.; while of all bilateral, frontal headaches 75 per cent. are due to eye-strain. In other sections herein it is shown that the ciliary and other eye muscles always endeavor to bring about effective vision and that in abnormal states of the refraction, particularly, this constant effort results in symptoms, prominent among which is the headache in question. These attempts irritate not only the third nerve nuclei but the center for the trigeminus; the end filaments of the latter on the forehead suffer, so that there is not only a peripheral aching noticed by the patient but a duller pain referred to the eyeballs and the parts behind them. In the very chronic cases, also, the whole front of the head aches. The pains of eye-strain are invariably bilateral.

The *exciting cause* of ocular headache is chiefly some form of near work that requires long continued use of the muscles of accommodation and convergence, such as reading, sewing, stenography, embroidery, drawing, painting, music, writing, cardplaying, typewriting, etc.

The site of the headache is very important. In the order of frequency this is supra-orbital, deep orbital, fronto-occipital and temporal. A unilateral, supra-orbital headache or a hemicrania of any kind is not commonly due to eye-strain.

The pains do not always follow immediately upon indulgence in excessive near work; they are sometimes not noticed until the early morning. As a rule, however, the eyes and head commence to ache after a certain number of minutes or hours of close work and with such regularity that the sufferer himself attributes it to some trouble with the eyes. Astigmatic, hypermetropic, and heterophoric patients also suffer when called on to use their eyes much for distant vision. An evening at the theatre or an afternoon in shopping is often responsible for an ocular headache, as these occupations reach the weak points in the ocular apparatus. In the latter case the necessity for keeping a lookout in all directions to avoid collisions with fellow-shoppers in a crowded store, with pedestrians on the pavement and with men, women and vehicles on street crossings, the close examination of fabrics—often in a poor light—all these efforts make large demands not only on the general nervous energy, but particularly on the extrinsic and intrinsic muscles of the eye. When the latter are handicapped by muscular anomalies or refractive errors, the shopper usually goes home with a headache. In the same way, riding in a railway-train or street-car, with the moving panorama viewed from the car window, is especially trying to defective eyes. Doubtless church, concert and theatre headaches are also due to efforts by abnormal eyes to stare at distant objects, while the cerebral centers are meantime further irritated by rebreathed air and unshaded lights.

Along with the headache are almost always other signs and symptoms that proclaim the ocular nature of the trouble. After reading for a time, lines and letters run together or become mixed up. The conjunctiva of the eyeball gets red from hyperemia of its vessels and the lids burn, smart and itch.

It must not be forgotten, however, in the diagnosis of ocular headache, that the eye, so far as symptoms and the results of inspection go, sometimes seems to be free from disease. There is an ocular headache, but no apparent disease of the eye. A patient may have a purely ocular headache although the vision is normal or even above normal, and although many of the asthenopic symptoms just detailed are wanting. It is, strange to say, usually the person with unusually good distant vision, or who at twenty years old has had it, that complains of eye-strain. The short-sighted person cannot distinguish objects in the distance, but he does not often suffer from headache.

Imbalance of the extrinsic muscles (heterotropia, heterophoria), (see these headings) is also a cause of ocular headache, and it is always desirable to apply the tests for this condition in the diagnosis of eye-strain.

The general practitioner should bear in mind that supra-orbital headache also results from several forms of nasal "catarrh." Hypertrophic rhinitis, deviations of and growths from the septum, polypi, mucous and purulent collections in the various sinuses, all produce frontal headaches. The chronic, frontal headache of nasal disease differs from ocular headache in that the former continues during the night, or gets worse when the patient takes "cold," while a purely ocular headache is not usually made worse by a simple coryza and ceases when the patient has retired and the lights in his room are extinguished; in other words, there is no headache when there is no ocular strain. (See, also, Vol. III, p. 1821 of this *Encyclopedia.*)

Alex. R. Tweedie (*Ophthalmic Review*, p. 326, Nov., 1909) comments on the paper of Snydacker (*Klin. Monatsbl. f. Augenheilk.*, June, 1909) partly as follows: The author found 799 headache patients out of 2,000 who had applied for treatment. Amongst this series were 55 in whom the headache was found to be entirely attributable to either acute or chronic empyema of the accessory sinuses of the nose. The real origin of the symptoms in some of these cases he did not at first diagnose, and he suggests that there are many instances where the oculist may overlook the true source of troubles which at first sight appear referable to some disability of the eyes and for which the patient seeks his aid.

The greater proportion of these cases he maintains will be found to be dependent on inflammatory affections of the frontal sinus alone, or combined with a similar condition of the anterior ethmoidal cells; it is only infrequently, he says, that empyema of the maxillary sinus or of the sphenoidal sinus comes under the notice of the oculist, as affections of these cavities do not usually produce symptoms referred to the eye.

With these data before him Snydacker submits that the oculist should have some knowledge of rhinology, not so much in order that he may undertake the treatment of such cases, but rather that he may be able thereby to transfer them to the care of the nasal surgeon or summon him in consultation when difficulties in diagnosis arise.

He believes that every headache limited to one side, not being of the character of migraine, should excite suspicion in this direction, especially if it can be accurately localized. Although pain from an inflamed sinus may be referred to other situations it is generally the case that the area immediately over it is tender when one of these cavities is occluded.

The oculist should always test the sensitiveness of the frontal and supra-orbital regions when the patient complains of headache, as under these circumstances the frontal sinus is often at fault.

All headaches which appear to date from an attack of influenza or severe cold should cause the oculist to suspect the nasal sinuses.

In the case of a headache which comes on suddenly and is pulsating in character the nose should be submitted to examination.

A headache which recurs periodically should occasion careful investigation into the condition of the nose, especially when it usually begins on rising in the morning, lasts a few hours and gradually decreases in severity, disappearing altogether in the evening. Such headaches are often due to frontal sinusitis, and the explanation of these phenomena lies in the fact that the natural ostia of this sinus are in the most dependent position when the head is upright, thus favoring the discharge of any pathological products, whilst drainage ceases when the patient is recumbent.

If the oculist has good reason to suspect the headache to be caused by some nasal lesion he should make careful inquiries as to the presence of any nasal discharge and particularly as to whether such, if present, is limited to one side. The discharge may occur anteriorly and necessitate the use of many handkerchiefs daily, or be complained of as accumulating in the back of the throat. Further, if the oculist himself wishes to make an examination of the interior of the nose, improvement of the symptoms after the intra-nasal application of adrenalin points to the headache having a nasal origin, whilst transillumination and radiography will both at times be of assistance in establishing a correct diagnosis. Whether or no the oculist should adopt these methods of examination is a matter, Syndacker considers, for each himself to decide.

Emphasis is laid on the fact that in headaches arising from affections of the nose the symptoms are often described as being worse the first thing in the morning and improving later on in the day. Some patients suffering in his respect will even state that they wake with the headache or are awakened by it, and although the author rightly assigns as a reason for this state of affairs the recumbent position and altered relation of the ostium to the cavity in the case of the frontal sinus, the same cause will also intensify headaches due to most other nasal affections.

Robert Sattler (*Ohio State Medical Journal,* April 15, 1909) makes his first subdivision of this subject, the ocular, the sole cause of headache. These cases are generally first seen by the oculist, and are usually promptly relieved by accurate optical correction. Heredity is chiefly responsible for the eye deformities present.

He next considers the ocular an associate, but wholly latent, cause of headache. These cases are usually first seen by the general practitioner or specialist in another line. He says that while lenses may benefit some, with a large number the optical correction, prism exercises, etc., are mainly justifiable as part of the general treatment for the other causes in evidence, or to aid these as possible suggestive measures in the moral management, which is of equal or greater importance in these cases.

He then discusses the ocular as a dominant and active associate cause. He believes that optical and other special treatment will relieve head pains due to inherent or acquired ocular causes, and that share of the general nervous tension, depression or extreme exhaustion which the eyes contribute, but questions whether the more uncommon headaches of hysterical origin, such as migraine, circular headache, habitual headache, etc., are more than favorably modified by the ocular treatment which may be indicated. He warns against assuming an ocular cause for head pain of grave central or other origin, and urges a more rational and searching diagnostic interpretation of the general symptoms of head pains and the other causes which create them.

This article stands out in striking contrast with those loose and semi-hysterical accounts widely disseminated in this country, that ascribe every headache to the ocular apparatus as its *fons et origo mali* and its uniform treatment in the form of a pair of glasses. As a consequence discredit is being cast upon effective diagnosis and upon the

careful measurement of refractive and oculo-muscular errors as one
of the most effective means of curing or relieving a well-defined class
of headache.

The various forms of *supra-orbital neuralgia* may usually be detected by their periodicity, by the tenderness at the supra-orbital notch
and soreness of the skin along the course of the nerve, by their being
almost always paroxysmal and unilateral and by the absence of asthenopic symptoms.

A class of practically incurable ocular headaches is that arising
from a combination of eye-strain and organic disease of the retina,
choroid, or ciliary body. The headaches from iritis, glaucoma, and
other acute diseases of the eye, are to be recognized by the presence
of the affections themselves.

It is probable that the hereditary form of **Migraine,** so far as
ocular treatment is concerned, is very rarely cured by ophthalmic
remedies. It is also doubtful whether acquired sick headache is much
influenced by attention to the eyes—and this is true even of those cases
in which eye symptoms (ocular pains, scintillating scotomata, asthenopia, etc.) are also present.

The treatment of ocular headache should be directed first of all
to the relief of the eye-strain, especially the correction of the hyperopia, astigmatism or the accommodative anomaly, by means of glasses.
Any local inflammation should be allayed; thus it not uncommonly
happens that diseases of the lids may prevent a complete cure of the
headache even after a correction of all refractive and muscular errors.

It should also be borne in mind that any departure from health
may affect the eye and so act as a predisposing cause of ocular headache. Prominent among the conditions that intensify or invite ocular
headache is insomnia, whatever be its origin, and one may be well
assured that complete relief from the chronic pains in the head is
very uncertain if the patient's sleep be disturbed or insufficient, even
if the other factors in their production receive proper attention.

Dyspepsia in all its forms, but especially the toxic form, due to
too much eating and too little exercise, is a frequent accompaniment
of frontal headache and should receive quite as much attention as the
purely ocular symptoms.

Excessive indulgence in tobacco and alcohol among male patients,
and tea and coffee among female sufferers, should not be overlooked.

Of local applications the simplest, most effective and least harmful
is the use of very hot or very cold fomentations. The patient may be
allowed to try both hot and cold water, choosing the one that seems

to him more useful or more grateful. Take a medium-sized towel, folded to measure twelve inches long by four wide. Grasp an end in each hand and dip into a basin of cold (40° F.) or hot (130° F.-150° F.) water. Bending over the basin, press the dripping towel gently against the closed eyes, forehead and temples. Repeat the applications in this way every fifteen seconds for five minutes, stopping them if additional pain or discomfort be produced. Do this every hour, or oftener, while the headache lasts.

Soothing collyria relieve the headache, sometimes, by their action on the congested conjunctival vessels: Borax; acid. boracic, āā. ʒss; aqua camphoræ, f. ʒss; sol. adrenalin. (1:5000), ad. f. ʒii. Drop into the eye every hour or two.

Another effective collyrium, to be used in the same way as the foregoing, is: Chloreton, 0.10; sodii boratis, 0.50; aquæ dest., 30.00.

The headache may often be dissipated by using the following mixture, to be rubbed over the forehead and temples; or a towel, wet with one part in ten of ice water may be laid over the closed eyes, and over the forehead, while the patient is lying down: Spirit of lavender, alcohol, of each 3 fluid ounces; spirit of camphor, 1 fluid ounce.

The following liniment is also effective: Chloroform, f. ʒi; spts. camphor; tinctur. aconiti, āā. f. ʒii.

Headache, Sick. See **Migraine, Ocular relations of.**

Headband trial frame. CALIFORNIA TRIAL FRAME. See Vol. VI, p. 4732 of this *Encyclopedia*.

Head injuries, Ocular symptoms from. Lesions of almost any portion of the intra-cranial visual organs may follow both direct and indirect injuries to the head. For the ophthalmologist an important section of this subject is discussed under **Military surgery of the eye.** Others will be found under **Injuries of the eye.** Here it may be said that in fractures of the base of the skull that pass through the optic foramen, the optic nerve is likely to be injured, either from tearing or compression or from hemorrhage into its sheath. As Swanzy (*System of Diseases of the Eye*) has said, blindness either complete or partial, is present in such cases from the first, but it is only after a time that optic atrophy can be recognized with the ophthalmoscope.

Fractures of the base of the skull which pass through the optic foramen are relatively frequent. Thus Hölder found that in eighty-eight fractures of the base the optic foramen was involved in fifty-four. Blows on the forehead, or supra-orbital margin, are sometimes followed by amaurosis, which used to be referred to injury of the supra-orbital division of the fifth nerve. We now know that the lesion is organic damage to the optic nerve at the optic foramen, by reason of the concussion transmitted along the roof of the orbit, which causes fracture of the bone, or rupture of membranes or of blood-vessels. But falls and severe blows on the head, apparently without fracture of the base, are sometimes followed by blindness, and at a later period the optic nerve becomes atrophied. Probably in these cases the optic nerve has been momentarily compressed and contused in the optic foramen, in consequence of the concussion. Transient blindness following head injuries is often caused by hemorrhage into the sheath of the optic nerve.

Elze (*Wochenschr. f. Therapie des Auges,* Oct. 1, 1908) details two cases illustrative of diplopia due to head injuries. In the first case, six months before the examination there had been concussion of the brain, with symptoms indicating labyrinthine disease and involvement of the semicircular canal on the left side. The subjective symptoms were diplopia and tinnitus. There was homonymous diplopia in all directions, with no change in the relative distance of the two images. The fundi were normal except for a slight pallor of the left optic nerve (not atrophied). Color perception was somewhat subnormal.

In the second case the history and symptoms were similar. No spontaneous diplopia, but with Maddox rod and double images close together, widening on lateral deviation to the right or left.

That the ocular disturbance is due to changes in the semicircular canal and not to labyrinthine disease is shown in a case reported by the author, in which the auditory nerve was greatly damaged in its peripheral distribution and was not accompanied by any ocular symptoms.

Casey Wood (*Practical Med. Series, Eye,* p. 181, 1909) has also had two patients with diplopia following head injuries without traumatism in or about the orbital region. In one instance the patient fell from a second story window to the pavement below. He was unconscious for three days and on awakening noticed that he could not see as well as before. Central vision was affected about equally in each eye, being two-thirds of normal, with ability to read Jaeger 8 only. Before the accident he had been able to read fine print. No glass helped his vision, but in the course of a month his sight improved both for distance and near. The double vision persisted and examinations disclosed a paresis of the external rectus.

In the second case the patient had an almost complete unilateral third nerve paralysis following a blow upon the back of the head. In this instance, also, vision deteriorated after the injury but slowly improved, but the double vision persisted, although after six months it slightly improved.

Head-light. The employment of head-lights and similar means of illuminating various ocular organs is fully described and depicted in Vol.

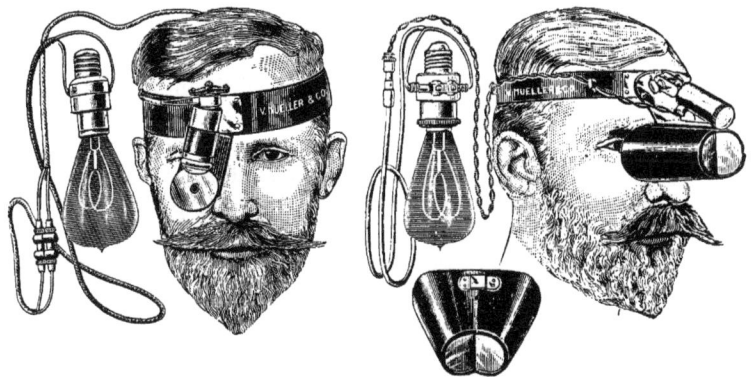

Kierstein's Electric Headlight.

This device is combined with the ophthalmoscope mirror for use in intraocular
operations and with the Berger loupe for corneal and anterior chamber operations.

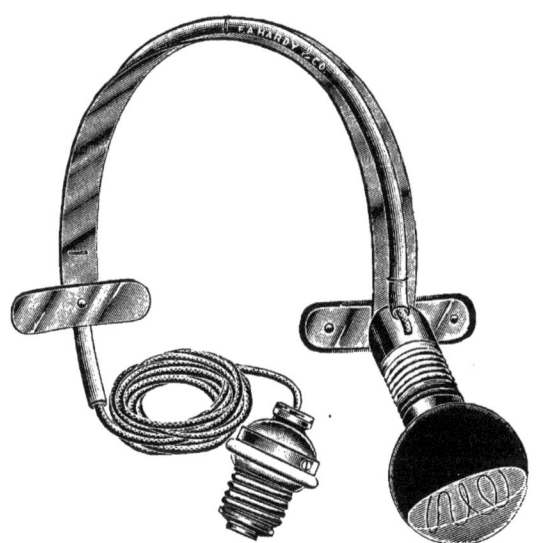

Stucky's Head-Light.

VI, p. 4601, of this *Encyclopedia*. Here it may suffice to depict a few
more simple but effective devices of the same variety. See the figures.

Headlights, Railway. The influence of these powerful lights upon the eyes both of railway employes and of the public is of sufficient importance to be considered under a separate heading. The matter is discussed under **Dazzling; Electric ophthalmia; Illumination; Glaring; Eyes of soldiers, sailors and railway employes** and to some extent under **Conservation of vision,** but in addition it may be said that Newcomb (*Ophthalmic Record,* March, 1912), who has investigated especially the dazzling effects of the electric headlight of locomotives, concludes that it interferes with correct reading of signals.

When the line of vision is opposed by high power headlight the distinctness with which the signals can be observed varies with the lateral distance of the signal from the headlight, greater interference taking place with high candle power headlight, and tapering off to no interference with oil headlights. In the cases of electric headlights the interference was so great that the average distance at which the signals could be correctly read was reduced to such an extent that high speed trains under the usual air line pressure, would not have been able to come to a full stop before reaching the signal. High candle headlights on approaching trains have no influence on the accuracy with which signals may be read, providing there are no opposing headlights of high candle power and the signal lights are burning properly. If any of the signal lights are not burning, false signals are obtained with the high candle power lights which are apt to be read as true signals. The zone of these false signals obtained with the electric and acetylene headlight approaching signal is situated between 1,500 feet and 400 feet from the signal. With approaching oil headlights no false signals are obtained. With acetylene and electric headlights, representing a high candle power headlight, false signals are obtained. None of the headlights tested sufficiently illuminated the track to avoid striking small objects and for large objects would result only in being able to reduce the speed at which they would be struck. Only the electric headlight sufficiently illuminates the track to warn of its approach to an observer when an observer is screened from the direct rays of the locomotive headlight and is looking across the tracks. It is difficult to make an approximate estimation of the distance of any of the headlights tested from the observer, when in their direct rays.

Head-tilting. Unnatural poses of the head due to ocular defects are generally the result of heterophoria or heterotropia.

Weeks (*Text-book,* p. 567) believes that the habit of tilting the head to one side or the other is a very common one. It occurred in the private practice of the writer in about 25 per cent. of the patients who consulted him for errors of refraction or of the extrinsic ocular muscles. Gould (*American Medicine*, 1904) has also drawn attention to the fact that astigmia may cause head-tilting when the axis of the astigmia in both eyes inclines from the vertical or horizontal, a few degrees "in the dominant eye alone, in the same direction for both eyes." The object of this tilting of the head is to render the axes vertical, or nearly so, in the interest of better vision.

Health resorts for diseases of the eye. See **Mineral** waters in eye diseases.

Hearing, Color. A synonym of chromatic audition. See, also, **Color music.**

Heart disease, Eye symptoms in. CARDIAC LESIONS AND OCULAR SYMPTOMS. Apart from retinal thrombosis and embolism—both of which will be found treated under their various captions—there are remarkably few ocular lesions directly produced by affections of the heart. Diseases of the circulatory system are briefly discussed by Parsons (*Pathology of the Eye*, p. 1254, Vol. IV). He says that v. Schulten has shown that the blood-pressure in the ophthalmic artery is only a few mm. Hg. below that of the carotid. Considering the very different blood supply of the eye it would be unwise to apply this result to man. Nevertheless, we may be sure that the arterial pressure is far above the normal intra-ocular pressure. It would not be surprising, therefore, if the pulse wave was transmitted to the central artery of the retina, and could be observed ophthalmoscopically. This, however, is seldom if ever the case under normal circumstances; and it is doubtless due to two causes: (1) The intraocular pressure reduces the pulsation, and the increase of pressure which accompanies each pulsation is spread over the whole volume of the contents of the globe, and is transmitted to the plastic sclerotic; (2) such pulsations as survive this diminishing effect are too small to be observed in these small vessels by ordinary ophthalmoscopic magnification.

Two types of *arterial pulsation* occur pathologically: (1) A true pulse wave, accompanied by locomotion of the vessels; (2) an intermittent flow of blood, or pressure pulse. In the latter, the arteries fill with blood only with the heart beats, being empty between them; it is only visible upon the disc. This type of pulsation is a pure pressure phenomenon, and is caused by any considerable increase of intra-ocular tension with normal or lowered blood-pressure, as in glaucoma; or by any considerable diminution of blood-pressure with normal intra-ocular tension, as in syncope, orbital tumors, etc. The true arterial pulse occurs in cases of aortic regurgitation or aneurysm, in Graves' disease, etc.; it is not confined to the optic disc. It is equally a pressure phenomenon, but the differences of pressure are smaller.

Capillary pulsation is seen only in aortic regurgitation as a systolic reddening and diastolic paling of the disc.

Venous pulsation occurs in three forms: (1) The normal negative venous pulse; (2) the positive venous pulse; (3) the transmitted centripetal venous pulse.

The normal venous pulse occurs in 70 to 80 per cent. of people; it is negative or diastolic, *i. e.* the veins are narrowed when the arteries are dilated. It is generally absent in lower animals. It can only be seen upon and near the disc. It is probably caused in exactly the same manner that the venous pulse is caused in the intra-cranial sinuses. There "the brain, as is shown by the cerebral pressure gauge, is lifted up by the stroke of the arteries at its base, and is thrown against the cerebral veins." In the eye the incompressible vitreous corresponds to the brain, but the sclerotic will also yield slightly to the shock, and so the pulsation in the veins will be less marked. In this manner each systole of the heart produces a dilation of the central artery, which is transmitted through the vitreous to the central veins, leading to a constriction, with diminished outflow of blood. This is the classical explanation of **D**onders. The constriction manifests itself first at the disc, and hence first affects the termination of the veins there, damming back the blood in the smaller veins. Moreover, this is the spot where the venous pressure is lowest, and it therefore responds most readily and most completely. The increased intra-ocular tension induced by the cardiac systole does not act equally and simultaneously upon the whole of the veins, leading to constriction and more rapid outflow of blood, as was suggested by Coccius. But there are other important factors which must be taken into account. One of these is direct pressure of the artery upon 'the veins during their course in the optic nerve, before entering the eye. Moreover, the response of the wall of the eye to the increased pressure will be most marked at the disc, where, although the nerve substance is incompressible, the lamina cribrosa contains much elastic tissue, and where there is a normal exit of lymph. Further, there is a tendency to a transmitted wave, caused by the high extra-vascular tension inside the globe, so that there may normally be some transmission of the pulse through the capillaries into the veins. More important in man is the relationship to the intra-cranial circulation, though this factor can be of little importance in most animals. Helfreich thinks that the venous constriction occurs before the cardiac systole, and may continue awhile during it. He attributes this to the blocking of the cavernous sinus during the systole, and its expansion during the diastole. If, however, this were the sole cause, we should expect to find actual dilation of the veins during the systole, and not constriction. Probably Haab is right in attempting to reconcile Helfreich's theory with that of Donders. It seems most likely that what happens is this: The intra-ocular effect of the cardiac systole is constriction of the veins; at the same moment the blood is dammed back from the cavernous sinus. It cannot flow back into the eye, but the communication with the facial and other veins tends to relieve the pressure. Soon after the diastole has commenced, the pressure in the orbital veins is still high and the blood is streaming through the intra-ocular capillaries and the veins dilate.

Parsons further says that the positive venous pulse commences with the auricular and continues through the ventricular systole. It is due to tricuspid regurgitation, and is permitted by the normal insufficiency or absence of the valves of the jugular veins.

The transmitted centripetal venous pulse is an accentuation of the normal tendency of the pulse wave to progress through the capillaries into the veins, owing to the intra-ocular pressure. It is due to a venous congestion with or without increased *vis a tergo*.

The degree of distension of the retinal vessels varies considerably under normal circumstances, and greatly under pathological conditions. Brief reference will be made here only to variations due to causes lying outside the eye. Uhthoff has examined the eye of the same side during ligature of the common carotid artery; there was slight transitory paling of the disc and narrowing of the retinal arteries; the transitoriness of the effect is due to the free anastomosis of the cerebral arteries through the circle of Willis. Permanent disturbance in such cases is caused by complications. During syncope there is narrowing of the arteries with or without narrowing of the veins, and arterial pulsation may arise.

Venous congestion is seen in its most pronounced form in congenital disease of the heart with stenosis of the pulmonary artery and patent foramen ovale; there may be retinal hemorrhages. Usually the arteries are also distended unduly. Generally venous congestion from various causes seldom produces much change in the retinal veins. Compression of both internal jugular veins causes slight retinal venous congestion and disappearance of venous pulsation, which recurs on deep respiration. The condition of the retinal vessels varies in epileptic fits: so-called retinal epilepsy is probably a complicated condition in which papillitis plays a part.

The object of *treatment* in *valvular diseases of the heart involving the eyes* is to aid the organism in maintaining the balance of compensation or in restoring it after it has begun to fail. It is unnecessary to discuss the treatment of the different valvular lesions separately; for the manifestations of the different single and combined heart lesions are in most cardinal respects similar, that is, in nearly all cases there is hypertrophy and dilatation of different portions of the heart, myocardial and arterial degeneration with changes in the blood pressure and ultimately venous stasis and cardiac dropsy in different organs.

The ophthalmologist is particularly interested in the correction of venous stasis, anemia, hyperemia and increased peripheral tension about the ocular apparatus resulting from cardiac lesions, hence the treatment of these particular manifestations of valvular disease alone will be discussed here. The above conditions rarely develop unless there is failing compensation. Absolute rest in bed is here a prime condition for restoring the balance of compensation. It is difficult, as a rule, to persuade patients in early stages of decompensation to go to bed, but it is absolutely essential that the situation should be fully explained to them and they be compelled to comply with this order. Rest in bed to be efficacious should be continued for weeks. The results obtained are frequently brilliant and very often one will be able to get along well without the use of any other treatment. The diet should consist of milk and cream, a little fresh fruit, an egg or two a day, a little meat and some cereal. The administration of liquids should be considerably reduced. Cold applied continuously or intermittently to the precordial region is a valuable adjuvant to the treatment. If compensation is not restored within a week or ten days by this simple expectant plan or, if the patient is seen for the first time when decompensation is far advanced and edema and congestion of different organs are present, then it may become necessary to use heart tonics.

The main effect of *digitalis* is exerted upon the ventricles, stimulating them to increased contraction, provided the heart muscle is not in an advanced stage of decompensation. Digitalis also raises the peripheral blood pressure and at the same time slows the action of the heart. Finally, by causing an increased determination of blood to the heart muscle, it improves the general nutrition of the heart. The dose is very important, for large amounts of the drug frequently produce an effect that is exactly opposite to that exercised by small doses, that is, they reduce the force of the systolic contractions and, in lethal doses, cause arrest of the heart in diastole. Its action is tardy as it is slowly absorbed, so that a day or two may elapse before the effect of the drug becomes apparent; hence there is always danger of cumulative action, especially as the excretion of digitalis is as slow as its absorption. Finally, the personal equation must be considered, some individuals showing a marked susceptibility, others an equally remarkable tolerance to its action. It is important, therefore, always to begin with small doses and during the first days of its administration to carefully watch the heart, the pulse and the blood pressure for signs of digitalis poisoning. It is claimed that some of the pure principles of digitalis possess only a cardiac action without the disagreeable local or general effects. Most of these principles, however, are quite uncertain in their action and vary much in strength. Their use should be reserved, therefore, as a rule, for those cases that display an absolute intolerance against the ordinary preparations of digitalis. Sometimes a case of valvular disease comes under observation for the first time with a very slow and intermittent pulse, great muscular weakness and certain gastric and cerebral symptoms. If, on inquiry, it is found that such a patient has been taking digitalis for a long time, it is always well to tentatively stop or greatly reduce the use of the drug in order to rule out the possibility of chronic digitalis intoxication. For a heart that is alarmingly slow as a result of digitalis poisoning 1-200 grain of atropin hypodermatically should be given as an antidote.

Digitalis and the whole group of which it is a member is contraindicated in any case of failing compensation in which the heart muscle has begun to degenerate, notably in advanced myocarditis and fatty heart. In diseases of the aortic valves digitalis should be given with the greatest care. Extensive atheroma or fragility of the arterial walls is also a contra-indication to the use of digitalis; for here the increased pressure may lead to rupture of the vessel walls.

Of the many preparations of digitalis a fresh infusion or the tincture are, from a practical point of view at least, best. Of the former the dose is 1 to 2 fluid drams (4 to 8 cc.), of the latter 5 to 15 drops (.03 to 1 cc.) three times a day. Occasionally patients do not react properly to the infusion or the tincture. In such cases the use of the powdered leaves in doses of from 1 to 4 grains (00.3 to 00.07 gm.) is indicated.

The glucosides, digitoxin, digitophyllin, digitalin and digitalein have been somewhat used, but it is unnecessary in the great majority of cases to have recourse to these preparations. For failing compensation strychnia may occasionally be used. As it acts chiefly upon the vasomotor center in the medulla and the general nervous system, it slows the heart beat by its stimulating effect upon the cardio-inhibitory nerves. It should never be used as a heart tonic when arterial tension is high. Caffein, another useful drug, strengthens the heart muscle, raises the peripheral blood pressure and increases diuresis.

This drug should never be given when the peripheral blood pressure is high, nor should it be used in very excitable individuals, nor in alcoholics. It is particularly valuable as a substitute for digitalis in cases in which the heart muscle is beginning to degenerate or has degenerated, because caffein presumably exercises its effect not upon the heart muscle directly but upon the nervous apparatus governing the heart beat. In extreme cases of cardiac failure, in which no time is given to gradually strengthen the heart by the use of heart tonics, it becomes necessary to have recourse to such drugs as camphor, ether and ammonia as emergency measures.—(A. C. C.)

Heart reflex. See **Oculocardiac reflex.**

Heat, The ophthalmic relations of. Heat may be defined as one of the forms of energy associated with molecular movement. In a popular sense it is the cause of the sensation called warmth. *Temperature* is that state of a body which determines how heat will pass between it and other bodies. See **Diathermy,** p. 3956, Vol. V, of this *Encyclopedia.*

Heat in eye surgery is generally applied in the form of moist applications.

Dry heat is sometimes used, but its action does not seem to be as effectual in promoting the absorption of the products of ocular inflammation as the moist forms. Various appliances and methods of using dry heat have been recommended, all possessing their advantages and disadvantages. A simple and easy plan is to take an ordinary saucer and place it in an oven until it is too hot to handle. It should then be wrapped in a piece of flannel, which has also been well heated, and applied over the eye and surrounding parts, previously filling in the depression around the eyeball with warm cotton wool. The whole dressing should then be kept in place by a bandage.

Several surgeons have devised methods for applying heat directly to the eyeball. For example, Ostwalt (*Annales d'Oculistique,* March, 1905) has invented an appliance, called a thermerophore, which essentially consists of an elastic bulb, a spiral tube, and a soft rubber cup (with attached thermometer) large enough to fit over the orbit. Fresh air is driven by the bulb into the spiral tube, which is placed over a Bunsen burner, and the air heated by this means is then forced into the rubber cup. The dry, super-heated air can be borne at a temperature of 100°, 150°, or 175° C. Treatment, given once or, occasionally, twice a day, is continued for about half an hour. The apparatus is intended to be used by the patient himself. Golesceano (*Recueil d'Ophtalmologie,* July and August, 1905), on the other hand, attains a similar end by adopting a somewhat different plan. He applies heat to the eye by means of hot vapor. His apparatus consists of a dome-shaped boiler, connected with one branch of a double-channeled tube, of which the second branch is connected with a hand-bellows. Vapor from the boiler passes through the peripheral part of this tube, while cold air from the pump is forced through the central division. The vapor is led into a funnel-shaped mask fitted over the patient's orbit. The steam has a temperature of 40° to 45° C. Applications number from one to four daily, and are continued on each occasion for from five to ten minutes. Ostwalt and Golesceano agree in finding the direct application of heat (dry or moist, as the case may be) useful in such superficial affections of the eye as blepharitis, phlyctenular keratitis, interstitial keratitis, and various forms of iridocyclitis. Roughly, then, the applications are indicated for the relief of pain and for the cure of chronic inflammations of the eyelids, cornea, or uveal tract.

The well-known Leiter's coils, made of lead tubing of a convenient size and supplied with tapes for application to the ocular region, are also quite effective as a means of supplying heat (or cold) to the eye. The reservoir is placed sufficiently above the level of the recumbent patient's face to permit of an easy trickle of water at the required temperature through the leaden coils, to be then received by a vessel placed beneath the bed or couch.

Hot, moist applications may be applied by means of pieces of flannel, or gauze, of several thicknesses wrung out of water as hot as can be comfortably borne. They should not be too large, although of sufficient size to completely cover the front of the eye. They should be changed quickly as soon as they show signs of becoming cool.

Hot water may also be applied with a small towel, or ordinary wash cloth, folded about three inches wide by eighteen inches long. The patient is directed to hold one end of the towel in each hand and, dipping it into water as hot as can be borne, to apply it to the closed lids and parts surrounding the eye. It is applied to the ocular region and held there a moment, the application being repeated for the length of time desired. Hot applications to be of any therapeutic value should be used every hour or two (depending upon the severity of the case) and for ten or fifteen minutes at a time. The temperature of the applications should be as high as can be endured, 115° to 125° F. On account of the danger of scalding, the skin of the lids and surrounding parts should be protected by anointing it with vaseline, or some simple ointment, previous to making the application.

Hot applications are valuable in most deep-seated inflammations of the eyeball to promote the absorption of exudates, for the stimulation of the circulation and for the relief of pain. They are especially indicated in ocular headache, iritis, cyclitis, keratitis and corneal ulcer.

The Japanese "hot-box"—the small hand-warmer to be obtained in any of our "Oriental" art stores—is a favorite instrument for applying dry heat to the eye. It is readily obtained, quite effective and gives out a uniform supply of caloric for an hour or two.

A. Duane advises hot (not simply warm), moist compresses in all painful and inflamed conditions of the anterior portions of the eye except when cold seems indicated or is not well borne. In cases of uveitis, etc., he thinks it is advantageous to apply hot water directly to the eyeball, drop by drop, using a solution (saline or boric acid) of 110°-145° F., or higher, as the patient develops tolerance.

Hot water bags are made of convenient size and shape for application to the ocular region. They afford one of the most cleanly means of applying dry heat and of securing rubefaction. When covered with flannel or wrapped in cloth they retain the heat much longer and are much less liable to produce burns. The possibility of this accident should always be kept in mind; the bag should not be used when it is too hot to be borne for half a minute against the cheek.

O. A. Griffin (*Trans. Am. Acad. of Oph.*, p. 140, 1906) uses in aggravated and prolonged acute inflammatory diseases of the eye a small rubber bag through which either hot or cold water can be syphoned. To make the application more effective (by a retention of the applied temperature) a double layer of moistened gauze, about two inches square, is first placed over the affected eye and the water bag then put into position and retained in place, if desired, by means of a tape or string. Single or double bags are used, depending upon whether one or both eyes are affected. To retard the discharge of water and thus prolong the duration of application, and also to produce a distension of the bag, a tiny opening is made at the end of the discharging tube by inserting a bit of hard rubber tubing which contains a minute passage through which the water escapes. The arrangement is completed by placing two pitchers of like capacity at the proper height to produce a slow and steady flow of water from the upper to the lower vessel. When the upper one is nearly empty, it is only necessary to pinch the tubing or elevate the discharging end and pour the water from the lower into the upper pitcher to keep the apparatus running properly. The stream will flow from thirty to sixty minutes, depending upon the relative height of the pitchers and the size of opening in the discharging tube. By timing the process, the attendant may know exactly when to change the water, and the compress may be applied steadily and indefinitely without disturb-

ing the eye or the patient, which is very important, especially when
the patient is sleeping and rest is essential.

If hot applications are indicated, heated water is used instead and
kept at a uniform degree by occasional additions of hot water. In
the writer's experience, unless pain demands a continuous application, the most satisfactory results are secured when the compress is
employed intermittently, fifteen or thirty minutes elapsing between
applications.

After the apparatus is properly arranged, the appliances for which
may be obtained in any ordinary home, it requires little or no attention and is a rational method of employing heat or cold in the treatment of acute inflammatory disorders of the eye, inasmuch as the temperature is uniform, the water bag is light and conforms to the surface beneath, the compress is applied directly to the area desired, the
patient is not chilled or drenched by escaping water, and the application may be used indefinitely without disturbing the patient.

In these days of the universal employment of electric lighting this
forms one of the most valuable sources of thermal treatment. A very
good method of using it is that described by Maddox. He uses a half
to seven-tenths ampere current passed through a very fine wire which
is wrapped around a roll of canton flannel. The current can be taken
from an ordinary lighting wire and controlled by a transformer. The
employment of dry heat he believes is especially indicated in rheumatic affections of the eye and in certain forms of glaucoma. The
electric hat-iron may also be used in the manner suggested by Maddox. This appliance can be purchased at most dealers in electric supplies and is a handy and effective means of applying dry heat to the
ocular region.

Waldmann's (*Ophthalmology*, Vol. II, p. 160, 1914) application of
diathermia is by means of an apparatus which has an oscillatory frequency of about three million per second. He places a suitably
shaped thermometer in the conjunctival sac before beginning the
treatment, and applies the electrode outside a moist layer of
cotton which is laid on the closed lids. Cocain is not necessary
and should be avoided, since lack of corneal sensibility may
lead to the use of excessive temperatures. If the patient complains
of pain from the heat, the temperature can be immediately reduced
by weakening the current. He reports the successful use of diathermia
in a variety of conditions, including vernal conjunctivitis, trachoma,
episcleritis, and hypopion from penetrating injury of the eyeball. In
a case of interstitial keratitis, two weeks after onset, after three treatments the eye became paler, photophobia and lachrymation ceased,

and the infiltration became smaller. Marked improvement followed the use of diathermia in a fully developed case of interstitial keratitis; and in a case of diffuse corneal opacity from a past attack of the same disease, there was an appreciable clearing of the cornea with distinct gain in vision. In a case of central infiltration of the cornea with ulcerative degeneration, which had resisted treatment with atropin, dionin, and a mercurial salve, twelve treatments with diathermia were followed by improvement in vision from 5/60 to 5/30 and diminution in the size of the infiltration; while the ulcerated surface was covered with epithelium after three sittings. Waldmann emphasizes the fact that by means of diathermia greater heat can be applied without injurious effects than in any other way.

In Qurin's (*Ophthalmoscope*, Vol. 12, p. 686, 1914) experience the highest temperature which could be attained in the human conjunctival sac was 43.6 C. Although it has been found that the animal cornea will tolerate a temperature of 45 C. without harmful results, yet the excessive sensation of heat prevented the use of such a temperature in applying the treatment to human beings. Experiments as to the diathermic behavior of the orbital tissue in comparison with the conjunctival sac showed the conjunctival temperature to remain in every case from one to two degrees lower than that of the deeper orbital structures. The most remarkable result of the use of diathermia, as described by Qurin, was in a case of bilateral optic atrophy in disseminated myelitis of many years' standing, in which the vision of the weaker eye rose from counting fingers at five meters to 6/24, with an increase in the visual field. This was after diathermia had been used for four weeks. The condition had not retrogressed after an interval of six months.

For the more convenient application of the treatment, Qurin has devised an apparatus whose basis is a padded head-band somewhat similar to the band used for head-mirrors. To this are attached, with facilities for adjustment, a positive electrode which is brought into contact with a moist pad over the eye, a thermometer which registers the temperature in the conjunctival sac, and a negative electrode which is applied to the back of the neck.

Best (*Münch. Med. Woch.*, Vol. 61, p. 1722, 1914) regards diathermia as superior to hot compresses in the treatment of corneal herpes, episcleritis, sclerotising keratitis, iritis, and cyclitis. He also considers it useful in retrobulbar optic neuritis and paralysis of the ocular muscles. It is contraindicated in anesthesia of the skin of the lids, in the presence of changes in the ocular vessels, in arterio-sclerosis, and in glaucoma.

Emanuel describes an electric warming apparatus for the eye. The heat-producing wires are enclosed in an appropriately shaped aluminum capsule, which is to be applied over a moist compress of cotton or gauze. The apparatus is furnished with a rheostat so that it is possible to regulate the amount of heat. See, also, **Heliotherapy.**

Heavy daturine. A term applied by Ladenburg to a mixture of atropine and hyoscyamine which he obtained from *Datura stramonium.* It fuses at about 114° C.

Heber. (G.) Levator.

Hebetudo visus. (L.) Asthenopia.

Hebra's salve. See **Diachylon ointment.**

Hechenberger, Johann Georg. A Tyrolese physician, of but slight ophthalmologic interest because of his *"Ueber eine Wichtige Nosologie und Therapie der Exsudativen Augenhaut-Entzündungen"* (Innsbruck, 1840). The dates of his birth and death are not procurable.— (T. H. S.)

Hecht. (G.) A pike.

Hecquet, Philippe. A physician of but small ophthalmologic importance who was born at Abbeville, France, Feb. 11, 1661. He studied at first theology in Paris; later, medicine at Rheims. Soon after leaving Rheims, he practised for a time in his native town. Tiring, however, of the uncongenial atmosphere of this place, he removed to Paris. Being there forbidden by the "Faculty" to engage in practice, he accepted a position as medical attendant in a religious foundation at Port-Royal-des-Champs. When 33 years of age he attacked his medical studies anew, received his license in 1696 and his doctorate in 1697. So highly honored was he, after a time, by the Faculty, that, in 1712, he was elected Dean. In 1727 he withdrew to a Carmelite cloister, where he lived the ascetic life until his death, which occurred April 11, 1737.

Hecquet wrote a large number of works, all of which were, at least in greater part, relevant to systematic medicine only. In one of his books (that entitled *"Remarks on the Abuse of Purgatives and Bile at the Beginning and the End of Diseases,"* Paris, 1724) he takes the ground that the lens is seated, not immediately behind the pupil, but in the middle of the eye, and, furthermore, that a cataract is a membrane lying between the pupil and the lens, and is formed of corrupted and inspissated "humor." These opinions, which had come down from the ancients, and were, even at the date of Hecquet's book, becoming decidedly antiquated, evoked from Petit three well-written letters, which are almost classics in the history of ophthalmology.—(T. H. S.)

Hectargyr. One of the organic compounds of arsenic like hectin and atoxyl, and producing, like them, lesions of the optic nerve in some instances where full doses are given.

Hectin. A preparation of arsenic which, like atoxyl (q. v.), is used in the treatment of lues. Several cases of optic involvement have been observed following full doses of this drug.

Valude (*Ann. d'Ocul.*, Vol. 146, p. 272, 1912) saw optic atrophy develop in a man 74 years of age who was receiving hectin in the treatment of lues. Small doses caused no symptoms, but doses of 8-20 cg. caused temporary defect in hearing and seeing. One year later vision was considered normal for the patient's age. He was then started on a series of injections of hectin without knowledge of the previous use of the drug. After the third injection there were blindness and deafness. Under injections of strychnin hearing returned but vision did not improve and later optic atrophy was present. Valude thinks that it would be best not to use this drug in cases in which the optic and auditory nerves are not quite healthy. Hallopeau and Dainville (*Rec. d'Opht.*, Vol. XXXIII, p. 218, 1912) report, that a few hours after the seventeenth local injection of hectin for recent chancre, vision became obscured; but it cleared up by the next morning. Another injection was given and again vision was impaired, but recovery soon followed.

Hedonal. METHYLPROPYLCARBINOLURETHANE. This is a white powder soluble in cold, but more soluble in hot, water. It is a hypnotic and used in mania, chronic alcoholism and, occasionally, in ophthalmic diseases.

Bielski (*Viestnik Ophth.*, Vol. 30, p. 135, 1913) reports on anesthesia obtained by the intravenous injection of hedonal, which he had resorted to in seven cases of cataract extraction. He considers it indicated when local anesthesia will be insufficient, and chloroform or ether is contraindicated. Three hundred cubic centimeters of 0.75 per cent. sterilized solution of hedonal are injected. The precaution of excising the portion of the vein in which it is injected to prevent thrombosis, he thinks unnecessary. The sleep produced lasts from 30 to 90 minutes.

Heermann, G. A well-known ophthalmologist of Tübingen, Germany. He was born at Blomberg, Lippe-Detmold, in 1807, became an assistant at the Insane Asylum in Siegburg in 1833, and from 1835 to 1840 was privat docent and assistant at the Academic Hospital in Heidelberg. In 1840 he removed to Tübingen, where he became professor extraordinary. He was a brilliant diagnostician and therapeutist. His more important writings are as follows: 1. *Ueber die Bildung der Gesichtsvorstellungen aus den Gesichtsempfindungen.* (Hanover, 1835.) 2.

Ueber das Studium der Psychischen Medicin auf Universitäten, als das Nächste Erforderniss ihrer Förderung. (Heidelberg, 1837.)

He died in Rome in the spring of 1844.—(T. H. S.)

Hefa cells. These minute bodies are generally supposed to be modified blastomycetes. Hanford McKee (*Ophthalmoscope*, p. 410, July, 1914) gives a complete account of them in a review of Stiel's article (*Archiv f. Augenheilk.*, August, 1913) on certain relations of trachoma to blastomycosis.

Lodato, by using Mann's method, found in the infiltrated adenoid layer and inside the trachoma follicles little bodies which Addario believed were blastomycetes. Stiel began his examinations in 1910. He found oval or round forms which were intensively stained, and which often had a double-bordered membrane. He also found similar formations in the protoplasm of large epithelioid cells. With the Giemsa stain, the hefa cells, which stain intensely, are the only ones that will be recognized. With tubercle bacillus stain, bands of hefa cells lying one by another will often be found in trachomatous tissue. These bands are recognizable as well by low as by high magnification, and are undoubtedly hefa, as they show many budding forms. Stiel's method was as follows: The material was taken from the upper transition fold with a sharp instrument, so that epithelial and sub-epithelial tissue was obtained. This was smeared thinly on cleaned glass slides, dried in the air, and fixed and stained with carbol-fuchsin solution and heat. After some minutes, the slide was decolorized with Ebner solution, and washed and counter-stained with a solution of methylene blue. It is most important that the decolorizing be done properly. Here the hefa cells will be found red in a blue background.

Stiel also obtained hefa colonies from trachomatous material on lakmus plates. The material was taken with a sterile ring knife from the epithelial and sub-epithelial layers of the granulations. Later he found it better to use Drigolski plates and slices of potato. The plates must be freshly prepared and free from air organisms.

The hefa colonies appear mostly after eight days. Their slow growth is attributed to the fact that they are fixed in the tissue and first must separate themselves, and, also, probably only some of the hefa present in the tissue begin to germ in this time. The colonies are very similar, and transference by means of Drigolski's plates is easy. The hefa colonies can be studied very well in their natural state by means of the hanging drop or the method of Nakanishi. On a clean glass slide one smears out thinly borax-methylene blue and allows it to dry. A cover slide is covered with a drop of distilled water mixed with hefa cells. This is put on the stained slide, the borders are closed with wax and the examination is made with the oil immersion lens. The hefa cells appear as round or oval bodies in different sizes with a simple or double-bordered membrane. The contents are not homogeneous. Most of the cells contain numerous colored granules or a larger colored mass which looks like a nucleus, while a more or less large border remains faintly stained. There are also within and outside the cells small opaque bodies which may be spores. Many of the cells are in a state of division, others have grown tube-like or taken irregular forms. Sometimes one sees formations which can only be explained as capsules. Stiel examined a number of school children suspected of having trachoma, and in the smear preparations, as well as in the sub-epithelial tissue, found numerous blastomycetes.

He also inoculated a pure culture of hefa into the conjunctiva of a blind adult and observed the appearance of transparent granulations in the transition fold, which disappeared after eight to fourteen days.

Hegar, Johann August. A German surgeon, of some slight ophthalmologic importance because of his Göttingen dissertation, *"De Oculi Partibus Quibusdam"* (Göttingen, 1818, 2 plates). Born at Darmstadt, Germany, in 1794, he received his medical degree at Göttingen in 1815, and, in the same year, as military physician, accompanied the English army on its expedition against France. Settling in Darmstadt, he there became, in 1817, Court-Surgeon, "with the character of a court-physician." He also became Privy Medical Advisor, and died June 3, 1882.—(T. H. S.)

Heiberg, Hjalmar. A distinguished Norse microscopist and ophthalmologist. Born at Christiania, Sept. 27, 1837, son of Prof. Christen Heiberg, he was from 1859 till 1863 assistant at the Imperial Hospital and Lying-in Asylum, and in 1863 and '64 studied his profession abroad. Returning to Christiania, he devoted himself to microscopy and ophthalmology. He died Sept. 25, 1897. His ophthalmologic writings are as follows: 1. Periferien af Tunica Descemeti og dens Indflydelse paa Accomodationen. 2. Om Gliomets Malignitet. (In collaboration with J. Hjort; also the same in von Graefe's *Archiv,* 1869.) 3. Zur Anatomie der Zonula Zinnii. (*Centralbl. f. d. Med. Wissensch.*, 1865.) 4. Ueber die Neubildung des Hornhautepithels. (*Med. Jahrbb. der k. k. Gesellsch. der Aerzte in Wien,* 1871.) 5. Ein Fall von Panophthalmitis Puerperalis Bedingt durch Mikrokokken. (*Centralbl. f. d. Med. Wissenschaften,* 1874.) 6. Tilfaelde af Hemiopi og Afasi. (*Norsk Mag. f. Laegev.*, 1874.) 7. Cyclopische Missbildung bei einem Kalbe. (*Ibid,* 1878.)—(T. H. S.)

Heiberg, Jacob Munch. A well known Norse surgeon and ophthalmologist. Born at Christiania, June 12, 1843, son of the general surgeon, Joh. Fritzner Heiberg, he was from 1867-69 Assistant at the Imperial Hospital and at the Lying-in Asylum, and for a time was Assistant to the Prosector. During the Franco-German War he served as military surgeon in Berlin hospitals. After the war, he studied in various cities, and then returned to Christiania, where he resided until his death. Here he founded an ophthalmic hospital, and was editor of the Norse *"Magazin f. Laegev."* He died at Christiania early in May, 1888.

Heiberg's chief (or only) ophthalmic writings are: 1. Om de Extrabulböse Svulster i Orbita. (*Norsky Magaz.*, 1873.) 2. Die Methodik der Ophthalmologischen Untersuchung, ein Leitfaden für Anfänger. (Christiania, 1875.) 3. Overplanting af Bindehuden fra en Kanin. (Christiania, 1875.)—(T. H. S.)

Heidelberg flower-paper. See p. 5228, Vol. VII, of this *Encyclopedia*.

Heidenreich, Friedrich Wilhelm. A distinguished German physician, who paid considerable attention to ophthalmology. Born at Rostall Sept. 2, 1798, he received the degree of Doctor in Medicine at Würzburg in 1821. After a year of further study, chiefly in Berlin, he settled in 1824 as general physician at Ansbach, where he practised until his death, Dec. 6, 1857.

His only ophthalmologic writing was *"Die Subcutane Blepharotomie gegen Subacuten Augenliderkrampf und Krankhafter Entropium"* (Ansbach, 1844).—(T. H. S.)

Heilanstalt. (G.) Sanitarium.

Heilbar. (G.) Curable.

Heilgeschäft. (G.) Medical practice.

Heilkunde. (G.) Therapeutics.

Heilmittel. (G.) Therapeutic agent.

Heilserum, Deutschmann's. See **Seropathy.**

Heilverfahren. (G.) Therapeutic treatment.

Heilwissenschaft. (G.) Therapeutics.

Heineken, Philipp Cornelius. A well-known German physician, who paid considerable attention to ophthalmology. Born at Bremen Dec. 6, 1789, the son of Johann Heineken, he received the degree of Doctor in Medicine at Göttingen in 1811. After a scientific journey through Hungary, Italy and France, he settled in 1813 as general practitioner in Bremen. His only ophthalmologic writing was *"Ophthalmobiotik, Regeln und Anweisung zur Erhaltung der Augen"* (Bremen and Leipsic, 1815).—(T. H. S.)

Heine's operation. Cyclodialysis. See **Glaucoma.**

Heisrath, Friedrich. A prominent ophthalmologist of Königsberg, Germany. The date and place of his birth are unprocurable. He practised at Königsberg for many years, and was known as a dexterous operator. His contributions to ophthalmic science and literature are chiefly on the subject of the surgical treatment of trachoma. He died July 12, 1904.—(T. H. S.)

Heister, Elias Friedrich. Born at Altdorf, Germany, the son of Lorenz Heister, he studied medicine at Helmstädt, Berlin, and Leipsic, received his professional degree at Helmstädt in 1738, and died a little over two years later, while traveling in Holland.

He wrote a diatribe against the great English oculistic charlatan, John Taylor.—(T. H. S.)

Heister, Lorenz. A celebrated surgeon and a noted ophthalmologist. Born the son of an innkeeper at Frankfort a. M. Sept. 19, 1683, he studied medicine at Giessen, Leyden and Amsterdam. He finally received his professional degree at Harderwyk, May 31, 1708, and, the following year, was made superior physician of the Dutch Army. In 1710 he became professor of botany at Altdorf. In 1720 he was called to the chair of surgery at Helmstädt, and here he worked for many years, dying April 18, 1758.

Not strikingly original, he nevertheless deserves his title of "father of scientific surgery in Germany," because of his open mind, his sound judgment, his numerous writings and the excellence of his literary style. He knew in great detail all the surgical literature which had been composed until his day, and, from this, he selected with well-nigh unerring accuracy whatever was really practical and valuable and set it forth so beautifully and charmingly, that it found at once a numerous body of readers.

Heister's *"Surgery"* appeared first in 1718. Other editions (all German) followed in 1724, 1731, 1745, 1747, 1770, 1779. Latin editions appeared in 1739, 1750 and 1759. The work appeared also at various times in Dutch, Italian, French, Spanish, and English.

Heister was a man of unflagging industry and well-nigh infinite scholarship. He read, wrote and fluently spoke a number of foreign languages, and, merely as incidental aids to the art of exposition, he acquired a pretty thorough knowledge of glass-cutting and of engraving on copper.

Ophthalmologically, Heister possesses importance because of his adoption and introduction into Germany of the (then) new and startling doctrine that a cataract is not, as had been taught by the ancients and those of mediaeval days, a deposit of inspissated "humor" in a (wholly imaginary) space between the pupil and the lens, but a hardening and clouding of the lens itself.

A memorial-tablet and effigy of Heister were erected in 1869 in the

Frankfort tavern in which the great man was born, and these strange mementos (unusual indeed in the case of physicians) are still to be observed in the old 17th century inn.—(T. H. S.)

Heitzmann's theory. The theory that the axis-cylinder of a nerve-fiber is ordinary connective tissue modified for the transmission of special impulses.

Helcophthalmia. (L.) An old term for ulcerative inflammation of the eyelids, conjunctiva, or cornea.

Heloophthalmuria. (L.) An obsolete term for a chronic ulcerative disease of the eye with a urine-like discharge.

Helcydrion. (L.) A small ulcer, especially one on the cornea.

Heliacal (Gr. hēlios, "the sun"), emerging from the light of the sun or passing into it. A star's heliacal rising is when it rises just before the sun.

Helical. See **Eyes of soldiers, sailors, etc., Examination of the.**

Helichrysum sanguineum. The root of this plant contains an aromatic oil, and has been used in chronic coughs, asthma, dysuria, and as an emmenagogue. The mildly astringent leaves were applied externally in eye diseases.

Helicoidal. Coiled so as to resemble a helix or snail-shell. Dor (*Clin. Opht.*, Vol. XVII, p. 620, 1912), believes there exists a special condition of the retinal vessels, a tortuosity of the retinal veins, to be distinguished from varix or passive venous stasis, which may be called helicoidal. This condition he supposed arose from altered pressure in the veins and arteries, with dilatation of some capillaries. He thinks it may be due to capillary obstruction by the red blood cells in polycythemia, or by white cells in leukemia. The occurrence of such vessels in the retina may indicate their simultaneous occurrence in other parts of the nervous system. This is rendered probable by the coexistence of nervous troubles and retinal lesions.

Heliochromic. Photographic.

Heliochromoscope. An instrument in which the triple images obtained by the heliochromic process may be viewed as one picture, showing the object in its natural colors.

Heliochromotype. A photograph in natural colors.

Heliochromy. The art of photographing in natural colors.

Heliography. A method of communicating swiftly between distant points by means of the sun's rays reflected from mirrors. Either successive flashes or obscurations of a continuous reflection of the sun's light may be combined so as to read like Morse's telegraphic system. Heliography may be used for geodetic measurement, or for military and other signaling. . The instruments which contain the mirrors are variously called heliograph and heliostat.　As far back as 1890 communication was established in Arizona by heliograph over a distance of two hundred and fifteen miles.　As early as the eleventh century A. D. Algeria possessed a system of heliographs.　Recently there has been a great development in heliography, or sun-telegraphy, for signaling messages between the sections of an army in the field, as during the British campaign in Afghanistan in 1880.　Drummond's and Begbie's heliostats and the heliographs of Mance and Anderson are favorably known.　A similar instrument called the heliotrope is used in making geodetic surveys for observations of very distant stations.— (Standard Encyclopedia.)

Heliogravure.　Photo-engraving; helio-engraving.

Helioid.　Resembling the sun.

Heliology.　The science of the sun.

Heliometer.　An instrument for the accurate measurement of small angles in the heavens, consisting of a telescope whose objective is cut into halves that may be slid past each other so as to form two images of any object toward which it is pointed.　The distance between two stars is determined by measuring the displacement of the halves of the objective necessary to cause one image of one of the stars to cover one image of the other star.

This optical instrument was invented by Savary and Bouguer in 1743-48.　As improved by Dollond, the object-lens of the instrument is in two halves, each of which will form a perfect image in the focus of the eye-piece.

Of important heliometers those of Yale College, the Hüffner Observatory, Vienna, and the Cape of Good Hope may be mentioned. That of Yale College has an object glass of six inch aperture and ninety-eight inch focal length.

Heliophag.　A name given to the animal pigment-cell, as being a supposed absorber of the radiant energy of the sun's light and heat.

Heliophilous.　LEUCOPHILOUS.　Attracted by sunlight.

Heliophobe.　One who is sensitive to the light or heat of the sun.

Heliophobia.　Fear of the sun's light or heat.

Helioscope.　A telescope for observing the sun without injury to the eyes, by means of blackened or tinted glass, or mirrors that reflect only a part of the light.

Heliosis.　A sun-bath; also, sunstroke.

Heliostat.　An instrument provided with clockwork, by which sunbeams may be steadily directed to one spot during the whole day.

Heliotherapy.　The therapeutic use of the light and heat of the sun. The employment of "sunbaths" has been especially exploited as part of the attractions of health resorts and sanitaria, but that there is a scientific side to this form of therapy there can be no doubt. It also has a useful, though indirect, application in some diseases of the eye.

The more valuable therapeutic uses of sunlight and the sun's heat are set forth by Henry Dietrich (*Jour. Am. Med. Assoc'n*, p. 2229, Dec. 20, 1913). The use of the sun's rays as a therapeutic agent is very old. C. E. Rogers says that some years ago, while traveling in the tropics of Central America, he observed a peculiar custom among some of the Indian tribes. Occasionally he would see one lying naked on the ground for hours at a time in the fierce rays of the midday sun. He learned that this was their method of treating consumption and rheumatism. The custom is an old one, having been practised before the Spanish invasion and can be traced all along the western coast of the South and North American continents. In the old world Herodotus as early as 484 B. C. describes the sun-bath, and the Romans built solaria on their houses for the purpose of utilizing the sun's rays. It was then lost sight of therapeutically until toward the end of the eighteenth century, when it was used to treat cancerous ulcerations.

Downe and Blunt first showed that *sunlight retards and inhibits the growth of bacteria.* Dieudonné found that direct sunlight kills typhoid bacilli in one and one-half hours; daylight in eight hours; arc-light (800 candle-power) in eight hours, and incandescent light in eleven hours. Arc-light is rich in ultra-violet rays. Tubercle bacilli are killed by the sun's rays in five hours at the seashore; in four hours at an altitude of 2,800 feet, and in three hours at an altitude of 5,000 feet. Diffuse light requires about double the time to produce this effect. This action is principally due to the chemical rays, though all rays have a bactericidal action. The ultra-violet rays also act on the ferments and toxins. Diphtheria toxin quickly loses its toxic property under the influence of these rays, while the antitoxin is less affected by them. Small-pox vaccine is but slightly altered by sunlight or diffuse light, but greatly so by ultra-violet light.

The *action of light on the human body* varies according to the intensity, the altitude and the individual. Sunlight in passing through the atmosphere to the earth loses a great deal of its energy, the loss depending on the position of the sun in the sky, the density of the air strata traversed and the amount of moisture and foreign matter in the air. The chemical rays show the greatest, the heat rays the smallest loss. The light intensity in the higher altitudes is much greater than in the lowlands, and this difference is particularly marked in winter. According to Dorno and Weber, Davos (altitude 5,000 feet) at noon in winter has four times the amount of light that Kiel (sea-level) has, while this difference is only half so great in summer. In about the same manner the volume of the ultra-violet rays increases with the increase in altitude. The difference in the ultra-violet ray's intensity in higher altitude in summer and winter, however, is comparatively small, while in the lowlands it is great.

The effect of light on the body is not as yet fully understood, but we may say when the body is exposed to sunlight for a period of time there results: (1) increased pigmentation, (2) increased growth of hair; (3) increased metabolism; (4) increase in number of erythrocytes; (5) local hyperemia; (6) decrease in number of respirations; (7) increase in depth of individual respiratory act; (8) fall of blood-pressure, and (9) stimulation of nervous system.

Under the influence principally of the ultra-violet rays, pigmentation takes place on those parts of the body exposed. This is as a rule preceded by an erythema of varying intensity, according to the strength of the light. The pigmentation is characterized by an increase of the pigment granules in the epithelial cells, as well as in an increase in the number of chromatophoric cells, which are probably epithelial cells which have migrated into the connective tissue. This pigmentation by some is considered a protective process on the part of the body against the ultra-violet rays. Others hold that it transforms short-waved, chemical rays into long-waved rays, which have a deeper penetration. A combination of the two views is probably more nearly correct. It is very important in practice, as Rollier states that prognosis and rapidity of healing are as a rule proportionate to the degree of pigmentation. This pigment absorbs the violet rays, but not the red.

All rays of light penetrate the human body, the violet or chemical rays possessing this power to a less degree than the heat rays.

Lenkei says that only about a hundredth part of the light falling on the body penetrates it 0.5 cm., but some rays reach a depth of from 5 to 6 cm. That light penetrates the thickness of the hand is proved by the experiments of Oninus. When light penetrates the skin, practically all the chemical rays are absorbed by the blood. This is a striking fact and probably some day will help explain the good results of heliotherapy. When we consider that exposure to light causes a local hyperemia, the amount of energy absorbed by the blood must be enormous. Von Schlaffer has also shown that blood during exposures to light absorbs light energy, which, in the dark, it can again transfer to a photographic plate. Is it not possible, as he says, that it can also surrender this accumulated energy to the internal organs, and thereby influence their function and possibly pathologic processes?

Rollier rarely sees acne or furunculosis on pigmented skins, and during an epidemic of German measles noticed that all the well-pigmented children were free from eruption and even in those wearing jackets the eruption only appeared on those parts of the body not exposed to the sun-bath.

Rollier considers a general exposure of the body as fundamental and the local exposures as only secondary in importance. The dry, invigorating air of the higher altitudes is also called to assist the solar energy. This it does by increasing the action of the skin, thus aiding elimination, drying up wounds when present and increasing the general tone of the body. The treatment then is really a combination of light and fresh air. When light is not available the air-bath is used alone. According to Saake, mountain air also contains many more radio-active emanations than the air in the lowlands. Furthermore, in higher altitudes the differences in temperature in the shade and in the sun are very great.

Finsen by his great work established many scientific facts and again brought the subject prominently before the medical profession, and established it as a clinical method. The French school under Bonnet and the surgeons Ollier and Poncet, of Lyon, observed and reported the good effects of heliotherapy in chronic joint-affections. The application of the method was at this time confined principally to the warm, sunny climate along the Mediterranean, until Bernhard, of Samaden, Switzerland, began using it on the high plateau of Graubunden. He first treated granulating wounds, and later extended its use to surgical tuberculosis and now gives the following indications for heliotherapy: I. Wounds: (1) traumatic in which primary healing is not probable as in case of those caused by blasts or crushing injuries; (2) due to circulatory disturbances, as ulcus cruris, mal perforans; (3) burns and frostbites; (4) infected wounds. II. Tuberculosis of the skin and serous membrane. Tuberculosis of the lymph-nodes, bones, joints and others. III. Carcinoma of the skin. IV. Specific ulcers with little tendency to heal. V. Leukemia, pseudoleukemia, tuberculosis of larynx and lungs.

In 1903 Rollier established the first sanatorium for the systematic treatment of surgical tuberculosis at Leysin, Switzerland, and since then he has erected two more at the same place, so that he can now accommodate 450 patients. These sanatoriums are located respectively at altitudes of 1250, 1350 and 1500 meters (about 3800, 4100 and 4500 feet). Two hundred beds are reserved for children.

Bardenheuer, assistant to Rollier, in a study of the blood, gives the following data:

During from the first to the third day of treatment, the red corpuscles usually increase about 500,000, and the white 3,000, the maximum in increase being reached about the third day. The leukocyte count in closed cases runs about 10,000, in cases with mixed infection from 13,000 to 17,000. He has found that cases in which the maximum increase in erythrocytes requires much more than three days are those offering a poorer prognosis. When healing starts there is a slight decrease in the number of erythrocytes.

Cases of tuberculosis of the hip, spine, lower extremities and peritoneum require immobilization in bed until healed; that is, until long after all pain has ceased and roentgenoscopy shows that the focus is healed. This, however, requires months and often a year or more. It is in cases of long duration particularly that we observe the better effects of treatment carried on in high altitudes over those in lower altitudes, for the former patients owing to the invigorating action of the mountain air, retain a good appetite, and with a good diet often take on weight. Not only that, but an increased tonus of the tissues, especially in children, is frequently seen. At lower altitudes loss of appetite and the depressing action of the heat interfere with the systematic treatment.

Rollier has discarded the use of all non-removable appliances for immobilization as antagonistic to the principles of heliotherapy. By their use, no matter how skilfully made, the activity of the skin is greatly reduced; exposure to sun and air is impossible, metabolism decreases and atrophy results. These factors tend to prevent healing and if healing does take place, the functional result is, in many cases, a poor one. All appliances for immobilization are therefore removed daily during the period of exposure, except occasionally in the case of very refractory children with spondylitis. In these cases he cuts large fenestra into the jackets. In general he applies extension apparatus, splints, bandages and removable corsets of celluloid. In many cases of spondylitis, a corset or jacket made of heavy material, which is in turn fixed to the mattress, is employed. Ambulatory appliances usually made of celluloid, so that they can be removed and treatment continued at home, are used only after the tuberculosis is healed to protect the newly formed bone.

Medication is rarely resorted to; children, however, receive cod-liver oil.

Cold abcesses unless interfering mechanically are given ample time to become absorbed. This occurs in a fair percentage of cases. Under all circumstances the rupture of an abcess is to be prevented, as a mixed infection is practically unavoidable and makes the prognosis so much worse. If necessary, they are aspirated and injected with iodoform, 10 per cent., in oil or glycerin, to guard against mixed infection. This is done even daily if necessary; every means and effort are used to avoid spontaneous rupture. If the patient has or develops a sinus, it is covered, when not exposed to the sun, with an alcohol dressing to prevent infection as much as possible. Sinuses, no matter where located, when exposed to light, first show an increased secretion, then gradually dry up, the granulations become healthy and complete healing is frequently seen. According to Bernhard, the scars resulting are firmer, yet more elastic, than when heliotherapy is not employed, and consequently produce less contraction.

The high fever due to mixed infection drops, large open wounds and ulcerations heal with a minimum of deformity, and thickening of joint capsules and exudates are likewise absorbed in many cases.

Franzoni, an assistant of Rollier, has recently published an interesting article on the behavior of bone sequestra under the influence of light. As a rule from three to five months are required for a sequestrum to form and free itself from the surrounding tissues. Heliotherapy increases the speed of evolution of the sequestrum and causes its spontaneous expulsion. Rapid and firm healing follows. By this method, only the necessary portion of bone is eliminated, and no new wound surfaces are created, as in the case of sequestrotomy. Franzoni has observed that when cloudy days intervene a sequestrum near the surface has retracted deeper into the cavity, to be fully expelled after further exposure to the sun.

The analgesic effect of the sun's rays is seen in almost all cases. In rare cases the symptoms become exacerbated but soon abate, and all cases show a marked lessening and more frequently an absence of pain after a short period of treatment. This, in turn, helps the patient by allowing him plenty of rest and sleep, the exposure to the sun being conducive to sleep itself.

In many cases of joint tuberculosis he finds a far better functional result after the use of heliotherapy than experience with other methods would lead one to expect. This he considers as characteristic of the use of the sun and air treatment. Passive and active movements are not employed.

In a certain number of non-tuberculous lesions heliotherapy renders unquestionable service. Various kinds of ulcer, varicose ulcers, atonic ulcers and certain forms of gangrene of the skin, are remarkably amenable to the solar treatment. Aismes, in his thesis, showed that heliotherapy is very efficacious in the treatment of fractures with delayed union, in osteosynthesis, bone grafts and the post-operative treatment of osteomyelitis. In some cases of burn also healing seems to be hastened by this treatment.

Among the constitutional diseases in which the solar treatment is capable of conferring benefit are: chlorosis, anemia, pre-tuberculous anemia, scrofulosis, rickets, chronic rheumatism, malaria and, lastly, advanced age and cachexia in which the languishing functions are greatly stimulated by the solar rays.

Heliothermometer. ACTINOMETER. An instrument for measuring the intensity of the sun's heat rays.

Heliotrope. A movable mirror, reflecting the light of the sun, used for signalling.

Heliotroper. A man employed to operate heliographic instruments.

Heliotropism. When a seedling plant is placed in a transparent vessel of water within reach of the light of a window, the stem and leaves gradually bend towards, and the roots from, the light. The shoots and leaves of nearly all plants turn towards the light and the turning of the sunflower towards the sun is familiar to every one. In the case of organs which are positively heliotropic the growth of the side next to the light is retarded, and that of the opposite side is increased; the result of these combined actions is a concavity on the former, and a convexity on the latter, thus causing a curvature toward the light. In the case of roots these actions are reversed.

Animal heliotropism is said to be the instinct possessed by animals which enables them to recognize their situation and to direct their movements with reference to the source of light.

Negative heliotropism is defined to be in plants the property of turning away from the light; in animals, the instinct by which the anal extremity is directed toward the source of light.

Transverse heliotropism is defined by Frank' to be a sort of heliotropic irritability peculiar to dorsiventral organs of plants by virtue of which such organs exhibit a strong tendency to assume a horizontal position when exposed to vertical lines.

Heliotropium hispidum. (L.) Erysipelas-plant; an astringent and antiphlogistic species growing in the East Indies and tropical America; used in gum-boils, pimples, ophthalmia, and venomous bites.

Helium. (He), an element of atomic weight, 4.0. It was first identified an element in the sun by its spectrum, but was not isolated until 1895, when Sir William Ramsay obtained it from the mineral cleveite. It is one of the lightest gases known, is colorless and insoluble in water. It was first liquefied by Professor Onnes, at Leyden, in 1908, and is very inert. It occurs in many radio-active minerals such as thorianite and monazite, in the waters of many thermal springs, and in the atmosphere of which it forms about four parts in a million. Recently it has been demonstrated that the X-rays emitted by radium are positively charged helium atoms.—*(Standard Encyclopedia.)*

Hellebore, as an ophthalmic remedy in antiquity, included both *Helleborus niger* and *H. viridis.* The black variety was called by Pliny "melampodium." "Veratrum" was applied indifferently to either the white or the black. The black variety was employed for caligo (q. v.) while the white was especially esteemed for clouding of the pupil. Before the use of hellebore, the patient had to abstain from wine for a week and to eat "sharp" food; while on the day immediately preceding the use of the drug he had to fast and vomit. Under no circumstances was either the white or the black variety to be taken on a cloudy day.—(T. H. S.)

Helleborein. $C_{37}H_{56}O_8$. This poisonous agent is a glucoside from *Helleborus niger.* It is a yellowish powder, soluble in water and alcohol. It is said that 3 or 4 drops of a solution containing in each drop 1-125 gr. (0.0005 grm.) will produce complete anesthesia, without irritation, of the cornea, lasting half an hour.

Helleborus fœtidus. Like *helleborus niger,* one of the sources of helleborein. A few cases of transitory amblyopia, with mydriasis and photophobia, have been observed after the ingestion of various hellebore preparations.

Helligkeit. (G.) Brightness. Illumination.

Helligkeitsempfindung. (G.) Sensation of brightness.

Helling, Georg Lebrecht Andreas. Born at Gross-Salze, near Magdeburg, Feb. 23, 1763, he received his medical degree in 1801 at Frankfort-on-the-Main. He settled in Berlin, Germany, where, after years of constant effort, he succeeded in securing a practice. In 1804 he delivered a course of private lectures on diseases of the eye. He invented a number of plastic operations on the eye, as well as several ophthalmic instruments. He died Nov. 23, 1840. His ophthalmologic writings are as follows: 1. Beobachtung eines Nachstaars. *(Jour. f. Chir.,* 1800.) 2. De Fistula Lacrymalis. *(Dissertation,* 1801.) 3. Merkwürdige Erfahrung an einem am Grauen Staare Blindgeborenen. *(Hermstädt's Bulletin,* Vol. II, 1803.) 4. Beobachtung über die im Letzten Kriege 1813 and 1814 bei den Preussischen Soldaten Gleichsam Epidemisch Gewordene Augenkrankheit. (Berlin, 1815.) 5. Heilung der Umkehrung der Augenlider nach innen mit Concentrirter Schwefelsäure. *(Hufelands Jour.,* 1815.) 6. Über die Augenkrankheit der Preussischen Soldaten. (Berlin, 1816.) 7. Krankheits- und Hailungs-geschichte einer Ungewöhnlich Grossen Exophthalmia Fungosa. *(Rust's Mag.,* 1817.) 8. Guter Rath über die Beschaffen-

heit, Auswahl der Brillen, etc. (Berlin, 1819.) 9. Ueber die Anwen-
dung des Kadmii Sulfurici gegen Hornhautverdunkelungen. (*Rust's
Mag.*, 1820.) 10. Praktisches Handbuch der Augenkrankheiten nach
Alphabetischer Ordnung. (2 vols., 1821, '22; 2 copper plates.)—(T.
H. S.)

Hellman, Johann Caspar. A German ophthalmologist. Born at Halle,
County Minden, in Westphalia, May 22, 1736, he seems to have studied, for a time at least, in Magdeburg. At all events, he became official
physician to that city, and there died, Mar. 21, 1793. He is said to
have had an enormous practice, and to have been a remarkably skilful operator. He wrote but a single work, "*Der Graue Staar und
dessen Herausnehmung, nebst Einigen Beobachtungen*" (Magdeburg,
1774). This was highly prized by numerous contemporaries.—(T.
H. S.)

Helmbold's test. This means of detecting the ocular malingerer is a
variation of Barthélémy's test (q. v.) except that two charts are employed, one with ordinary test types and the other with the letters
printed reversed. The latter are intended to be read by reflection
from a mirror.

Helmholtz, Hermann Ludwig Ferdinand von. The discoverer of the
ophthalmoscope, and, thereby, though not an ophthalmologist, the
most important personage of all the ages in ophthalmology. He was
born at Potsdam, Germany, Aug. 31, 1821. His father was August
Ferdinand Julius Helmholtz, who had been a lieutenant in the German Army, and who, afterward, giving up his original profession of
theologian, because of conscientious scruples, secured a position as
teacher of the classical languages at the Potsdam Gymnasium in 1820.
The mother of the subject of this sketch was Caroline Penne, the
daughter of a Hanoverian artillery officer, one of whose ancestors
was the illustrious William Penn, founder of Pennsylvania. She and
August Ferdinand Julius Helmholtz were married in 1820, immediately after the appointment of the young artillery officer to the Potsdam Gymnasium.

August Ferdinand Julius Helmholtz was a writer of much ability
(consult, for examples, his "*Early Development of the Hellenes*" and
his equally lucid and interesting "*The Arabs as Described in the
Hamaseh*") and he also seems to have been an instructor of the very
highest rank. However, his constitution, always feeble, had been
seriously impaired by his military life, and, in consequence, he was
ever in straitened financial circumstances.

Hermann, the eldest son and the subject of this sketch, was born
at Potsdam in 1821—just thirty years before the publication of the

''*Augenspiegel*,'' and only twenty-nine years before the discovery of the instrument itself. Two sisters came soon after—Marie and Julie, and, in 1831, a brother, Otto. Two other brothers, Ferdinand and Heinrich, were born soon after Otto, but died in infancy.

Hermann was a frail and feeble infant, and not much stronger as a lad and youth. Perhaps the greater portion of his time, at least until his seventh year, was spent in bed. At the age of seven, however, he was sent to the Potsdam Normal School, where his masters were considerably astonished at the progress which he had already made in geometry. This rather advanced condition of affairs was due, as it seems, to geometric toys with which the sickly child had been amused at home by his scholarly and no doubt rather over-zealous father. However, at the Potsdam school the boy increased considerably in stature, and a little in health and strength—as well, of course, as in the learning of his masters.

From the very beginning, he was, like almost every genius, mentally one-sided. Though an excellent reasoner, he was ''hampered by the want of a good memory for disconnected facts.'' ''This showed itself,'' as he himself declared in after life, ''in the difficulty which I still remember of distinguishing between left and right; later on, when I got to languages in my school-work, it was harder for me to learn the vocabularies, grammatical irregularities, and idiomatical expressions, than for the others. History, in particular, as it was taught in those days, was quite beyond me. It was a real torture to learn prose extracts by heart. This defect has of course increased, and is a nuisance in my old age. I found no difficulty in learning the poems of the great masters, but the more labored verses of second-rate poets were far less easy.''

He was strong in mathematics, stronger still in physics, and strongest of all, it is interesting to know, in optics, whose problems were never hard enough to suit him. In fact the lad had fully decided to become a physicist when his father (on account, as it seems, of the family poverty) declared for medicine instead. After a severe competitive examination, he entered the Royal Medico-Chirurgical Friedrich-Wilhelm Institute in October, 1838, being seventeen years of age. To Surgeon-General von Wiebel his father wrote: ''I recommend this good boy,* my dearest treasure, on whose education I have expended my best energies, to the fatherly care of one who is so valued for his goodness.'' At the Friedrich-Wilhelm Institute young Helmholtz

---

* ''Of all the great and good men I have had the good fortune of coming in contact with, I have admired none more than Helmholtz.''—Hermann Knapp.

received a medical education gratis, with the understanding that, after his graduation, he was to serve as surgeon in the Prussian Army.

While at the Friedrich-Wilhelm Institute, Hermann Helmholtz formed a remarkable friendship with Brücke and du Bois-Reymond, each of whom was two years older than himself. Both these friendships were maintained until, many years after, they were broken by the hand of death. He also here became acquainted with Johannes Müller, Gustav Magnus, Kirchoff and Virchow.

In 1842 Hermann received his degree, his dissertation being "De Fabrica Systematis Nervosi Evertebratorum." Some four weeks earlier he had been appointed house-surgeon at the Charité. The following year he was military physician at Potsdam, and, in 1848, instructor in anatomy at the Academy of Art and the Anatomical Museum, in Berlin. In 1849 he was made professor of physiology and general pathology at Königsberg (during his residence at which place he discovered the ophthalmoscope) and in 1855 professor of anatomy and physiology at Bonn. Three years later he was called to the chair of physiology at Heidelberg. In 1871 he removed to Berlin in order to accept the chair of physics and the directorship of the Physical Institute, as well as the title of "Geheim Regierungsrath."

For the first few years of his residence in Berlin, he was assistant physician at the Charité and assistant surgeon in the Red Hussars Regiment at Potsdam. He never had a private medical practice, and he never practised ophthalmology as a specialty.

In 1877, when the Physico-Technical Institute was founded by von Siemens at Berlin, Helmholtz was chosen as its first director. In 1883, because of his many astounding discoveries in physical science, he was ennobled. Eight years later, the 70th anniversary of his birth was made an occasion for international rejoicing. Honorary degrees were conferred upon him by many universities; a Helmholtz medal was founded in his honor; the German Kaiser sent to him an autograph letter of congratulation, and the Kings of Sweden, Italy, and other countries conferred upon him the insignia of numerous high orders.

To recite the achievements of von Helmholtz in detail would be to exceed by far the limits of this sketch. We may, however, recall to the reader his greatest and most far-reaching performances. Von Helmholtz it was who secured the acceptance by the scientific world of the doctrine of the conservation of energy (*"Erhaltung der Kraft,"* 1847); who discovered a way to measure the angle of aperture in a microscope; who first declared that electricity consists of atoms—a theory of most enormous consequences; whose *"Sensations of Sound"* and *"Physiological Optics"* altered forever the subjects of optics and acoustics; who gave "to Hertz the inspiration to find experimental proof of Maxwell's electric waves," a proceeding which led to the invention of wireless telegraphy; and, finally, who, by his own unaided invention of the ophthalmoscope, uttered the *fiat lux* of ophthalmology.*

A part of the success of von Helmholtz was due to his happy domestic life. He married, Aug. 26, 1849, Fräulein Olga von Velten, who bore him a number of children and who died in 1859. In 1861 he married Fräulein Anna von Moll, by whom he also had several children and who outlived him. Of his first wife he wrote: "I enjoyed the purest and highest happiness that marriage can give one; it was too beautiful for this world." His second marriage would seem to have been quite as happy. All his children were affectionate and dutiful toward him, and a source of the greatest joy and consolation in times of sickness or other distress.

In 1893 von Helmholtz, at the earnest request of Hermann Knapp, of New York, attended the World's Fair at Chicago, and made a number of journeys to the western portions of this continent. On his way back to Bremen, he met with a painful accident, from which, as it seems, he never recovered completely.

In the words of his wife, as she wrote on board the Saale, October 14, 1893: † "In defiance of superstition, we embarked late on Friday, the 6th, started at 7 a. m. and at once got onto the edge of a cyclone which stood by us all the time—warm, misty, depressing. I suffered unspeakably till today; your father, well, energetic, and particularly kind and dear about my sickness, told me on Thursday, as on all the other days, what he had been talking about with our nice captain, and then took Kuno Fischer's *Schopenhauer* into the smoking-room —while I lay more wretched than ever. Then Professor Klein came in, and broke to me that your father had fallen down the companion, and was bleeding from forehead and nose, and that two doctors were with him; and then led me into the ship doctor's cabin. There lay your father covered with blood, but he appeared to be conscious, and was able to answer all questions. At first they feared an apoplectic stroke, which I never believed for a moment, but I think one of his old and long-forgotten swoons must have suddenly come upon him.

---

* For evidence of Helmholtz's astounding literary productivity, see the extensive bibliography at the close of this article.
† This passage, as well as a number of the facts in various parts of this sketch, I take from Koenigsberger's *"Hermann von Helmholtz,"* translated by Frances A. Welby (Oxford, at the Clarendon Press, 1901).

Evidently he had become unconscious before the fall; since he did not put his hands out to protect himself, but fell heavily on his face.''

Helmholtz and his party arrived in Bremen Oct. 17, and, after a week of attention there at the hands of Bardeleben and Renvers, he was able to return to Berlin. On the following New Year's Day, he learned of the death of his old friend, Hertz, an occurrence which served still further to prostrate him. He still performed considerable work, but was never himself again. On July 11, he wrote a very lucid letter, in which he recommended that a certain prize, of 15,000 marks, should be awarded ''to Heinrich Hertz, who died at the commencement of this year. I think all our contemporaries will agree as to the value of his discoveries and their scientific results. The circumstance of his death does not, as I interpret the statutes, preclude the allotting to him of the prize, since his life was prolonged into this year,'' etc. On the following day came the beginning of the end.

''On the morning of the 12th,'' said Wachsmuth in a letter,* ''I was summoned from the Reichsanstalt. Helmholtz had crossed the vestibule, but suddenly became incapable of going farther; the servants sprang forward, led him back into his room, and put him on the sofa. The paralysis, due no doubt to some increasing cerebral hemorrhage, crept on slowly. In the forenoon he was still able to talk calmly about all necessary arrangements, and I wrote a number of letters at his dictation. The first physician who came was Bardeleben, followed by Gerhardt and Leyden, but Helmholtz himself knew too much about medicine not to grasp the situation fully. Then came a time of wandering and lucid intervals, with anxious nursing, reminiscences of America and the Falls of Niagara,—lastly a decided improvement.''

On July 18, his wife wrote to her sister: † ''His thoughts ramble on confusedly, real life and dream life, time and scene, all float mistily by in his brain—for the most part he does not know where he is—thinks himself traveling—in America—on the ship, and so on. I was obliged to bring him the pictures of Niagara. It is as if his soul were far, far away, in a beautiful ideal world, swayed only by science and the eternal laws. Then his surroundings jar on him, and he gets confused and wanders.''

So he lingered until Sept. 8, when, at last, after many sufferings, he passed away, in the afternoon, at a little after one o'clock.

On Dec. 14, a memorial ceremony was held at the Singakademie in Berlin, at which were present the Emperor, the Empress, the Empress

---

* Koenigsberger, *op. cit.*, p. 429.
† Koenigsberger, *op. cit.*, p. 429.

Frederick, and a very large number of other distinguished persons. An eloquent discourse was delivered by his old-time friend, Wilhelm von Bezold; and that master of the violin, "the soul-refining" Joachim, played, with sublime organ accompaniment, Schumann's Abendlied, which had been a favorite selection of the great departed.

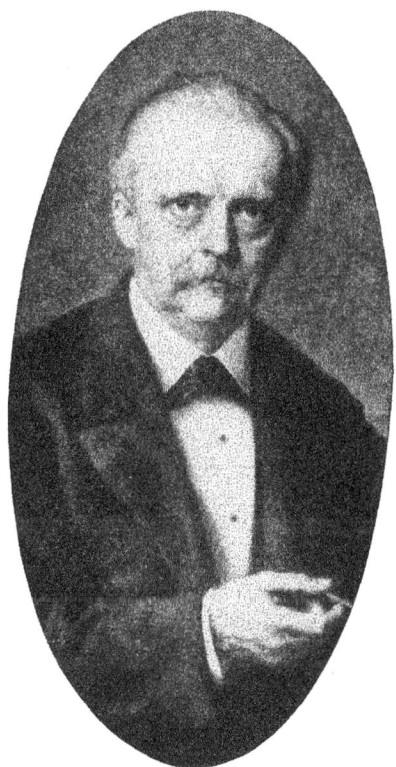

Hermann von Helmholtz.

At the suggestion of the Emperor, a "public memorial," in the form of a monument of Helmholtz, was erected in front of the University Building in Berlin. Toward the expense of this the Emperor himself contributed 10,000 marks. The monument was unveiled June 6, 1899.

The following reminiscences of Helmholtz are taken from an address by Casey A. Wood, made before the Minnesota Academy of Ophthalmology and Oto-Laryngology, at the Annual Meeting, Oct. 13,

1911: "I feel like apologizing to you for choosing what may at first glance seem a time-worn subject, but in explanation let me advance the undoubted fact that in the constellations that bedeck the medical firmament, the star that shines for us physicians and ophthalmologists, with a particularly clear and steadfast light is that of Helmholtz. I do not make this assertion because he invented more useful and practical instruments, and elucidated more problems in ophthalmology than any other man, but because he combined, to an extent found in few men of science, the virtues of the specialist with the best qualities of the all-round medical man.

"One naturally thinks of Helmholtz as a great physicist, a famous mathematician, or a learned exponent of the pure sciences; he was indeed all these, but in his well-known lecture on 'Thought in Medicine,' delivered before the Institute for the Education of Army Surgeons, he refers in most enthusiastic terms to his work in hospital and to his graduation as a physician. 'I am glad,' said he, 'that I am able to address an assembly consisting almost altogether of medical men. Medicine was the intellectual home in which I grew up; and even the emigrant best understands, and is best understood by, his native land.' In the same paper he says, 'I consider the study of medicine to have been that training which preached more impressively and more convincingly than any other could have done, the everlasting principles of scientific work; principles which are so simple and yet so easily forgotten, so clear and yet always hidden by a deceptive veil.'

"In another relation than that of medicine, we may, I think, claim Helmholtz as one of ourselves. Although born at Potsdam (in 1821) he was a lineal descendant, on his mother's side, of William Penn, the great Quaker, who founded Pennsylvania. Moreover, his immediate ancestors came from Hanover when it was English territory, and his grandmother spoke the English language. I leave it to you to decide, with McKendrick, whether it is possible that 'something of his calm, reserved, self-possessed manner may have come through the maternal line from the old Quaker statesman who made his mark on the new world.'

"Helmholtz stood for sobriety and simplicity in living. He was a quiet but effective example of the democracy in science, and, although the most social and kindly of men, he had no time for the ordinary distractions of society. It is true that conditions in his own country rather emphasized this Spartan attitude; it is always easier to make a national virtue out of a national necessity, but, after all, the temperamental virtues and the simple life go not unnaturally together.

"I think I have elsewhere related my experience of the style observed by the various teachers in the *Physiologisches Institut* at Berlin when I was first a student in that school of learning a quarter of a century ago. Every now and then one of the teachers would invite his colleagues and some of the students to a modest repast—generally known as a *Microscopische-Bier-Versammlung*—at which we talked, ate sandwiches, drank beer, and then talked some more, not only about the special matter in hand, but about everything else under the sun. The simple, almost primitive character of the material entertainment, contrasted with the elaborate and priceless quality of the spiritual and mental food, made an enduring impression on my mind. Looking back on those happy, care-free days, I believe at the time it was more the unobtrusive informality of these meetings,—if I must use the word, the frugality of it all,—that I remember most decidedly. Truly the greatest are often the simplest of men. Just think of it: we listened, in their hours of ease, to the conversation of Helmholtz, Du Bois Reymond, König, Fritsch, Gad, and a dozen others at that time less widely known, but since become famous.

"I wonder what importance you as the medical advisers and citizens of a free state attach to the waste of life, of money and of energy that goes on all about us, and, for the matter of that, in the bosom of our own families. None of us wishes to be regarded as a croaker or even to rank as a Jeremiah, but what in the name of Hygeia, or any other goddess, is the meaning of it all? Is it a passing phase in the development of a new world, to be corrected by time and experience, or are we going to seed prematurely, to be finally purified into the Gehenna of nations? Personally, I do not 'despair of the Republic,' but I cannot help thinking that it is foolish to mistake mere display for effectiveness, to accept lavish expenditure in lieu of high thinking, to substitute the shadow for the reality. Of course, the difficulty generally is, how, in the face of serious obstacles, to live our own lives properly, yet how can *we* consistently and effectively criticize that deplorable waste and extravagance in public and private life that we, better than anyone else, know to be abundant everywhere, unless we demonstrate the faith that is in us by simple and hygienic habits?

"I am sure that Helmholtz was not a mere ascetic. Although a tireless worker and a deep student, he liked the good things of this world, but he fervently desired, first of all, to bring them within the grasp of others; and he believed that it is mainly through the appreciation of scientific discovery, advanced education, and rational living that the general level of mankind would be raised to higher things, that more solid satisfaction is to be derived from a dollar rationally spent in the public service than from ten cast into the ditch of selfish enjoyment. But to attain this Nirvana the individual must begin early, the nation must begin early, must keep it up and keep always at it. The price of personal and national advancement is that of liberty—everlasting vigilance.

"We have heard a good deal about the story of the simple life in recent years, and we know that it is only the revival of that gospel preached by philosophers when Babylon and Thebes were young, and long centuries before Rome was founded or Paris dreamed of, but I attach some importance to the knowledge that Helmholtz thought it worth while to champion it, and that he did what he could to foster plain living in conjunction with exalted thought.

"During his long and eventful career Helmholtz, in pursuance of the belief that the salvation of the race lies chiefly in the rational application of painfully acquired knowledge, found time to give popular lectures to those he thought would appreciate them. These lectures were prepared with great care and were fully illustrated, often by experiments. The text of these lectures, both in the original and in their translation, is a model of literary style, while the subject-matter is inspiring and instructive. I have long felt that, as medical men, we have been very derelict in our duties as teachers and as guides of public opinion. . . .

"Finally, gentlemen, I would like to speak of a characteristic of Helmholtz that, developed more or less in many great men, is sufficiently uncommon to be worthy of comment. Perhaps, also I think of it because I once played a minor part in the exhibition of this quality of the master. I refer to his scrupulous and kindly regard for the failings, claims, and rights of others. You will recollect that although Helmholtz was undoubtedly the first to give an intelligent and complete explanation of the mechanism of accommodation, he declared when the papers of Cramer were laid before him some time after the publication of his own researches, that the Dutch observer and not Helmholtz should have the honor of the discovery, that he had done little subsequent to Cramer's solution of the main problem to elucidate the theory. Again, Helmholtz's discussion of the claims of those who had *almost* invented the ophthalmoscope, as well as his attitude toward those who subsequently improved upon the first model, are couched in the same terms of praise of their efforts, with but few remarks about his own.

"As most of you know, Helmholtz visited this country in 1893, the year before his death. Among the receptions and dinners in his honor a banquet was given in Chicago, and because, I suppose, I had been one of his students,—for I had no other claim upon the distinction,—I was asked to speak at the dinner upon a subject connected with the history of ophthalmology. Owing to the noise and confusion attendant upon dining and wining several hundred doctors, and because of the distance I was placed from him, I am sure Helmholtz did not hear one-tenth of the sentences I was doing my feeble best to deliver. He must have noticed my predicament, for a good part of his reply to the toast we drank to his health was taken up by a reference to the labor I must have undergone in preparing such a fine speech, and to the reward that awaits every young man who intelligently studies the works of the Fathers in medicine. Of course, the praise was undeserved, and nobody knew it better than myself, but the incident shows, as his whole life demonstrated, the sort of man he was—learned and kindly, successful and generous, endowed with all great qualities; but simple, modest, and true. Indeed, he seems to me to have exemplified Bayard Taylor's dictum that

> " 'Fame is what you have taken,
> Character's what you give;
> When to this truth you waken,
> Then you begin to live.' "

The writer cannot conclude this sketch without presenting a passage from du Bois-Reymond regarding the physical appearance of his friend, von Helmholtz: "For those unacquainted with him it may be said that the external aspect wholly corresponded with the greatness of his mind. His skull was immense, but perfect in form; his splendid eyes did not betray the efforts they had endured unscathed in subjective experiments, while the delicacy and refinement of the lower half of his face revealed the subtlety of his intellect. He was of a dark complection, above the middle height, and powerfully built with a noble bearing."

Strange to say, the epoch-making *"Beschreibung eines Augenspiegels,"* important as it is in ophthalmology, has never, until recently,* appeared in the form of a translation either in English or any other language—a curious fact which has been referred by some to a supposed obscurity of Helmholtz's style in this one little volume at least, and, by others, to the sheer inherent difficulty of the subject. Those who have actually read the classic will probably agree with the present

---

* An English translation by the present writer first appeared in January, 1916, in the form of a small volume for private circulation only. It will also appear in full, in this *Encyclopedia*, under the caption **Ophthalmoscope.**

writer, that both these suppositions are, in greater part at least, erroneous.

A bibliography of Helmholtz's ophthalmologic writings (only) is as follows:

1. Description of an Ophthalmoscope for the Investigation of the Retina in the Living Eye. (Berlin, Förster, 1851.)

2. Theory of Compound Colors. (*Poggend. Annal.*, LXXXVI, 1852.)

3. On Brewster's New Analysis of Solar Light (*Berl. Monatsb.*, Poggend. Annal., LXXXIX; (Trans.) *Phil. Mag.* [4], IV, 1852.)

4. On the Scientific Researches of Goethe. (Lecture at Königsberg, 1853. Eng. Trans., *Pop. Sci. Lect.*, Series I, 1853.)

5. On a Hitherto Unknown Alteration in the Human Eye During Accommodation. (*Berl. Monatsb.*, 1853.)

6. On the Composition of Spectral Colors. (*Poggend. Annal.*, XCIV, 1855.)

7. On the Sensibility of the Human Retina to the most Refrangible Rays of Solar Light. (*Ibid.*, XCIV, 1855.)

8. On the Accommodation of the Eye. (Graefe's *Archiv*, 1855.)

9. On Human Vision. (Königsberg, Lecture, 1855.)

10. On the Explanation of Lustre. (*Nieder-Rh. Sitzungsber.*, 1856.)

11. The Telestereoscope. (*Poggend. Annal.*, 1856.)

12. Textbook of Physiological Optics. Part I. (1856.)

13. On the Subjective After-Images of the Eye. (*Nieder-Rh. Sitzungsber.*, 1858.)

14. On After-Images. (*Karlsruhe, Naturf.-Versammlung*, 1858.)

15. On Color Blindness. (Heidelberg Society, 1858.)

16. On Contrast Phenomena in the Eye. (Heidelberg Society, 1860.)

17. Textbook of Physiological Optics. Part II. (1860.)

18. On the Horopter. (von Graefe's *Archiv*, 1864.)

19. Remarks on the Form of the Horopter. (*Poggend. Annal.*, 1864.)

20. Handbook of Physiologic Optics. Part III (final). (1867.)

21. The More Recent Developments in the Theory of Vision. (*Preuss. Jahrb.*, XXI, 1868. Eng. Trans., *Pop. Sci. Lect.*, Series II.)

22. The Relation of Optics to Painting. (Eng. Trans., *Pop. Sci. Lect.*, Series II. 1868.)

23. On the Signification of the Convergent Position of the Eyes for the Purpose of Determining the Distance of Objects seen Binocularly. (*Berlin Physiol. Soc.*, 1878.)

24. Handbook of Physiological Optics. (Second Edition, 1885-1895.)

25. On the Intrinsic Light of the Retina. (*Physical Society*, 1888.)

26. An Attempt to Extend the Application of Fechner's Law in the Color System. (*Zeitsch. f. Psychol. u. Physiol. d. Sinnesorgane*, II, 1891.)

27. An attempt to Apply the Psycho-Physical Law to the Color Differences of Trichromatic Eyes. (*Zeitsch. f. Psychol. u. Physiol. d. Sinnesorgane*, III, 1891.)

28. Shortest Lines in the Color System. (*Berlin Academy*, 1891.)

29. Electromagnetic Theory of Color Dispersion. (*Wiedemann's Ann.*, XLVIII, 1892.)

30. Additions and Corrections to the Essay: Electro-Magnetic Theory of Color Dispersion. (*Ibid.*, XLVIII, 1892.)—(T. H. S.)

Helmholtz, Lines of. Those normal to the plane of the axes of rotation of the eye.

Helmholtz's chess-board. The so-called, hyperbolic, chess-board of Helmholtz is a well-known optic device, which is described and pictured under **Chess-board of Helmholtz.**

Helminthiasis. The condition produced by worms that infest the human intestinal tracts. Parasites producing eye symptoms receive attention under their single and appropriate captions.

On the basis of sixty cases Campos (*Brazil. Med.*, 1914, Nos. 3, 4, 5, 1914) discusses acute hemeralopia as seen in Brazil. He finds it is not merely a symptom of some toxic condition, but a true retinal lesion dependent on defect in the nutrition of the retina—a toxic injury of the pigment epithelium. His patients were mostly children of 2 to 7 years of age, anemic, asthenic and apathetic. Most of them suffered from *helminthiasis,* and treatment of this condition brought about rapid cure.

Helminthology. The science of intestinal worms, of their effects, etc.

Helminthoma. A term for a disease of the skin thought to be due to the presence of animal parasites, at a time when it was supposed that such parasites originated by spontaneous generation in vesicles, boils, or tumors in the skin.

Helosis. Plica polonica. An obsolete name for inversion of the eyelids, strabismus and ''eye-spasm.''

Helvella esculenta. One of the least poisonous of the mushrooms, but known to have produced mydriasis and immobility of the pupils. See **Toxic amblyopia.**

Helvolous. Dull reddish-yellow; tawny.

Hem. (F.) A dry cough.

Hemachromatosis. Blood staining, e. g., of the cornea.

Hemachroses. (L.) Diseases in which the color of the blood is changed, as in those causing cyanosis.

Hemacytometer. An instrument used in counting the corpuscles of blood.

Hemadynamometer. An instrument for measuring the force of the blood-current. It consists of a U-shaped tube, one arm of which contains mercury, the other and longer arm being graduated. The shorter arm is inserted into an artery. The height to which the mercury rises in the other arm represents the blood-pressure. In normal man this is equal to about 6˚ inches of mercury.

Hemalaun. A well-known (nuclear) stain (discovered by P. Meyer), of value for laboratory purposes. It is made as follows: One gram of hematein is dissolved in 50 cubic centimetres of 90-per-cent. strength alcohol by warming. This is added to a solution of 50 grams of alum in 1000 cubic centimetres of distilled water. A crystal of thymol may be added to prevent the growth of fungi. For staining, wash the sections in water; stain for from five to fifteen minutes; wash in water for from ten to twenty minutes; dehydrate in 95-per-cent. strength alcohol; clear in carbol-xylol. Balsam.

Hemalops. An old and obsolete term for an extravasation of blood into the eye; a condition in which every object appears of a blood-red color.

Hemalops externus. (Obs.) An extravasation of blood outside the eyeball, beneath the conjunctiva. ·

Hemangioma. An angioma made up of blood-vessels, as distinguished from lymphangioma.

According to Parsons (*Pathology of the Eye*, p. 18) these tumors are either capillary or cavernous. Capillary hemangiomata are either congenital *(capillary nevi)* or acquired *(telangiectasis)*. In either case they consist of capillaries, increased in size and number, and closely aggregated. *Cavernous nevi* are circumscribed and composed of thin-walled veins and sinuses, bound together by a small amount of cellular connective tissue. The walls often consist simply of endothelium lying on the connective tissue. A few small arteries open into the sinuses without the intervention of capillaries.

Hemangiomata are usually seen in the eyelid and conjunctiva although they also affect the iris, choroid, retina and orbit. See these various captions.

P. H. Adams (*Trans. Oph. Society U. K.*, Vol. XXXII, p. 389, 1912) reports a typical case occurring in the conjunctiva. A woman, aged

36 years, for about four years had noticed a red spot slowly growing just above one cornea. On examination a nearly circular patch, about 1/6th in. in diameter, the details of which were obscured by hemorrhage, was found, and associated with it was a large subconjunctival hemorrhage extending half way round the cornea. Some six weeks later, when the hemorrhage had almost disappeared, the patch was found to be prominent, to have fine red vessels at its centre, and to be surrounded by purplish veins. It was sensitive to pressure. The growth was eventually excised, and was found to include vessels of two kinds:—(1) large blood spaces, and (2) capillary vessels. The structure indicated that the tissue was a fibrous angioma.

Hemanthus toxicarius. In the human subject the ingestion of this South African poison plant has produced mydriasis.

Hematemesis. The ejection of blood from the stomach by vomiting is most common in carcinoma and gastric ulcer; congestion of the stomach or neighboring portions of the alimentary canal from various causes; and certain conditions of the blood, as in yellow fever, purpura, and typhus. The resulting anemia leads, in certain cases, to visual disturbances, especially to optic lesions. See **Hemorrhage, Amblyopia and amaurosis from**; also p. 292, Vol. I, of this *Encyclopedia*.

Hematidrosis. Bloody sweat. Ephidrosis cruenta. Chromedrosis. A sanguineous perspiration caused by the extravasation of blood into the coils and ducts of the sweat-glands, whence it is carried to the surface, mixed with sweat. See, also, p. 2206, Vol. III, of this *Encyclopedia*.

Hematinometer. An apparatus, consisting of a vessel with parallel glass faces 1 cm. apart, for estimating the amount of the hemoglobin in the blood. This is done by comparing a specimen with a test solution of known strength contained in the vessel.

Hematischesis. Obsolete. The stopping of a hemorrhage or of a hemorrhagic discharge.

Hematitic. Of a dull red color.

Hematochrosis. Any disease characterized by discoloration of the skin. A discoloration of the skin.

Hematochysis. (L.) A synonym, according to Willis, of hemorrhage.

Hematocytometer. An instrument for measuring the number of corpuscles present in the blood. The hematocytometer of Malassez consists of a cell in a microscope-slide, which can be made to contain a precise amount of the blood which before examination is diluted with a specified amount of water. The surface of the cell is divided into squares, each of which corresponds to a certain volume of the diluted blood. The number of corpuscles present in each square is found by counting under the microscope.—(Foster.)

Hematoidin. Probably a derivative of hemoglobin, although hemo-toidin contains no iron and is soluble in chloroform. It is seen in blood-staining of the cornea and similar conditions.

Hematoma, Ocular. Blood-clots or consolidated hemorrhagic deposits may form, especially as the result of direct or indirect injury, within many of the vascular tissues of the eye.

In most cases of hematoma of the conjunctiva (the commonest form) a dark-red swelling begins to show itself in the conjunctiva to the outer and lower portion of the ball and half a centimetre from the corneal edge. This increases slowly in size, and at the end of a

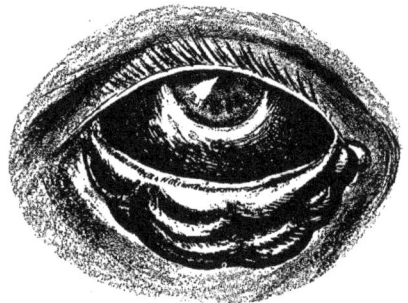

Hematoma of Lower Lid and Conjunctiva.

month or so has attained nearly the dimensions of a pigeon's egg. The inflammatory symptoms are not severe.

The rarer forms of hematoma are of the *optic nerve sheath* and *orbit.* Rollet (*Révue Gen. d'Opht.*, Feb. 1908) reports three cases of the former condition resulting from fracture of the skull, all of which were subjected to microscopic examination, and two were examined with the ophthalmoscope before death. In one of the latter the fundus was normal. In the other case the retinal arteries appeared thread-like, and the disk was surrounded by a blackish ring or halo. Oishi (*Arch. f. Augenh.*, LXI, Pt. I, 1908) reported two cases, one of spontaneous hemorrhage occurring in diabetes, the other with fracture of the base of the skull. Both were examined with the ophthalmoscope and microscopically. They presented numerous retinal hemorrhages, and the dural sheath was found distended with blood, causing a swelling just back of the eyeball, such as is seen with choked disk. In a case reported by Williamson, ten days after being struck on the brow with a brick there was absolute blindness, dilated pupil, a large hemorrhage at the upper outer side of the optic disk, and a small one in the margin of the macula. Muetze (*Ann. of Ophth.*, April, 1908) has also mentioned one in which vision had been reduced to recognition of hand movements and there was marked blanching of the disk a few weeks after injury. But several months later vision had risen to 10/20.

Hematoma of the orbit is often difficult of recognition. Valli (*Ann. di Ott.*, Vol. 42, p. 65, 1913) reports a case of a girl of five years who suddenly, and without known traumatic cause, developed a swelling of the left parietal region, which rapidly extended over the whole head and to the left orbit, producing an enormous exophthalmos. A physician was not called for four days, at the end of which time the eyeball protruded four-fifths outside the orbit. There was no pulsation. Skin punctures over various parts of the swelling, together with the use of compressive bandages, gave issue to about 400 gm. of blood; and with reduction in the general swelling the exophthalmos also subsided. The child was rachitic, and the parents stated that on previous occasions very slight traumata and falls had given rise to bloody swellings, which had lasted as long as a month. Two relapses of the hematoma occurred in the course of the next four weeks, but the exophthalmos was completely recovered from, although the eye was permanently damaged as the result of a perforating corneal ulcer with iris prolapse.

Hematomma. (L.) Another spelling of hematoma.

Hematophthalmia. (L.) A more correct form of hemophthalmia.

Hematopsia. A synonym of hemophthalmia—an extravasation of blood into the subconjunctival tissues of the eye.

Hematoscope. An instrument for observing the spectroscopic properties of the blood. It consists of two plates of glass, which touch at one end, but are distant half a millimetre at the other. A drop of blood is introduced into the space between the plates, where it can be conveniently studied with the spectroscope. The thickness of the layer can be varied at will by approximating or separating the plates.

Hematospectroscope. An instrument for ascertaining the proportion of hemoglobin in the blood by spectroscopy. It consists of the graduated chamber of a hematoscope and a Browning's spectroscope. The less hemoglobin in the blood the thicker the layer from which the spectrum is obtained. Hénocque has compiled a table from which the quantity of hemoglobin may be calculated by the depth of the blood stratum.—(Foster.)

Hematoxylin. See **Delafield's hematoxylin.**

Hematuria. The discharge of blood with the urine, usually from disease of the kidneys or bladder. It is rather a symptom than a disease, and although of some gravity it is not very often directly fatal. When profuse or long continued it may, from the general anemia, lead to changes in the optic nerve. See **Hemorrhage, Amblyopia from**; also, p. 292, Vol. I, of this *Encyclopedia*.

Hemeralopia. DAY-BLINDNESS. The confusion of this term with nyctalopia is referred to on page 3777, Vol. V, of this *Encyclopedia*.

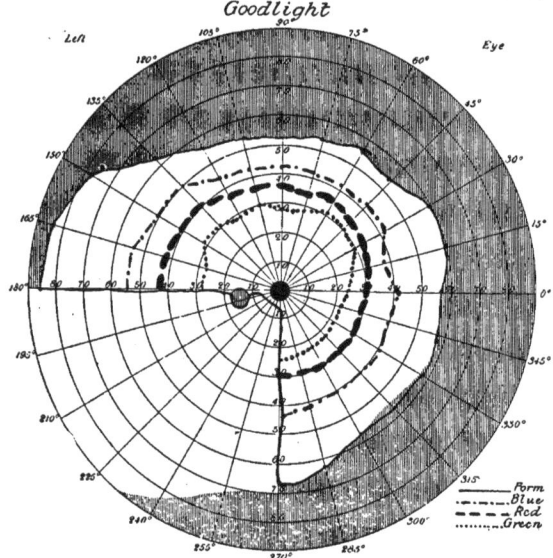

Field of Vision in Family Hemeralopia with Quadrant Anopsia. Good Light.
(Bordley.)

In addition it may be said that Leonard Guthrie (*British Med. Journ.*, July 31, 1915), honorary secretary Nomenclature of Diseases Committee of the Royal College of Physicians, also discusses the proper meanings of hemeralopia and nyctalopia. He goes back to Hippocrates, Galen, and Aristotle in the course of his investigation and declares that he is not prepared to agree to the proposal made by certain distinguished ophthalmologists, and suggests that if it is necessary to provide a word which implies vision by day but blindness by night, it should be "hemeropia," and not hemeralopia.

John Tweedy (*Brit. Med. Journ.*, Aug. 10, 1915) points out that many years ago he and Dr. Greenhill determined, in connection with the preparation of Quain's *Dictionary of Medicine,* that nyctalopia means night-blindness, and that the College of Physicians had accepted this view.

Bordley *(Johns Hopkins Hosp. Bull.,* Vol. XIX, No. 210, 1908) reports as a family of hemeralopes a group of cases traced to five generations, in which night-blindness was congenital, progressive,

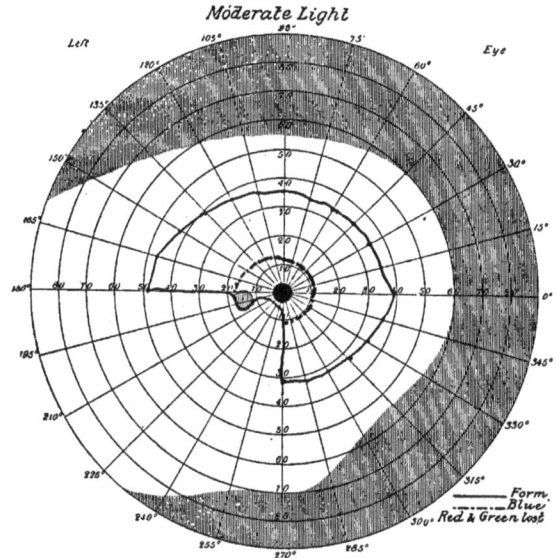

Field in Night Blindness. Moderate Light. (Bordley.)

and associated with defect of the lower temporal quadrant of each visual field, as shown in the figures. There was progressive, concentric contraction of the fields and they were greatly narrowed by diminished illumination. Death occurred at middle age within about one year after becoming entirely blind.

Von Haearenschwand *(Arch. f. Augenheilk.,* LXXIII, p. 133, 1913) has reported his observations on *idiopathic epidemic hemeralopia* in 54 men of the same regiment, of Polish and Ruthenic nationality. They were small, delicately built, but strong, between 22 and 24 years old, of marked Slavic type. Excepting seven they all had been at home working on farms, where they lived chiefly on vegetables. The majority came from large families. In many of these several children had died in early infancy of unknown diseases. In the older cases the hemeralopia had developed a year before, in the

more recent ones a few weeks previously. Twenty-two noticed a
sudden, the others a more gradual, development. Physical strain
and glaring by the sun aggravated the condition. Nine were emmetropic, 30 hypermetropic, 13 slightly myopic. The fundus presented
in general no pathological changes. In six the disc was slightly discolored and the retinal veins lighter (anemic fundus). The visual
field in daylight was normal for white, contracted for blue, in the
dusk also for white. Four men had red-green blindness. Wassermann's reaction was positive in four.

The general examination revealed one peculiar condition: Fifty-
one out of the 54 men had enlarged lymphatic glands at the neck,
arm pit and groins, but no changes of the spleen. Microscopically·
the blood showed an augmentation of the small lymphocytes, the
large mononuclear cells and the forms of transition, a decrease of
hemoglobin to 60 per cent, and poikilocytosis. As the nourishment
was good and plentiful, and the same as of the other regiments of
the same garrison, who underwent the same physical exertions and
were in equal manner exposed to glaring of the sun, the author
attributes the affection to individual predisposition from hereditary
influences. This was evident from the swelling of the lymphatic
glands and the increase of lymphocytes. He considers as the elicit-
ing element for hemeralopia the slight degrees of anemia, indicated
by the decrease of hemoglobin and the poikilocytosis. Such anemia
may disturb the functions of the retina, especially if combined with
external influences, as physical exertion and glaring of the sun.

An investigation by circular letter of an *epidemic of acute hemeralopia* in Saxony during April and May, 1912, was undertaken by
von Hippel (*Klin. Monatsbl. f. Augenheilk.*, May, 1913). Although
the malnutrition and glaring reported cannot fully explain the etiology of hemeralopia, they are certainly of great importance as the
success of the treatment with better nourishment, cod liver oil, iron
and quinine, and the wearing of dark goggles proved.

In a case of severe keratomalacia, which is rather frequent in that
region, the two older children of the same family, aged 4½ and 5½
years, had marked xerosis, but nothing was said about hemeralopia.
If this could be proved by further reports it would suggest a toxic
or auto-toxic etiology of epidemic hemeralopia with xerosis, since
the elimination of such substances by change of nutrition is of the
greatest therapeutic importance in keratomalacia. Von Hippel says
that a defective formation and abnormal consumption of a substance
in the retina, perhaps of the visual purple, must be the cause of
hemeralopia. The accumulation of this substance is kept under

certain limits of noxious influences, but if by removal of one or the other of these a sufficient accumulation of the substance is possible, the function returns.

Ishihara (*Klin. Monatsbl. f. Augenheilk.*, May, 1913) also studied the same problems in his own country. He observes that the excellent therapeutic effect of cod liver oil in xerosis, hemeralopia and keratomalacia, observed especially in Japan, is so far unexplained. Mori considers the scarcity of fat in the food or a diminished absorption of fat by the intestines as the cause of xerosis of the conjunctiva. Upon the supposition of a diminution of fat in the blood, the writer ascertained the percentage of fat in a quantity of blood withdrawn from each of two patients with xerosis and hemeralopia 18 hours after the last meal, and again after recovery, and found it more or less diminished. It is, however, independent of the general nutrition and the amount of the food for the weight of the body showed no essential differences both times. Ishihara saw xerosis in patients who were well nourished and in whom the physical examination revealed normal conditions. A single dose of from 10 to 15 cc. cod liver oil sufficed for the cure of a case of hemeralopia.

Subsequently the same writer made a series of experiments in xerosis of the conjunctiva with hemeralopia with various fats, especially oils, e. g., of eel and olive oil. The effect of all these fats was striking, whence he concludes that hemeralopia, or xerosis of the conjunctiva, is due to lack of fat in the blood. This explains its occurrence in general malnutrition, diseases of the liver, diarrhea, etc., although the direct relations between these etiological elements and the disease itself are still unknown. Ishihara surmises some relation between the formation of the visual purple and the fats. Finally, he once more emphasizes that cod liver oil must be considered a specific against xerosis with hemeralopia.

C. Hess (*Archiv. of Ophthalm.*, Sept., 1912) examined twelve hemeralopes and finds that there is a distinct, sometimes a marked, diminution of sensibility to high light strengths in almost all examined. This is instanced in the cases of those who say that they are able to look at the sun better than most people, and that they can see only stars of greater light strength, e. g., Venus and Jupiter, but cannot see others, even with a telescope; there is a diminution of sensibility to red, both with spectrum red and that of a red glass; and foveal vision is not normal. Hess has devised a special instrument for testing this, and with it finds that in one case foveal vision for red required six to eight times the illumination that he himself required, whilst for blue the multiple was 800. Hess does not consider that we know whether an imperfect formation of visual purple plays a part in hemeralopia.

Finally, Oguchi (Graefe's *Archiv. f. Ophth.*, Vol. 81, Part 1, 1912) reports three very rare cases in which the symptoms closely resembled those of retinitis punctata albescens, or rather that form of retinitis punctata albescens in which hemeralopia is the only functional disturbance. Instead of isolated whitish specks, however, a diffuse grayish white coloration of the fundus was observed. Two were of consanguineous parentage.

. Regarding the ophthalmoscopic picture in these cases he claims: The fundus may show a complete or partial grayish-white coloration of variable intensity; the most careful search failing to reveal pigment spots or white specks. The papilla and vessels are absolutely normal. In contrast to the grayish-white fundus, however, they appear very dark and prominent. The macula lutea likewise appears abnormally dark by contrast, and the macular vessels unusually distinct. This appearance could be brought about, he thinks, by the presence of a thin layer of connective tissue between the retina and choroid, or by approximation of whitish specks, but since no anatomic study has ever been made, it is best to consider the affection apart from other diseases.

Hemeralops. A person affected with hemeralopia.

Hemeropia. A substitute term for hemeralopia, suggested by Leonard Guthrie.

Hemerotyphlosis. (L.) An old term for nyctalopia.

Hemiablepsia. A synonym of hemianopsia.

Hemiachromotopsia. The loss of color-sense in the half-field. A lesion may be such as to destroy only the color-sense, leaving the form-sense and light-sense intact. See **Hemiopia.**

Hemiamaurosis. A term applied by Hjort and Otto to a form of temporary blindness in which hemiopia is associated with amblyopia in the other half of the field.

Hemiamblyopia. See **Hemiopia.**

Hemianesthesia. Anesthesia of greater or less extent on one side of the body. When strictly limited, it is usually due to a disease of the white substance of the brain on the opposite side, in the posterior portion of the internal capsule, just outside the optic thalamus. See, also, **Hysteria.**

Hemianopia. See **Hemiopia.**

Hemianopsia. The opposite of hemiopia (q. v.). If the blind half be toward the same side in both eyes, it is called *homonymous;* if on opposite sides, it is known as *heteronymous* hemianopsia. It may be complete or incomplete, according to the involvement being of one-half the field or merely of a sector of it. It may be absolute or relative, as the blind field is totally or partially blind. The hemianoptic field usually shows an indenture at the point of fixation corresponding to the overlapping of the nerve-supply to the macula.

The right optic tract contains all the nerve-fibres going to the right halves of both eyes. Its division would cause half-blindness on the opposite side of the field of vision. Those on the nasal side decussate to the right half of the left eye. Those on the temporal side continue forward on the same side.

Longitudinal division of the chiasma would cut off all the fibres to the nasal halves of the retinæ, and produce bitemporal hemianopsia—blindness to the right for the right eye and to the left for the left eye. Pressure on the third ventricle or enlargement of the pituitary gland may be the cause. A lesion of the chiasma laterally would cause blindness on the temporal side of the retina. In rare instances bilateral blindness in the nasal fields has been produced by corresponding lesions on each side affecting the non-decussating fibres. A double temporal or nasal blindness can occur only in diseases of the chiasma. The chiasma may be the seat of tumors or syphilitic growths or may be pressed upon through the third ventricle in hydrocephalus. Gouty changes and interstitial hemorrhage have been observed. Migraine and hysteria may cause temporary hemianopsia. Superior and inferior, or altitudinal, hemianopsia is very rare. The optic tract may be involved by traumatism, hemorrhage, softening, basilar tumors, or thickening in multiple sclerosis. One eye may be entirely blind from degeneration of, or from injury to, the optic nerve, or from tumor, aneurism, basilar fracture, or caries of the sphenoid bone. —(J. M. B.) See **Hemiopia.**

Hemianopsia, Pseudo-. A term proposed by W. B. Lancaster (*Boston Med. and Surg. Journ.*, June 12, 1913) for those cases in which the visual fields are not unlike in extent and distribution those classified as true hemianopsia, but are of wholly different origin; for example, in chronic glaucoma and in retinal or choroidal lesions symmetrically disposed in the two eyes. These should not be classed as cases of true hemianopsia.

Hemianopsia, Quadrant. See **Hemiopia,** at the end of the section.

Hemianoptic pupil-symptom of Wernicke. See **Hemiopia.**

Hemicephalous monsters. See **Monsters.**

Hemicerebrum. Half brain, or cerebral hemisphere. The cut in the text shows the relative position of the various cortical centers.

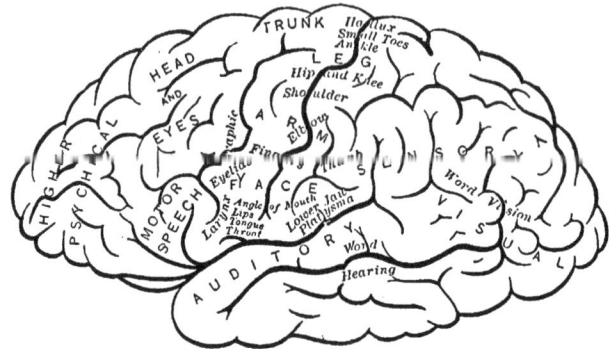

Lateral Aspect of the Left Hemicerebrum, Showing the Cortical Centers. (Nagel.)

Hemicircle. A semicircle.

Hemicrania. See **Migraine**; as well as **Headache, Ocular.**

Hemicrania ophthalmica. (L.) Ophthalmic migraine.

Hemicylindrical. Having the form of half of a cylinder, axially divided.

Hémie. (F.) Deterioration of the blood in general.

Hemierythropsia. The condition in which there is red vision in one-half the field. It is often hysterical or hystero-traumatic.

Hemihypesthesia. (L.) Impaired sensibility limited to one side of the body.

Hemikinesia. A synonym (suggested by C. von Hess) of the so-called (Wernicke) *hemiopic pupillary reaction* (q. v.), or hemianopic pupillary inaction, for the diagnosis of a lesion in the path of the optic radiations.

Hemikinesometer. An instrument devised by Hess for studying retinal sensibility—especially for applying the hemianoptic pupil reflex.

Hemiopalgia. Pain on one side of the head and in one eye.

Hemiopia. HEMIAMBLYOPIA. HEMIAMAUROSIS. HALF-SIGHT. HEMIANOPIA. HEMIOPSIA. HEMIOPY. HEMIABLEPSIA. HEMIANOPSIA. Hemiopia, or half vision, is the older term for hemianopia. Hemiopia and hemiopsia refer to the seeing-half of the retina; hemianopsia and hemianopia to that part of the field not seen.

This symptom commonly results from a focal disease affecting the chiasma, the optic centers or tracts, especially in syphilis, embolism, tubercle, tumor, cerebral softening and injury. It may also be due to sphenoid or ethmo-sphenoid disease, acromegaly, diabetes, migraine, hysteria, elephantiasis, myxedema and other diseases.

For further consideration of this important symptom see Vol. III, p. 1832, of this *Encyclopedia;* as well as **Examination of the eye;**

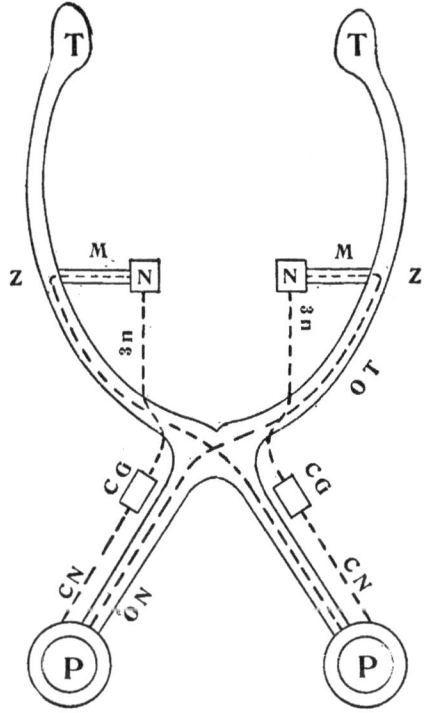

Diagram of Wernicke's Pupil Symptom.   (Ball.)

P, The pupil. T, Center for vision. *ON,* Optic nerve. *OT,* Optic tract. *M,* Meynert's fibers from *Z* (the geniculate body) to *N* (the nucleus of the third nerve). Thence by the third nerve to *CG* (the ciliary ganglion) and by the short ciliary nerve *(CN)* to the sphincter pupillæ *(P)*. A lesion beyond *Z* would not disturb the pupillary reflex. *3n,* Third nerve.

also **Pituitary** body; **Brain tumor; Acromegaly; Neurology of the eye; Migraine; Hysteria,** and **Perimetry.**

If the lesion exists anywhere between the cortical centre and the chiasma, for example, in the right optic tract, the nerve-fibres going to the right half of each retina will be cut off, and the left fields of vision will be cut out—left homonymous hemianopsia. If the lesion is in the chiasma, the decussating fibres to the nasal side of the retina

. will be involved, and the opposite fields may be blind—bitemporal hemianopsia. If the lateral fasciculi of both sides of the chiasma or both optic nerves should be coincidently involved, the temporal halves of the retinæ would be cut off and binasal hemianopsia would result.

Hemianopsia due to a lesion of the optic radiations is generally associated with symptoms such as word-blindness, mind-blindness, word-deafness, alexia, dyslexia, paraphasia, hemianesthesia, and astereognosis. Cortical hemianopsias are not generally associated with visual or auditory aphasias. Visual hallucinations may occur in the blind fields in cases of hemianopsia and must not be mistaken for the visual hallucinations of insanity. They are supposed to be due to an irritation of the visual-memory centre.

By means of the hemianoptic pupil-symptom of Wernicke a differential diagnosis between lesions of the tract and the cortical centre may be made. If the pupil responds to light thrown on the amaurotic retina, the lesion is back of the geniculate bodies. The presence of this reaction indicates that the pupillary nerves which accompany the optic tract as far as the geniculate bodies are not involved. There the afferent pupillary nerve leaves the tract by way of Meynert's fibres to become the efferent impulse to the pupil, going first to the gray matter of the aqueduct of Sylvius, then to the third-nerve nucleus, and from there through the short root of the ciliary ganglion to the ciliary ganglion and the short ciliary nerves to the sphincter pupillæ. If the lesion is in the path of the pupillary reflex, the pupil will fail to react.

A lesion peripheral to the chiasma will cause loss of direct light reflex in an amaurotic eye, and loss of consensual light reflex in the other eye. The consensual reaction is preserved on the blind side. A lesion of the chiasma, such as a sagittal section, will cause a loss of both the direct and consensual reactions when the blind or nasal half of the retina is illuminated. If the optic nerve of one side be destroyed at the same time, there will be a reaction only when the temporal half of the retina of the sound side is illuminated, and a consensual reaction will occur on the blind side.—(J. M. B.)

Clifford Walker (*Trans. Oph. Sec. A. M. A.*, June, 1913; also, *Jour. Am. Med. Assocn.*, Sept. 5, 1914) has made elaborate experiments on and observations of the hemiopic pupillary reaction—both of the Wernicke test proper and of its modification by Wilbrand, the so-called hemianoptic prism phenomenon. See page 4621, Vol. VI, of this *Encyclopedia*.

Heddacus (*Inaug. Dissert.*, Halle, 1880), after reporting his findings as to the pupillomotor relation of blind and seeing retinas, advanced the half-sided or hemiopic pupillary reaction as an aid in determining whether the lesion producing the hemianopsia was central or peripheral to the basal stem ganglion cells, and gave one case in which the reaction was observed.

Wernicke published (*Fortschr. der Med.*, Vol. I, p. 49, 1883) an elaboration of the reaction, mainly on theoretical grounds, as a certain method of locating a hemianoptic lesion anterior or posterior to the corpora quadrigemina, which was considered the sole point of deviation of the pupillary reflex of the oculomotor nerve.

In this reaction it was assumed that the entire retina was pupillomotoric since it seemed to react promptly to a beam of light thrown on the pupil from any part of the field, though it was known that the macular retina was far more active than the peripheral retina; secondly, that pupillomotoric activity persisted in the entire blind area of the retina if the lesion was posterior to the reflex arc, since this was apparently found to be the case in totally blind eyes; thirdly, that it was possible to stimulate isolated areas of the retina only, without materially affecting the macular and other regions.

In 1899 Wilbrand became convinced that the Wernicke hemiopic pupillary reaction was a practical failure, and decided that a new method to the same end was desirable, and proposed his hemianoptic prism phenomenon. With one eye covered the hemianoptic patient was told to concentrate attention on a small white point on a black wall. A strong prism was then suddenly placed before the eye, throwing the image on the blind retina. If the eye instantly moved so as to fix on the point again, the lesion was central; otherwise it was peripheral to the basal stem ganglion. Likewise if the prism was suddenly interposed, throwing the light on the seeing retina, the eye instantly moved to fix the image again; but when the prism was suddenly removed the eye would once more jerk back to fix the point or not according as the lesion was central or peripheral. While he found positive or central cases verified at necropsy, he found no negative or peripheral cases. One case of acromegalic bitemporal hemianopsia failed to give the negative test presumably, he thought, because there was some light perception left in the defective field. The test may be made binocularly in homonymous cases. Wilbrand himself did not argue the presence of a definite reflex arc in this phenomenon, but subsequent observers have postulated such an arc; for instance, Behr (*Archiv. f. Ophthalm.*, p. 340, 1910) locates the afferent branch in Bernheimer's fibres which are supposed to have about the same course as the pupillomotoric fibres.

Walker has devised an apparatus (depicted on pp. 4623-4-5, Vol. VI, of this *Encyclopedia*) for the more effective application of this test. In Walker's clinical experience, the hemiopic pupillary reaction has failed in chiasmal lesions of dyspituitary origin, of rather rapid onset and rapid recovery after operation. The occurrence of pseudo-refixation throws serious doubts on the presence of a definite reflex arc in the prism phenomenon.

Walker holds also that a weak hemiopic pupillary reaction may be masked by the pupillomotor light when observed consensually. Light and dark adaptive phenomena, in addition to dispersion light, seriously complicate the hemiopic pupillary reaction. The hemiopic pupillary reaction is definitely present in anterior lesions, when examined by the rotary shutter method. The hemiopic pupillary reaction is also present in cases having every clinical evidence of being purely posterior cases, although necropsy examination is necessary to prove absolutely that there is no involvement of the optic tract or primary ganglion centers. Although it may be concluded from the examination of these cases that the peripheral retina does possess a weak pupillomotor sensitiveness, there is no evidence that the hemiopic pupillary reaction has any topical diagnostic value.

A. Saenger's method (*Ophthalmic Record*, Aug., 1910) of applying the test of Wilbrand, as demonstrated by the former during a visit to the United States, is as follows: The patient is requested to fix a white point on a large black surface and direct his attention to it. In this way all other impressions on the retina are excluded. The patient takes his seat at a distance of 30 to 50 cm., immediately in front of the white point. Suddenly two prisms of equal degree are brought before both eyes, the apices being turned towards the heminanopic defect. In this manner the white point is directed towards that side of the retina which is not perceptive. The bases of the prisms must be parallel.

If a cortical hemianopia exists the patient will quickly change the direction of sight and move the eyes until the fovea is directed to the object. This proves that there exists a reflex independent of the cerebrum, and on the opposite side; that the optical route between the retina and corpus geniculatum laterale is free. If the disease is situated in the tractus opticus the eyes make no movement to fix the object, but remain quiet.

The *blind visual field in hemianopsia* is discussed by J. Gonin (*Annales d'Ocul.*, CXLV, p. 1, 1912), the following being an outline:

Bard has maintained that in so-called absolute homonymous hemianopsia the sensation of light is never entirely abolished from the blind field; and Bard's conclusions have been accepted by Rochon-Duvigneaud in his description of hemianopsia in the *French Encyclopedia of Ophthalmology*. Gonin therefore discusses one by one the experiments upon which Bard based his argument. Speaking generally, it is urged that, in judging the ability of the blind retinal area to receive light impressions, Bard failed to take into account the play of light and shade on objects in the room, or on the patient's nose; although such indirect effects of the illuminant would be sufficient to indicate its general position to the healthy part of the retina.

One of Bard's tests consisted of throwing on to the cornea from the blind part of the field a feeble light from a mirror placed at a distance. According to Gonin the patient's declaration that the light was increased in this direction depended upon illumination of the corresponding side of the nose. In another test, made in the dark-room, a candle was brought from behind into the blind field; in this case Gonin attributes the positive results to a diffuse illumination of the sclero-corneal limbus. A hemianopsic patient will have acquired superior power of localization by means of such subtle indications. As a control test Gonin "canalized" the light through a long tube, concentrating it by means of a convex lens inside the tube; the patient then·became unable to detect the light. Gonin concludes that we are not justified in surrendering the classic conception of an absolute hemianopsia.

Lohmann (*Archiv f. Ophthalm.*, 80, 2, p. 270) attempts an explanation of the well-known fact that in cases of *lateral hemiopia the power to bisect a horizontal line is almost entirely lost,* the centre being usually placed nearer the end corresponding to the blind side of the field.

Two explanations have been suggested, one depending on alteration in the action of the eye-muscles on account of loss of sensory regulation in respect of movement towards the blind side, the other on a physiological observation of Feilchenfeld's that the portion of such a horizontal line, which corresponds to the larger half of the field—in health, the temporal—is underestimated. Both views are rejected by Lohmann in favor of an explanation, also due to Feilchenfeld, that the error is due to the fact that peripheral portions of a horizontal line correspond to larger visual angles than more central portions of equal size. This can be shown for the normal eye, for if it is attempted to bisect a horizontal line while fixing one end of it the central half is made too small, as in hemiopia. The arrangement of the sensory elements along a meridian of the retina is such that, while having the same functional value, they are more closely placed in the central than in the peripheral parts.

Attention is also directed towards a less known disturbance of absolute localization found by the author in two cases of hemiopia. A vertical line was drawn and the subject was required to continue it, a screen being interposed so that he could not see his hands. Both were right-sided hemiopia and in most cases an error of 2 to 5 cm. to the left side was made. This error is due to loss of optical control of movement and depends on the loss of field, though probably not entirely. These two varieties of visual disturbance are terminal rather than cortical or sub- or trans-cortical.

For bitemporal hemianopsia to be produced by traumatism, it is necessary that the injury should affect solely the crossed fibres of the optic chiasm. Bietti (*Ophthalmic Year-Book*, p. 301, 1914) summarizes eight cases of this condition previously reported in the literature. In a new case which he is able to record, the patient was a man of 21 years, who was injured by a fall and remained comatose for twelve days. There had been profuse hemorrhage from the mouth, and hemorrhage from the ears. The visual acuity when the patient came to the clinic was R. 5/50, L. counting fingers at one meter. The pupils were equal, and both reacted to light and convergence. Each visual field showed a typical temporal hemianopsia, with a sharply vertical line of demarcation, but in the right eye passing five degrees beyond the vertical at the fixation point. The right disk was of normal color, the left pale throughout, with narrowed arteries. The left field rapidly diminished in size and finally disappeared completely, and the right nasal field became somewhat contracted. The vision of the right eye improved from 5/50 to normal, and this fact leads Bietti to believe that the nerve disturbances were mainly due to a hemorrhage which at first compressed the chiasm, and also involved the fibres of the left papillomacular bundle. The disturbance of the crossed fibres of the chiasm, as affecting the left eye, was later followed by progressive atrophy of the direct fibers. The slight secondary contraction of the visual field of the right eye also suggests some degeneration of the direct fibres to this side, but the lesion seems to have been limited for some time to the crossed fibers.

H. M. Traquair (*Edin. Med. Journal*, p. 197, Sept., 1913) has made a practical contribution to the study of *bitemporal hemiopia* in which he finds this sign is much more common than present statistics show. He believes that the frequency with which it is found depends upon the method of examination used, and regards the use of small objects and of Bjerrum's method as essential. . He claims that there are two chief types of bitemporal hemiopia of which the scotomatous type is characterized by early loss of direct vision. Typical cases show regular progression of the defect around the fixation point. This field is associated with active lesions, or lesions active during the presence of the scotoma.

The non-scotomatous type is associated with good vision for a long time.

The field changes occur slowly, affecting the quadrants in the same sequence, the defect diminishing in intensity from periphery to centre.

The *relations of the pituitary body* to *giantism, acromegaly and hemianopsia* will be found under the first named caption. Uhthoff (*Bericht der oph. Gesellsch.*, 1907) gives his experience as follows: "I have met with about 40 cases of temporal hemianopia from disease of the optic commissure; 7 undoubted cases (with 3 autopsies) associated with anomalies of growth, i. e., 18 per cent.; acromegaly in 1 case; giant growth and acromegaly in 1; dwarfishness in 1; general corpulence with moderate giant growth in 2; general corpulence with retarded bodily growth in 1. I am, however, inclined to think that this percentage would have been higher if, when I began my inquiries, I had paid more attention to the question of general trophic disturbances in temporal hemianopia. "

Examination of the literature of the subject shows that general corpulence in consequence of tumors of the hypophysis occurs most frequently in young people. Uhthoff is of opinion that tumor of the hypophysis in the young undoubtedly leads to general disturbances in growth (dwarfishness or giant growth), not infrequently accompanied by general corpulence, but without actual acromegaly.

Uhthoff expresses his opinion that the phenomena of cretinism, cachexia strumipriva, and myxedema associated with pathological conditions of the thyroid gland are not strictly comparable to the phenomena of dwarfishness, general corpulence, etc., resulting from tumor of the pituitary body. In the first named conditions, disturbances of vision with optic atrophy, temporal hemianopia, etc., are rarely if ever seen. In the latter they are constantly present.

A. Levy (*Ophthalmic Review*, p. 304, Oct., 1910), in discussing Best's essay on hemiopia (*Archiv f. Ophthalm.*, Vol. 74), considers the fact that in *many hemianopic fields the line of division is an exact vertical one*, and in others it has a curve avoiding the macula region. This peculiarity appears to prove that the optic fibres travel differently in different parts of their course, and it is assumed that in the beginning of the optic tract the fibres from each half are exactly divided, so that an interruption here will cause a hemianopia with a vertical division. Later the macula fibres are divided so that from here to the cortex an interruption can no longer totally destroy one-half of the field, but the macula is spared.

This question has also a physiological interest, for the disease might bring to light the physiological line of division which separates the course of the fibres of the two halves of the retina, and Hering has used the fact of the semi-decussation of the optic nerve as proof that our optical sensations of space are congenital and that there exists a congenital connection between corresponding points of the two retinæ, while others have held that the correspondence of the two retinæ are based upon individual experiences and practice. If therefore it can be shown that the hemianopia line of division cor-responds to the physiological line of division this would be an addi-tional proof of Hering's theory, and for this purpose only hemianopias with vertical lines can be used, and these are rare.

The conclusions which Best thinks himself justified in drawing from his investigations are as follows: In tract hemianopias the border line runs vertically through the fixation point without avoiding the macula. This border line coincides with the physiological line of separation of the two halves of the retina. In tract hemianopia the hemianopic pupil reaction is obtained, and not in cortical hemianopias. The hemianopic error of measurement is also found in normal eyes in indirect vision. The apparent shortening of the periphery in indirect vision is due to the fact that judgment is based not upon the actual size but upon the relative visual angles. This, however, is compensated for if differences in depth can be appreciated.

Bearing on this point, an unusual case (with post mortem report) of *bilateral hemianopsia with preserved macula* is published by Rönne (*Klin. Mon. f. Aug.*, 53, p. 470, 1914). In a woman, aged 66, bilateral hemianopsia suddenly developed with preserved macula so that a visual field with a radius of 2° remained, V=6/18; fundus normal. The sight half of the visual field was successively restored, leaving a left-sided hemianopsia with a macular preservation of 1° and V=6/6. The autopsy revealed softening of the whole lingual lobe, the lower half of the cuneus, parts of the apex of the occipital lobe and fusiform lobe of the right hemisphere, extending to the splenium of the corpus callosum. In the left hemisphere there was a small pigmented cica-trix in the inferior longitudinal fascicle just in front of the entrance of the visual path into the external geniculate body, 6.5 cm. before the occipital apex. Rönne assumes that the apoplexy in immediate

proximity of the left visual path produced by distant action transient right hemianopsia, which, later, disappeared after absorption
of the hemorrhage. Naturally the peripheral and macular fibres of
the path were influenced, the former so intensely that their function
was temporarily abolished. In the latter, essentially on account of
the pre-existing higher function of the macula, the effect was only a
decrease of vision to about 6/18, which would correspond to destruction of about 7/8 of all the macular fibres.

Rönne (*Klin. Mon. f. Aug.*, Sept., 1911) had before this held that
the so-called macular preservation represents only a part of the

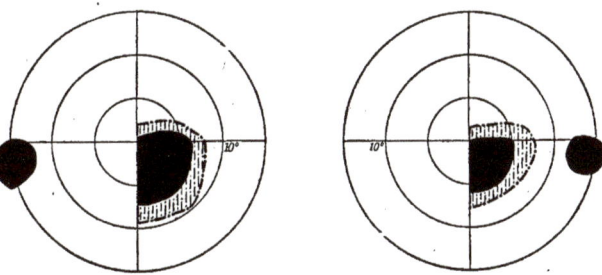

Hemianopic Central Scotoma. (Rönne.)

defective half of the visual field, due to the magnitude of the supposed
macular center in proportion to the corresponding part of the retina
and area of the visual field, whereby the chance is greater that a
part of the macula is spared than of the periphery. The writer
further assumes that the macula only appears to escape more frequently than the periphery, because it is the place where a remaining
function can be longest proved. A similar decrease of vision in the
whole half of the visual field, a hemiamblyopia, must in a certain
number of cases bring the periphery below the threshold of excitation, but leave the macula free.

Twenty cases of hemiopia have been examined by Behr (*Archiv
für Ophthalm.*, April, 1909), with especial reference to *Wernicke's
sign* and that of *Wilbrand's prism-reflex-conjugate-deviation*. A
study of these and of the literature of the subject brings him to the
following conclusions: The hemianopic pupillary inaction is with
proper investigation demonstrable in every case of tract-hemianopia
accompanied by large, absolute field defects. The absence of reflex
eye movements in Wilbrand's prism test is also proof of a tract-
hemianopia. A degeneration of the optic tracts, descending from an
intracerebral focus, leads to a secondary degeneration of the basal

tracts through the primary optic centers and with it to a bilateral atrophic papillary pallor only when the hemianopia is developed in early childhood. The optic atrophy is most pronounced on the same side of the nerve head as the field defect. In these cases the eye with the greatest peripheral field takes over the visual act; the other becomes more and more amblyopic and assumes the position of muscle rest. The remaining visual field contracts to the area surrounding fixation (macular preservation). Failure of this in intracerebral hemianopia is the exception, and there is great likelihood that in pure tract-hemianopia this preservation is the rule. Moreover the question as to the place of division of the macular fibres has not been definitely settled. There is a certain fixed relation between the central visual acuity and the preservation of the maculæ. Normal vision always indicates preservation while an involvement of them is accompanied by a reduction of from one-half to one-third. A pupillary difference with a difference in the width of the palpebral fissure (the name of the hemianopia corresponding to the side with the greatest width) renders probable the diagnosis of a lesion of the tract of the opposite side. Further observations are necessary for confirmation. In a relative intracerebral hemianopia the adaptation on the seeing and on the half which is restricted in its function is equal. The paracentral adaptation in these cases is normal. There is no necessity for the assumption of an isolated color center within the optic perception area. A typical color hemianopia has no diagnostic localization value. The visual memory area lies in one hemisphere in the occipital or temporal lobe. In the vast majority of cases of disturbance of orientation associated with hemianopia the lesion with the greatest likelihood has been located in the left hemisphere. It is a center in the narrowest sense of the term. The quality of a visual field defect (expressed through the smallest observable perimetric object) permits of a fairly accurate conclusion as to the degree of the disturbance of the visual fibres. The nasal retinal half, has a greater pupillomotor excitation than the temporal. The periphery of the retina also has pupillomotor properties. Through a positive result with the prism test of Wilbrand in cerebral hemianopia proof is afforded of the existence of a subcerebral reflex arc for automatic eye movements.

Casey Wood (*Ophthalmic Record*, p. 111, March, 1908) reports *heteronymous hemiopia* in a case of probable tumor of the pituitary body without acromegaly, myxedema or giantism. The patient was a woman, aged 39, in apparent good health. There was no indication of lues or of any other general disease except acute articular rheumatism in childhood. The only ancestral eye anomaly was the fact that her father became blind at 40 years of age and had so remained until his death. The patient does not now complain of any trouble except slight nervousness.

When 18 years of age she had diphtheria, after which there set in the naso-pharyngeal pareses so common in the early history of the

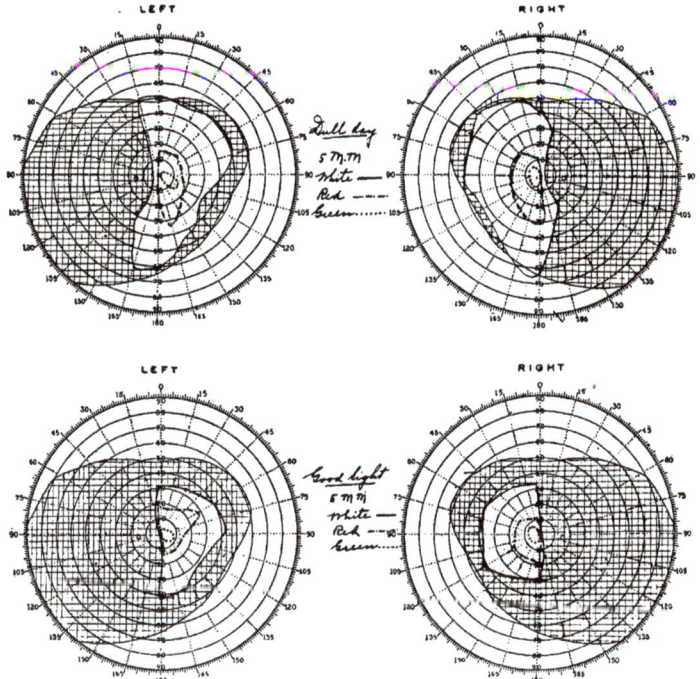

Probable Tumor of the Pituitary Body without Giantism, exhibiting a Binasal Hemiopia. (Casey Wood.)

disease. Her vision for near was very decidedly affected at that time, and she also says that she was deaf, speechless and could not walk for over a month. Since the diphtheria her health has not been robust, although she has had no serious disease.

Her eye troubles set in with dimness of vision, noticed especially when she tried to read. She found that there was a sudden disability in that direction beginning with a sense of strain after reading or sewing for a few minutes—always worse at night. After a while she noticed that she could see better by turning her head to one side, or by reading a few words ahead of the place that she desired to see.

This trouble she thinks has been getting slowly worse in spite of the fact that her hypermetropia (about 1.25 D.) has been corrected with glasses, which she now wears constantly. The eyes themselves are perfectly quiet, there being no visible congestion of the anterior vessels and the patient does not complain of any discomfort apart from a sense of strain and blurring.

Her vision is 20/100 and words of J. 6 in the left eye; 20/200 and words of J. 10 in the right eye, all eccentrically. The pupillary reactions and the tension are practically normal. The fundus, otherwise normal, shows a diffuse gray-white decoloration on both optic nerves. The central vessels showed no abnormality. The fields of vision for white and colors exhibit a well marked heteronymous hemiopia, with decided, rather regular limitation of the periphery. The nose and other neighboring cavities were carefully examined, and with the exception of hypertrophy of the middle turbinal on both sides, were found to be free of disease. A blood count showed hemoglobin about 90 per cent., red blood corpuscles, 4,250,000; white blood corpuscles, 9,600. Urinalysis negative.

A skiagram showed a very evident enlargement of the sella tursica with a faint shadow in the same neighborhood that probably represents an enlarged hypophysis.

Under large and repeated doses of the iodides improvement set in and persisted as long as the patient was under observation. The improvement in her visual fields is easily recognized in the accompanying perimeter charts. A fact worthy of note is that her Jaeger is practically the same as at the first examination, namely, words of J. 6 left eye, and J. 12 in her right eye, eccentrically; on the other hand, her distant vision has improved to 20/50 minus, eccentrically, and has remained about the same (20/200) in the right eye.

A case of macular hemianopsia, described by Wilbrand, is reported by Posey (*Oph. Record,* May, 1908). The visual defect involved the right lower quadrant of the central portion of the field of vision, extending about 10 degrees from the fixation point. It was noted after an attack of dizziness, with confusion of mind and speech. There was difficulty in reading, which subsequently became less without material change in the field. Posey points out that cases of this sort were noted over ten years ago by Mills, who holds that the macular center of one side is more or less representative of the macular fields of both eyes.

F. Krauss (*Ophthalmic Record,* p. 28, Jan., 1910) furnishes an instance of monocular *hemiopia due to ethmo-sphenoidal disease.* In Krauss's case (see the figures) the salient features are that there was a chronic sinusitis for many years, which had latterly caused depression of spirits and intense headache. Removal of the turbinate body of the ethmoid bone, and the opening of most of the ethmoidal cells gave great relief and improvement. Purulent discharge continued freely from the frontal and ethmoidal cells of the left side, while those

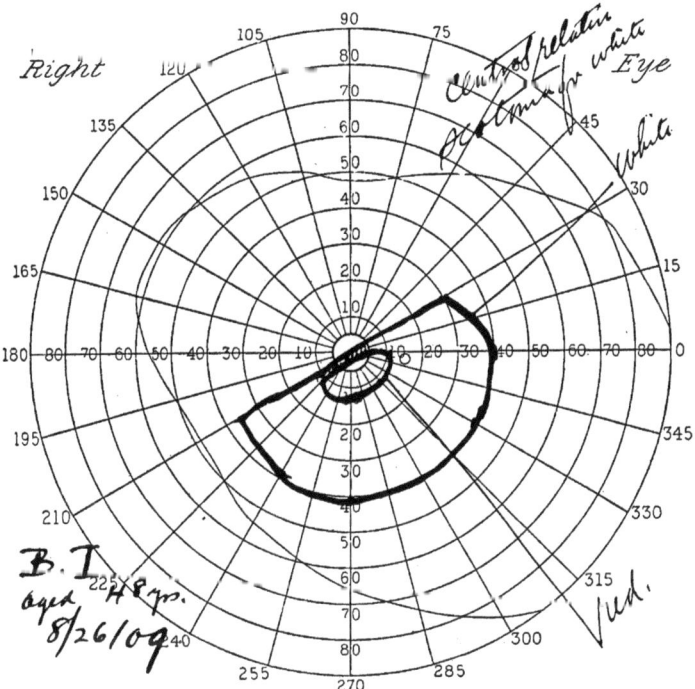

Monocular Hemianopsia, due to Ethmo-sphenoidal Disease.
First chart. Before treatment. (Krauss.)

of the right side secreted to a lesser degree. Four months later the patient became conscious of a relative central scotoma in the right eye and on the apparently least affected side. This was transient. It recurred with greater intensity six weeks later and rapidly extended until the upper half of the field of the right eye was affected. The scotoma was absolute for red and white. The fact that the upper half of the field should be affected, and that at a slight angle, conforms exactly with that portion of the optic nerve nearest to the spheno-ethmoidal region. The accompanying perimeter charts indicate the progress of the case.

An instructive case of *bilateral, homonymous hemianopsia after labor* is reported by Endelmann (*Archiv f. Augenheilk.*, p. 177, 1912). A woman, aged 32, without constitutional affections, suddenly became blind after being delivered of triplets. Gradually some improvement took place, leaving a complete right-sided, and incomplete left-sided,

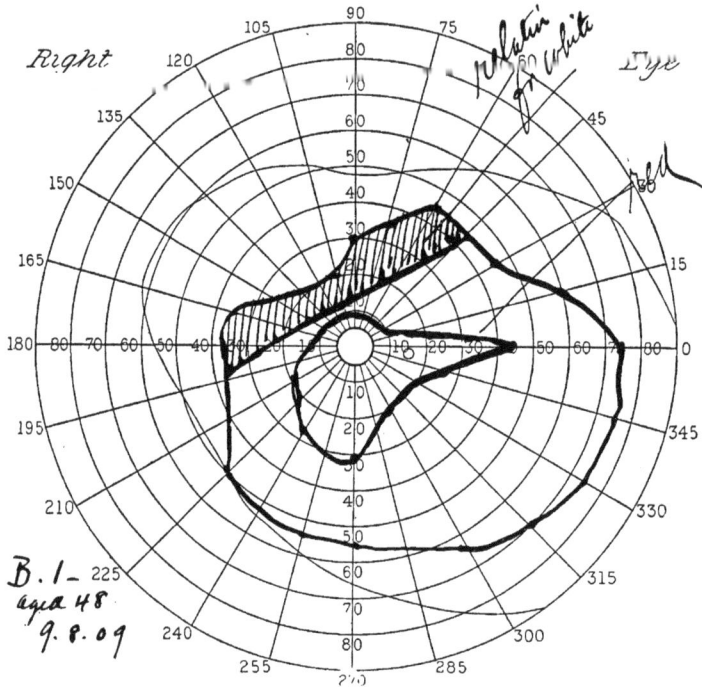

Monocular Hemianopsia, due to Ethmo-sphenoidal Disease. (Krauss.)

homonymous hemianopsia, with wrong projection and faulty concep-tion of the size of objects, amnesic aphasia, alexia and agraphia, and visual hallucinations. The preserved visual field had the shape of small central islets. The ophthalmoscopic condition and pupillary reaction being normal and other symptoms wanting, there were, in the opinion of Endelmann, only two possibilities with regard to the etiology, viz., thrombosis of the cerebral arteries and encephalitis from auto-intoxication during the puerperal state. The marked psychic symptoms seemed to favor the second hypothesis.

The affection was, according to the symptoms, localized in the parieto-occipital lobe and the left angular gyrus, the center for letters.

The alexia alone could be attributed to a lesion of the white sub-cortical substance, but the simultaneous agraphia indicated that also the cortex was affected and that it was a cortical alexia. In similar cases of Bauer, Chevallereau, and Meyer, the labor was of greatest importance for the origin of the disease, but the immediate causes of the cerebral affection varied, viz., nephritis, acute anemia of some

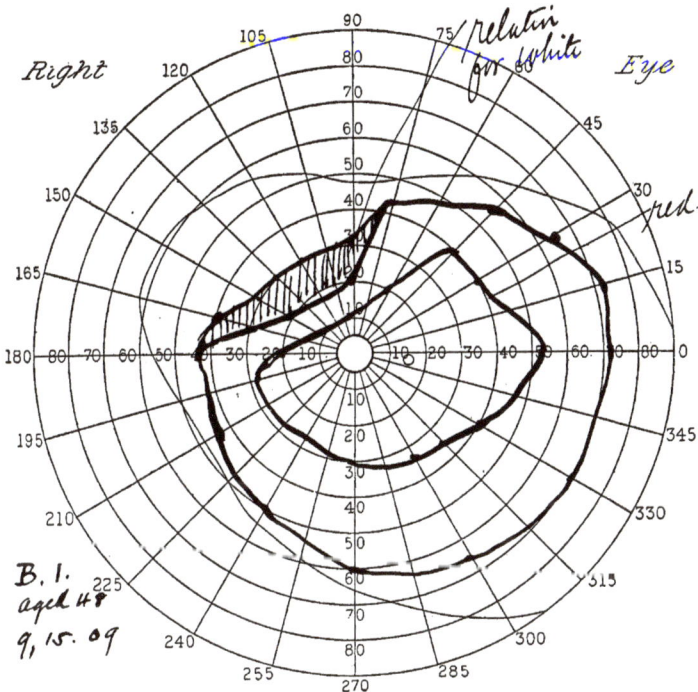

Monocular Hemianopsia, due to Ethmo-sphenoidal Disease. (Krauss.)

portions of the brain after profuse hemorrhages, and the assumption of an embolic process in the brain. The faulty appreciation of the size of objects and the wrong projection were explained by disturb-ance of the constant relation between centripetal excitation and cor-tical perception of motion by the hemianopsia.

A case (male, æt 34) of probable *cerebral syphilis* with *hemianopsia* resulting in partial recovery is reported by W. E. Bruner (*Practical Med. Series,* Eye, p. 162, 1913). There had been no trouble with his eyes until he had difficulty in reading the telephone book. There was no ocular discomfort and no headache. His general health was good.

Vision, O. D.=6/6, O. S.=6/9. Ophthalmoscopic examination: O. D. media clear, disk round, slight physiologic cup, hyperemic with edges hazy, retina striated, high-colored and granular, especially in the macula, entire fundus slightly hazy and irritable looking. O. S., same condition.

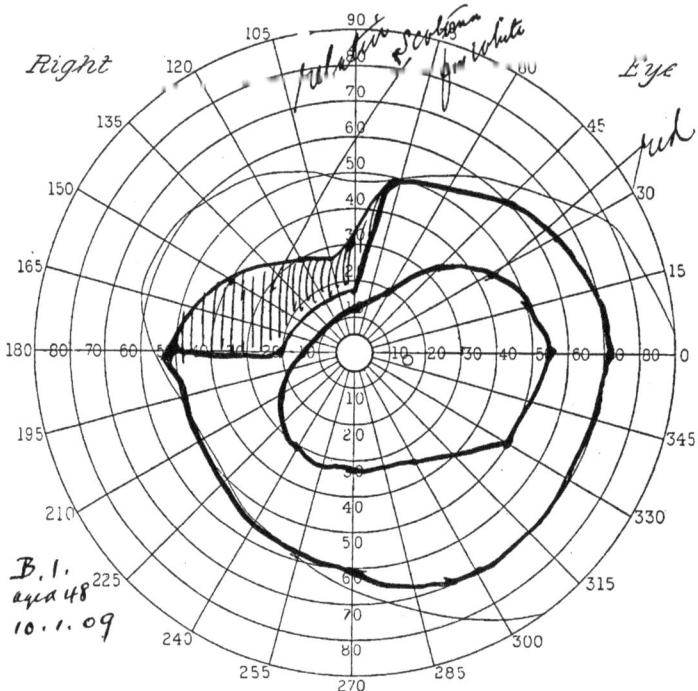

Monocular Hemianopsia, due to Ethmo-sphenoidal Disease.   (Krauss.)

Two months later ophthalmoscopic examination showed the temporal half of the right disk slightly pale, the left more hazy but of good color, and the vessels normal. Examination with the perimeter showed a small scotoma to the nasal side of fixation in the left eye. The right eye is normal with no scotoma. The pupils are equal and respond to light. The knee-jerks are +. He denies venereal history; smokes moderately.

Examination of the fields shows a right-sided homonymous hemianopsia. The patient was put upon iodalbin in increasing doses. Several days later he confessed that he had had syphilis six years previously.

The blur gradually lessened. Vision, O. D. 6/5, O. S. 6/6 +. The blind area became smaller in each eye.

Four months later the eyes were feeling better and stronger; the fundi normal except that the nerves were possibly a little pale in the deeper layers. The fields showed further contraction of the blind

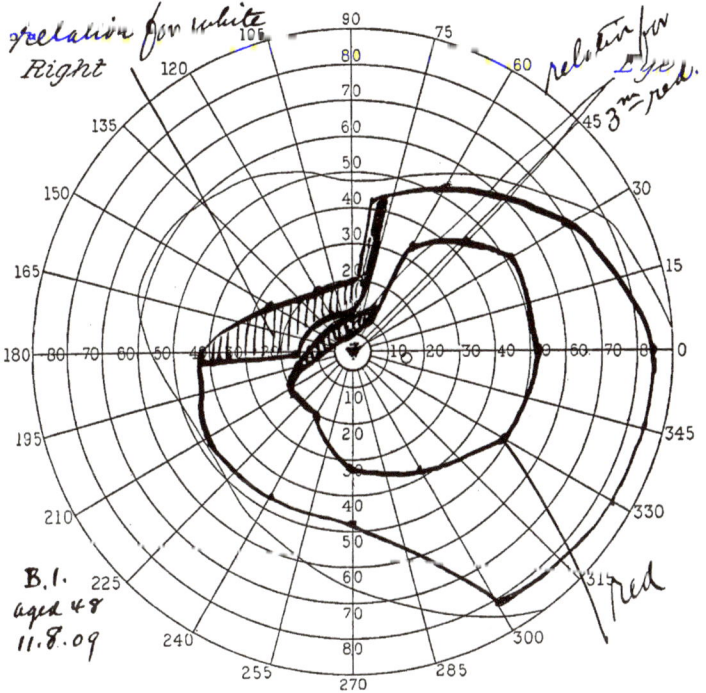

Monocular Hemianopsia, due to Ethmo-sphenoidal Disease. (Krauss.)

area. The fields continued to improve, although the scotomas were about the same, but did not trouble him so much.

For a year he took mercurials most of the time, with occasional intermissions when he was given potassium iodid or iodalbin. Vision, O. D. 6/5, O. S. 6/5. The ophthalmoscope shows the central portion of the nerve pale.

Over four years after the attack of blurring he is feeling very well; the eyes give him no trouble whatever, and he is working hard. He is still taking mercury at intervals. Seven months ago he had a Wassermann test made with negative result, and again within a few

weeks, with the same result. Vision, O. **D.** 6/5, O. S. 6/5, accommodation 0.50 pp., 17 cm. The outer limits of the form field are normal
in each eye and the blind area is practically the same as at the last
visit or as the last chart shows. The pupils are equal and respond
to light. Ophthalmoscopic examination shows the central portion of

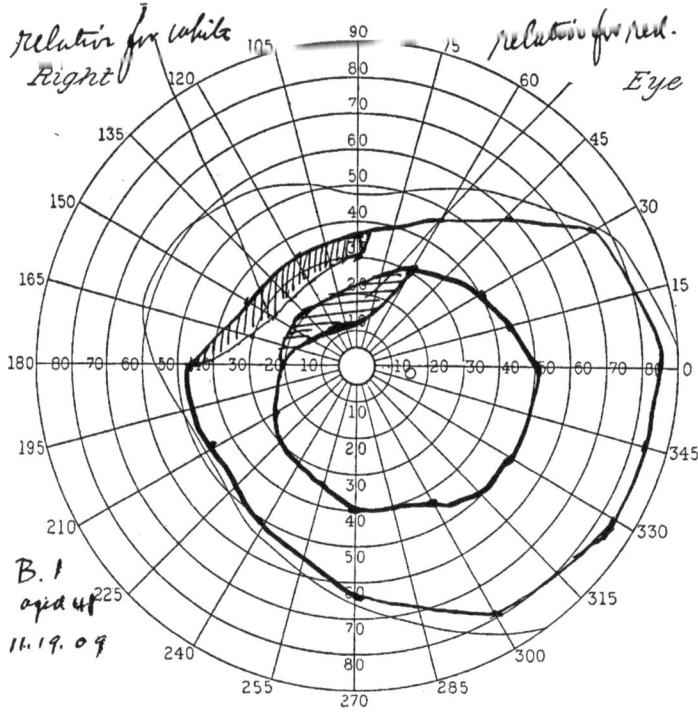

Monocular Hemianopsia, due to Ethmo-sphenoidal Disease. (Krauss.)
Final chart.

the right nerve pale, but not so the left. The vessels are normal in
size and the fundi perfectly normal in other respects. As it is now
several years since the attack of hemianopsia, it is evident that the
present scotomas will in every probability remain permanently. There
have been absolutely no other indications whatever of any cerebral
disease or disturbance of the nervous system.

Permanent hemianopia occurs in migraine but it is very rare. A.
W. Ormond (*Ophthalmic Review*, p. 193, July, 1913) describes two
cases and mentions three others. Similar instances are reported by

Thomas (*Journ. Nervous and Mental Diseases,* 1907) of Boston. Both occurred in women. The histories, illustrated by figures in the text, are in brief as follows:

"The first, Elizabeth W., æt. 33, comes from a large family, two members of which died from tuberculosis and one brother (younger) has had attacks of sick headache all his life; her parents are alive but her mother had a severe left-sided cerebral hemorrhage eighteen months ago. The patient has been for more than ten years subject

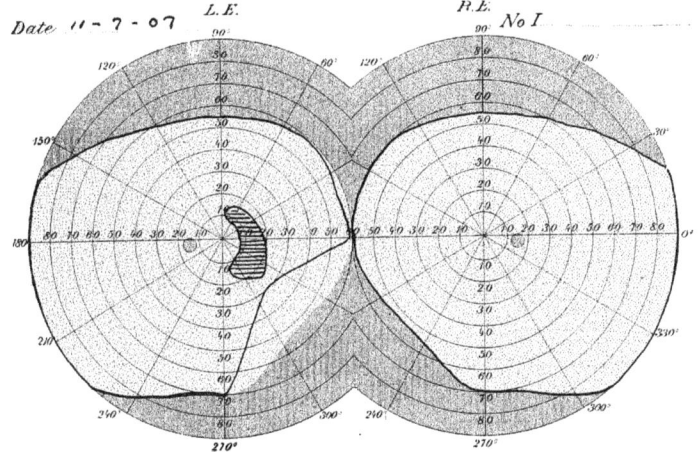

Fields of Vision in Bruner's Case of Luetic Homonymous Hemiopia. Early development of the (unilateral) scotoma. First chart.

to migraine of a severe kind and previous to that had had headaches of less severity. During the more severe attacks her sight had been defective, no evidence obtains that the defect of sight was other than an intolerance of light and neither scotoma nor hemianopia seem to have been noticed. On September 26th, she had an unusually severe attack of migraine lasting three to four days; the photophobia was extreme but when she recovered she noticed that she could not see anything on her right side. The patient's heart, lungs and kidneys are quite healthy and there is no loss of power in arms or legs; her speech has not been interfered with, neither has she any amnesia.

"The fundus was perfectly healthy and her central vision 6/6 with proper correction; the ocular movements were unaffected and the hemiopic pupillary reaction was not obtained. The defect in the right field of vision was not absolute; she was conscious of light when a very strong electric globe was placed on that side. The headaches have not been so severe since she lost her sight, although she has had frequent attacks. The following February her condition was unaltered.

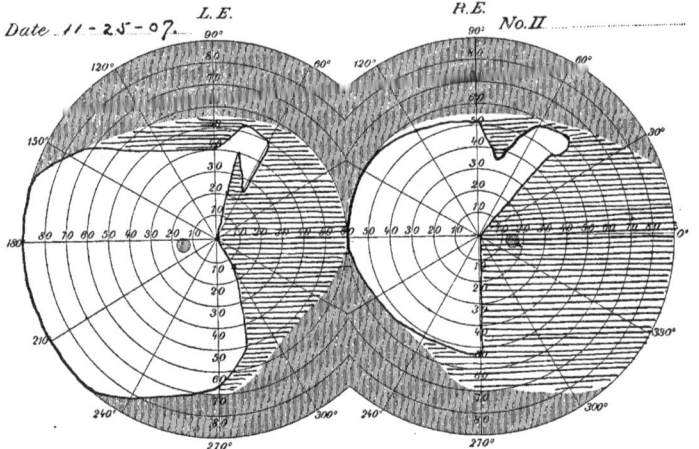

Fields of Vision in Bruner's Case of Luetic Homonymous Hemiopia.
Developed scotomata. Second observation.

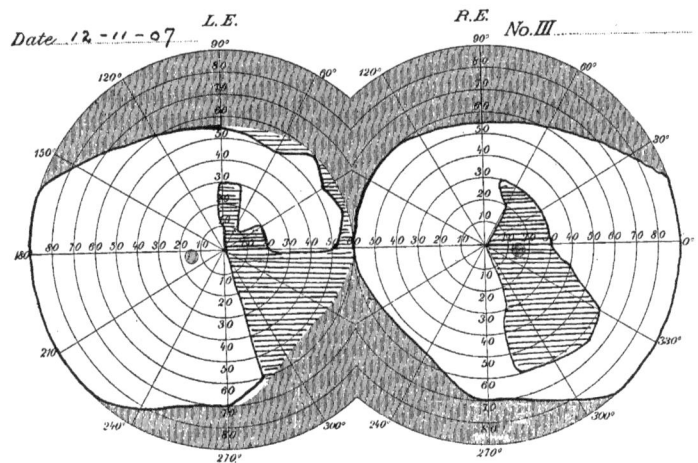

Fields of Vision in Bruner's Case of Luetic Homonymous Hemiopia.
Third observation.

"Second case. Mrs. E., æt. 32, had been subject to bilious headache for many years, which seem to have started when the patient wa.

about 18 years old; her four sisters have also been subject to attacks
of bilious headaches since childhood. The patient was at the time

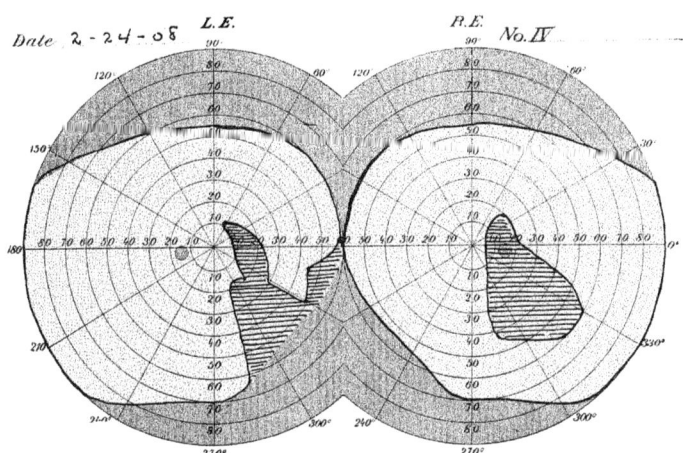

Fields of Vision in Bruner's Case of Luetic Homonymous Hemiopia.
Fourth observation.

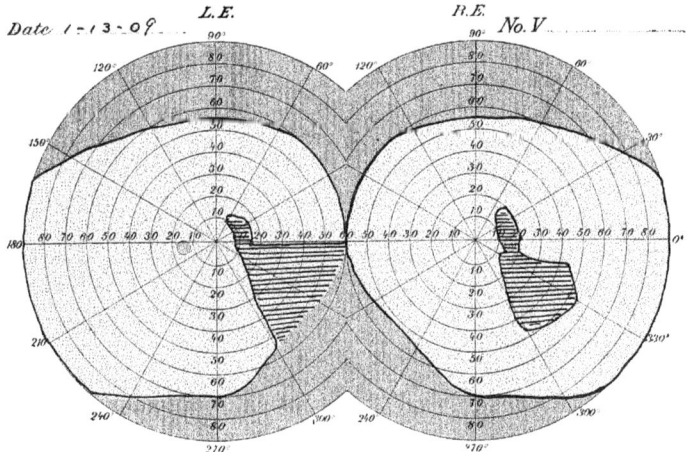

Fields of Vision in Bruner's Case of Luetic Homonymous Hemiopia.
Final observation.

three months pregnant, and seemed to be in usual health; she is a
strong, healthy-looking woman. July 20th, 1912, the patient had a
headache followed by sickness and again on July 27th, and August

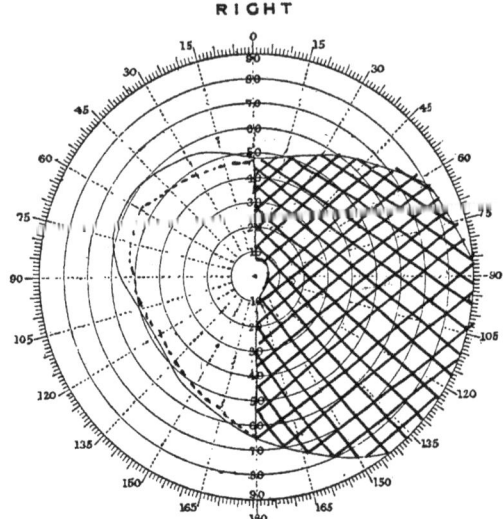

Permanent Hemianopia, after Attacks of Migraine.   (Ormond.)

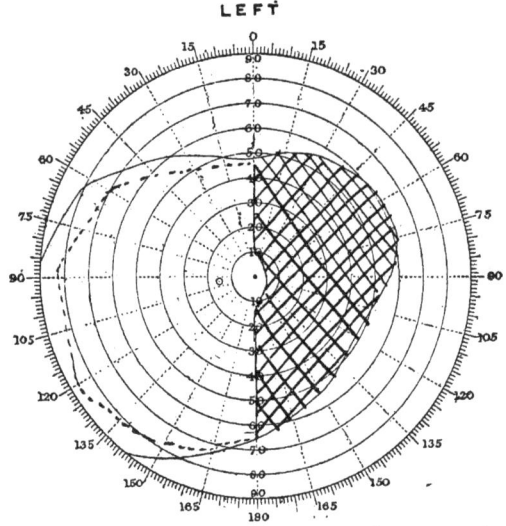

Permanent Hemianopia, after Attacks of Migraine.   (Ormond.)

3rd. On August 4th, 1912, she awoke with the headache still present. She then noticed that she could not see anything on her left side
although she had 6/5 vision in her right eye and 6/6 in the left.
Wassermann reaction was negative; there was no albuminuria and
her physician could find nothing abnormal in her general medical
condition. The hemianopia involved the left side of her field of vision
and was homonymous. The knee-jerks were present and there was

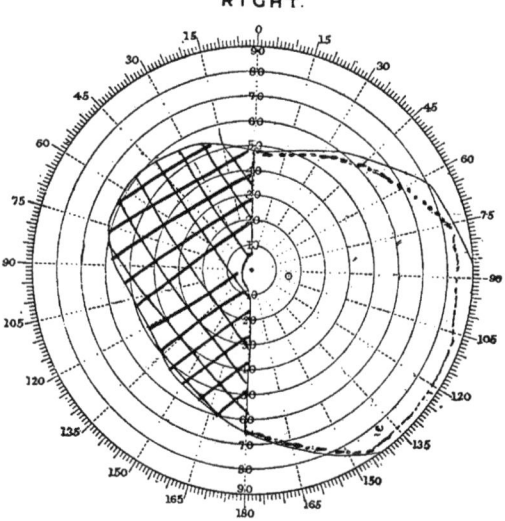

RIGHT.

Permanent Hemianopia, following Attacks of Migraine. (Ormond.)

no loss of sensation; the fundus oculi showed no change and the
hemiopic pupil was doubtful. March 31, 1913, she still could not see
at all on her left side. The perimeter showed that the hemianopia
remained as before.''

Sir William Gowers (*British Med. Journ.*, Dec. 6, 1909) records a
similar case in the following words: ''A woman of 29 had been subject to migraine as long as she could remember, always on the right
side of her head; during the fourth month of her second pregnancy,
an attack of her customary pain was followed by left-sided weakness
with ataxy of the hand, permanent left hemianopia and impairment
of sensibility on the left side. Pregnancy often involves an increased
proneness to blood coagulation; there was no heart disease nor albuminuria.''

These cases suggest that simple migraine may be followed by permanent lesions involving the cortical area. As far as can be ascertained
none of these patients were suffering from any recognizable cardiac
or vascular disease, and all were younger than the age at which such
conditions would be likely to exist.

L. C. Peter (*Ophthalmology,* Vol. IX, No. 3, April, 1913) refers to
the case of *double inferior hemiopia,* reported by Uhthoff, thought to
be caused by symmetrical disease of the optic nerves, as the only

LEFT

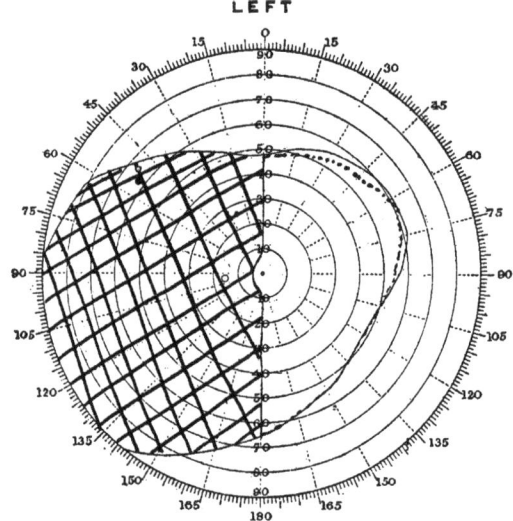

Permanent Hemianopsia, after Attacks of Migraine. (Ormond.)

binocular case of altitudinal hemiopia in literature. Unilateral cases
are reported by Russell (basilar bone tumor), Sailer (rheumatic retrobulbar neuritis), and Krause (ethmoidal disease). The author adds
one unilateral and one bilateral case. The first case was due to local
disease—embolism of the inferior retinal arteries—and the macular
region was not involved.

The second patient, a woman, aged 41, had a paralysis of the left
external rectus muscle in December, 1905, which disappeared under
the use of mercury. In April, 1906, a supposedly leutic affection of
the nose developed. In September, 1907, she found that her vision
was affected in the upper half of the field of each eye. Central vision
was 20/30, without scotomata, but with a defect including most of
the upper half of the field in each eye. In 1908 central scotomata
were present. In 1912 this defect persisted, with general contraction

of the remaining halves of the fields, with pallor of the lower halves of the nerves and slight contraction of the arteries. There was a slight difficulty of speech and occasional mental confusion. Wassermann not taken. History negative. The lesion was thought to be a gumma of the inferior part of the chiasm.

The history of a patient, aged 65, with *bitemporal hemianopsia* and well-marked *acromegaly* is given by S. D. Risley (*Oph. Record,* September, 1912). The symptom-complex pointed to disease in the pituitary region and x-ray study showed an enlargement of the sphenoid, the anterior and posterior clinoid processes bending toward each other, forming an incomplete foramen, but left the presence of any enlargement of the soft parts, or the presence of a tumor, in doubt. The patient regarded herself in good health, had no pain, but suffered an uncontrollable drowsiness. She was first seen in October, 1910. In December, 1911, and February, 1912, there was no notable change in her condition. In March, 1912, she died of an intercurrent lobar pneumonia. An autopsy showed at the base of the brain a large tumor 5 cm. in length and 5 cm. in width and 9 cm. thick, oval in shape, resting on the frontal lobes, anterior to the optic chiasm and compressing both optic nerves, making a distinct concavity in the mesial aspect of the frontal lobes. Lying in front of the chiasm, it was slightly separated from it. On the lower surface of the tumor, near its middle, was a smooth, cup-shaped depression 2x2½ cm. in depth caused by the projecting posterior ethmoidal cells. The tumor was well encapsulated, finely nodular on the surface and the capsule very vascular. In the anterior fossa in front of the sella turcica the floor of the skull was raised in an irregular manner, in an area the size of a small walnut. The bone here was thin, porous, dark in color and when chiseled away the posterior ethmoid cells were found to contain a large amount of thick, yellow, purulent material. The tumor seemed to have entirely replaced the pituitary body. The brain otherwise showed nothing abnormal. The tumor proved to be, on examination, a highly vascular spindle-celled sarcoma. In the sections made no trace of the pituitary body was found.

F. R. Cross (*Trans. Ophth. Society U.K.,* Vol. XXXIV, 1914, p. 200) gives details of eighteen cases of *homonymous hemianopsia,* complete or partial. Two of the cases were of traumatic origin. Many of the others seem to bear out the points elsewhere (Bradshaw Lecture, Royal College of Surgeons of England, 1909) suggested by the author that hemianopsia may occur without of necessity being an early symptom of brain mischief; that a number of the patients may retain their ability of doing useful work; that they may remain free from other evidence of disease for many years; and that the common cause in localized cases is likely to be embolism of a twig of the calcarine artery.

In *quadrant hemianopsia*—where one-fourth (or thereabouts) of the field of vision is obscured or blinded—the cause is often injury and not infrequently military traumatisms.

Monbrun (*Ophthalmic Year-Book*, p. 300, 1914) adopts the view that the upper segment of the optic tract and of the external geniculate body corresponds to the upper quadrants of the retina, and the lower segment to the lower quadrants of the retina. He also regards the optic radiations as being differentiated into an upper bundle corresponding to the upper quadrants of the retina, and a lower corresponding to the lower quadrants of the retina, and considers that the upper quadrant of the retina is projected on to the upper lip of the calcarine fissure and the lower part of the cuneus, while the lower part of the retina is projected on to the lower lip of the calcarine fissure and the upper part of the lingual lobe. Crisp's (*Oph. Record*, Vol. 23, p. 426, 1914) case of *apoplectic quadrant anopsia* occurred in a woman of 42 years, of robust health and negative history, who came complaining of a cloud over the upper nasal corner of the right visual field. The disturbance came on with severe headache and a sense of dizziness. The right field in the quadrant complained of was contracted about half way to the center. The left field was normal. Four months later the outline of the field was the same. In a case of *apoplexy with anopsia* of both right lower quadrants, studied by Winkler (*Arch. d'Opht.*, Vol. 34, p. 191, 1914), he found complete destruction of the dorso-lateral part of the sagittal strata of the left hemisphere.

Hemiopsia. A synonym of hemiopia.

Hemiopy. Hemiopia.

Hemioscope of Prato. This is one of the numerous modifications of the Fles box (q. v.) or pseudoscope. See Vol. II, p. 1185 of this *Encyclopedia*.

Hemiplegia. (L.) Motor paralysis of one lateral half of the body. It is usually limited to the muscles of the arm, leg, and face. Some of the muscles may not be affected at all, or may be only temporarily weakened.

As Swanzy (*System of Diseases of the Eye*, Vol. IV, p. 586) maintains, *the orbicular sign* is one which may be noticed in some attacks of apoplexy with hemiplegia, after consciousness has returned. It consists in this, that the hemiplegic person, who during health has been able to close each eye separately, and who even now can close both eyes together, or the eye on the sound side alone, is unable to close the eye on the paralyzed side by itself. This sign usually passes away after a short time. Sometimes with this sign it may be noticed that, when both eyes are closed, the eyelids on the paralyzed side are brought together with some effort, and that the other muscles of the upper part of the face supplied by the seventh nerve are somewhat wanting in power.

If the lesion implicate the pyramidal fibres in the crusta, along with the roots of the third nerve, then the well-known symptom of crossed hemiplegia is produced,—more or less complete loss of power in the third nerve on the side of the lesion, with hemiplegia and paralysis of the lower part of the face of the opposite side of the body. The paralysis of the cranial nerve is usually complete, but it is possible even for one muscle alone to be paralyzed. Leube, for example, has published (*Deutsch Archiv für klinische Medicin*, XL., 2, S. 317) a case of disease of the peduncle in which the levator palpebræ alone had lost power, ptosis with hemiplegia of the opposite side of the body being the only localizing symptoms; and a similar case has been recorded by Rickards (*British Medical Journal*, I, p. 774, 1886).

Hughlings Jackson has pointed out that the localizing value of crossed hemiplegia depends chiefly on the hemiplegia and the paralysis of the cranial nerve coming on simultaneously. If they occur at different times, they may be due to two distinct lesions, neither of which may be in the crus; for the hemiplegia may be due to a lesion in the hemisphere, and the third-nerve paralysis to a basal lesion of earlier or later date. But cases have been observed in which, with a lesion in the crus, the third-nerve paralysis preceded the hemiplegia by a considerable interval.

When the lesion causing this crossed paralysis is a tumor, hemianopsia from pressure on the optic tract underlying the peduncle is liable to be an associated symptom.

In about 40 per cent. of the cases of *cerebral hemiplegia* there are, according to Klippel and Weil (*Wien. Klin. Wochenschr.*, Jan. 10, 1913), differences in the size of the pupils. In hemiplegia this difference begins when coma sets in. In comatose hemiplegia the wider pupil is on the side of the cerebral lesion, that is, on the opposite side to the paralyzed side. In cases of hemiplegia without coma, the dilated pupil is on the paralyzed side, and on the opposite side of the cerebral lesion. There are, however, exceptions to this rule.

It has been proven experimentally that strong irritation of any part of the cortex of the brain produces a dilatation of the pupil, while a weak irritation may produce contraction or dilatation.

Generally speaking, in all cases of coma, in sleep, in narcosis and in various forms of intoxication there is contraction of the pupils. In hemiplegia with coma, the pupillary difference is brought about by the contraction of one pupil. In cases of hemiplegia without coma the difference of the pupils is brought about by the dilatation of one pupil. In the first case contraction is produced by inhibition on the part of the affected hemisphere of the brain; in the second case, the pupillary difference is produced by an excitation of the affected hemisphere. A pupillary difference in coma indicates organic hemiplegia, and excludes hysteria.

Contraction or dilatation of the pupil on the paralyzed side is important from a prognostic standpoint, as it indicates whether the affected hemisphere has the ability to react upon irritation or not.

Hemiplegia alternans. (L.) Crossed hemiplegia.

Hemiprosoplegia. (L.) Paralysis of one side of the face.

Hemiscotosis. Blindness of one-half of the retina.

Hemisine. One of the numerous (proprietary) suprarenal preparations, found to be more irritating and less satisfactory than adrenalin or suprarenalin.

Hemisphere. The half-globe, often spoken of in reference to the half-segment of the eyeball; thus, the nasal hemisphere, or the temporal hemisphere.

Hemispherical illuminator. A name given by Wenham to a hemispherical lens attached to the under side of a (microscopical) slide for projecting rays of great obliquity upon the object.

Hemispheroid. Half of a nearly spherical figure.

Hemispherule. Half of a minute sphere.

Hemistomum spathaceum. In making a study of exophthalmia in the roach Jugeat (*Hyg. de la Viande,* Vol. VIII, p. 229, 1914) found a number of these fish that had lost one or both eyes, the exophthalmia having been apparently recent. Other specimens presented a more or less accentuated lesion of the crystalline lens which in some had retained some of its transparency, while in others the opacity was complete. A microscopic examination of the lens revealed a peculiar, active, mobile parasite, which was recognized as *Diplostomum volvens,* (Mordmann), larva of the *Hemistomum spathaceum,* a trematode frequent in aquatic birds. The author points out a possible danger in eating this variety of fish.

Hemitropic. HEMITROPOUS. Half turned round.

Hemlock. *Conium maculatum.* The juice of the stem of this plant, in the form of a collyrium, was anciently esteemed, according to Archigenes, Dioscorides and Pliny, as a remedy for "summer epiphora,'' and, in fact, for any affection of the eyes accompanied by pain. Archigenes especially recommends hemlock juice for profuse discharges from the eyes, because of its very decided astringency.— (T. H. S.)

Hemmung. (G.) Inhibition.

Hemochromometer. HEMOMETER. COLORIMETER. HEMOGLOBINOMETER. An instrument for estimating the amount of hemoglobin in the blood, by comparing a solution of the latter with a standard solution of picrocarminate of ammonia. See Vol. IV, p. 2395 of this *Encyclo- pedia.*

Hemoglobinometer. See **Hemochromometer.**

Hemolysin. A substance, generally of bacterial origin and produced in the body, capable of destroying red corpuscles. It is formed in the body of an animal into which red corpuscles of another animal have been introduced, capable of dissolving the red corpuscles of the animal from which the blood was derived. The hemolysin which destroys cells of the animal's own body is called an *autolysin;* that formed by the injection of blood from the same species is an *isolysin;* that from another species, a *heterolysin.* See **Bacteriology of the eye;** subsection, at the end, *Immunity.*

For example, Epalza (*Klin. Mon. f. Aug.,* 54, p. 90, 1914) agrees with Neisser and Wechsberg that hemolytic action is the characteristic difference between pathogenic and non-pathogenic staphylocci. He studied this methodically on the eye by growing staphylococcus albus in clear cultures from normal conjunctivæ. Out of 17 strains 9 showed immediately after being taken from the conjunctiva an hemo- lysis on the blood agar plates. All 8 cultures, which showed no hemolysis on the plate, were inoculated into the vitreous of rabbits. After a few days the experiments on the blood agar plate was re- peated with clear cultures of the strains taken from the vitreous with the result that two strains showed now hemolysis. Hence it is beyond doubt, that saprophytic staphylococci are biologically changed by inoculation into the eye, especially the vitreous body, and may acquire new properties.

Hemometer. HEMADYNAMOMETER. The names generally given to Fleischl's instrument for measuring the amount of hemoglobin in the blood. It consists essentially of a wedge of ruby glass through which a beam of lamp-light is made to pass. The tint of the latter is compared with that of a suitably diluted specimen of blood, and from the thickness of the wedge required to produce an equality in the shade of the tints compared, the amount of hemoglobin is deduced. See **Colorimeter.**

Hemophilia. HEMORRHAGIC DIATHESIS. These names are applied to a constitutional peculiarity which manifests itself in a tendency to excessive bleeding when any blood-vessel is injured. In those who suffer from it (bleeders) a slight bruise may cause extensive extravasation of blood; a small cut, an enucleation of the eye or the extraction of a tooth may lead to dangerous or even fatal hemorrhages. The condition is strongly hereditary; and though it seldom affects women is often transmitted in the female line.

Scurvy, hemophilia and purpura constitute a category of diseases of obscure etiology that are grouped under the general name of the hemorrhagic diathesis. The three disorders are more or less related to one another; hemophilia in most cases being attributable to an hereditary transmission of a tendency to bleed and being a permanent condition, whereas scurvy and purpura are always acquired; the former appearing endemically, the latter sporadically; the former usually as the result of malnutrition, the latter rarely dependent upon definite external conditions. Even in scurvy and purpura, however, one is almost forced to the conclusion that a congenital predisposition to hemorrhages exists.

For the ophthalmic surgeon this disease is important. "Bleeders" are troublesome patients; and any means that can be adopted to allay the tendency to hemorrhages must be welcomed. A member of a bleeder family should for some time preceding any contemplated operative inroad, however slight, be placed on a diet as described under scurvy. Alcoholic beverages, tea, coffee, condiments and spices should be reduced.

Here again lemons are the most popular remedy and there is no question in regard to the power in some cases of citrates of potassium and sodium to reduce the hemorrhagic tendency. Mineral acids, sulphuric acid in particular, deserve a trial; dilute sulphuric acid may be given in doses of ten to fifteen drops in water several times a day, or sulphate of magnesium or sodium may be administered instead. Ergot, hydrastis, opiates are all advised but are of indifferent value.

As a preliminary to an operation, or during an operation, if intractable hemorrhages should develop, subcutaneous injections of gelatine or coagulose may be tried. The greatest care should of course be exercised that the gelatine solution is altogether sterile, on account of the danger of a tetanus infection. From 5 to 200 c.cm. of a 2 to 3 per cent. solution of gelatine in normal salt solution, heated to the body temperature, may with impunity be injected under the skin. This occasionally stops the bleeding. Calcium chloride that has been recommended on the supposition that the coagulability of the blood, owing to a calcium deficit, is reduced, is of no value. Surface hemorrhages should be treated with adrenalin chloride and other local styptics according to ordinary surgical principles.—(A. C. C.)

As one of numerous examples of hemophilia in its ophthalmic relations Berger (*Woch. f. Ther. u. Hyg. des Auges,* Nov. 28, 1912) reports a case in which some hours after a simple tenotomy in a five-year-old boy, examination revealed an enormous hematoma of the conjunctiva and orbit (external hemophthalmos). In spite of the continuous use of ice compresses, bleeding continued for three days, resulting in a profound secondary anemia, with thready pulse and subnormal temperature. On the fourth day the bleeding ceased.

Hemophthalmia. (Obs.) An effusion of blood into the interior of the eye, either into the anterior chamber, vitreous, or between the coats of the eyeball; also a hemorrhage beneath the conjunctiva.

Hemopia. (L.) Hemiopia.

Hemorrhage, Amblyopia and amaurosis from. This matter has already been discussed on page 292, Vol. I of this *Encyclopedia.* It may, however, be further said here that a number of recent cases have been reported but it is a question whether they have thrown additional light on this important and in some respects obscure subject. Among these are clinical reports and papers by C. B. Welton (*Illinois Med. Journ.,* p. 572, Nov., 1912); F. P. Calhoun (*Ophthalmic Record,* July, 1913); James Moores Ball (*Interstate Med. Journ.,* p. 531, June, 1913); Géhard (abstract in the *Ophthalmic Year-Book,* p. 302, 1914); and G. H. Grant (*Archives of Ophthalm.,* p. 234, May, 1914), to which the reader is referred.

Hemorrhage into the orbit. In the vast majority of cases hemorrhage into the orbital cellular tissue is caused by traumatism, either direct or indirect. Instruments or foreign bodies thrust into the orbit must necessarily cause bleeding. Blows upon the eyeballs or head, or fracture of the skull involving the orbital bones, may permit of an outpouring of blood into the cellular tissue. The condition rarely occurs spontaneously, and may then be due to hemophilia, scurvy, deterioration of the blood-vessels, or to too great a rise of blood-pressure incident to coughing, sneezing, straining, etc. Once liberated within the orbit, the course of the blood is determined by the layers and processes of the orbital fascia. It extravasates in the direction of least resistance, which is generally forward, and in a short time comes to view under the conjunctiva of the eyeball or eyelids.

According to the amount of hemorrhage, the symptoms will vary from those scarcely noticeable to marked proptosis, limited ocular movements, great subconjunctival accumulation of blood, and pressure injury to muscles and nerves, including the optic nerve, with perhaps loss of vision.

The diagnostic value of subconjunctival hemorrhage after injury, in determining fracture at the base of the skull implicating the orbital bones, has depreciated somewhat since the demonstration a number of times by autopsy of traumatic orbital hemorrhage without fracture. Evidence of orbital hemorrhage is, notwithstanding, a valuable sign and serious symptom after head-injury, and makes basal fracture at least probable. Sometimes the blood escapes into the nose, indicating fracture of the ethmoid bone.

A few cases of spontaneous subperiosteal orbital hemorrhage in infants suffering from malnutrition have been reported by Spicer, and a so-called traumatic subperiosteal blood-cyst has been observed by Baquis, which disappeared within four days. Denig reports a case of subperiosteal blood-cyst situated behind the lachrymal gland, extending toward the orbital roof, where it had caused perforation into the anterior cerebral fossa. The patient had received a severe orbital injury ten years before.

Insomuch as the optic nerve is always jeopardized by orbital hemorrhage if extensive enough to cause considerable pressure, the prognosis should be guarded quoad visus in the presence of pressure symptoms.

Absorption takes place in from three to six weeks and may be aided by hot fomentations. A pressure bandage may be indicated in certain cases, and, when the proptosis is so extensive as to prevent closure of the lids, the cornea must be carefully guarded. The use of the bistoury for the purpose of liberating the blood may be advisable when the bleeding has been excessive, but in ordinary cases it seems to be of doubtful efficacy, as extravasations are not often relieved by incisions.—(J. M. B.)

As a means of controlling hemorrhage deep in the orbit, due to an aneurysmal varix, Gifford (*Oph. Rec.*, Vol. 23, p. 94, 1914), uses a sterilized cylinder of wood ¾ of an inch in diameter and about 3 inches long. After applying a swab of iodoform gauze dipped in Monsel's solution to the apex of the orbit, he presses down firmly with the wooden cylinder, packs gauze tightly around it, and then applies a firm bandage, over which is placed a second bandage of elastic flannel. This device stopped the hemorrhage in his case after tying the bleeding vessels and compressing both common carotid arteries had been tried without success.

Hemorrhage, Intracranial. CEREBRAL APOPLEXY. See **Neurology of the eye**; as well as **Hemiplegia**.

Hemorrhages, Ocular. Apart from bleedings that occur into various tissues of the visual apparatus as the result of operations and other forms of traumatism ocular hemorrhages are generally divided into *(a)* epibulbar or subconjunctival hemorrhage; *(b)* anterior chamber bleedings; *(c)* hemorrhages into the uveal tract; *(d)* vitreous bleedings; *(e)* preretinal or subhyaloid hemorrhages; *(f)* retinal hemorrhages; *(g)* bleedings into the optic nerve sheath; *(h)* orbital hemorrhages. Many of these are treated under such captions as **Choroidal hemorrhage; Conjunctiva, Hemorrhage into the;** while still others it is proposed to consider in this section.

Subconjunctival or epibulbar hemorrhage. This form of bleeding assumes two aspects, generally trivial but sometimes of serious import. They usually follow coughing, sneezing, straining at stool, etc. As de Schweinitz (*Ther. Gazette, Apr.* 15, 1914) says, startling in appearance but practically always harmless are the extensive *subconjunctival hemorrhages* which occur during paroxysms of whooping-cough in children. Often bilateral, they may occupy the entire epibulbar surface and even force their way into the lids. Absorption is usually prompt, and visual disturbance in the absence of intraocular changes most unusual, if it ever occurs.

Subconjunctival and often recurring hemorrhages or ecchymoses, which occur in elderly persons in association with general vascular disease, appear also in comparatively young persons—that is to say, in persons between forty and fifty years of age, whose blood-pressure is pathological, and who may or may not have an associated nephritis. Sometimes they replace the retinal lesions of chronic nephritis; often they precede them. Usually they occur during sleep, and are more frequent in the left than in the right eye. They may occur at comparatively short intervals; sometimes the periods between the extravasations comprise weeks or months. An interesting association is recurring subcutaneous ecchymoses of the lids. Very small bluish or purplish spots, looking like small bruised areas, appear, and like their congeners in the conjunctiva they come and disappear quickly, and they have exactly the same significance. Occasionally subconjunctival hemorrhages and subcutaneous lid ecchymoses alternate.

In the presence of any of these hemorrhages, thorough cardio-vascular and renal examination is strongly indicated, and will often be rewarded by finding abnormal blood-pressure or renal disease, even in persons who are apparently in perfect health; serious renal disorder is sometimes latent, and even in an advanced grade may be compatible with mental and bodily vigor.

Hyphemia or anterior chamber hemorrhages are generally recurrent in type and may be a symptom of, or at least occur in association with, purpura, certain toxemias, and diabetes. In the last-named instance not infrequently an iritis complicates the state of affairs. Like the sub-conjunctival hemorrhages, these rarer manifestations in the anterior chamber are recurring, coming and disappearing quickly. A patient with iritis which is associated with recurrent hemorrhage into the anterior chamber should be carefully examined for the presence of sugar in the urine. Less frequently hyphemia is a symptom of general arteriosclerosis.

Intrauveal tract hemorrhages and their associated vitreous changes. Hemorrhage into the vitreous chamber is seen in anemia, nephritis and diabetes, arteriosclerosis, and as the result of the absorption of certain toxins, the source of the blood being either the vessels of the choroid, ciliary body, or retina. If the ciliary body is the source, the hemorrhage bursts through the hyaloid into the vitreous and is there readily detected, either in its fresh state, or at a later period in the form of various types of vitreous opacity.

An interesting and important group of cases are those which relate to young persons, generally male adults, who are the subjects of spontaneous hemorrhage into the vitreous, often associated with hemorrhage in the retina. These patients generally are constipated, their circulation is irregular, and they suffer from epistaxis. The gouty diathesis was supposed by Hutchinson to be the cause of this distressing condition of affairs, which sometimes, and, indeed, not infrequently, leads to permanent blindness. Recent investigations indicate that of importance as an etiological factor in these circumstances is tuberculosis, and that the active agent is a tuberculous toxin.

De Schweinitz further finds that some of the best therapeutic results have followed the persistent use of tuberculin injections, especially if these are proliferating retinal lesions. It must be remembered also that anomalies in the coagulability of the blood may account for many of these lesions, and in these circumstances the administration of calcium salts is worth a trial, and intravenous injections of human blood serum have been used.

Naturally all of these hemorrhages may be caused by syphilis, and therefore in circumstances like these the patient should be subjected to all modern tests—Wassermann, etc. Even in the absence of syphilis iodides are of service, as also is mercury. So-called auto-intoxication must be corrected, and diaphoresis is of service.

For *choroidal* hemorrhage see Vol. III, p. 2130, of this *Encyclopedia*.

Intraocular hemorrhages of retinal origin and position. These constitute an important, indeed, the most important, group of ocular hemorrhages. Their causes, based on the classification of Dimmer, may be grouped thus:

(a) Hemorrhages caused by changes in the composition of the blood and the tissues of the blood-vessel walls; pyemia, septicemia, ulcerative endocarditis; diseases of the liver, spleen, kidney; atheroma of the vessels, and angiosclerosis of the retinal vessels; loss of blood (menorrhagia, hematemesis, especially if there is carcinoma of the stomach, the so-called cachectic hemorrhagic retinitis); anemia (simple and pernicious); hemophilia, purpura, and scurvy; diabetes and gout; tuberculosis; malaria and recurrent fever. Naturally, in certain types of syphilitic disease of the retina hemorrhages are an associated condition, particularly in the so-called syphilitic retinitis with hemorrhage, but hemorrhages in syphilitic retinitis are of comparatively rare occurrence.

(b) Hemorrhages caused by disturbances of the circulation; hypertrophy of the heart and stenosis of the valves; thrombosis of the central vein of the retina and embolism of the central artery; suffocation, compression of the carotid; and hemorrhages in the newly-born, a not infrequent complication, and from menstrual disturbances.

(c) Hemorrhages caused by sudden alteration of intra-ocular tension, for example after iridectomy, which do not come now into discussion. Interesting are those hemorrhages which occur after large cutaneous burns, and those which follow compression of the thorax and of the neck and blows upon the head.

(d) Hemorrhages caused by certain toxic agents—for example, phosphorus, chlorate of potassium, serpent virus, and the reabsorption of toxins, of bacterial origin, from the intestinal tract.

These hemorrhages may be in any layer of the retina, may remain in their original position, or burst through the limiting membrane and fill the vitreous. By preference they are found along the course of the vessels. The macula is a favorite seat. An unusual type of hemorrhage is the so-called *preretinal extravasation,* which lies between the internal limiting membrane of the retina and the hyaloid membrane of the vitreous, and which is not a little prone to make its way into the vitreous.

Corneal hemorrhage. Apart from blood-stain of the cornea (see page 1228, Vol. II of this *Encyclopedia*) this condition is obviously rare, even as a result of injury. DeBeck pictures a hemorrhage into the substantia propria, reproduced in the text. Occasionally blebs form on the corneal surface and into these extravasations of blood may occur.

Relapsing juvenile or adolescent *hemorrhages into the vitreous* call for more than passing comment. In addition to tuberculosis of the choroid and ciliary body as a cause Noll (*Zeitschr. f. Augenheik.*, p. 548, 1908) attributed the condition to three causes: anomalies of the blood, e. g., in pernicious anemia, leukemia, oxaluria; disturbances of circulation, frequent at the age of puberty; local vascular diseases, perivasculitis, from general affections, as pernicious anemia, lues, leukemia, malaria, sepsis, intoxications, amyloid, glycogenous, hyaline or sclerotic degenerations, and hemophilia.

Gehrung (*Practical Med. Series,* Ophthalmic volume, p. 117, 1910) believes that hemorrhage into the vitreous body during adolescence

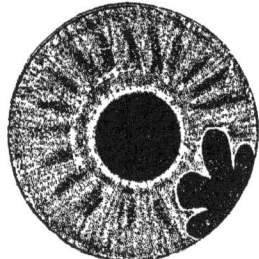 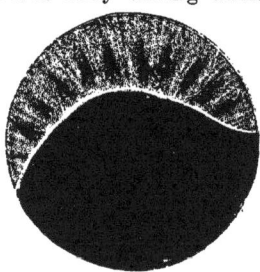

Hemorrhage into the Cornea. (DeBeck.)

is quite frequent, and owing to the danger of recurrence, and tissue changes in the eye, is a dangerous condition, worthy not only of patient, careful, and exhaustive treatment after the occurrence, but also of prophylactic measures. He also thinks that in this connection the too rapid development of children should cause solicitude. Rapid changes of temperature and prolonged exposures to heat or cold are etiological factors. Menstrual disturbances, undue sexual excitement and abuse, cardiac disease, dyscrasia, malnutrition, errors of refraction, all causes of eye-strain, hereditary diseases and tendencies, vascular diseases, anemias, abnormal (premature?) development, or malformations, all mental and physical causes of sudden and rapid fluctuations of the blood-stream and tension are causative factors in this form of intra-ocular hemorrhage. Bleeding may be from the retinal vessels or from the vessels in the region of the ciliary body, not from the sheath, etc., of the optic nerve. Glaucoma is rather the result than a causative factor of these hemorrhages. The treatment should be medicinal if possible, the knife to be used only as a dernier resort. Attacks in women usually follow menstrual disturbances. When there is epistaxis which suddenly ceases we have a danger signal of hemorrhage. Males are more liable to intra-ocular hemorrhage than women, normal menstruation being apparently a safeguard. The age from puberty to manhood, is a danger period. Anemic conditions predispose to attacks.

E. A. Davis (*Trans. Amer. Ophth. Society,* Vol. XIII, Part 1, 1912) reports a case in which beyond the fact that he had lost flesh during the previous four months and that he did not look well, a thorough examination of the patient, a young man of 22 years, revealed no abnormality. Wassermann was negative. The tuberculin test was positive. Repeated and extensive hemorrhages occurred in both eyes, and there was a most pronounced peri-vascularitis, especially affecting the veins, followed by proliferating retinitis, vascular veils, and vitreous opacities, with almost total loss of vision in the right eye and vision reduced to 20/40 in the left. Treatment either by absolute rest, or with moderate exercise, appeared to produce no influence whatever on the recurrence of the hemorrhages, and the credit for any good result obtained seems to have been due to open-air treatment, tuberculin injections, and general hygiene, although a note at the end of Davis' paper tends to throw doubt even upon these methods, inasmuch as a detachment of the retina occurred later still in the left eye, reducing vision to the counting of fingers at 10 feet.

That tuberculosis was an etiological factor seems certain from the decided reaction to tuberculin. Davis thinks that auto-intoxication is also a factor, from the facts that there had been indigestion, that there was at times a large excess of indican in the urine, and that at one time there was an acute desquamative involvement of the kidneys, lasting between two and three weeks. Davis notes that the hemorrhages seemed to come from the retinal veins and arteries, and not from the choroidal veins. The patient's blood-pressure and blood tests were normal throughout.

Ligature of the carotid for recurring vitreous hemorrhage should be chosen as a therapeutic last resort. G. S. Derby's (*Practical Med. Series,* Eye, p. 73, 1908) case was not benefited. However, three others have been saved from hopeless blindness by the operation. Mayweg's patient one and one-half years after the operation had vision of 20/40. Axenfeld's first case twenty-six months after operation had vision of 6/12; and the later case six months after operation vision of 6/9. Such a procedure would be unjustified except, as in these cases, both eyes were involved, and repeated recurrences took place in spite of careful treatment.

Angelucci has tried thyroid feeding in four cases of recurrent vitreous hemorrhage with good results. From an experimental study of the action of hemolytic serums and blood dissolving substances, especially saponin, upon the eyes of lower animals, Sattler concludes that it is not yet practicable to use a hemolytic serum in the human eye, because of the severe inflammatory processes excited by it. He objects to saponin in the therapy of intraocular hemorrhage. Experimenting by the introduction of sterile normal tissues and emulsions thereof into the vitreous he found that they cause inflammation of the rabbit's eye and their presence is opposed by phagocytosis, encapsulation or extrusion.

Kyrieleis (*Klin. Monatsbl. f. Augenheilk.*, p. 513, 1908) reports a case in which the left eye of a healthy full blooded man, aged 19, without any other affections, especially of the circulatory apparatus, had gradually become totally blind from relapsing intraocular hemorrhages and the right eye seemed to be doomed to the same fate. Kyrieleis resorted to five venesections at intervals of from 8 to 10 days, drawing about 250 grams of blood each time, kept the patient in bed and gave him iodid of potassium. No new hemorrhage occurred within the next seven years. R. V. rose to 1/x and everything remained well for a year.

Except in cases of extreme anemia, hemophilia and senile cachexia, he recommends venesection in relapsing ocular hemorrhages, and, if not successful, as a last refuge the ligature of the common carotid.

Kyrieleis thinks venesection has several advantages over ligature of the carotids; under aseptic precautions it is a perfectly harmless procedure and it may be repeated without damage as often as required. Venesection decreases the tension in the vascular system, but must be combined with long-continued rest in bed and non-irritating diet (in order to prevent increased heart action), while iodine should be given internally.

Preretinal, semilunar, or subhyaloid hemorrhage, was first fully described by Hotz, of Chicago. Probably the first pathological examination of this interesting condition was made by Fisher. Exception was then taken to his statement that the extravasation was situated beneath the limitans interna, on the ground that that membrane, being formed from the expanded feet of the fibres of Müller, could not be stripped off in the manner described. Further observations, however, have shown that this theoretical objection has no weight, and have fully confirmed the original description. The occurrence of hemorrhage in front of the limitans is extremely exceptional, and seems to occur only when the extravasation is not at the macula, but near the disc.

Komoto (*Klin. Monatsbl. f. Augenh.*, Vol. L. i., p. 309, 1912) reports a case in confirmation of Fisher's observation. In a man aged

17, four days before his death from purpura, radiate and round hemorrhages were present, and in the left eye there was a small hemorrhage at the macula. After death a large dark hemorrhage, measuring 7 mm. by 10 mm., was found at the left macula, as well as some smaller extravasations elsewhere. Microscopically the blood was found to be covered on its vitreous aspect by a thin, homogeneous membrane, directly continuous on both sides with the limitans interna. The retina showed only slight changes—edema, some loosening of the nerve fibre layer, and degeneration of a few nerve fibres. The blood corpuscles had partially sunk into the lower part of the extravasation. The vitreous was normal. The deeper parts of the cavity were lined with fibrin, and Komoto suggests that the fluidity of the blood in these cases is due to defibrination.

The connection between arterial blood pressure and *retinal hemorrhage* has been studied by Fox and Batroff (*Ophthalmic Record*, Oct., 1908). They report, in 100 cases, the ocular diagnosis, general diagnosis, blood pressure, hemoglobin, red and white blood corpuscles, and condition of the urine. In 80 per cent. they found the blood pressure abnormally high. In 40 per cent. the retinal hemorrhage was associated with chronic interstitial nephritis; in 27 per cent. with arteriosclerosis, and in 13 per cent. with parenchymatous nephritis. In five out of six cases of anemia, and in the two cases of diabetic retinitis, the blood pressure was subnormal. They urge the value of venesection as a means of reducing the blood pressure, to decrease the tendency to hemorrhage, and to promote absorption of the clot. In one case of acute glaucoma where the other eye had been lost after an iridectomy, the removal of twenty ounces of blood from the arm reduced the pressure from 265 to 150 mm., allowing the performance of a successful iridectomy.

Rochon-Duvigneaud in reporting two cases of leukemic retinitis calls attention to the value of blood examination in all cases of retinal hemorrhage.

Straub (*Klin. Monatsbl. f. Augenh.* May, 1908) investigated the subsequent history of 15 cases of retinal hemorrhage after a period of five years. Ten of these whose ages varied from 49 to 68 years, furnished six cases of death by apoplexy, while two younger and three older patients escaped this fate. Straub concludes that the prognosis of retinal hemorrhages is particularly bad between 45 and 65 years of age.

Best (*Zeitschr. f. Augenh.*, Dec., 1908) recommends thyro-therapy for intraocular hemorrhage for the reasons that extirpation of the thyroid in animals causes arteriosclerosis, the injection of thyroid diminishes the blood pressure and he hàs seen a case of hemorrhage in a patient who had undergone extirpation of the thyroid and presented slight cachexia strumipriva.

Hemorrhage into the sheath of the optic nerve. Although hemorrhage into the subdural and subarachnoidal spaces of the optic nerve has been described by Magnus, de Wecker, and others, there is no evidence to show that it exists as an idiopathic affection. There are no reasons for believing that hemorrhages situated at the border of the optic disc, or in the vitreous humor, are indicative of apoplexy of the optic-nerve sheath (Gonin). Intervaginal hematoma may occur after cerebral apoplexy or following trauma. In such a case there will be rapid and great loss of vision. Early ophthalmoscopic examination may show nothing abnormal, or may give a picture resembling that which is found in embolism of the central retinal artery. At a later date the disc will be atrophic.

Dupuy-Dutemps (*Ann. d'Oculistique,* March, 1914) reports two cases of bilateral hematoma of the sheaths of the optic nerves due to penetration of intra-cranial sub-arachnoid hemorrhages into the intervaginal space. In the first case, which was traumatic, ophthalmoscopic examination, thirteen hours after the accident (fracture of the skull), showed the presence of slight edema of the discs with indistinctness of their edges, dilatation of the veins, and a number of small, scattered retinal hemorrhages. In the second case, which was non-traumatic, diffuse vitreous hemorrhages on both sides made it impossible to see the fundus details.

The pathological examination showed in both cases that the intervaginal hematoma did not extend towards the globe farther than the anterior part of the cavity, and did not pass the scleral barrier; that the blood did not penetrate into the trunk of the optic nerve, but infiltrated the connective tissue around the central vessels, forming a continuous sheath which accompanied them into the orbit, thus constituting a path of propagation of the ecchymosis which had not been previously described; that there was edema of the discs without any inflammatory reaction; and that the retinal hemorrhages originated locally and had no continuity with the hematoma.

Dupuy-Dutemps believes that the ophthalmoscopic signs usually ascribed to hemorrhage into the sheaths of the optic nerve (ischemia, late peripapillary hemorrhage, and secondary pigmentation) have not been found in any case in which such a hemorrhage has been definitely proved, and are in complete disagreement with anatomical and physiological facts. The sudden spontaneous unilateral intervaginal hemorrhage, which is often assumed clinically as the cause of sudden amaurosis, has never been demonstrated, and even if it exists, must be exceedingly rare. Except in cases of direct traumatism compli- cated by wounds of the nerve, hematoma of the sheaths is always con- secutive to traumatic or spontaneous meningeal hemorrhage. Its only physical signs are congestion of the disc with more or less marked edema, dilatation of the veins, and retinal hemorrhages, variable in number and extent, due to vascular ruptures in the retina. The oph- thalmoscopic lesions occur very early, and should appear as soon as the hematoma is formed. Their cause seems to be the venous stasis set up by the compression to which the central vein is exposed in its passage through the intervaginal space. It is possible, however, that there may be a complete absence of ophthalmoscopic changes.

Dupuy-Dutemps considers that, apart from the speculative interest of the question, it is important to establish the ophthalmoscopic signs which may accompany meningeal hemorrhage, since their recognition may furnish an indication for an early decompression operation. See, also, **Hemorrhage into the orbit.**

Hemorrhagic cataract. (Obs.) A form of cataract in which hemor- rhage is apt to occur at the time of the operation for its extraction, with percipitate escape of the lens, with or without the vitreous.

Hemorrhagic diathesis. See **Hemophilia.**

Hemorrhagic glaucoma. See **Glaucoma.**

Hemorrhagic retinitis. See **Hemorrhages, Ocular**; also, **Retinitis.**

Hemorrhoids. PILES. Frequent bleedings from hemorrhoids may di- rectly, as the result of anemia, lead to visual disturbances. On the other hand, when the hemorrhage is not too frequent or too copious it may be beneficial in certain eye diseases. For instance, a chronic, progressive glaucoma may be relieved by this means; and it may take the place of the ordinary form of blood abstraction for a number of ophthalmic affections.

Hemorrhoscopia. (L.) Examination of the blood with the hemato- scope.

Hemoscope. An instrument for observing the spectroscopic properties of the blood. It consists of two plates of glass, which touch at one end, but are distant half a millimetre at the other. A drop of blood is intro- duced into the space between the plates, where it can be conveniently studied with the spectroscope. The thickness of the layer can be varied at will by approximating or separating the plates.—(Foster.)

Hemosiderin. Two definitions are usually given for this agent: *(a)* a preparation containing the iron of the blood; *(b)* a dark-yellow pigment containing iron found in various phagocytic cells of the blood.

Hemostasis in eye surgery. For a full account of this important subject see p. 142, Vol. I of this *Encyclopedia.*

To this may be added a brief description of Mark Stevenson's
(*Ophth. Record,* February, 1913) useful hemostatic lid clamp.
Proper sized rubber tubing, such as is used on the eye wires of spectacles (or a little larger) is pulled over the metal arms; the tissues are
then not cut and very little pain is caused. In addition the pressure
of the elastic rounding rubber surface serves better to constrict the
blood vessels than the flat metal arms. The instrument is larger than
the Wilder V-shaped one and shaped like the letter U, somewhat
similar to one of the arms of the old models of lid clamps. Stevenson
has a o had the set screws made so that the pressure of the blades
can be regulated from either side, permitting easy use of the instrument on either the upper or lower lids of either eye.

Hemostatic. Capable of checking hemorrhage.

Hemostatic glaucoma. A name for the inflammatory forms of glaucoma.

Hemostatics. STYPTICS. See p. 660, Vol. I of this *Encyclopedia.*

Hemostatin. This agent is one of the numerous proprietary remedies
resembling suprarenalin or adrenalin. It is used in about the same
manner, closely resembles the action of these remedies but presents
no practical advantage over them.

Henbane. See **Hyoscyamus niger.**

Hen-blindness. A popular name for night-blindness.

Henle, Friedrich Gustav. A famous German anatomist, physiologist
and pathologist, who devoted considerable attention to the anatomy
and physiology of the eye. Born at Fürth July 19, 1809, he received
his medical degree at Bonn Apr. 4, 1832, presenting as dissertation
"De Membrana Pupillare, Aliisque Oculi Membranis Pellucentibus."
After further study at Paris and Berlin, he became docent in the latter university from 1838 till 1840. In the last-named year he was
called to Zürich as Professor of Anatomy and Physiology. From
1852 until his death (May 13, 1885) he was Professor of Anatomy
and Director of the Anatomical Institute at Göttingen.

Henle's chief ophthalmologic writings were: 1. Bemerkungen zur
Anatomie der Retina. (Müller's *Archiv,* 1839.) 2. Zur Anatomie
der Thränenwege und zur Physiologie der Thränenbildung. (*Zeitschr.
f. rat. Med.,* 1865.) 3. Zur Anatomie der Krystallinse. (*Göttinger
Nachrichten,* 1878.) 4. Zur Entwicklung der Krystallinse und zur
Theilung des Zellkerns. (*Archiv f. mikr. Anatomie,* Bd. XX, 1883.)—
(T. H. S.)

Henle, Glands of. Near the point where the tarsus joins the fornix, the conjunctiva is studded with papillæ separated by tubular depressions. These depressions are called *Henle's glands,* although their glandular nature is denied by many anatomists.

Henle, Layer of. See **Henle, Glands of**.

Henna. This ancient cosmetic is made from the leaves of *Lawsonia alba* powdered and made into a paste. It is still used by the Egyptian Mohammedan men and women for dyeing their finger-nails, palms of the hands, soles of the feet, eyebrows and hair an orange-red color. It is the *camphére* (camphor) of the Scriptures. It contains tannic acid, and has also been employed internally and locally in leprosy, skin diseases and in granular ophthalmia.

Henning, Friedrich. A Swedish physician, who devoted considerable attention to ophthalmology. Born in 1767 at Woten, he received the medical degree in 1788 at Greifswald. In 1799 he settled at Barth, in Swedish Pomerania, and was made assessor at the Royal Swedish Sanitary College. He died in 1840.

Henning's only ophthalmologic writing is *"Commentatio Medico-Chirurgica de Ptosi"* Leipsic, 1788.—(T. H. S.)

Henosis. (L.) (Obsolete.) A growing into one. The uniting together of the eyelids.

Henry the Minstrel. He was also called "Blind Harry" and "The Northern Homer." His surname is not known. He was born blind about A. D. 1361, but became a very learned man, traveled about the country as a beggar, reciting his own poems, and was very well known all over Scotland. His most important composition is "The Battle of Biggar." The place, date, and cause of his death, are alike unknown.—(T. H. S.)

Henry, Thomas. A British apothecary and physician, who devoted considerable attention to ophthalmology. Born at Wrexham, North Wales, Oct. 26, 1734, he practised at Kentsford, in Cheshire, later at Manchester. He was a Fellow of the Royal Society and of the Medical Society in London, and died June 18, 1816.

Henry's only ophthalmologic writing is "Case of a Person Becoming Short-Sighted in Advanced Age" (*Mem. Manchest. Soc.*, V, 1790). —(T. H. S.)

Hepar. (L.) The liver; also an old term for an alkaline sulphide.

Hepatic disease, Ocular relations of. There are very few genuine diseases of the liver that produce eye symptoms. As Lawford (Norris and Oliver's *System*, Vol. IV, p. 684) points out, if an hepatic disease is accompanied by jaundice, the subjective symptom of yellow vision (xanthopsia) is occasionally noted. This phenomenon is present in a very small percentage of cases; Hirschberg reported five in one thousand. It is most frequent in catarrhal jaundice, and is usually noted as an early symptom. The explanation formerly given, and generally accepted, that the sensation was due to a yellow tint of the refractive media has been called in question, and it is suggested that the symptom may be the expression of a toxic effect upon the retina. It is almost certainly a peripheral lesion, and in some of its features is analogous to the yellow vision of santonin-poisoning (Knies).

The altered condition of the blood which is present in jaundice, from whatever cause, may lead to retinal hemorrhage. Litten (*Zeitschrift für klinische Medicin*, Vol. V, Pt. 1) especially has drawn attention to the (according to his investigations) frequent occurrence of blood extravasation in the retina in almost every variety of hepatic disease in which jaundice is present. Junge (*Würzburger Verhandlungen*, Vol. IX, S. 219) and Stricker (*Berlin. klin. Wochenschr.*, 1874) have also recorded observations upon the occurrence of retinal hemorrhage in hepatic jaundice.

Landolt (*Archiv für Ophthalmologie*, Vol. XVIII, Pt. 1), a few years ago, published some observations upon two cases in which disease of the liver, of the cirrhotic type, and retinitis pigmentosa coexisted. He considered that the hepatic and the retinal disease were closely connected, and that the structural changes in the liver and in the retina were in many ways analogous. More recently Hori (*Archives of Ophthalmology*, Vol. XXVII, No. 6) has reported the case of a man, aged forty-nine, who died of cirrhosis of the liver; he was greatly emaciated and jaundiced. There were ophthalmoscopic signs of disease of the choroidal vessels, but no obvious changes in the retina; the visual fields were contracted and the man was night-blind. Post-mortem examination revealed signs of a chronic inflammation of the uveal tract.

Further evidence is necessary before Landolt's views as to the relation between hepatic cirrhosis and disease of the choroid and retina can be accepted in their entirety.

Eales (*Birmingham Medical Review*, 1880) described a group of cases of recurrent hemorrhage in the retina, and into the vitreous from the retinal vessels, associated with epistaxis, in young males in whom chronic constipation and high arterial tension were present. Eales held that constipation was in part due to inactive hepatic functions, the main factor in the production of the retinal hemorrhage in these individuals.

Herabgekrümmt. (G.) Curved downward.

Herausdrängen. (G.) A squeezing out (as of trachoma follicles).

Herausschneiden. (G.) Excision.

Heraustreten. (G.) Protrusion.

Herauswachsend. (G.) Exuberant, proliferating.

Herauswenden. (G.) Eversion; turning outward.

Herbalist. One who collects or deals in plants and herbs, or an irregular practitioner who uses herbs only.

Herba ocularia. The plant *Euphrasia officinalis,* var. *pratensis.*

Herba ophthalmica. (L.) The herb *Euphrasia officinalis.*

Herbe à l'ophthalmie. (F.) Euphrasy or eyebright (q. v.). Its use was recommended by the old herbalists both outwardly and inwardly, in powder and in decoction, for diseases of the eyes. It is still a domestic eye remedy.

Herbe-aux-sorciers. (F.) Datura stramonium.

Herbe-du-diable. (F.) Datura stramonium.

Herbeiführend. (G.) Causative.

Herbert's bacillus. INTRAEPITHELIAL CAPSULATED BACILLUS. This bacillus is not unlike *Bacillus mucosus capsulatus* in appearance but differs in being difficult to stain.

Herbert's operation. WEDGE-ISOLATION OPERATION FOR GLAUCOMA. SMALL FLAP SCLERECTOMY. Frank Todd (*Trans. Am. Acad. Oph. and Oto-Laryng.,* p. 377, 1914) has invented an instrument intended to secure all the benefits of this operation and yet to avoid its difficulties.

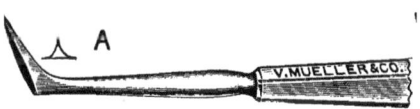

Frank Todd's Leech-bite Sclerotomy Knife.

It consists of a knife which makes a leech-bite incision, i. e., three lines proceeding from a central point, thus producing three flaps, an incision very difficult to close. While this incision remains open and allows satisfactory filtration under the conjunctiva from the anterior chamber, no scleral tissue is removed, and weakening of the sclera does not take place, so that there is less liability to protrusion of the ciliary body into the opening than where a large opening is made, as with the trephine, when a portion of sclera is removed.

In performing the operation with this instrument a conjunctival flap may be dissected up or the knife may be shoved under the conjunctiva well above the margin of the cornea. The point of the knife may then be slid along between the conjunctiva and sclera until it reaches within 2 or 3 mm. of the cornea when it should penetrate the sclera and enter the anterior chamber, being as quickly withdrawn. If prolapse occurs, iridectomy is performed. See, also, page 5521, Vol. VII, of this *Encyclopedia*.

Herbstliche Bindehautentzündung. (G.) Autumnal conjunctivitis.

Hereditary ataxia. See p. 662, Vol. I and p. 5161, Vol. VII, of this *Encyclopedia;* as well as **Heredity in ophthalmology.**

Hereditary cataract. See **Cataract, Hereditary**; as well as **Heredity in ophthalmology.**

Hereditary central retinitis. This is a name proposed by Cargill (*Ophthalmoscope,* Vol. X, p. 62) for **Leber's disease** (q. v.)—familial optic atrophy—mainly because of the fact that the morbid changes usually begin in the retina. See, also, **Familial eye diseases,** and **Heredity in ophthalmology.**

Heredity in ophthalmology. HEREDITARY EYE DISEASES. HEREDITY IN RELATION TO THE EYE. As the application of Mendel's rules of heredity to the transmission of human anomalies, deformities and diseases has stimulated ophthalmologists to investigations along these lines, a brief notice of this original and indefatigable investigator seems most appropriate. Johann Gregor Mendel was born July 22, 1822, in Silesia, Austria, and was of German descent. He was ordained a priest of the Roman Catholic Church in 1847. Recognizing the scientific mind and ability of the young priest, the Church sent him to the University of Vienna, 1851-53, to study natural and physical science. After this he became a successful teacher. He spent eight years of steady application to pea-crossing experiments, which were carried to definite, final conclusions, carefully recorded and systematically tabulated. In his lifetime his work apparently failed to influence biologists, and he died, in 1884, unrecognized by the world of science. But his courageous prophecy, "meine Zeit wird schon kommen," has been fulfilled, and his great contribution to heredity is now the foundation stone of that fast developing science.

The headings **Congenital anomalies,** as well as **Familial eye affections**; **Leber's disease** and other minor captions should be read in conjunction with this section.

D. B. Hart *(Phases of Evolution and Heredity)* gives a clear and concise exposition of the Mendelian laws, and considers that Mendel's researches on variation in plants and the distribution of the contrasted characters in the crossed plants, constitute the greatest single contribution yet made to the science of evolution. At the same time Hart gives credit for the epoch-making work of **D**arwin and the exhaustive labors of Weismann. As the edible pea has the advantage of being self-fertilizing and having many varieties, Mendel chose it for his experimental work. He selected seven varieties of this pea, each with one contrasted character, as shape of seed, color of seed-skin, shape of pod or height of plant. The results of the experiments made by crossing a tall plant of six to seven feet with a dwarf variety of one to one and one-half feet, are very striking. The pollen of either parent plant is dusted on the stigma of the other selected parent, the cross fertilized parent being protected from accidental fertilization, as by insects. There are no offspring plants of a size intermediate between tall and dwarf, in the second generation, but all are tall. Next, the peas were allowed to self-fertilize. The succeeding, or third, generation showed three kinds of offspring: talls, "somatic talls" and dwarfs, in the proportion of three talls to one dwarf plant. The dwarfs, self-fertilized, now bred true. Only dwarf plants resulted, however many generations were bred. The somatic talls (hybrids) gave, on self-fertilization, one-third which bred true to tallness, and two-thirds which as impure talls gave somatic talls, and also dwarfs; breeding true again in the ratio of 3:1.

Mendel described each of the contrasted and selected qualities tested in his cross fertilization, as "unit characters." He showed that these contrasted qualities did not blend in their consecutive generations, but appeared unaltered in definite ratios. The unit characters, called by him "dominant" and "recessive," are thus shown to be not blendable but antonomous. This fact is of the highest importance in heredity. It is also important to note that the determinants of a character may be secluded in the propagative part for one or very many generations. Their delayed appearance is attributed to recession, or atavism. The soma of the plant is the transient part, whose life is only for a generation; it is the propagative part that lives and transmits.

Further elucidation of Mendel's laws of heredity, by W. Bateson, may be found in *Brain,* Part 1141, 1906, and Mendel's *Principles of Heredity,* 1909.

Weismann (Clarendon Press, Oxford, 1891) states that heredity is the process which renders possible the persistence of organic beings throughout successive generations; depending on the continuity of the molecular substance of the germ plasma. This substance transfers its hereditary tendencies from generation to generation, at first unchanged, and always uninfluenced in any corresponding manner by anything that happens during the life of the individual who bears it.

A. Peters (*Lancet,* Jan. 13, 1912, p. 108) takes the ground that the study of heredity must be considered of much greater importance to ophthalmologists than has hitherto been the case. In no domain of

pathology has the collection of well authenticated, illustrative examples been so productive as in ophthalmology. The types of ocular
disease which display most clearly the influence of hereditary transmission are often more sharply defined and less obscured by extraneous influences than most types of bodily ailments. Peters believes
that the cause of all the hereditary malformations and diseases of the
eye is to be found in variation of the plasma, which had been "stamped
with the impression of inferiority."

The *Ophthalmic Year Book*, Vol. IX, 1912, p. 000, states that the
literature relating to the inheritance of ocular defects and conditions
is increasing rapidly. Over forty papers have been published in the
past two years, in which heredity is recognized as the essential causative factor of albinism, myopia, congenital squint, ophthalmoplegia,
nystagmus, vernal conjunctivitis, corneal opacities, blue sclerotics,
glaucoma, cataract, dislocation of the lens, optic atrophy, word-blindness and ptosis. To this list might be added retinitis pigmentosa,
congenital stationary night-blindness, color-blindness, iritis and
choroiditis.

To the late Edward Nettleship must be credited the most productive
investigations of the ocular effects of heredity that have yet been
made. Devoting all his time to this subject for many years prior to
his death, and while yet in his prime, he worked out many admirable
pedigrees and drew therefrom most important conclusions. Not only
did he investigate personally the living members of many affected lines
and the records of others, even to the tenth generation in one instance,
but he also tabulated the work of widely scattered observers in this
field; thus giving the scientifically certified statistics and comprehensive observations that furnish the fundamental requirement for the
study of heredity. Further, Nettleship inspired many of his English
colleagues to do similar work; so that it is not too much to say that
the largest and best classified genealogies bearing upon the relation
of heredity to ophthalmology have come from England, although close
observers in many countries have made very many valuable contributions to this subject.

W. Bateson (*Lancet*, Aug. 16, 1913, p. 451), in an address before
the International Congress of Medicine, speaks of the exceptional significance that the study of heredity must soon assume. The tendency
is to exhibit increasingly the definiteness and fixity of the laws of
descent. Whatever influences may be brought to bear by hygiene or
education, the ultimate decision rests with the germ cells as to man's
physical destiny. The re-discovery, in 1900, of Mendel's work, made
possible an analysis of the confusion, the paradoxes and the capricious

disorder of the phenomena of descent, and contributed to a right interpretation of special problems of pathology and anthropology. The
essence of the Mendelian principle is that in great measure the properties of organisms are due to the presence of distinct, detachable
elements, separately transmitted in heredity, and that a parent cannot
transmit to offspring an element which it does not itself possess. Some
of the ophthalmic conditions which commonly descend as dominants
are presenile cataract, ectopia lentis, ptosis, cryptophthalmos, coloboma, distichiasis, night-blindness and retinitis pigmentosa. Color-
blindness is one of the best examples of the descent of an abnormality
being limited by sex. The sons of color-blind males do not inherit the
peculiarity, and therefore cannot transmit it. The daughters of color-
blind fathers do inherit it; and though it does not appear in them,
probably all of them have the power of transmitting it to their sons.
Color-blind males are frequently seen, color-blind females very rarely.
Hurst first succeeded in determining the inheritance of the color of
the eyes, which had long puzzled anthropologists. He clearly showed
that the presence of pigment in the iris, giving brown or black eyes,
is a dominant; its absence, giving blue or gray eyes, is a recessive.

Congenital anomalies (q. v.) *when not clearly hereditary are not
included in this section.* The stigmata of syphilis are mostly omitted,
as the same abnormality is seldom transmitted in the direct line in this
disease. When two or more members of one generation have the same
defect it is considered a "family" disease even though it cannot be
traced to a preceding or succeeding generation. The result argues a
cause that is unescapable, although the difficulty of obtaining accurate
data further back than two or three generations usually conceals the
origin of the familial defect.

HEREDITARY ANOMALIES OF THE LIDS.

The writer has observed hereditary narrowing of the palpebral
aperture of one eye as a family trait, extending for three or four generations. Other familial peculiarities may be noticed by careful
observation of generations known in person, or by study of family
portraits or photographs.

Epicanthus. Double epicanthus running through two and three
generations is fairly common. Usually the development of the bridge
of the nose corrects the deformity by or before adult life.

Deformity of the inner canthus. The condition reported on by
A. S. Cobbledick (*Proceedings of the Royal Society of Medicine,*
March, 1913) seems to be a family defect, since the mother, one

brother, two sisters, and a child of the patient, had the same defect. The deformity in the patient himself, a man aged 39 years, consisted essentially in enlargement of the lacus lacrimalis, which, instead of being triangular in shape, was somewhat oval, so that the vertical and lateral measurements of the lacus were much greater than normal. The lachrymal papillæ were very prominent. There was marked flattening of the malar bone and smallness of the palpebral fissures, the latter partly from ptosis and partly from an abnormally short lateral measurement. An appearance of internal strabismus was thus produced. Epiphora was gradually getting worse. There were no other congenital defects.

Ectropion. H. A. Smith has personally told the author of ectropion of both lower lids occurring after forty years of age, which he had observed in a father and his seven sons.

Coloboma of the lid occurs rarely as a congenital, hereditary anomaly.

Ptosis. In a personal communication, S. Z. Shope has related a striking case of hereditary ptosis, affecting the right eye in five generations. One child only in a large childship was affected in each generation. A female showed this defect in the fourth generation of the affected line; only males being affected in the other generations.

H. R. Stilwill has mentioned to the writer a case of ptosis affecting a man, his daughter and her son.

Huetlemann (Graefe's *Archiv. f. Ophthal.*, Vol. LXXX, part 2) published his observations on congenital ptosis, with epicanthus, in three generations. Eight children out of eleven were affected. In only one case was there disturbance of other ocular muscles. The electric current showed absence or imperfect development of the levator.

Ptosis and ophthalmoplegia. A. A. Bradburne (*Trans. Ophth. Soc. of Un. Kingd.*, 1912, Vol. XXXII, p. 142) describes three types; first and most common, that in which the congenital defect is limited solely to the levator; second, a fairly common type in which ptosis is associated with epicanthus, and third, a form in which ptosis may or may not be present, but one or all of the ocular muscles are defective. He reports a family in which a varying degree of ptosis of one or both lids, accompanied by an almost complete loss of movement in one or both eyes, has been manifested for five generations. In this family tree are thirty-seven individuals, of whom fifteen are living. Of these thirty-seven persons, sixteen are believed to have been affected—eleven females and five males. Of the sixteen, seven

only are now living—six females and one male. These were all
studied by Bradburne, although they showed disinclination to have
a "family failing" investigated, as is often the case. The oldest
surviving member, a widow of seventy, distinctly remembers this
affection in her mother, grandmother, great aunt and two uncles.
An unmarried brother, aged eighty, is free from the ocular defect,
as are also a sister with her family of three girls and a boy. The

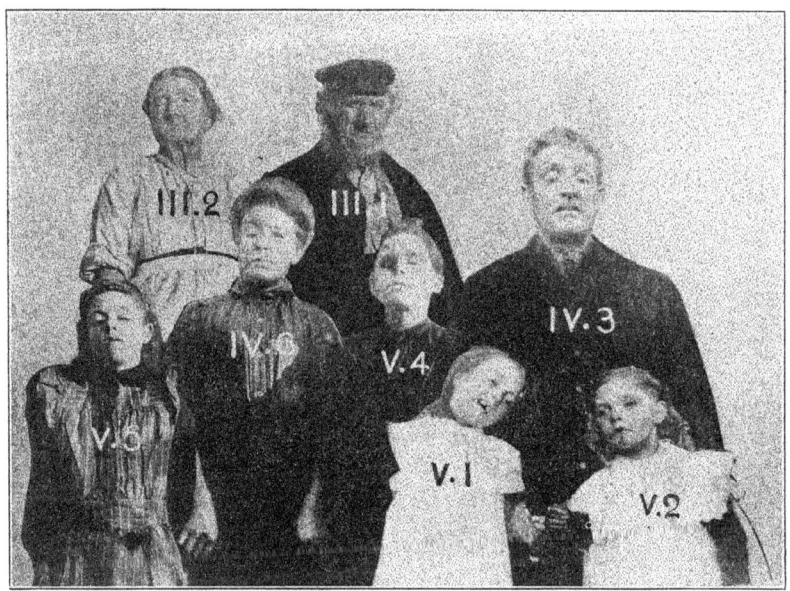

Group Illustrating Ophthalmoplegia with Ptosis. (Bradburne.)

widow has had eight children, equally divided as to sex. The first
two were unaffected males. The next two, a male and a female, were
both affected. The female died of bronchitis at eighteen months; the
male is alive and has two living daughters, and had a son who died
in infancy. All three children were affected. The fifth child of the
widow was a normal female, who died when one month old. The
sixth was an affected female, who has two affected daughters. The
seventh child, a female, and the eighth, a male, were both normal and
both died in infancy. The ptosis was complete in several right eyes,
and Müller's muscle was apparently absent in two cases. One
patient had a very white, cupped disk and semi-dilated pupils. In
the diseased members who reached adult life, the double disability of

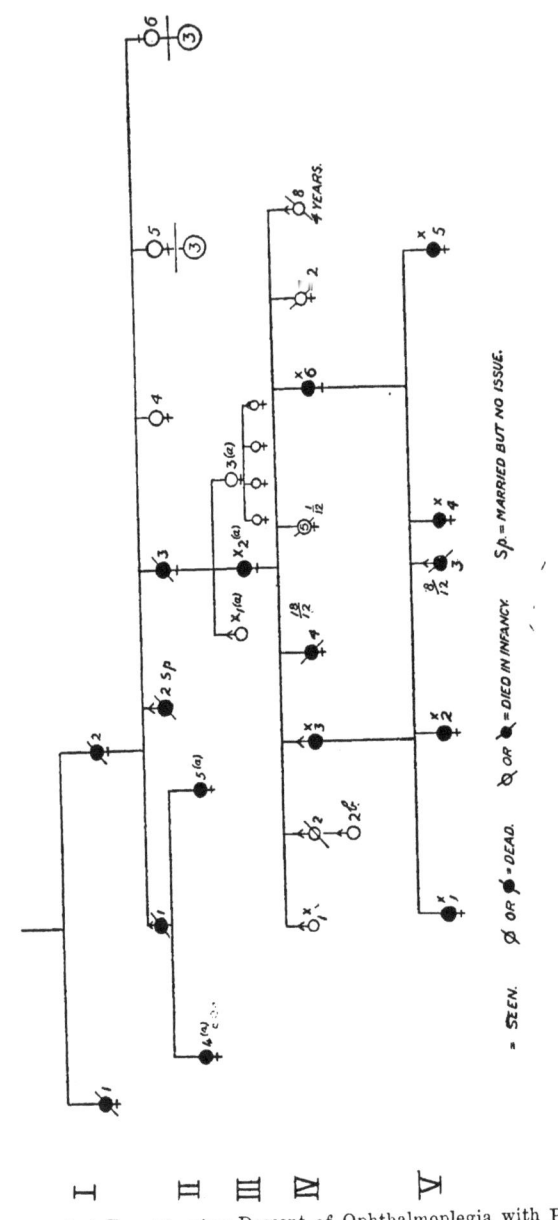

Genealogical Tree Showing Descent of Ophthalmoplegia with Ptosis.
(Bradburne.)

ptosis and immobility of the eyes was present. Bradburne states that the condition is congenital, non-progressive, not sex-limited, of continuous and direct descent, not replaced by any other affection, and unaccompanied by any of the common congenital defects, such as hare-lip, cleft-palate or faulty colored irides, though all possessed high-arched palates. The family showed no signs of degeneracy such as defective mental development, supernumerary fingers, or attached ear lobes. The affection was traced through five generations, covering the period from 1710 to 1912. In the first generation there were two affected individuals, both females; in the second, of six members equally divided in sex, two males and one female were affected. Of eleven in the third generation, only three were affected, all females. The fourth generation produced twelve individuals, of whom one male and two females were affected. In the fifth, only one male escaped out of two males and four females born. There has been no intermarriage, and the birth rate was not affected. Bradburne suggests that the condition may be one of reversion to a lower type, analogous to the shark, in which animal the ocular muscles are developed from three centers; or perhaps non-use of the eyes in some ancestors afflicted with ptosis may have been the original factor in the condition of muscle palsy.

HEREDITARY ANOMALIES OF THE GLOBE.

Microphthalmos. O. Stuelp (Graefe's *Arch. f. Ophth.*, 1913, Vol. LXXXVI, p. 136) records family congenital microphthalmos of high degree in eight out of fourteen children. The preceding and following generations showed no marked ocular defects. In the father, who was dead, syphilis could not be excluded. Of the eight children, four were blind and died in infancy; two being females, one a male, and the sex of the fourth being unknown. The living children, one woman and three men, were 46, 61, 59 and 57 years old, respectively. None of their children or grandchildren were affected. All indications from the histological and clinical examinations point to intra-uterine uveitis followed by phthisis bulbi, rather than a developmental anomaly.

Microphthalmos with and without cataract. Chr. Thomsen (*Woch. f. Therap. u. Hyg. d. Auges,* Vol. XVI, p. 326, July 17, 1913) calls attention to the association of cataract with microphthalmos in a family studied by him. The grandparents were blood relations, and the husband's great aunt was born blind. The husband's brother had double cataract and his children were very myopic. A sister had low vision. The husband had lamellar cataract but no microphthalmos. The oldest of his five children had normal eyes. Of the other four, two girls and a boy had microphthalmos and lamellar cataract in each eye, while another boy had lamellar cataract, without

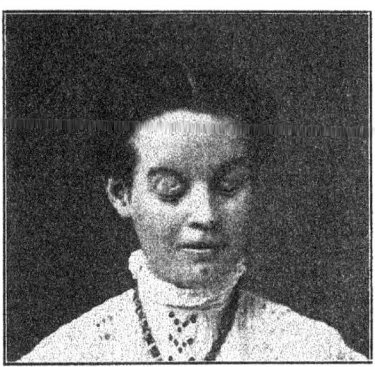

Coover's First Case of Cryptophthalmia, the Mother.

microphthalmos, in both eyes. All children having eye anomalies had slight nystagmus. The wife's family is said to have had no ocular abnormalities.

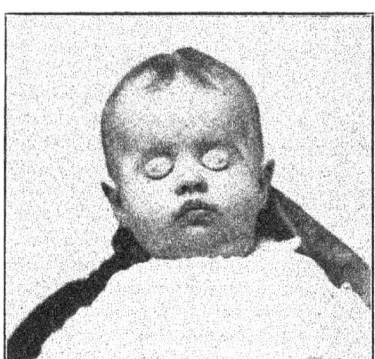

Coover's Second Case of Cryptophthalmia, the Daughter.

Microphthalmos and anophthalmos. F. B. Hofmann (*Klin. Monatsbl. f. Augenh.,* p. 594, May, 1912) finds that in white rats microphthalmos and anophthalmos are chiefly inherited from the mother.

Enophthalmos. In a personal report J. M. Foster has described an apparent binocular enophthalmos of 5 to 10 mm. in all members of a family for three generations, coming on after thirty years of age. He ascribed the recession of the eyes to absorption of the fat in the eye lids and orbits. The vision and muscle movements were not affected.

Cryptophthalmos. D. H. Coover (*Jour. Amer. Med. Assn.*, July 30, 1910, p. 370) has reported the unfortunate cases of a mother and child with bilateral congenital cryptophthalmos, as proved by orbital

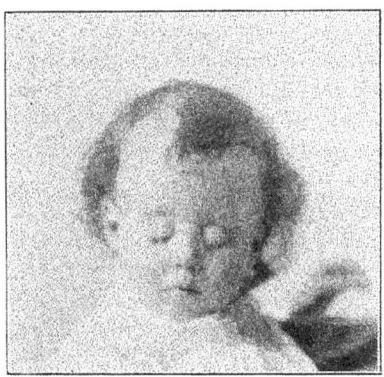

Coover's Third Case of Cryptophthalmia.

A male aged eighteen months. Rudimentary eyes somewhat larger than those of mother and first child.

dissection. Since that report another child has been born with the same anomaly. The father and four grandparents of these two children showed no such defects. Only once has consanguinity been recorded in association with this happily rare congenital defect.

Early in 1915 the third child, a male, was born to this couple. As far as the accoucheur could determine, in the dim illumination of a mountain cabin, the eyes and lids were normal.

Hydrophthalmos. Kayser (*Klin. Monatsbl. f. Augenheilk.*, Jan., 1914, p. 142) reports a family tree of 150 persons of whom 17 showed hereditary hydrophthalmos and megalocornea. The condition was congenital and unprogressive throughout life, with intact visual acuity. It illustrated the same type of heredity as color-blindness and hemophilia.

HEREDITARY ANOMALIES OF THE CORNEA.

Family degeneration of the cornea. L. Buchanan (*Ophthalmoscope*, Oct., 1911, p. 693) reported the case of a woman, aged thirty-six, showing this defect, and completed the previously noted histories of her two brothers, who had the same disease. One brother died of tuberculosis. The vision of the other gradually failed until he had to give up his occupation as an engine fireman. In the sister's eyes both corneas were similarly affected. The central area was hazy for a radius of about 2 mm.; around this was a ring of dotted opacity of 1.5 mm., and beyond this a clear ring to the periphery. The corneal microscope showed the central haze to be made up of very small bluish-grey dots. The vision was 4/00 in each eye, the tension and pupils normal, and the health said to be good.

J. Komoto (*Klin. Monatsbl. f. Augenheilk.*, Oct., 1909, p. 445) noted a father, son, daughter and nephew, who were all born with diffuse, non-vascular corneal opacities of a bilateral character. The son and daughter had congenital cataract, also. Neither syphilis nor tuberculosis could be detected.

Preobraschensky (*Zeit. f. Augenheilk.*, Vol. XXX, p. 78) has reported family corneal degeneration in three sisters.

Acquired symmetrical opacity of the cornea, of unusual type, has been observed by G. F. Libby (*Trans. Amer. Ophthal. Soc.*, 1914). It strongly suggested the family type of degeneration, but diligent search into the history revealed nothing of the sort for three generations. A symmetrical opacity 4 mm. to 5 mm. in diameter, a little to the nasal side of each cornea, more below than above the median line, was observed. It was whitish, with a faint-yellowish tinge, penetrated by a few fine blood vessels. The opacities seemed to arise from the deepest portion of the cornea, and extended through, but not between, the corneal layers. The distribution of the fibrils of the opacity resembled the petals of a chrysanthemum. The corneal epithelium was unaffected. Cholesterin crystals had appeared in the center of both areas. There was no elevation of the epithelium. The case is most unusual and interesting, and does not seem to correspond exactly with anything of the kind reported in the literature.

Lattice-form opacity. H. Freund (Graefe's *Archiv. f. Ophthal.*, Vol. LVII, part 2) reported fifteen cases of lattice-form opacity of the cornea, occurring in two families, and running through at least four generations. The opacity appeared at or after puberty, reaching its full development between thirty and forty years. Both eyes were involved, but not to the same extent. The opacity was thickest at the center, with a clear periphery. Both the superficial and deep layers were affected; and a chalky deposit appeared in the late stages. No constitutional disease was detected.

Family macular degeneration of the cornea. C. A. Veasey (*Trans.*

Amer. Ophthal. Soc., 1904, Vol. X, p. 387) recorded two cases of family macular degeneration of the cornea in a man of forty-one and his sister of forty-three years, and referred to Fehr's article on the subject in the *Centralblatt f. prakt. Augenheilk.*, Jan., 1904. The disease is described as a progressive opacity of both corneas, beginning at 10 or 12 years and leading to disability for work at about 30 years. The opacity consists of numerous fine dots which look like a diffuse opacity to the unaided eye. Intermingled are larger whitish dots and maculæ. The central area of the cornea presents a denser and more superficial opacity than the peripheral portion, where the opacity is deeper and less opaque. There is no vascularization. Progressive failure of vision and very slight irritation and photophobia are the chief subjective symptoms. The surface of the cornea is smooth, and sensation is unaffected. The etiology is undetermined and treatment ineffective. Fehr had reported three cases at that time, and Koerber one case. The man examined by Veasey had noticed beginning failure of sight at about the tenth year. At 46 years R. V.$=7/200$ L. V.$=6/200$. The lenses were clear. The sister's vision was first found to be impaired about the twelfth year of age. At 48 years V.$=1/50$ in each eye. In both patients the corneal conditions corresponded with the description given; in the sister the degenerative conditions were more advanced than in the brother. There were no other cases in four generations, so far as known.

Nodular degeneration of the cornea. Dunbar Roy (*Trans. Amer. Ophthal. Soc.*, Vol. XIII, p. 101, 1912) reports six cases of degeneration of the cornea ("nodular keratitis") occurring in the same family. This is a rare affection, and its etiology and pathology are obscure. As it is a non-inflammatory condition it is not, strictly speaking, a keratitis. Roy states that three cases constitute the greatest number known to have occurred in one family, as reported by A. McNab and Fehr. Roy's cases comprised a mother, aged 48, and five children ranging from 29 to 20 years of age. All presented the same clinical symptoms, except that they were most pronounced in the mother and barely perceptible in the youngest child. The central area of the mother's corneas was largely covered with numerous opaque, slightly projecting, dirty-grey dots of various sizes and shapes. When one was removed an indented, opaque surface was left. The mother's health had always been good and her eyes had been free from inflammatory disturbance. R. V.$=20/70$, L. V.$=20/50$. No treatment of any benefit could be devised. Roy considers that the general *family type* of corneal disease must be recognized whether it be called macular, nodular, grill-like, fenestrated, lattice, trellised or simply family

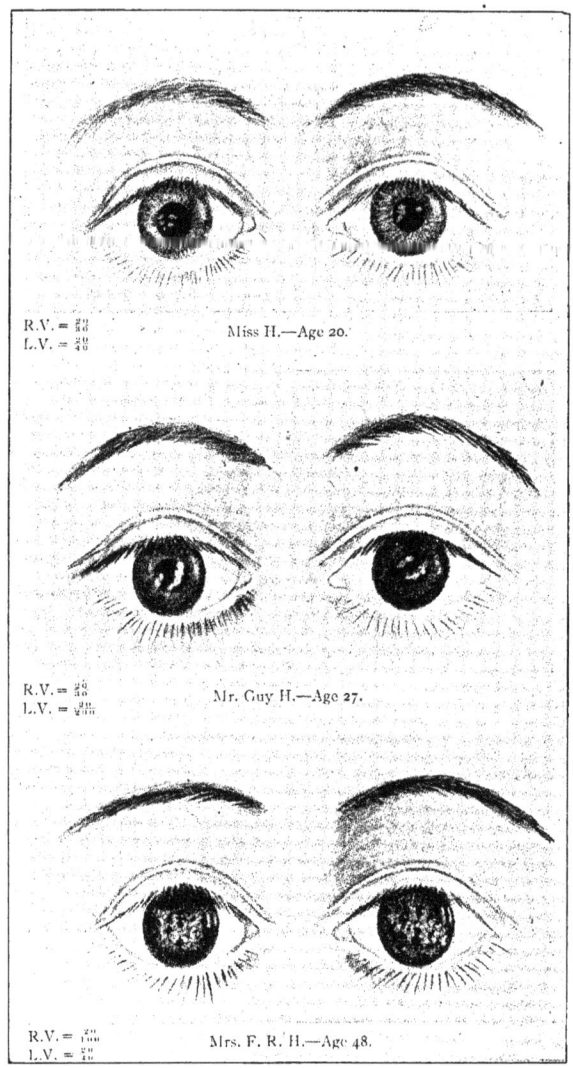

Three Cases of Nodular Degeneration of the Cornea.   (Dunbar Roy.)

degeneration of the cornea, and that they have much in common as to their pathology. Fleischer and Spitta observed 34 cases in the clinic at Tübingen. As Fleischer found only 59 had been reported up to 1905, the unusual number in his district suggests climate, environment or other local conditions as the possible cause of the disease. Intermarriage among affected families in a locality where

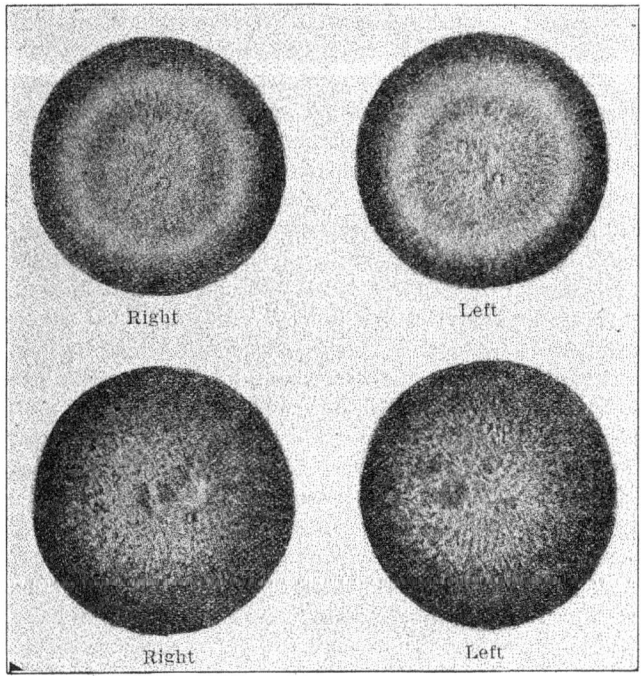

Degeneration of the Cornea in a Man and his Son. (Burton Chance.)

little new blood is introduced is probably a more important factor. Tuberculosis has been considered the cause in cases observed by John Green, Jr., Shumway and Zentmayer. This was excluded in Roy's cases, who points out that nodular keratitis of a tubercular nature begins with marked corneal irritation and inflammatory signs. He agrees with Fleischer that these cases represent a hyaline degeneration rather than any other pathologic process.

H. H. Folker (*Trans. Ophthal. Soc. of Un. Kingd.*, Vol. XXIX, p. 42) observed family degeneration of the cornea in three generations, eight cases, ranging from twelve to ninety-two years of age. All the affected areas were nodular, and both eyes were involved in each case.

Burton Chance (*Trans. Amer. Ophthal. Soc.*, Vol. XIII, p. 282, 1913) describes at length a nodular degeneration affecting both corneas of father and son sufficiently to cause blindness. The father, aged fifty-four and healthy, the first of his line to show the disease, stated that his sight had always been poor. Of two living children the daughter had healthy eyes. In early manhood the older patient had assisted his father in tuning and repairing organs, but in middle life vision had dropped to finger movements at one or two feet. The globes were well formed. At the center of each cornea and for two-thirds of the area of the cornea was a faint, almost circular disk of yellowish-grey, flocculent material. It was beneath the epithelium, which was intact and glistening, and seemed to lie between Bowman's membrane and the corneal stroma. Here and there were glistening points, like crystals. At the apex of the summit were two larger bodies, looking like bubbles, about 1½ mm. in diameter, which projected forward beyond the general surface of the cornea. These discoid areas terminated somewhat unevenly in radiations. At the center they showed condensation, outside of which was a partly transparent zone, while beyond this was another denser portion. The cornea between these areas and the limbus was normal.

The son, aged twenty-six and rather stunted, was married but childless. Poor sight was discovered on entering school at seven, which was much dimmer at twelve, and compelled abandonment of school at fourteen. Typhoid at twenty-five was followed by further diminution of vision. The corneas were much like his father's except that the discoid opacities were not so dense and showed a somewhat more pronounced reticulation. The disease was bilateral, without inflammatory signs, and confined to the central two-thirds of the cornea.

J. E. Weeks (*Archiv. of Ophthal.*, Vol. XLII, p. 179, March, 1913) has reported two patients with family nodular degeneration of the cornea; one the father, aged 56, the other a son, aged 23 years. Each had a punctate or short lined, elevated opacity of the cornea, gradually lessening in density towards the periphery, and terminating about 2 mm. from the margin of the cornea. The condition was the same in both patients except that it was more pronounced in the elder. The father's vision was 20/70, the son's 20/40. The affection was noticed in early youth in each case, and advanced very slowly, without inflammation. The father had three brothers and five sisters; two sisters and one brother had poor sight from some unknown condition. Besides the son mentioned there were two others; one 18 years old, with normal vision, while the other son had poor·vision from an unknown cause. Weeks defines the pathology as follows: "Opacification begins from the twelfth to the eighteenth year, and slowly increases in density. Males and females are equally affected. The opacity is greatest at the center, never reaching the limbus. It begins as minute dots or lines, which by transmitted light appear transparent."

HEREDITARY DISEASES OF THE SCLERA.

Blue sclerotics. H. Burrows (*British Med. Jour.*, July 1, 1911, p. 16) reports a family in which thirteen out of twenty-nine individuals, in four generations, showed this peculiarity. In every instance there was direct heredity from a parent who showed the same condition. The appearance of the sclera was described as pale China blue, and was very striking. The family illustrated the association of brittle bones with this condition. Nine of those with blue sclerotics had suffered fracture, in seven cases multiple fractures, from very slight violence. Of the sixteen members who had normal scleras, not one experienced a broken bone. Burrows accepts the theory of Eddowes of a deficiency in white fibrous tissue, to account for thin sclerotics and brittle bones; and mentions the fact that many people, especially when young, have a shade of blue in the sclera.

Adair-Dighton (*Ophthalmoscope*, April, 1912, p. 188) has reported "azure" blue sclerotics in nine persons, running through four generations, and transmitted directly through either parent. In the first generation, one out of two children, and in the second, one out of three children were affected. Six out of eight children in the third generation had this condition; and the only member of the fourth generation yet born, also showed it. Osteoporosis was shown by multiple fractures in five cases. It was thought that the blue color was caused by thinning of the sclerotics, due to a deficiency of fibrous tissue.

J. D. Rolleston (*British Jour. of Children's Diseases*, May, 1911, and *Ophthalmoscope*, Vol. IX, p. 321, 1911) reported a syphilitic mother who, with her male infant of five months, had blue sclerotics with embryontoxon at the margin of each cornea. Two brothers escaped, but the sister and their grandmother were affected. The child's father had syphilis. The child had a so-called spontaneous fracture of the humerus when only a few months old, but this may have been due to congenital syphilis. In the child the sclerotics were described as pale-blue, while in the other affected members they were of a leaden-blue.

Von Ammon, in 1841, first described blue sclerotics as a congenital disease, stating that the sclera was thin and almost transparent. The study of an excised eye with a blue sclerotic, by L. Buchanan, showed the cornea to be three-fifths, the sclera one-third of the normal thickness. Histologic examination demonstrated that the fibres of both cornea and sclera were of normal size but unusually few in number.

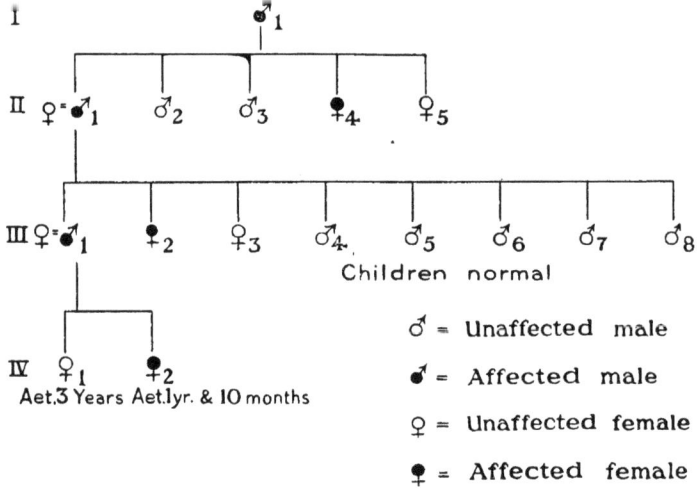

Hereditary Blue Sclerotics. (Cockayne.)

The anterior elastic lamina was entirely absent. Rolleston states that the hereditary transmission of blue sclerotics was first pointed out by A. Peters, who recorded cases in four generations. Typical embryontoxon occurred in four of his cases. Peters regarded the condition as due to sclerotics of abnormal thinness or transparency.

Sydney Stephenson observed blue sclerotics affecting twenty-one of thirty-two members in four generations of a family of syphilitics. Harmon followed this genealogy further, finding thirty-one out of fifty-five showed the same congenital peculiarity.

E. A. Cockayne (*Ophthalmoscope*, May, 1914, p. 271) examined a child of nearly two years, supposed to be suffering from rickets, and at once noticed the uniform blueness of the sclerotics. An inquiry into the family history elicited the fact that several other members exhibited this peculiarity, and that all had suffered from sprains and fractures of the bones. This family corresponds with those previously recorded, since the condition was first recognized by Eddowes in 1900, in that both sexes are affected and transmission only occurs directly through the affected members.

Bishop Harman has shown that the choroid is abnormally thin in cases of blue sclerotics, giving rise to Fuchs' colobomata, with an oval appearance of the optic discs. The fractures are known to depend on a deficiency of the supporting framework of the bones.

The defect probably affects the whole of the mesoblastic tissues of the body. Careful examination of all the tissues, especially of the muscles, ligaments, and fasciæ, are much needed to throw further light on the subject.

HEREDITARY ANOMALIES OF THE IRIS.

H. Drinkwater (p. c.) writes that he described the following cases of *hereditary aniridia* at a meeting of the North Wales Branch of the British Medical Association in 1907. ''The woman marked (1) in the illustration had been married twice. By (2) the first husband (17 years her senior) she had two children, both living and normal. By the second (3) she has had six children, all showing the same peculiarities as herself,—five shown in the chart, and one since. This I have not inserted as I have not seen the child and do not know its sex. I think it illustrates what I have termed, from a Mendelian point of view, *relative dominance*. All the cases that have aniridia, also show nystagmus and more or less corneal opacity.''

S. D. Risley has reported a man of 27 whose right eye had been lost in childhood, but whose left eye was aphakic, with entire absence of the iris. No rudimentary trace of that membrane could be discovered. The retina was detached and ruptured. The vitreous was fluid. With difficulty the patient could count fingers and see to walk about the ward.

It was discovered that in July, 1914, a cousin of the patient had been under treatment in the hospital, also with aniridia. Inquiry revealed the fact that the condition was prevalent in the family. The patient's mother had double aniridia, and he had a son and daughter both of whom were aniridic in both eyes. The patient belongs in the third generation. The condition of the eyes of John F., Sr., and his wife, is not known, but their son John F., Jr., had double aniridia, his wife having normal eyes. From this stock there were 117 descendants, 234 eyes. In the first generation, therefore, the male progenitor had double aniridia.

In the second generation there were four males and nine females, all of them suffering from double aniridia, giving a total of twenty-six eyes with this abnormality of development.

In the third generation, to which the patient belongs, there were thirty-two males and thirty-one females. The patient had but one eye in which the presence of the aniridia could be demonstrated, the other eye having been lost in childhood, and there were four male individuals, eight eyes, in which the condition was not known. The remaining fifty-five eyes had no iris. Of the thirty-one females, with sixty-two eyes, all had aniridia. The total number of eyes in the third generation was 117.

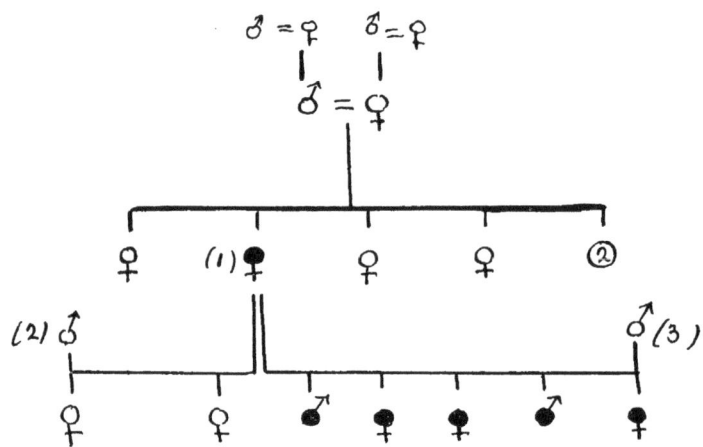

Drinkwater's Cases of Hereditary Aniridia.

In the fourth generation there were nineteen males known to have aniridia and two eyes known to have cataract; and twenty-three females with forty-four aniridic eyes, the condition of two eyes not being known. That is to say, in this generation there were forty-two individuals with seventy-six eyes in which the iris was absent, the condition of the remaining eight eyes not being known.

Summary. One son. 2 eyes (aniridic).

Second generation; male, four: 8 eyes; female, nine: 18 eyes.

Third generation; male, thirty-two: 55 eyes (condition of four individuals not known); female, thirty-one: 62 eyes.

Fourth generation; male, nineteen: 32 eyes, 2 eyes cataractous, 4 eyes not noted; female, twenty-three: 44 eyes (condition of two eyes not known).

Report has been made by T. K. Hamilton (*Ophthalmoscope*, May, 1903) of a father and three sons who showed congenital absence of the iris. The mother was highly hyperopic, but her eyes were otherwise normal.

Hereditary aniridia has been studied by **L.** Palmieri (*Ann. di Ottalmol.*, Vol. 41, p. 367) in a mother and two daughters. The mother had bilateral aniridia, cataract, nystagmus and glaucoma. Her 26-year-old daughter presented the identical conditions in both eyes, the glaucoma later becoming inflammatory. The 24-year-old daughter also exhibited all the four conditions named, without pain, however, in either eye.

Hereditary defect of iris. A. Thye (*Klin. Monatsbl. f. Augen-heilk.*, part 2, p. 374, 1903) has reported bilateral congenital defect of the anterior layer of the iris affecting father (aged 32 years) and son (aged 10 years) similarly, although the lesion was more extensive in the father's eyes. The other living child, a girl, had normal eyes; but an infant that died at six months had the same anomaly as the father, according to the statement of the observing and credible parents. Both father and son were physically sound except as to their eyes. Both had horizontal nystagmus, and the son had alternating divergent squint also. In the father's right eye the iris dilated only above and below, under atropin, giving a vertically oval pupil; in the left there was an operative coloboma above, and the pupil reaction was weak. Both pupils were somewhat displaced upward. His corneas were each but 10 mm. in diameter. The vision with cataract glasses was 6/18 partly in each eye. The son's pupils were displaced upward, somewhat, and their reaction to light was good. With correction of moderate hyperopia and astigmatism, R. V.=6/18 partly, L. V.=6/24 partly. The father showed operative aphakia in the left eye and mature cataract, which was later extracted, in the right. The son presented punctate opacities in the left lens. The anterior layer was absent from about one-half the surface of the father's irides, and about one-fourth of the son's, the remaining portion being unaffected. The pigment layer showed distinctly in this area; and in one spot in one eye of father and son the iris was entirely deficient, the lens opacity being seen through these openings. Both patients were decided blondes; and the grey-blue of the unaffected stroma made a sharp contrast to the brown, exposed pigment layer of the iris.

Thye referred to Manz's case of hereditary bridge-coloboma affecting two generations, and congenital anomalies or hereditary defects of the iris as described by a number of observers.

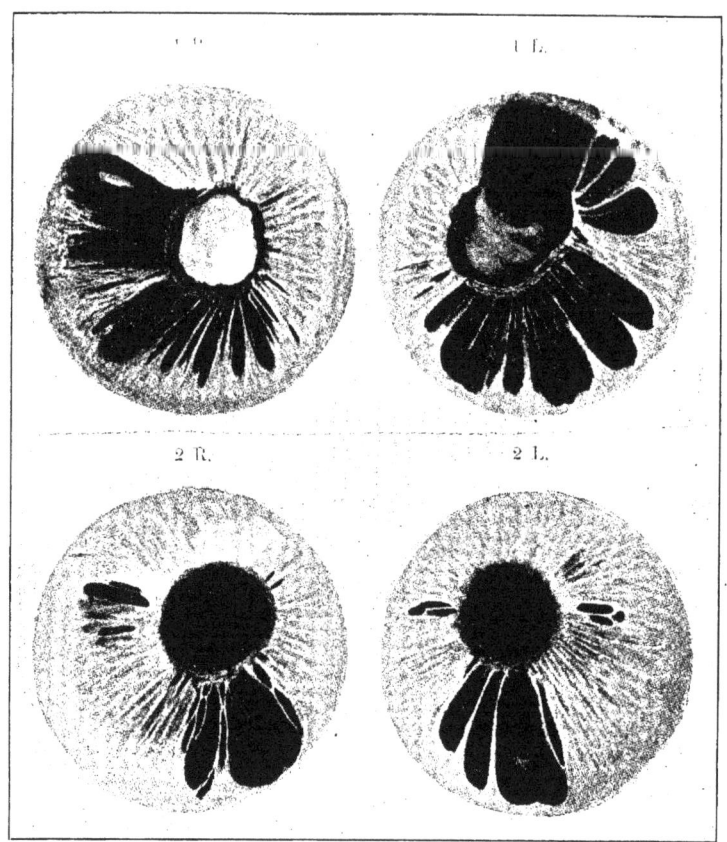

Bilateral Congenital Defect of the Anterior Layer of the Iris in Two Generations. (Thye.)

Heterochromia. A. M. Gossage (*Quarterly Journal of Medicine,* April, 1908, p. 341) mentions a family in which heterochromia of the iris tended to appear when one eye, always the left, was greyish-blue in color, with chestnut-brown patches. Of the offspring of the affected members of the family, 8 were affected and 22 free.

Coloboma. W. C. Posey (*Annals of Ophthalmology,* Vol. 12, Jan., 1903, p. 1) has described two cases of congenital coloboma of the iris affecting both eyes of a mother and, to a much less degree, the daughter's eyes. The corneæ and pupils were ovoid, at corresponding axes. There were also very large colobomata of the optic nerve and choroid of the mother's right eye and of the choroid only of her left eye. The daughter's right fundus showed degenerative retino-choroidal changes of a character and location to suggest the hered-

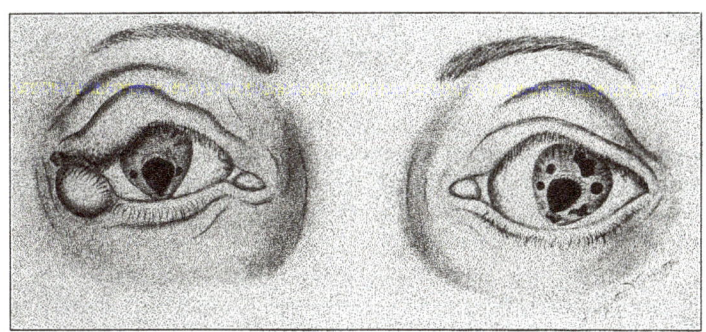

W. C. Posey's Cases of Hereditary Coloboma of the Iris.   (Mother.)

itary influence of her mother's defect.   Her left fundus was normal. See the illustrations.

Plange (*Klin. Monatsbl. f. Augenheilk.*, Oct., 1912, p. 490) reports a girl of fifteen years, in whom the anterior surface of the iris was absent in several places in one eye; while in the other there was only

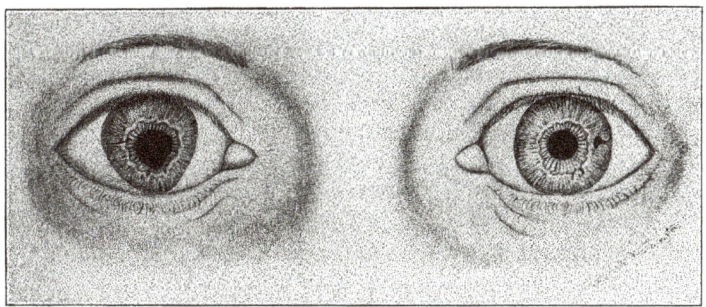

W. C. Posey's Cases of Hereditary Coloboma of the Iris.   (Daughter.)

rudimentary development of its ciliary portion, with numerous separations from the underlying tissues, which were adherent to the posterior surface of the cornea at the root of the iris.   Diffuse corneal clouding and cataract were present in each eye.   The father of the child presented identical anomalies.

Family anisocoria. Paderstein (*Klin. Monatsbl. f. Augenheilk.*,

Vol. Ll, p. 105, July, 1913) reports a family, of which all five members showed a difference in the size of the pupils, with normal reaction. The difference was very pronounced in the mother, a daughter of fourteen and one of nine years; less in the father, and very slight in a daughter of eleven years. In the father syphilis could not be excluded, but examination of the others resulted in negative findings. Blood tests were not made. Paderstein believes the condition should be considered a family congenital anomaly.

The writer has seen a medical man with anisocoria, the right pupil being larger than the left, and the relative difference being maintained in varying illumination. He stated that his adult sister has the same anomaly, only her left pupil is the larger. The doctor's only child, its mother, grandparents and, so far as known, its great grandparents had pupils of equal size.

Iridocyclitis. E. Ehrensberger (*Ophthalmic Review*, 1912, Vol. XXXI, p. 241) has reported recurring iridocyclitis ("moon-blindness") in four pedigrees of horses, in Switzerland, in which the number of affected offspring varied from 64 to 86 per cent. While this disease seems to be an acquired condition influenced by the environment of an unhealthy soil, yet through some special susceptibility, as the transmission of a lowered resistance, heredity appears to be an important factor in its production. Horse breeders carefully avoid introducing an affected stallion or mare into their stables.

HEREDITARY ANOMALIES OF THE LENS.

Cataract. E. Nettleship (*Royal London Ophthal. Hosp. Reports*, Vol. XVI, part 3) traced senile and juvenile cataract through 167 families, three to six generations being affected; and studied 238 cases of congenital cataract. In one family thirty members in four generations showed the defect. The transmission was direct, from one or both parents to offspring, rarely skipping a generation. In some families he noted a striking tendency for the cataract to appear at about the same age, generation after generation; but on the whole it appeared or ripened earlier. In four out of ten families affected, the parents of children with complete congenital cataract were first cousins.

B. L. Millikin (*Amer. Jour. of Ophthal.*, March, 1903) observed fourteen cases of hereditary cataract in three families. In two it was traced through three generations. In one family cataract developed during early childhood for three generations, being bilateral in each case.

J. A. Campbell (*Jour. Ophthal., Otol. and Laryngol.*, April, 1913) has noted five cases, consisting of the father, two sons, one daughter and a niece, each of whom developed cataract in both eyes between the ages of 25 and 29. The members of the family were remarkable for their size and perfect physical development. The author operated upon both eyes of the two boys and one eye of their sister with perfect visual and cosmetic results. The father was 72 years of age and had been operated upon when he was thirty. In both eyes there had been an upward iridectomy. The pupils were small, drawn upward and dimmed by dense, spider-web-like lines. R. V. w.+8 sph. was 15/100, L. V.=light perception. The vision of the right was improved to 15/50 by a needling. The cousin of this group was a woman of 40. She was paralyzed and bed-ridden, when a girl had "sore eyes," and the right eye was removed. The left eye had been blind for a number of years, and showed constant nystagmus, chronic conjunctivitis, with an atrophied nuclear cataract; light perception nil. No ancestral history could be obtained, as the patients had emigrated to this country when very young.

Congenital cataract. E. Nettleship and F. M. Ogilvie (*Trans. Ophthal. Soc. of Un. Kingd.*, Vol. XXVI) collected twenty cases of hereditary congenital cataract among 150 members, in a family history covering seven generations. The time of appearance of the cataract ranged from 10 to 82 years. In every case the inheritance was direct, from parent to child.

Zonular, or lamellar, cataract. A. Collomb (*Archiv. d'Ophtal.*, Vol. XXXI, p. 549, 1911) has reported zonular cataract in two and probably three generations of the same family. In six children of the supposedly third generation one was slightly affected, while two showed pronounced cataract, and three were unaffected.

J. S. Manson (*Trans. Ophthal. Soc. of Un. Kingd.*, Vol. XXXII, p. 45, 1912) has recorded hereditary lamellar cataract occurring in four consecutive generations, affecting six males and seven females, all living. The cataract was transmitted in all cases by affected females. Three members of the pedigree in different generations had a congenital deformity of the little fingers; but only one person showed both the digital and lenticular abnormality. A study of this pedigree revealed no connection between cataract and absence or scantiness of pigment in the iris stroma.

Juvenile cataract. E. Nettleship (*Trans. Ophthal. Soc. of United Kingdom*, 1912, Vol. XXXII, p. 337) reported a pedigree of 129 individuals, seventeen cases showing what he termed "presenile or juvenile cataract," and five presenting one or more vacuoles in their lenses.

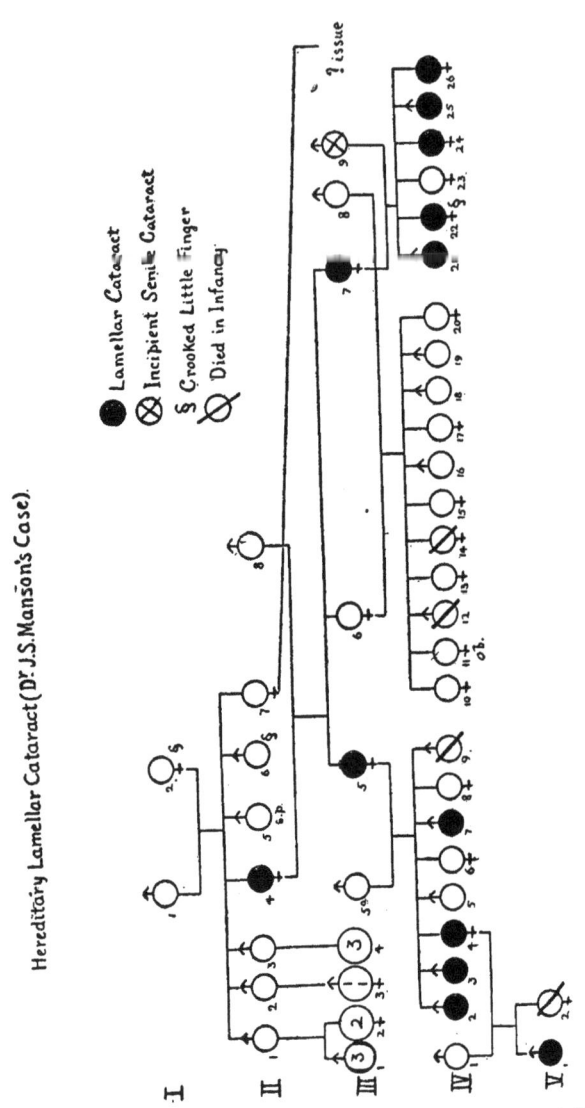

Genealogical Tree Showing Descent of Lamella Cataract and Digital Deformity.
(Manson.)

In one case only was cataract diagnosed as early as eight years. In the entire series a posterior polar opacity probably formed either before birth or within the first few years. Scattered cortical opacities formed during childhood, leading to general cataract in middle life. The cataract was not characteristically lamellar nor did the polar opacity resemble discoid or coralliform cataract. The operative results were very good. Evidently in this pedigree the occurrence of the cataract was not associated with lack of pigment in the stromâ of the iris, as only one-fourth had blue or grey irides.

Discoid cataract. E. A. Dorrell (*Trans. Ophthal. Soc. of Un. Kingd.*, Vol. XXXI, p. 157, 1911) reports a mother, aged 45, and four out of seven living children, all of whom showed discoid cataract.

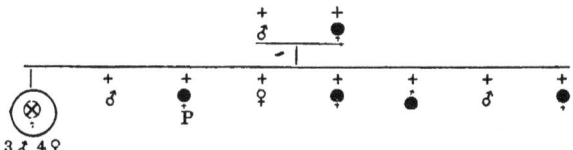

3 ♂ 4 ♀

+ Examined.   ♂ Male *nil.*   ♂ Male affected.   ♀ Female *nil.*
● Female affected.   ⊗ Dead, nothing known.   P Patient.

Genealogic Tree Showing Descent of Discoid Cataract.   (P. Smith.)

The children ranged in age from 21 years to 4 months. Seven children had died young, of whom nothing was known. The father was unaffected. Of the affected children, Ethel, aged 21, showed discoid cataract of Ogilvie's "first variety," Violet, aged 11, discoid cataract of less density and more granular in the center; Walter, aged 6 years, moderately dense discoid of the first variety in the left eye, but in the right the opacity was so transparent as to be barely detected, and corresponded to Ogilvie's "second variety;" Ivy, aged 4 months, presented a translucent discoid cataract in each eye.

In the *Ophthalmic Review*, Nov., 1909, pp. 341-2, Priestley Smith has a chart containing an extensive pedigree of congenital discoid cataract, consisting of 6 generations of a family named Forman, settled in Leicestershire. The family belongs almost exclusively to the laboring class, some are farm laborers, and some coal miners. On the whole they are a healthy family; many have dark hair, like the Coppock family (see this *Encyclopedia*, Vol. V, pp. 3316-3322) but there are to be found some with light hair, both among the affected and unaffected.

The cataract was in all cases found to be discoid and post-nuclear, the size varying and thus producing different degrees of visual impairment.

John Forman, the progenitor, was known to be troubled with a peculiar weakness of his sight all his life, so that he had to shade his eyes to see well; of his two brothers the elder had good sight and left many descendants among whom no defect of the kind had been known; the younger brother died without issue. John Forman had 14 children, and several of these had large families. The number of his descendants was 113, and of this number information was obtainable as to 102, and out of these 26 were affected with discoid cataract; of the 26 affected, 24 have been examined. Excluding unaffected childships, and also from affected childships persons about whom no

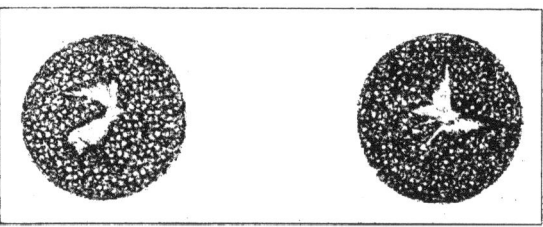

Unusual Types of Punctate Cataract.   (Holloway.)

information was forthcoming, we have 51 cases remaining, of whom 26 are affected; this equals 50.9 per cent.; 15 male and 11 female. With one exception every affected person who has had offspring has transmitted the disorder, the exception being in the case of a man who has at present only one child.

The form of cataract which affects this family has, therefore, the character of a dominant according to the Mendelian theory.

Hereditary punctate opacities. The writer has observed numerous peripheral punctate opacities in the outer fourth of the lens, of identical appearance, in a mother, aged thirty-seven, and her daughter of twenty years. Except for errors of refraction these eyes were not otherwise affected. Correcting lenses gave normal vision.

Anterior polar cataract with punctate opacities. T. B. Holloway (*Ophthalmic Record*, Aug., 1913, Vol. XXII, p. 407) reports a peculiar anterior polar cataract, with diffuse punctate opacities of a robin's-egg-blue tint involving the anterior and posterior cortex of the lenses. All three children were affected: a sister of 28 years, two brothers of 24 and 31 years, respectively. The fundus was normal in each case. The sister had a comma-shaped central posterior polar cataract in both eyes, much smaller than the anterior polar opacity. The vision was from $\frac{1}{4}$ to $\frac{1}{2}$ of normal in the different patients. Heredity was not evidenced unless a paternal aunt of sixty years, with "bad eyes," had lenticular degenerative changes. Holloway also mentions two brothers, Russian Jews, aged 12 and 11 years, with greyish dots centrally grouped in the deeper cortical layers of the lenses, forming a disk the concavity of which was directed forward, and apparently 5 mm. in diameter. The nucleus was clear, and the eyes normal except for the lenticular opacities. The vision was 6/12 in each eye. Both parents and three sisters showed no pathologic changes. Holloway regarded all these cases as congenital, but was uncertain whether they were stationary or progressive. They are of the family type of disease.

Posterior polar cataract. W. F. Matson has personally reported to the writer binocular posterior polar cataract affecting two daughters of a man who had suffered from defective vision all his life, but without a history of traumatism or inflammatory disturbance. One of these daughters had no children; the other had two daughters and a son, both girls showing the mother's defect in each eye. Numerous efforts to secure the boy for examination have failed. In a letter to Dr. Matson, E. Nettleship stated that these cases of hereditary posterior polar cataract were the first to which his attention had been drawn.

Bishop Harman (*Ophth. Review,* Aug., 1909, pp. 244-45) shows charts of pedigrees of three families with eye defects. 1. Posterior polar cataract: The lens defect took the form of a mass of opacity in the posterior layers of the lens proper. In one case the opacity extended to the nucleus, and in another projected from the front of the lens through the pupillary opening, so forming a true "axial cataract." In the first generation no defect could be discovered from the available evidence. In the second generation two were affected. Both married and had affected children; the elder had five children, three being blind; the younger had three children, all blind. Of this third generation one had married a woman who had previously born a normal child to another man. Eight children were born; two were blind and four had minor eye defects. All were dwarfed both in stature and in mind. 2. Anterior polar cataract and microphthalmia: The globes were very small, corneæ measuring 7 mm., with marked squint, nystagmus, and minimal vision. In the first generation a woman, the condition of whose eyes was not traceable, married twice. It is interesting to find that in each childship she had an affected child. One of these affected children married a woman from a normal family; of their eight children, two are blind. Two of one child-ship—one affected and one not affected—died insane. 3. Lamellar cataract: A boy of 14 was found to have bilateral cataract, slight in one eye, marked in the other. His teeth were honey-combed in the extreme. The boy's father had identical defects, and both had suf-fered severely from fits in the first year of life. Investigation of the connections of the family showed that no lens defects had appeared in any member in any branch; only it was found that the man's children had feeble viability, for of five only one survived the second year.

Harman thought that a germ-plasm transmission of defect could not certainly be held to explain such a likeness in father and son. Similarity in conditions of life might be sufficient, but the point could only be decided if and when the boy had progeny. Of the other two histories, there could be no doubt that the transmission of a germ-plasm defect was responsible for the inheritance of the eye conditions.

Ectopia lentis. F. W. Marlow (*Archives of Ophthalmology,* Sept., 1903) has reported six cases of congenital dislocation of the lens occur-ring in one family, and traced abnormality of the eyes, probably of this nature, through five generations. In only one of these six cases was the lens used in the act of vision. The others used the aphakic part of the pupil. From one of his patients, aged twenty-two, Mar-low removed one eye on account of buphthalmos. It had been en-larged since birth, and staphylomatous for four years previous to its removal.

In a family that had been under observation six years J. S. Hos-ford (*Trans. Ophthal. Soc. of Un. Kingd.,* 1911, Vol. XXXI, p. 50) observed that six out of seven children had congenital dislocation of both lenses, the exception being the eldest, aged 21 years. Two chil-dren had been seen by Hosford a few weeks after their birth. Of the twelve dislocated lenses, one was displaced upwards, two outwards, two inwards, and seven upwards and outwards, the corectopia gen-erally corresponding in direction. The lenses floated in the vitreous in every instance. The parents, uncles and aunts were healthy, the family history was negative as to syphilis, gout and tuberculosis, and no relatives were known to have any malformations of the eyes or other parts of the body.

Dehenne and Baillart (*Bull. de la Soc. Fran. d'Ophtal.,* p. 227, 1911) give a genealogic tree of double congenital luxation of the lens. Four generations were affected. All of the six descendants of the first recorded case showed the same anomaly. The sexes were about equally divided as to the numbers involved.

J. Strebel (*Archiv. f. Aug.*, 78, p. 208, and *Ophthalmology*, Vol. XI, pp. 790-91, July, 1915) describes the history of a family, studied in Eichorsts' medical clinic, which showed through four generations an hereditary transmission of a specific predisposition to acquired rheumatic valvular affections through the mother; and besides, in the third and fourth generations, an hereditary propagation of congenital diseases of the aorta through the father, where the rheumatic and infectious elements were not conspicuous. The simultaneous occurrence of congenital ocular affections (ectopia lentis, ectopia pupillæ and myopia), partly from embryologic causes, excluded any doubt of the hereditary character of the heart lesions. Then O. Steiger reports thirty-five cases of interesting local and general correlations, observed at Haab's eye clinic.

A. R. Gunn (*Ophthalmoscope*, Apr. 1912, Vol. X, p. 193) reported seventeen out of twenty-two children, the offspring of an affected and unaffected parent in five families, all of whom showed bilateral and complete congenital dislocation of the lens, without coloboma of the uveal tract. The sexes were about equally affected, and the ratio of affected to unaffected children was about 3:1. The condition was not a Mendelian recessive, for in two families it acted as a pure dominant. The lens was well-developed and clear in the three children examined, and floated in the vitreous. In three adults examined small pupils and posterior synechia prevented a satisfactory inspection of the interior of the eye, but the absence of the lens was demonstrated. Whether the suspensory ligament was ruptured or congenitally absent could not be determined by the reporter.

G. G. Lewis (*Archiv. of Ophthal.*, May, 1904) noted hereditary dislocation of the lens affecting sixteen persons in six successive generations.

Congenital aphakia. S. Toufesco (*Ann. d'Oculist.*, Aug., 1904) has reported a case of congenital aphakia, and collected fifteen other cases previously recorded. Most of the cases showed other abnormalities of the eye. Toufesco expressed the belief that, as a rule, the absence of the lens was due to a process of degeneration and absorption of the previously formed lens, rather than a fault of embryonic development. See, also, **Coppock cataract.**

HEREDITARY DISEASES OF THE OPTIC NERVE.

Hereditary optic atrophy was first described by T. Leber (Graefe-Saemisch *Handbuch*, Vol. V) in 1871, whence it has been called "Leber's disease." It is an affection of the papillo-macular bundle of neurons, is evidenced by a central scotoma and ends in optic atrophy of varying degrees.　In 1877 Leber added to his previously reported cases, collecting a total of fifty-five in sixteen families.

C. Behr (*Klin. Monatsbl. f. Augenheilk.*, p. 138, Aug., 1909) described an unusually early appearing bilateral optic atrophy which he classed as hereditary.　It occurred in six cases, and all were boys, affected in early childhood.　Other parts of the nervous system were involved.

Raymond and E. Koenig (*Rec. d'Ophtal.*, p, 65, 1909) have reported four family groups of optic atrophy, and point out their medico-legal'importance.　They cite cases in which compensation was claimed and allowed for optic atrophy ascribed to slight injury or to retrobulbar neuritis due to exposure.

V. Hanke (*Klin. Monatsbl. f. Augenheilk.*, June, 1903) had made a similar observation in the case of two brothers.

R. D. Batten (*Trans. Ophthal. Soc. of Un. Kingd.*, Vol. XXIX, p. 144) reported two cases in one family, together with a cousin.　All were affected before twenty.　The family history indicated transmission through healthy mothers, as is usual in this disease.

Twelve cases of optic atrophy (*Royal London Ophthal. Hosp. Reports*, Vol. XVII) in one family were traced by W. I. Hancock through five generations.　Six cases recovered good sight.　Each affected person was a male, and the optic degeneration was transmitted through healthy daughters to grandsons of the affected male.

Arnold Knapp (*Archiv. of Ophthal.*, July, 1903) observed eight cases in three generations, being discovered at 6 years of age.　The disease was transmitted from the father to two sons and two daughters, and through one of these daughters to three of her sons.

In 1909 E. Nettleship (*Trans. Opthal. Soc. of Un. Kingd.*, Vol. XXIX) collected all published and many unpublished cases of this disease; in all 180 separate records, with references.　In 150 cases atrophy appeared between 6 and 67 years, the largest number occurring at about 20 years.　He gave a resumé and analysis of hereditary optic atrophy, together with a number of genealogic charts, and an abstract of all published cases in chronological order.　Nettleship characterized Leber's disease as an example of so-called "sex limited" inheritance, thus resembling color-blindness, the transmission being through apparently normal females and usually affecting only males. Consanguinity was rare; the only risk from it being when an affected male married a cousin who carried a latent liability, inherited either from her affected father or, through her mother, from an affected ancestor.

L. V. Cargill (*Ophthalmoscope*, Vol. X, p. 62) has reviewed the subject from Leber's time to the present, and has an important bibliography of various contributions to the study of this disease. As it seems probable that the primary pathologic changes are in the retina, the term "hereditary central retinitis" has been suggested. Cargill pointed out that light-perception has been retained in all cases; that, as a rule, the sight remained stationary after the rapid initial onset, and that improvement might be delayed for as long as one, two or even three years. Hence a hopeful, expectant attitude should be observed during that period. He found both eyes usually affected, and generally at the same time, and that the liability to the disease was hereditary. It occurred most frequently in males, usually about the age of twenty years, and was transmitted by unaffected females.

A. Lutz (Graefe's *Archiv f. Ophthal.*, Vol. LXXIX, p. 399) considers the principles of heredity in connection with some pedigrees of hereditary optic atrophy, and myopia associated with a brown iris in a family in which this occurred as a dominant, while a blue iris occurred as a recessive character.

J. Taylor and G. M. Holmes (*Trans. Ophthal. Soc. of Un. Kingd.*, Vol. XXXIII, pp. 95 and 116, 1913) record two families showing familial optic atrophy. In the first, three out of four living male children were affected, two sisters being unaffected. The parents had good vision. Beyond them the family history was not obtained. In the second family, three out of six males had the visual defect of Leber's disease, while the four females were not involved. The parents had no known atrophy. Two of the mother's sisters were married: one had a healthy son who begat four healthy children; the other had seven children, four females, three males, all of the latter showing family optic atrophy. One of these daughters had an affected son. The chief points of interest are: (1) The visual affection occurred only in males but was transmitted through females. (2) In many cases the initial failure of vision was sudden and did not progress after four weeks. In others the onset was slower and more gradual. No marked improvement in vision occurred in any case. (3) Peripheral contraction of the visual fields was noted in several cases, and in two patients complete blindness developed in one eye only. (4) When more than one member of the family was affected the younger members developed the disease at an earlier age. (5) One case showed cataract in early life, another died from orbital tumor, and several members of one family had migraine. (6) Two sons of another branch, through the female line, showed a peculiar visual disturbance, probably due to some congenital defect.

Taylor and Holmes discuss the signs of organic nervous disease that may be associated with optic atrophy of the family type, indicating the necessity of differential diagnosis between this disease and tabetic atrophy, retrobulbar neuritis, diabetes, poisoning by lead,

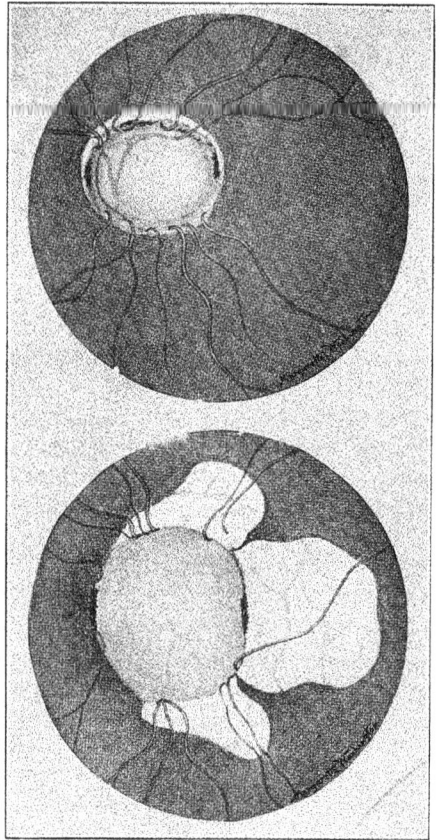

Binocular Coloboma of the Optic Nerve.   (Crampton.)

carbon bisulphide or other organic or inorganic substances, or papilledema from increased intracranial pressure or renal disease. Leber pointed out that hereditary optic atrophy is often found in families with a neuropathic taint, in which headache, vertigo, tremors, numbness of the limbs and such symptoms occur. Rarely have associated organic lesions been recorded, however. From a group of seven cases, Taylor and Holmes concluded that the most common physical signs were absence or diminution of the deep reflexes, especially the ankle- and knee-jerks; numbness or tingling of the limbs; dull, aching pains; some analgesia, anesthesia or loss of station; occasionally slight sphincter troubles, and some mental disturbance early in the disease. An important bibliography is appended to the treatise.

A. S. Worton (*Lancet*, p. 1112, Oct. 18, 1913) records eleven cases occurring in three generations. All the affected persons were males, from 9 to 32 years of age. Of four cases personally examined, two had retained practically normal vision, but with some deficiency of the light sense; in another the vision equalled hand movements only, while the fourth was under treatment for optic neuritis. Of six living cases not examined one was said to be blind, one to have bad sight, two said to have improved, and of the other two nothing was ascertained. When improvement in vision occurred it was before twenty years. After describing the disease Worton says that it is regarded as primarily a retinal affection, the resulting neuritis being of the ascending type. The all-important predisposing cause of heredity seems to imply an inherent instability of the neural elements of the retina, especially affecting the macula as consisting of the most highly specialized cells. A depression of the general vitality would serve to precipitate an attack.

F. Mügge (*Zeit. f. Augenheilk.*, Vol. XXV, p. 236) has reported four cases occurring in two families. The first family consisted of five sons and one daughter. The first and third sons were affected. The vision of one was found to be impaired when he entered school. At twenty three his disks were pallid, especially the temporal halves. The right field of vision presented a sector defect for colors, above, and a central scotoma. The left field was not taken. The other affected child showed failing sight at twelve years. At nineteen there was characteristic pallor of the disks. The color fields were slightly contracted. In both cases some permanent improvement in vision followed strychnine injections. In the second family the two older of the three sons were affected. One, aged 27, discovered poor vision in the left eye at 17 years of age. Two years later the other eye began to fail. The patient became almost blind, but after prolonged use of electricity vision rose to about 5/30. There was contraction for color and absolute central scotoma. The disks were white and vessels narrowed. The other brother discovered one eye to be almost blind at 26 years. The other eye became involved two weeks later. The disks were red-gray and swollen, with peripheral edema. Later, atrophy occurred.

Other articles on hereditary optic neuritis or atrophy to which reference may be made are those of E. Guzmann, in the *Wien. Klin. Woch.*, Vol. XXVI, p. 139; Onishi, in the *Nippon Gank. Zasshi*, Nov., 1913, with 5 illustrations; S. Takashima, in the *Klin. Monatsbl. f. Augenheilk.*, Dec., 1913, p. 714, and **L. P. Marques**, in the *Sem. Med.*, Jan. 9, 1913, Vol. XX.

W. E. Bruner (*Trans. Amer. Ophthal. Soc.*, Vol. XIII, p. 162, 1912), presents *X-ray studies of the spheroid in optic atrophy of the Leber*

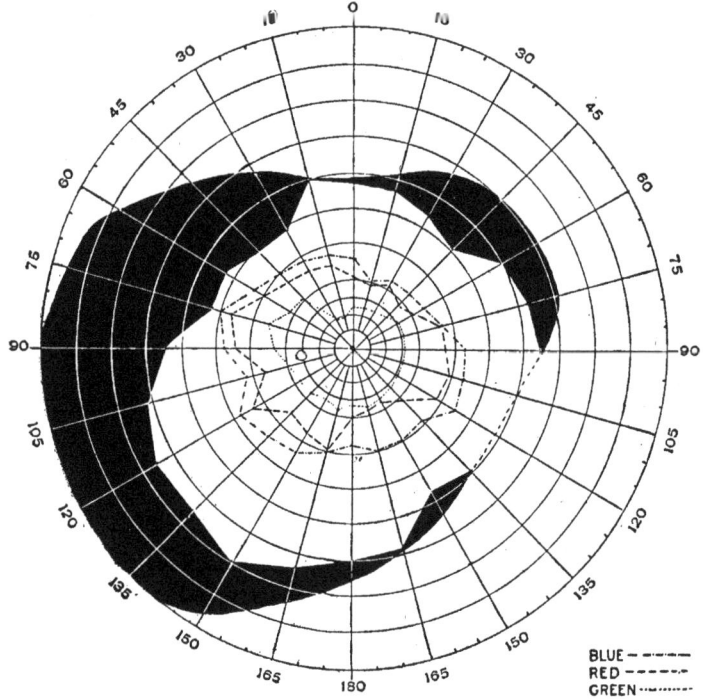

BLUE — —·—·—
RED — — — — —·
GREEN ····—····—

Crampton's Binocular Coloboma of the Optic Nerve.   Left Eye.   Form and Color Fields.

type. The sphenoidal cells were much enlarged in his first patient, a male adult, and the walls were very thin, but there were no evidences of retention beyond a little clear serum in one sinus.; Brain tumor was suspected. Decompression showed an edematous brain, but was attended with no benefit. Despite all treatment the patient's vision steadily declined and the fields contracted. A sister and a nephew affected with this disease showed considerably enlarged sphenoidal cells. Another sister and the mother, both unaffected, showed much smaller cells than the affected members of the family. With one exception normal individuals examined showed sphenoidal cells that were much smaller than the patients with optic atrophy. Bruner suggests the advisability of studying other patients thus afflicted, to

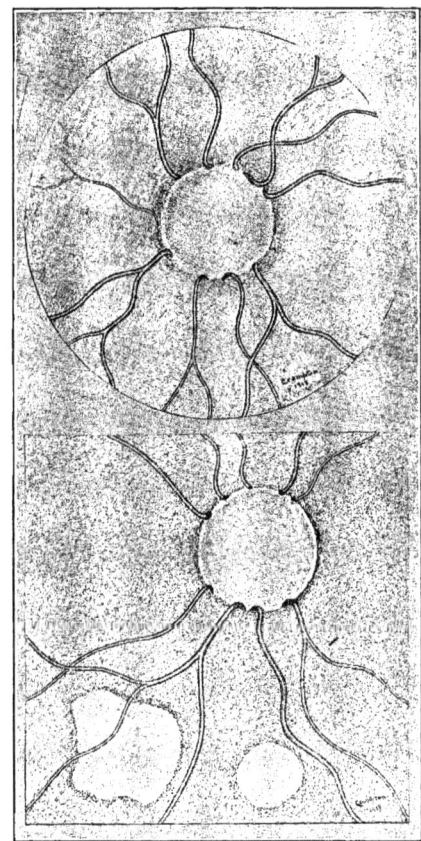

Binocular Coloboma of the Optic Nerve. (Crampton.)

determine the relation, if any, between enlarged sphenoidal cells and familial optic atrophy. He points out that these cells do not attain their full size until puberty, normally, and that their development is often delayed until late in life.

Coloboma of the optic nerve. G. S. Crampton (*Trans. Amer. Opthal. Soc.*, Vol. XIII, p. 451, 1913) reports two cases of binocular coloboma of the optic nerve in the same family. The first case was that of a

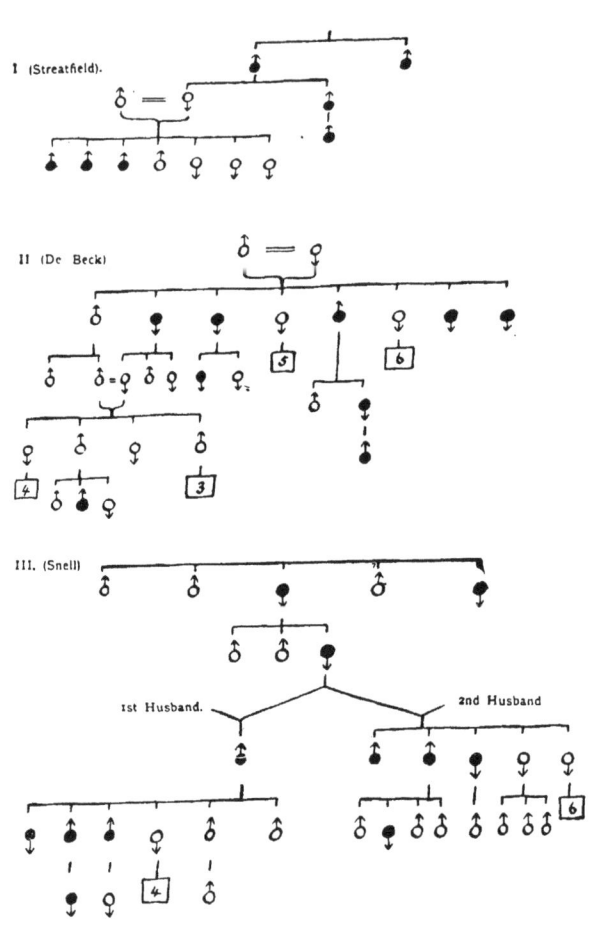

Geneologic Trees Showing the Descent of Ocular Colobomata. (Hird.)

youth of twenty who had been blind in the right eye since birth. This pupil was enlarged and nictitation was excessive and involuntary. The right fundus presented a striking appearance. The papilla was replaced by a large, almost round, sharply defined scleral aperture which seemed about two and a half times the size of the normal disk, although myopia of six diopters no doubt accentuated the size. The aperture was remarkable for its thin, clearly cut edges. Equally clean cut were three larger, wing-like, grayish-white, choroidal faults which enclosed the disk on its temporal side. The rest of the fundus was apparently normal. The left eye was everywhere normal except that the disk, which was somewhat enlarged, was transversely oval and deeply excavated, with a sharply-defined, broad scleral ring. The vision was 6/6 with low myopic correction, and there was a slight reduction of the field of vision. The second case, a sister of the first, was five years of age. She had congenital convergent squint of the right eye, and active lateral nystagmus. Both disks were replaced by deep, round apertures with sharply-defined and apparently undercut margins. The vessels appeared about the edges of the pseudo-disk. In the lower part of the right fundus there were two colobomata, one of which was circular and pearly-white, and about two-thirds the size of the disk. The other was a slightly larger, irregular coloboma of the choroid, with pigmented margins.

R. B. Hird (*Ophthalmic Review*, Vol. XXXI, p. 162, 1912) gives an exhaustive treatise on the various colobomata of the eye. He believes that heredity plays a very important part in these conditions, although in many cases hereditary tendency cannot be traced. He reproduces tables in which the condition was traced through several generations. Hird is of the opinion that colobomatous eyes are more liable to inflammation and disease than normal eyes, and finds that colobomata are frequently associated with other ocular defects.

HEREDITARY ANOMALIES OF RETINA.

Macular degeneration. A. **D**arier (*Clin. Opht.*, Vol. XX, p. 3) describes and illustrates progressive familial macular degeneration in two females out of four living children in one family. The pictures show the fundus changes at intervals of 15 and 20 years. In another family with seven children, three of the six boys were affected. The changes are pictured at an interval of 21 years. Vision was gradually reduced to as low as 1/10 in some cases and 1/50 in others.

Atrophic and pigmentary changes occurred in and about the macula. Darier refers to Stargardt's article (*Zeitschr. für Augenheilk.*, Sept.,

1913, in which three members of one family, aged respectively 45, 43 and 38 years, were affected. It was noticed at 10 years in the first case, and at 14 in the other two. The condition was progressive and all had absolute central scotoma. The first case and the third had extensive maculo-choroidal atrophy. In two cases the atrophy surrounded the disk.

Glioma. H. De Gouvea (*Annal. d'Oculist.*, Vol. CXLIII, p. 32) has recorded an instance of heredity in glioma. The father had the right eye removed, when two years old, for glioma. This diagnosis was confirmed by the microscope. At twenty-one he married a woman whose family history was good in reference to neoplasms. They had seven children. Of the first two, both girls, one had glioma of the retina at five months, the other at two years. Another female child developed glioma at five months. The other four children escaped this form of malignant sarcoma.

Retinitis pigmentosa. Of 976 families (pedigrees) affected by this disease, which is incurable and usually leads to practical blindness, E. Nettleship (*Royal London Ophthal. Hosp. Reports,* Vol. XVII, p. 4; *Trans. Ophthal. Soc. of Un. Kingd.*, Vol. XXIX, p. 95, 1909) found heredity without consanguinity in 230, consanguinity without heredity in 226, and both these factors in 32 affected families. In half of the recorded cases there was no information as to consanguinity or heredity so that the above findings should be based on 488 families fully investigated. It has not been proved that consanguinity can originate retinitis pigmentosa, as Liebrich thought, even though the offspring of cousins show it with striking frequency; but intermarriage does surely act as an intensifying cause by increasing an hereditary tendency. A family has been reported in which twenty males and eighteen females were affected by retinitis pigmentosa in seven generations.

The disease has skipped even three generations and then reappeared with undiminished force.

Nettleship has called attention to one type of heredity which affects the sexes in about the same proportion, and another in which the males only are affected, but the disease is transmitted through the female line alone. He considers that consanguinity of parents emphasizes and even originates hereditary taint. It has also been noted by him that certain families seem subject to varying diseases of the eye, one member having glaucoma, another cataract, a third detachment of the retina or gouty inflammation; and that probably this sometimes indicates an hereditary imperfection of the whole eye, comparable with certain defects of the nervous system.

S. Snell (*Ophthalmic Review,* Jan., 1903) has traced a family history of 67 descendants, 28 showing night-blindness and other evidence of pigmentary degeneration of the retina; males and females being affected in about equal proportions. The disease affected five generations, skipping none. It was transmitted through both males and females, and consanguinity was not proven. Night-blindness made its first manifestations in early childhood, and was complete at 40 years.

Aubineau (*Annal. d'Oculist.,* June, 1903) has reported three out of five of the children of second cousins affected by retinitis pigmentosa;

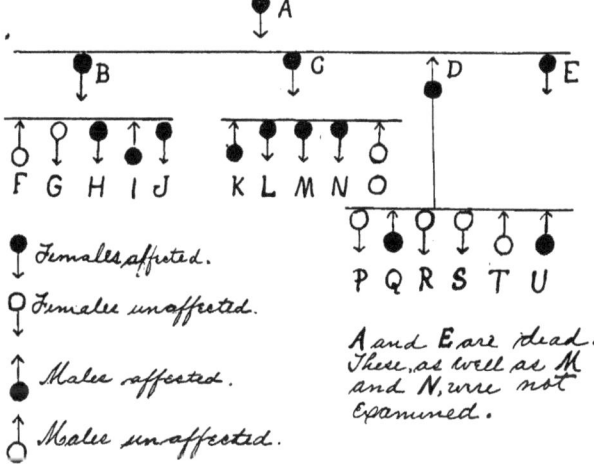

Genealogical Tree Showing Descent of Retinitis Pigmentosa. (Oliver.)

and the case of two affected brothers, whose parents were first cousins. The averages of many observers who have collected data indicates that consanguinity is a factor in fully 25 per cent. of all cases of retinitis pigmentosa.

W. C. Posey had under observation two generations of a family affected by retinitis pigmentosa, it is said, for two centuries. Posey and A. C. Sautter (*Ophthalmic Record,* p. 682, Dec., 1908) have urged that consanguineous marriages should be more generally discouraged by the profession and prohibited by law.

G. H. Oliver (*Ophthalmoscope,* Vol. XI, July, 1913, p. 407) records the hereditary transmission of retinitis pigmentosa to two generations, from a night-blind grandmother to thirteen of her twenty descendants. All her children had it, and nine out of sixteen of her grandchildren.

Oliver examined all but four on the pedigree and found retinitis pigmentosa in ten cases, and felt assured that it was present in the four cases that were reported to him as having the disease. Consanguinity and syphilis were excluded as etiologic factors.

In the *Royal London Hospital Reports* for Jan., 1914, Vol. XIX, p. 130, C. H. Usher gives the most elaborate treatise on the inheritance of retinitis pigmentosa that has yet been published. It consists of 107 pages, 40 genealogic trees, and 6 charts of the visual fields, and a bibliography, with 125 references. He quotes the opinion held by Hutchinson that there could not be the slightest doubt that retinitis pigmentosa was remarkably hereditary, and Landoldt's view that it was almost always hereditary. Usher found that of 35 affected individuals subjected to a Wassermann test, 28 were negative and 7 positive. In 27 out of 40 pedigrees the original case of retinitis pigmentosa was given the Wassermann test. It was negative in 23, positive in 4, and not made in the 13 remaining pedigrees. He suggests that the value of his grouping is diminished by the possibility of a person having had syphilis although the test gave a negative result; and that an individual with retinitis pigmentosa may acquire syphilis. Of 69 examined cases of retinitis pigmentosa, 42 were males, 27 females, a preponderance of males as usual. In 63 cases the onset of symptoms occurred before 12 years in 34 individuals. Thirteen, and possibly 15, of the 69 examined cases were mentally affected; there were 11 deaf mutes and six had no light perception at from 41 to 67 years of age. Of 48 cases examined as to refraction, myopia was found in 18, hyperopia or emmetropia in 28 persons, anisometropia in two. In one case coloboma of the iris was present, in another lamellar cataract, hyaline bodies on the optic disk in three cases, dislocated lens in one case, nystagmus in nine cases. Brothers and sisters of the cases of retinitis pigmentosa showed ocular and bodily defects of structure or functions. In only five out of 53 cases were the fields of vision unimpaired. Night-blindness was present in 57 cases, absent in 2, and not noted in the other 10 cases. Five eyes in three individuals that were found, on first examination, to be without pigment in the retina, showed typical appearances of retinitis pigmentosa on subsequent examinations. Of 21 cases who married (11 males, 10 females) 16 had 91 children, and there were 11 miscarriages. In no instance did a parent with retinitis pigmentosa have a child with the same disease. In 41 marriages of the parents of the original case, consanguinity occurred 9 times. Usher states that it is exceptional to find affected individuals in more than one childship of a pedigree, and refers to Nettleship's figures of 1.72 per family.

Chorio-retinitis. W. Pöllot (Graefe's *Archiv. f. Ophthal.*, Vol. LXXX, p. 379) reports a typical hereditary chorio-retinitis pigmentosa, transmitted from the grandfather through his twin daughters to two sons of each. One son of each daughter was slightly affected, showing only hemeralopia and small scotomas. The other two sons were severely affected. Some of the pigment deposits lay deeper than the retinal vessels, and there were several areas of choroidal atrophy. No intermarriage of blood relations was shown.

A. Lutz (*Klin. Monatsbl. f. Augenheilk.*, p. 699, May-June, 1911) has described what he terms hereditary familial chorio-retinitis. Four

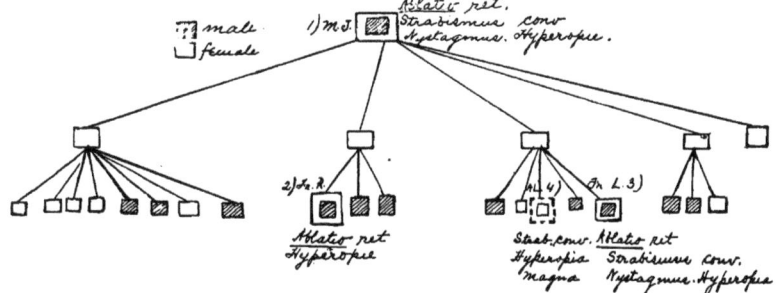

Genealogical Tree Showing the Descent of the Detachment of the Retina.
(Pagenstecher.)

out of six sisters were affected. The other two sisters and the three brothers escaped. The parents and, so far as could be learned, their ancestors, were not affected. There was no consanguinity. In each case the disease appeared in the eleventh or twelfth year, progressed rapidly and reduced vision to 3/60 or 1/60 in a few months. Both eyes were affected. In the posterior part of the fundus there were fine yellowish-grey dots, with minute pigment deposits between them. The light sense was reduced. Except for the ocular disease the patients were healthy.

Retinitis punctata albescens. D. Zani (*Ann. di Ott.*, Vol. XLI, p. 66) records two cases, a brother of twelve years and his sister aged six, in a family of five children. Hemeralopia, lowered vision and white dots in the fundus were observed. In the boy's eyes the white spots were seen in the periphery and about the disk, while in the girl's fundus they were only in the periphery of the retina and were smaller.

A family came under the notice of J. van der Hoeve (*Klin. Monatsbl. f. Augenheilk.*, April, 1913) one member of which had retinitis punctata albescens, another retinitis punctata albescens combined with a typical retinitis pigmentosa, while a third presented a number of albinotic patches in the fundus. These three were deaf-mutes. Of the three remaining members, one had an albinotic fundus, the second was hemeralopic and had albinotic conditions in the fundus periphery, while the third had normal eyes and ears. Among the other relatives there were cases of dwarfism and idiocy.

Detachment of the retina. H. E. Pagenstecher (Graefe's *Archiv. f. Opthal.*, Vol. LXXXVI, p. 457, 1913) reports detachment of the retina with hyperopia, affecting a man and two of his eleven grand-sons. Eight granddaughters escaped. One granddaughter and one of the affected grandsons had convergent strabismus, and the other affected grandson also had nystagmus, like the grandfather. The second generation was unaffected. It contained one unmarried and four married persons. Pagenstecher refers to Alt's paper (*Amer. Jour. of Ophthal.*, p. 355, 1888) concerning detachment of the retina in three successive generations of a family.

HEREDITARY DISEASE OF THE CHOROID.

Doyne's choroiditis. In the *Ophthalmic Review*, p. 31, Jan., 1900, R. W. Doyne depicts the fundi of four members of a family having this variety of choroiditis. The appearance is one of guttate choroiditis affecting the disc-macula region, the spots being closely grouped, separated sometimes by pigmentation, but more often by none. The disease comes on in adult life, and there appears to be no special family diathesis associated with it.

HEREDITARY GLAUCOMA.

E. Nettleship (*Ophthalmoscope*, Sept. and Oct., 1906) suggested the probable disproportion in size between cornea, ciliary region and lens in inherited primary glaucomas. Three to five generations have been affected; the most extensive invasion being nine out of twenty-two persons in two generations. Anticipation, i. e., the tendency for the disease to appear at an earlier age in succeeding generations, or in the younger members of the same generation, is very marked in some of the cases of glaucoma where heredity can be proved. The child may have both compensatory myopia and glaucoma.

Primary glaucoma. Priestley Smith (*Ophthalmic Review*, Vol. XXXI, p. 289, 1912) states that primary glaucoma sometimes occurs in several members of a family, appearing in two or more generations, and in two or more members of one generation. He thinks a special liability to it may be inherited. Three instances are related in which hereditary glaucoma was associated with well-marked smallness of the cornea. In one eye excised the globe was exceptionally small. He advises measuring the corneal diameters in all cases of glaucoma to determine the frequency of the association of short diameters with hereditary glaucoma. As the cornea attains its full diameter before the tenth year, Smith thinks that it might be possible to prognose hereditary glaucoma or lack of liability to it in the children of a glaucomatous parent or parents.

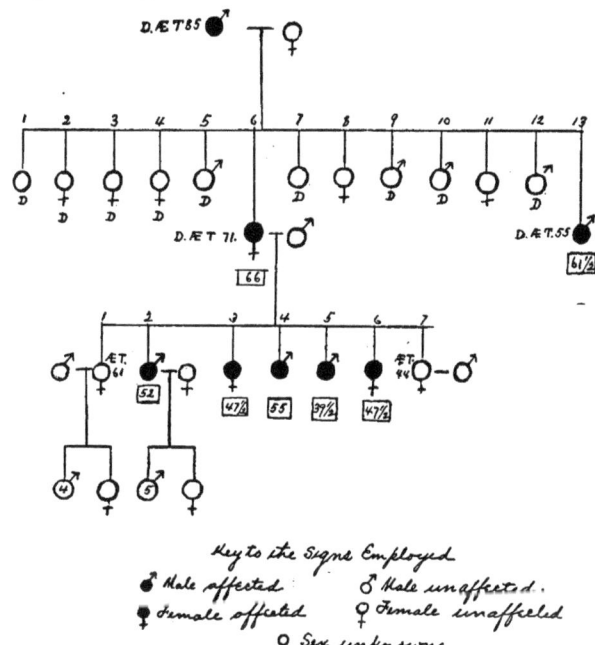

Genealogical Tree Showing the Descent of Primary Glaucoma. (Lawford.)

Generations are indicated by Roman numerals; members of a childship by Arabic figures. The numbers enclosed in squares show the age at which definite glaucomatous symptoms were first noticed.

J. B. Lawford (*Royal London Ophthal. Hosp. Reports,* Vol. XIX, p. 42, 1913) records a family in which three generations showed eight members affected by primary glaucoma. The first generation showed one affected male; the second, an affected male and female out of thirteen children, and the third, three affected males and two females out of ten children. The disease had not yet appeared in the fourth generation. Measurements of the cornea in three members were 12, 12 and 12½ mm., respectively, in both corneas. Lawford established, from analysis of available evidence (*Royal London Ophthal. Hosp. Reports,* Vol. XVII, p. 57) that hereditary primary glaucoma is usually continuous in descent, not skipping a generation to reappear in the next; that anticipation is frequently observed; that it occurs both in the acute and chronic form, and that it may be transmitted by, and inherited by, either sex.

F. P. Calhoun (*Trans. Amer. Med. Asso.*, 1914) reports three generations of one family affected by hereditary glaucoma simplex. Of sixteen individuals, eight exhibited glaucoma; two were amblyopic, with doubtful glaucoma, and six were unaffected. Bad sight was first detected at 11, 12, 13 (2), 14, 17, 21, and 29 years, respectively. The early cases showed reduced vision, elevated tension and contracted fields, without ophthalmoscopic nerve-changes, but in those of longer standing atrophic change and cupping had taken place. In five of the cases thirteen operations were performed on nine eyes. Scleral trephining gave better results than iridectomy or sclerectomy with iridectomy; and the tonometer was found as invaluable in studying the progress of the disease as the thermometer in a febrile condition. Calhoun finds hereditary glaucoma simplex exceptionally rare beyond the second generation, and that only four families are recorded. In his own cases he found no peculiarities, serious illness, or common ailment except malaria; although "anticipation" was prominently displayed. Calhoun notes (1) the early age of the development of hereditary glaucoma, with a decided tendency for it to appear earlier in succeeding generations ("anticipation"); (2) the importance of the smallness of the cornea and globe as a factor; (3) the small part played by general diseases, other than gout and so-called rheumatism, in the causation, and (4) the equal liability of the two sexes as to transmission, with the males showing a greater liability to inheritance.

HEREDITARY AMETROPIA.

Myopia, hyperopia and astigmatism are undoubtedly hereditary defects. Myopia in one parent may be overcome by hyperopia in the other. The writer observed a case of eight diopters of myopia in each of the mother's eyes being counteracted, as an hereditary influence, by emmetropia or hyperopia in the father's line, so that the four children of these parents were emmetropic. Fleischer (*Trans. of 34th Ophthal. Congress of Heidelberg*) found, in a German village where myopia was especially common, that fifty per cent. of the children in seventeen families in which one parent was highly myopic, developed myopia. In another family in which both parents were myopic, all the children manifested the same error. The parents of eighty families in this village had normal eyes in each instance, as did their offspring.

Although myopia is often regarded as a simple error of refraction, grave complications may arise which altogether overshadow the original condition. Myopia is frequently inherited. In a series of 687 cases examined by Claud Worth (*Medical Press,* Mar. 14, 1906) 33 were malignant and 654 were uncomplicated. Of the latter, 56 per cent. gave a family history of myopia, while of the former in only 24.25 per cent. was evidence of heredity found. In one family, whose pedigree was shown, nearly all the males were myopic and none of the females; but the myopia was transmitted through the female line. In all cases examined the amount was about the same, viz., 10 to 12 D. with some astigmatism. The fundi showed crescents, but grave complications were wanting. Curiously enough in this family all the healthy eyes were blue, and all the myopic ones were brown. Night-blindness was only admitted in one family. The statistics of the 687 cases are as follows: Of 313 with no family history of myopia, 163 were males and 150 females. Of 374 with a family history of myopia, 228 ·were males and 146 females. This showed that the usual preponderance of myopia in men was increased in those in which myopia was hereditary. Of the 374 cases in which a family history of myopia was obtained, in 159 the parents were myopic, but the myopia was present in uncle, aunt or grandparent of the other cases. The fault was on the mother's side in 104 cases, on the father's side in 33 cases, and on both sides in 32 cases.

In a report of a case of hereditary nystagmus Casey Wood noted that in the patient's family for four generations the brunettes had invariably nystagmus and myopia; the other members had blue and healthy eyes.

J. A. Wilson (*Brit. Med. Jour.,* Aug. 29, 1914) has tabulated some details of 1,500 consecutive cases of hereditary myopia:

Age Groups. Years.	No. of cases.	Females.	Males.	Av. amt. of myopia. Dioptres.	Percentage of females.
8 and under.....	90	54	36	4.5	60
9–12	227	135	92	3.7	59
13–15	172	102	70	4.2	59
16–20	215	140	75	4.9	65
21–30	318	218	100	5.6	68
31–40	224	163	61	5.9	72
Over 40	254	180	74	6.4	70
Totals	1,500	992	508		

These cases were ophthalmologically selected, and may not represent the relative distribution of these conditions in the general population, but intrinsic evidence may be found bearing on the question
of heredity.

In this table there are 992 females and only 508 males—that is,
there are nearly two females to one male.

His method of classification gives the following results:

```
Grandparents myopic ........................ 54
Mothers myopic ........................... 369
Fathers myopic ...........................254
                                                      —677
Brothers or sisters myopic .....................164
Uncles or aunts myopic ....................... 31
Cousins myopic ............................. 9
                                                      —204
```

In 204 cases the evidence of heredity was collateral and the transmitting parent was not disclosed. Nevertheless the mother obviously
played the larger part in the transmission of myopia.

Myopia was transmitted:

```
From father to son in....................... 79 cases
From father to daughter in...................149 cases
From mother to son in .......................111 cases
From mother to daughter in ..................231 cases
```

These figures do not include all the myopic members of the various
families, for probably both sons and daughters have been omitted;
but, taken as they stand, the fathers transmitted myopia to two daughters for one son, and the mothers also transmitted myopia to two
daughters for one son.

There is evidence of heredity in 58 per cent.; keratitis is classed as
the cause of the myopia in 12 per cent.; cases in which evidence of
heredity is unobtainable, 30 per cent.

Arranged according to the amount of myopia:

```
Low myopia—i. e., up to 3 D......Females 425; males 243
Medium myopia—i. e., 4 to 6 D....Females 249; males 113
High myopia—i. e., 7 to 12 D.....Females 217; males 112
Very high myopia—i. e., over 12 D.Females 101; males  40
```

The following figures indicate the percentages of the cases in these sections that present evidence of heredity; cases due to keratitis are, of course, excluded:

Low myopia ....65 per cent.
Medium myopia ....66 per cent.
High myopia ....67 per cent.
Very high myopia ....67 per cent.

Tscherning's statistics are well known. They were obtained from the examination of 7,523 Danish conscripts, and among these he discovered 627 myopes—that is, 8 per cent. He classed the conscripts as educated and uneducated. In the educated class he had 2,336 persons, and among these he found 420 myopes, or 17 per cent. In the uneducated class he had 5,187, and among these he found 207 myopes, or 4 per cent. The myopia in the educated class was mainly of low degree, and in the uneducated class was mainly of high degree. These figures may or may not apply to present conditions, and may or may not apply to this country; but the inference is that near-work is the cause of low myopia and determines its presence or absence.

Wilson believes that when myopia is clearly hereditary, it exists in all degrees—high and low—but that low degrees are more frequently hereditary than high degrees. High myopia makes its appearance before school-work begins, and therefore must be due to heredity.

Worth has reported several families in which the males alone were affected and where the myopia was transmitted by unaffected females, but these he thinks are pathological curiosities.

Crzellitzer (*Soziale Hyg. und Med.*, No. 14-15) analyzed 330 families affected with more than six diopters of myopia. Male and female members appeared to be equally involved as to the hereditary factor. In 30 per cent. of the cases there was myopia of both parents, in 20 per cent. of the father alone, and in 17 per cent. of the mother alone. Transmissibility of myopia seemed to diminish in later children.

Crzellitzer (*Berlin. Klin. Woch.*, Vol. XLIX, p. 2070) has collected further data, making records of 525 families with high myopia, and 99 with high hyperopia. Consanguineous marriages were strikingly frequent. Girls inherited the tendency to these errors of refraction more often than boys. He points out the urgent need of accumulating reliable records on the subject of the inheritance of ametropia.

G. Bogatch (*Klin. Monatsbl. f. Augenheilk.*, p. 431, Oct., 1911) has reported three generations of a family of thirty-eight members. Eleven had progressive myopia; some with retinal detachment. In all the high myopia developed in early youth, with early blindness in some cases. Consanguinity was probably a factor, as the grandparents and parents of the most affected children were cousins. The grandparents were emmetropic. One of their daughters married a cousin. Five of their seven children were affected. There was also an hereditary predisposition to myopia, from diminished resistance of the sclera at the posterior pole of the eye, which consanguineous marriages emphasized.

G. Perrod (Ann. di Ott., Vol. XLI, p. 34) reports a father and his two children, male and female, with 8 to 18 diopters of myopia in one or both eyes. In another family there were 8 to 10 diopters of myopia in each of five individuals in three generations.

Krusius (38th Ophthal. Congress, Heidelberg, p. 73) made studies of school children, gathering data that convinced him of the certainty of the influence of heredity in causing ametropia, and that the mother exerted the greater influence. By means of photographs he pointed out the connection of myopia with a certain shape of skull.

Barrington and Pearson (Study of the Inheritance of Vision) as the result of their investigations, state that "neither school life nor any other influence save only heredity must be considered to be the cause of myopia."

Astigmatism. Based on ophthalmometric measurements in a large number of children and one or more near relatives, Steiger (Zeitschr. f. Augenheilk., Apr.-May, 1906) found corneal astigmatism inherited from one or the other parent in a large proportion of the cases.

Lucien Howe (Trans. Amer. Ophthal. Soc., Vol. XII, p. 1001, 1911) called attention to the fact that the eye of a child sometimes resembles that of a parent or other ancestor, not only in the kind of astigmatism but approximately in amount, and occasionally even in the meridian of abnormal corneal curvature. Howe discarded simple hyperopic astigmatism with the rule, as so common as to be almost normal, but gave striking examples of astigmatism against the rule in six families, and oblique astigmatism in two generations of one family. His cases indicated that a difference in corneal curvature represented by one diopter, or 0.13 mm. in radius, is transmitted from parent to offspring. The writer has several times observed one-fourth this amount of astigmatism other than with the axis vertical, in both parents and in one or more of their offspring; and is in accord with Howe's statement: "In the far-reaching effect of heredity there is perhaps no more striking example than this, in which a variation from the normal type to so small a fraction of a millimeter is transmitted from one generation to another."

Howe has also observed the inheritance of the same form of hetero-phoria in different members of the same family. He noted marked exophoria in four families, and similar instances have been observed frequently by others. The delicacy of the variations in structure or function in the affected muscles pointedly illustrates the potent in-fluence of the hereditary transmission of even slight defects.

Family exophoria. W. Reber (*Ophthalmic Record*, Vol. XVII, p. 621, 1908) studied seven families with fifty-six members, covering two generations. Of forty persons examined, thirty-four were exophoric. It was found in several instances that individual cranial peculiarities marked those particular members of such families who had "the same kind of headache or neuralgia as their mothers or fathers." Reber used a hatter's conformateur to obtain skull measure-ments in cases of family exophoria in males, and large calipers for females. The diagrams obtained and tables computed were of much interest. The great majority of heads measured fell into the long skulled class. Reber, like Howe, pointed out the minute changes in corneal curves and in the structure or function of the muscles, that are so strikingly handed down from generation to generation.

HEREDITARY HETEROTROPIA.

Different authorities have estimated squint to be hereditary in 33 to 70 per cent. of all cases. Heredity is especially marked in convergent strabismus.

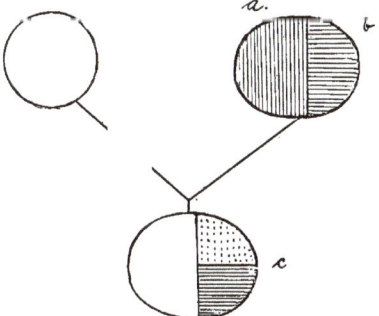

Chart Illustrating the Theory of the Transmission of Amblyopia but not of the Accompanying Strabismus.
a. Weak fusion center. b. Amblyopia. c. Amblyopia of various intensities.
(Bradburne.)

O. Von Sicherer (*Muench. Med. Woch.*, Vol. LIV, 24-25) traced convergent squint through four generations of one family.

A. Peters (*Lancet*, p. 108, Jan. 13, 1912) thinks that the mono-lateral amblyopia of hereditary strabismus may be "the result of an inferiority of the macular area, usually combined with an anomaly of refraction, which in turn may be due to a variation of the germ-plasm of hereditary origin." He further states "that if it should be proved that there are groups of cases of squint in which the hereditary principle is of prepotent influence . . . and that either con-genital amblyopia or the loss of the power of fusing the images . . . is a hereditary characteristic, little hope of improvement by orthoptic treatment can be held out."

In a personal communication to the writer, A. A. Bradburne writes: "Speaking of heredity I am endeavoring to prove that amblyopia which occurs in strabismus can be transmitted, and in these cases it is the presence of a good fusion faculty inherited from one parent which prevents the strabismus becoming manifest."

HEREDITARY NYSTAGMUS.

E. Clark (*Ophthalmoscope*, Sept., 1903) has noted this disease ex-tending through five generations, affecting 23 persons, all males. In each generation none of the daughters was affected; and only the eldest daughter transmitted the defect, and she to her sons only.

Radloff (*Klin. Monatsbl. f. Augenheilk.*, May, 1910, p. 276) described a new family group of miners' nystagmus, which is characterized by very regular undulatory oscillations, varying from 180 to 240 per minute. Vestibular nystagmus, on the contrary, is of the jerking type.

Lenoble and Aubineau (*Révue de Méd.*, March 10, 1911, and *Oph-thalmoscope*, Vol. IX, p. 802, 1911) have described a type of con-genital nystagmus, often affecting several generations of a family and associated in many cases with spasmodic movements of the head, limbs or other parts of the body. Relying upon the frequent co-existence with the nystagmus of myoclonic disturbances elsewhere, these authors name the condition "myoclonic nystagmus." Stigmata of physical or psychical degeneration are not rare in this affection, but in the greater number of cases it is not accompanied by any such defect.

The history of a man, aged 31, who had horizontal nystagmus, from early childhood, is furnished by Caspar. There was irregular and regular myopic astigmatism of the right eye; with correction V.=5/50; hyperopic astigmatism of the left eye; with correction V.=5/30. Excepting atrophy of the choroid around the optic nerve, the fundus was normal in both eyes. His 2 brothers and none of his 5 sisters; the 2 sons and none of the 5 daughters of his mother's sister, had the same affection. None of the 5 daughters of his mother's second sister, nor the son, nor any of the 5 daughters of the mother's third sister were affected. The history shows an hereditary transmission of nystagmus through the parents of the mother to the male descendants. Next to the great number of children, the predominance of the female progeny is remarkable. There was, probably, an hereditary syphilitic element.

In a lengthy treatise, illustrated by many genealogic charts, tables and summaries, E. Nettleship (*Trans. Ophthal. Soc. of Un. Kingd.*, Vol. XXXI, p. 59, 1911) discussed hereditary nystagmus based upon thirteen pedigrees of which four were new. They were divided into two groups: (1) As a rule the nystagmus was associated with head movement, and both sexes were affected by direct inheritance from either parent; (2) Here the nystagmus was without head movement, and males only were affected by inheritance through unaffected females, as in color-blindness and hemophilia. In the first group the nystagmus was horizontal, varying greatly in rapidity and extent, and the head movement diminished with age. Poor sight and marked ametropia, usually hyperopia and astigmatism, characterized both groups. Many cases were of the albino type. There was no evidence of general nerve disease or consanguinity. Color-vision was normal in all the cases examined. Nettleship stated that "In any consideration of the causation of nystagmus in general, I think we cannot but believe that, as in many other conditions, idiosyncrasy, a personal equation, must take a considerable share; and that such liability may, as is often true of other liabilities, be heritable. . . . It must be admitted that the share taken by the several factors in hereditary nystagmus needs further elucidation from neurology and physiology." In discussing this paper, W. Bateson declared it to be the most important of Nettleship's contributions to the study of hereditary diseases, and added that there were no known examples of a disease sex-limited to women, as in men.

W. Niccol (*Ophthalmoscope*, p. 224, May, 1914) states that during the last thirty years there have been recorded, under the name of "Hereditary or Congenital Nystagmus," a number of cases in which oscillation of the eyes was present, as an inherited characteristic, in individuals apparently otherwise normal. It is to the distinguished labors of the late Edward Nettleship, who collected and analyzed these records, that we owe chiefly our present knowledge of the condition.

The following example of inherited nystagmus came under Niccol's notice at the Birmingham and Midland Eye Hospital in January, 1914:

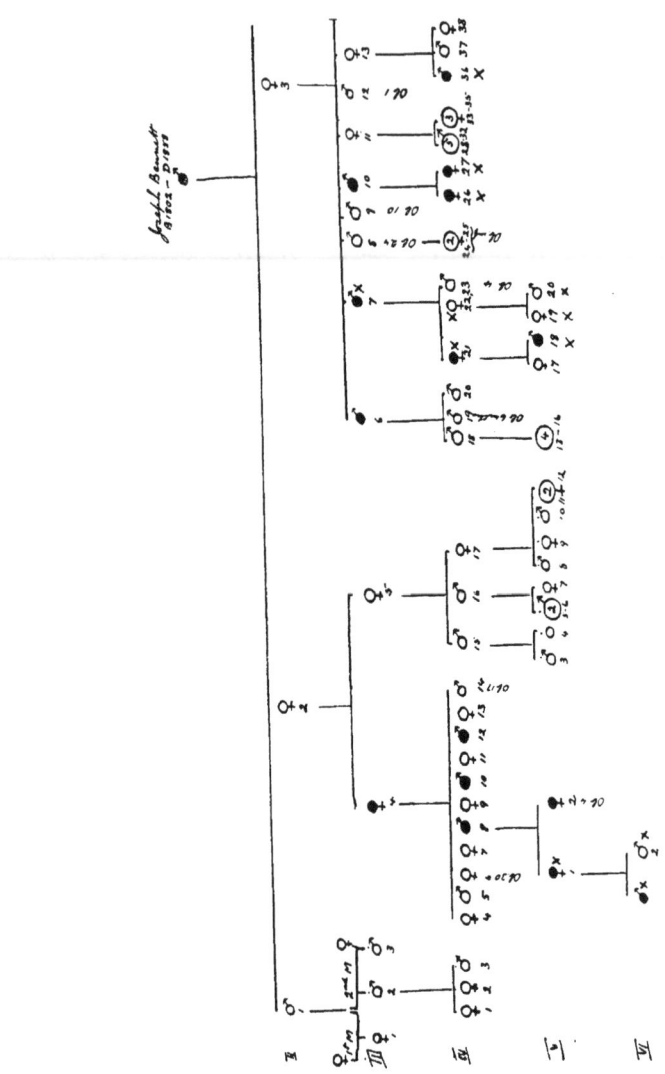

A Pedigree of Hereditary Nystagmus.   (Niccol.)

The patient was a laborer, aged 54 years, who came for advice regarding an erythematous condition of the eyelids. The striking feature which he presented, however, was a continuous oscillation of the eyes. This movement, he said, had been present ever since he could remember; also several other members of his family "worked their eyes" in a similar fashion, having inherited the peculiarity from their grandfather.

The nystagmoid movements were regular, rather slow, horizontal, and concomitant, and slightly increased in rapidity in the extreme lateral positions of the eyes. On ophthalmoscopic examination twitch-

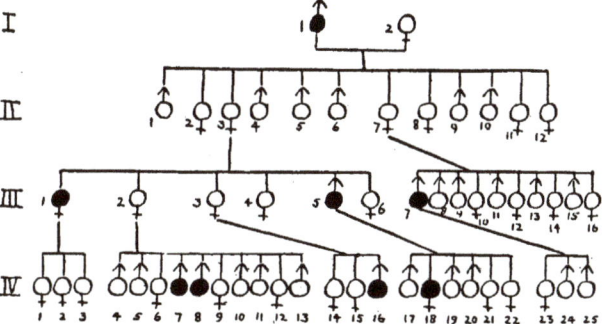

Genealogical Tree Showing Descent of Hereditary Nystagmus. (Nettleship.)

ing of the lids was produced, which increased and finally was accompanied by "shaking" movements of the head. His vision was much below normal (6/36 partly in each eye). This seemed to be due to myopic astigmatism. Correction with glasses gave improvement up to 6/18 only in each eye.

There were one or two small patches of choroidal atrophy close to the macula in each eye. None of these was exactly central.

This man was of rather poor physique, and was said to suffer from chronic bronchitis and dyspepsia; but there was no evidence of any organic nervous disease. He had never worked as a miner. The movements, he said, caused him no inconvenience as a rule. He was unconscious of them, and objects appeared to him to be quite steady.

In this pedigree the transmission was: From father to daughter in 6 cases. From mother to son in 12 cases. From mother to daughter in 2 cases. (In no case from father to son.)

This pedigree of hereditary nystagmus seems of value not only in furnishing additional evidence of the soundness of Nettleship's conclusions, but in showing particularly that the cases of hereditary nystagmus with head movements are related to the male-limited class, and will probably be found eventually to conform in their mode of descent with the Mendelian laws.

As regards the evidence of defective pigmentation, all that can be said is that a majority of the "nystagmists" examined were of rather fair complexion. There was no definite evidence of defective pigmentation of the retina or choroid in any case.

The "nystagmists" are individuals otherwise normal. They are of average physique and intelligence. In all cases examination of the knee-jerks, gait, etc., failed to show any sign of organic nervous disease.

There was no instance of a consanguineous marriage.

AMAUROTIC HEREDITARY AND FAMILY IDIOCY.

R. M. Smith (*Boston Med. and Surg. Jour.*, p. 370, Mar. 7, 1912) has reported two cases occurring, as usually reported heretofore, in Hebrews. The characteristic symptoms are a mahogany-red spot on a white or greyish background in the macular region, decreasing vision, progressive paralysis, mental deficiency going on to idiocy, nystagmus and drooling. All die before three years of age.

H. B. Sheffield (*N. Y. Med. Record,* p. 165, Jan. 27, 1912) has recorded the case of a Hebrew child of eleven months. It developed well the first six months; when it gradually became pale, flabby, less active physically and mentally, and developed the characteristic fundus changes, with blindness and idiocy. The child died of la grippe and pneumonia. An older brother and sister were normal.

In the *Ophthalmic Record,* p. 511, Nov., 1912, H. Gifford states that as opposed to the Tay-Sachs, or infantile form of family amaurotic idiocy, which begins in early infancy and almost invariably leads to death before the fourth year, Vogt pointed out in 1905 that there is a juvenile form beginning, not in infancy, but in early youth; leading slowly to blindness, frequently with paralysis, death after several years, and showing no predilection for the Jewish race. Gifford reports two children affected at 7 years, out of seven living children of mentally defective parents; and also mentions a set of five children which he thinks probably belongs on the outskirts of this group, though decidedly atypical. He gives a good abstract of cases reported by other observers, with a full bibliography and a note on the pathology.

V. Magnus (*Norsk. Mag. f. Laegevidensk.*, Vol. LXXIII, p. 1598) has reported a boy of seven with defective sight, motor disorders and optic atrophy, whose sister had died at fourteen after suffering blindness, paralysis and dementia. He also reported a case resembling typical amaurotic family idiocy of the infantile type occurring in a family of seven children, the other six being healthy. The parents were of old Norwegian peasant origin, without admixture of Jewish blood, were not related, and no nervous or mental disease had affected their families so far as their knowledge went.

Ochi (*Nippon Gank. Zasshi,* Nov., 1912, with Bibl.) reports a typical case of Tay-Sachs disease, the first reported from Japan. He made a microscopic study of the eye ball, and found the usual degeneration of the ganglion cell layer and atrophy of the nerve fiber layer.

In the *Archives of Pediatrics,* Vol. XXX, p. 825, Nov., 1913, A. Hymanson reports six cases of Tay-Sachs disease. In the first two cases studies in metabolism showed that it was not disturbed. A complete post mortem examination of one of these cases was made, with microscopic findings. The next two cases were unique in that two brothers were married to sisters, and their parents were first cousins. Several of their children were afflicted with amaurotic family idiocy. In the last two cases the disease affected twins. Death occurred between seventeen and twenty-four months in each case; and all were of Jewish parentage. Hymanson stated that while the infantile form was usually seen among Hebrews, the juvenile type of the disease is far more common among Gentiles. He expressed the opinion that it is the duty of every physician to discourage the marriage of near kin, and also of persons in whose family there is a neuropathic taint. A good bibliography is added to this article. See also p. 5155, Vol. VII, of this *Encyclopedia.*

HEREDITARY BLINDNESS.

Clarence Loeb (*Trans. Amer. Acad. of Ophthal. and Oto-Lar.,* 1908) has reported a family in which every member for five generations was affected with cataract, and also six families, headed by blind parents, in which seventeen out of thirty-one children were blind. He thinks that about two per cent. of all blindness, and ten per cent. of congenital blindness, is hereditary. In optic atrophy he noted a marked tendency to transmission through a healthy mother to a blind child. It is his opinion, and that of a large number of ophthalmologists to whom he addressed inquiries on this subject, that the marriage of a person afflicted with hereditary blindness should be advised against and, if possible, legally prevented.

The United States census of 1900 showed 64,763 inhabitants were blind. Of this number 2,527 were the children of cousins. Bemis traced 823 marriages of cousins, finding 85 blind (over 10 per cent.), and 145 deaf mutes.

In the *Journal of the Missouri State Medical Association*, Jan., 1913, p. 234, Loeb carries his observations and studies to further conclusions. He believes that evil hereditary influences, except from syphilis, cannot be averted. In three families in which both parents had cataract, 9 out of 15 children were affected. In another family with double heredity as to ophthalmoplegia and ptosis, 8 out of 6 children were affected, and in two families with retinitis pigmentosa, five out of the ten children were affected. In direct heredity with one parent affected, 57½ per cent. of the children were affected; in indirect heredity, 58 7/10 per cent.; in collateral heredity, 66 4/10 per cent. of the children were affected with various incurable diseases or defects of the eyes. He states that there are many cases of indirect heredity where the blindness has skipped one or more generations and reappeared in later ones. He found that of 64,763 blind in the United States, 65 per cent. had married; 2 per cent., or 842 of these individuals, were afflicted with some form of hereditary blindness; and one-half of their children he would expect to be blind. Loeb again advocates immediate attention to this problem; and urges that it should be made impossible, by the strictest legal regulations, for the marriage of a person afflicted with any form of hereditary blindness to take place.

HEREDITARY COLOR-BLINDNESS.

As a rule, color-blindness is transmitted through normal sighted mothers to affected sons, and is comparatively rare among women. E. Nettleship (*Trans. Ophthal. Soc. of Un. Kingd.*, Vol. XXXII, p. 309, 1912) has reported pedigrees departing from this rule. In the first family the maternal grandfather, the mother and all her four sons were color-blind, while her two daughters escaped. The grandfather, mother and one of her daughters had a little finger that was constantly flexed and adducted. The father and mother were not blood relations. Two other families were given in which both sexes showed examples of color-blindness; and of female twins, one only was affected although in bodily features they were almost indistinguishable. Nettleship also recorded two color-blind sisters, all of whose five sons were color-blind, while their two daughters were normal. In another family a color-blind man had two daughters with normal sight. They had three sons and six daughters. All the sons and three of the daughters were color-blind. Nettleship stated the belief that a color-blind female derived the defect from both parents, one being color-blind, the other "carrying" the defect; and that when a female has an heritable condition usually limited to males it is derived from both her parents,

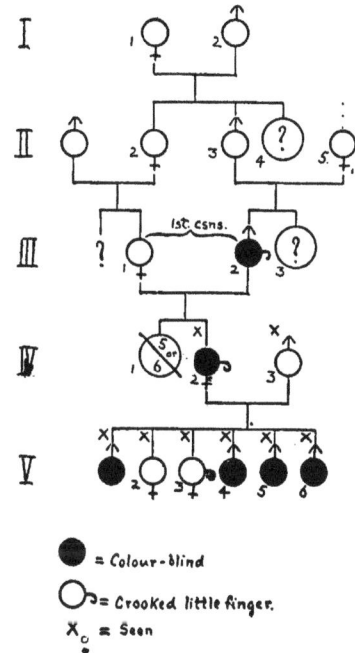

Genealogical Tree Showing the Descent of Color-Blindness. (Nettleship.)

the father showing it, the mother carrying it, latent or undeveloped, from a male ancestor.

C. H. Usher (*Trans. Ophthal. Soc. of Un. Kingd.*, Vol. XXXII, p. 352, 1912) records a pedigree showing the union of two unrelated stocks, both affected by color-blindness. A color-blind man of one family married a normal woman of the other family, who presumably carried the condition. They had two color-blind sons, one son and five daughters unaffected. Color-blindness appeared in twenty-two males in five of the seven generations affected, no color-blind females being discovered. Usher considered that this pedigree suggested that a color-blind male might transmit color-blindness to a son provided he married a woman, herself unaffected, who had a color-blind maternal grandfather. Further, that a female who was not color-blind, but had

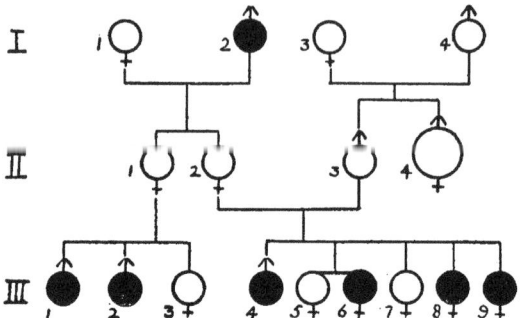

Genealogical Tree Showing the Descent of Color-Blindness. (Nettleship.)

a color-blind maternal grandfather and an unaffected father, could only have color-blind sons provided her husband was color-blind.

HEREDITARY STATIONARY NIGHT-BLINDNESS

Nettleship (*Trans. Ophthal. Soc. of Un. Kingd.*, Vol. XXVII, p. 269, 1907) supplemented Cunier's record of the awful perpetuation of night-blindness in the Nougaret family, between 1637 and 1838, by bringing this history down to 1907. He also further perfected this most remarkable record of a family hereditary disease.

The night-blindness affecting this clan has always been congenital and stationary. It is attended by no pigmentary change in the retina or other discoverable fundus abnormality. Vision is normal by day, but is lost out of doors on nights when the moon does not shine. The general health is uniformly good, and longevity is noticeable.

This pedigree numbers 2121 persons. Night-blindness has been recorded definitely in 135 cases; 72 males, 62 females, sex not recorded in one case. This is 6.36 per cent. of the whole genealogy. In 255 affected lines, about one-half each of the males and females showed this disease. It was rather oftener transmitted by the female line; probably because they oftener married into their own stock.

Invariably the condition was transmitted from night-blind parent or parents to offspring, without alternation. This tendency to night-blindness was emphasized by frequent intermarriage. Whenever, by marrying into other stock or by some kindness of nature, a Nougaret is born free from this disease, it never re-appears in his descent. Thus many branches of the family have been freed from this hereditary taint.

By the aid of parish registers, and slightly by tradition, this family and its hereditary disease have been accurately traced back to Jean Nougaret, a butcher, who was born about 1637, and brought night-blindness to a little isolated town of Southern France. Here this family has since dwelt, intermarried and multiplied, and here one-half its night-blind members have been born. This pecular disease was first noted by medical men in 1831, in one of Jean Nougaret's descendants.

In this family there is recorded a marriage between fourth cousins once removed. They had two daughters, both night-blind, who married normal husbands. One of these daughters had two night-blind children, and one that died at two months. The other daughter had one night-blind child, one normal, and one that lived but two months. Of course some Nougarets concealed their night-blindness as it became a bar to desirable marriages, at times. One woman is known to have concealed it from her husband for twenty years.

The conditions of isolation, a patois almost unintelligible in other parts of France, an occupation (grape culture) common to all, and the rare introduction of new blood into this community, still obtain almost to the same extent as for the 270 years in which this annoying hereditary defect has been handed down from generation to generation, largely through consanguinity. As Nettleship well said: "Such agencies have acted merely by facilitating marriage between distant cousins within the affected stock. One does not see why the disease should die out so long as those affected continue to marry within the stock, i. e., within the local population, which is nearly the same thing. . . . It is possible that examples of inheritance as extensive as that recorded might be found in many another isolated clan or tribe."

H. M. Langdon (*Ophthalmic Record,* Vol. XXI, p. 200, May, 1912) has reported a family of five in which the father and one daughter were affected by more or less helplessness in dim light. Corrected vision was 6/5, the fundi were of healthy appearance, and the fields were normal for form and color in a good light, with concentric contraction in diminished illumination. Henry's photometer showed the daughter's light-sense to be R. 3/5 and L. 2/5, while the father's was 3/5 in each eye. Langdon pointed out that only since the invention of the ophthalmoscope has it been possible to differentiate between pigmented retinal degeneration and the cases with no fundus changes known as congenital stationary night-blindness.

J. Bordley, Jr. (*Johns Hopkins Hosp. Bulletin,* Vol. XIX, No. 210) has noted congenital night-blindness in a group of cases traced to five generations. It was associated with defect of the lower temporal quadrant of each visual field. There was progressive concentric contraction of the fields, which were greatly narrowed by diminished illumination. Death occurred in middle life, about one year after total blindness booamo ootablichod,

Sinclair has collected eleven cases in a family of forty members, the disease affecting four successive generations.

Hereditary night-blindness with myopia. E. Nettleship (*Trans. Ophthal. Soc. of Un. Kingd.,* Vol. XXXII, p. 21, 1912) divided congenital stationary night-blindness into two varieties.. One is transmissible from generation to generation without a break, by either parent to children of either sex, which he called the "ambisexual variety." The other is confined to males, but transmitted only by mothers with normal sight, and the affected generations are therefore always separated by at least one generation. The second, or male sex-limited variety, is the subject of this treatise, which is illustrated by a pedigree chart and many visual fields taken under different degrees of light. The pedigree showed 21 affected by congenital night-blindness and myopia, out of 212 individuals, covering 6 generations. All were males who inherited the defect through their mothers. He believed this to be the largest well-authenticated record of this form of night-blindness extant, and stated that in no case of congenital stationary night-blindness had the eyes been examined microscopically. Clinically the two varieties agree in that the night-blindness dates from the earliest recollection, and is stationary. In the ambisexual form the eyes are normal in every respect except inability to see in dim light. In the male sex-limited cases that have been investigated there was always found myopia and notable defect of visual acuity with the best correction, considerable mental instability, nystagmus in a few of the worst cases, and normal fundus except for macular changes.

HEREDITARY WORD-BLINDNESS.

This defect, which is cerebral rather than ocular, has been traced by Stephenson through three generations. J. Hinshelwood reported four cases and pointed out, in 1907, that children with this defect never get a fair chance in public schools, but do very well with private instruction, when not subject to ridicule for their great backwardness in learning to read. In all respects but retention of words, the mentality is normal. Four years later Hinshelwood (*British Med. Jour.*, Mar. 18, 1911) reported two cases occurring in the second generation of that same family. One of these cases showed defective visual memory for both words and figures; though this investigator has shown, from his study of cases of acquired word-blindness, that the visual memory for words and letters is completely independent of that for figures. All of Hinshelwood's many cases of congenital word-blindness have ultimately been taught to read; showing that none were defective as to general intelligence.

HEREDITARY ALBINISM.

In 30,000 private patients Lagleyze (*Archiv. d'Ophtal.*, May-June-July, 1906) found 27 cases of albinism, mostly among people in an isolated province in the Argentine republic, where intermarriage had been practised to an extraordinary extent for nearly a century. These 27 cases occurred in 13 families; and 5 of these families produced 13 cases in children of first cousins, or of uncle and niece. The parents of five of these albinos were not related; and this point was not ascertained in the other nine. Lagleyze considers that consanguineous marriages are even more of a factor than heredity in causing albinism, and that a parent with partial albinism may have offspring showing complete albinism. In this way hereditary deficiency of pigmentation is intensified.

HEREDITARY DEGENERATION AND EYE LESIONS.

C. D. Camp (*Amer. Jour. of Med. Sciences*, p. 716, Vol. CXLVI, Nov. 1913) discusses the question of differentiating an hereditary characteristic from an acquired degenerative condition caused by a neurotoxin transmitted from parent to child, and thinks that hereditary degeneration may be due to disease or toxemia possibly preventable or amenable to treatment.

He suggests that when we find that one type of degeneration in a parent is followed by another type in the offspring, or when we note degenerative changes variously localized, it seems probable that something truly external is acting on the organism, attacking the weaker parts. He states that generally true heredity acts in a way which is distinctly opposed to degeneration. Quoting Lugaro: "Degeneration is a disturbance of physiologic hereditary transmission; it is a disease of the hereditary mechanism." Camp believes that degeneration is a result of disease of the stock, but a disease that may be curable. If that is true it is of great importance that it be generally recognized.

He reports the case of a child of 10 years with Friedreich's ataxia and pseudohypertrophic muscular dystrophy, with nystagmus on lateral deviation of the eye balls. The child's parents were healthy but his maternal uncle and great uncle had an affection similar to the patient's, coming on at the age of 10 years and causing death at 18 years. He also reports a child of 8 years with pseudohypertrophic muscular dystrophy showing well marked optic neuritis in each eye, which Camp believes to be hereditary. The child said he had three brothers with similar trouble. The family history was not obtained as the father deserted his family and the mother was dead.

INSANITY AND INHERITED EYE DISEASE.

E. J. Ledbetter and E. Nettleship (*Brain*, Vol. XXXV, p. 195, Feb., 1913) show an association between mental deficiency and ocular defects, the latter being partly developmental, partly morbid. The pathologic changes noted were chiefly detachment of the retina, based upon disease of the choroid, but with iritis and secondary cataract in some cases. Both the mental and ocular conditions are hereditary, and are probably due to a common underlying cause. The ocular changes were entirely different from those commonly observed in cases of cerebral and spinal disease; neither optic neuritis, optic atrophy, altered pupillary reflexes, nor ocular palsies were observed in this pedigree. Syphilis was excluded except in one doubtful case. No consanguinity. Tuberculosis in three cases, alcoholic excesses in about six. They believe that all the ocular and mental abnormalities began as intrauterine arrests. Small stature was frequent. Marriage between an insane man of one stock and an insane and blind woman of another stock was followed by mental and ocular disease in many of their descendants, as was to have been expected.

In the affected stock were found 65 individuals, 40 of whom were unsound in mind or eyes or so disabled as to need public care. The morbid conditions descended directly from parent to child in every instance with the possible exception of a tuberculous father who left an insane son. And unfortunately the fertility of the insane members was high.

INHERITED SYPHILIS OF THE EYE.

In the *Ophthalmoscope* for Dec., 1913, Vol. XI, p. 718, J. Igersheimer deals with the damage caused to the eyes by inherited syphilis, principally in childhood. Although the identical lesion is not transmitted, yet the effects of an heritable disease so far-reaching should be considered in a treatise on heredity. Of 27 nurslings between 2 and 18 months of age whom Igersheimer found involved by general syphilis, 6 had normal eyes, 21 showed pathologic changes. He considered syphilis to be a factor in the following eye diseases which he had studied with that point in view: conjunctivitis, keratomalacia, parenchymatous keratitis, pseudo-glioma, choroiditis or chorio-retinitis of the periphery of the fundus, optic neuritis, optic atrophy, nystagmus, dacryo-cystitis and ocular palsies. He found that nearly one-half of the cases of congenital syphilis who had parenchymatous keratitis, showed disease of the nervous system. Igersheimer and E. T. Collins have traced syphilis to the third generation; which suggests redoubled efforts as to the prevention or spread of this terrible scourge.

Oval cornea in hereditary syphilis. There have been very few observations of oval cornea, says Antonelli (*Rivist. Ital. di Ottal.*, April, 1913, and *Ophthalmoscope*, Dec., 1914) and yet the association of this condition with hereditary syphilis is well recognized. In one of the few preceding papers mentioned, the oval cornea, with long axis vertical, was found in connection with oxycephaly. This is specially interesting since it affords evidence that the "tower skull" is one of the stigmata of syphilis.

Antonelli, in the present paper, gives notes of five cases of oval cornea, all of whom were the subject of hereditary syphilis, and most of them the seat of parenchymatous keratitis.

There is a distinction to be drawn between the eyes which show crescentic patches at the sides (embryontoxon, or arcus fetalis) and these oval corneas of which Antonelli speaks; the former are the scars of intrauterine sclerosing keratitis, the latter are the result of arrest of development at a late stage of fetal life; this explains the frequent association with microcornea. The two conditions may co-exist; one of the cases referred to in the paper had a vertically oval cornea and a small patch of sclerosis of fetal date in the infero-temporal quadrant.

INHERITANCE OF ACQUIRED OCULAR DEFECTS.

This question is of interest, even though it has not passed the speculative stage. Tobias (*Klin. Monatsbl. f. Augenheilk.*, Apr., 1911) has recorded the instance of a mother with bilateral operative colobomata of the iris who gave birth to five children, the two youngest showing congenital coloboma of the iris and choroid. The eyes of the other children were normal. The operation on the mother had occurred four years before her marriage. In her right eye the coloboma was

below and in, in the left, up and in. One child had bilateral coloboma below, the other showed coloboma of the iris and choroid down
and in; suggesting to the reviewer's mind that failure of the fetal cleft
to close may have been the cause of the colobomata, rather than direct
inheritance of the effects of surgical interference. Weismann has
asserted that it has never been proved that acquired characters are
transmitted.

Conclusions. In all the diseases, defects or anomalies of the body,
no better or more sharply defined examples of heredity have been
found than in the human eye. The persistency of the transmission
of defective eyes in some families is very striking, although it is said
to be even more definite in animals of lower development than man,
and in plants. To quote Nettleship: "The Mendelian laws are seldom clearly and fully demonstrated in human beings, as the members
in a childship are so comparatively few, the ascertained genealogical
trees so short and imperfect, and the surrounding circumstances so
uncertain. It is very different from the data which can be obtained
and the inferences which can be drawn from well-planned botanical
cultivation or animal breeding."

The question of heredity can hardly be studied too closely. Its solution will depend on the accumulation of masses of reliable statistics
based on accurate observations by students the world over. To this
end ophthalmologists are urged to report *all* cases of family or hereditary disease which come under their notice. In this connection it is
gratifying to observe that in the past two years about as many articles
on this subject have appeared in ophthalmic journals as in the previous
ten or more years. Probably ophthalmology has contributed more to
the study of heredity than all other departments of medicine combined.

Through a continuous campaign of education and the development
of a public sentiment that will both demand the enactment and secure
the enforcement of laws prohibiting the marriage of the hereditary
blind, untold suffering and much economic loss will be prevented.
Attempt should now be made on every suitable occasion to discourage
the marriage of blood relations and of a person with an inherited
defect that will cause physical disability or mental distress in the offspring. It is to be hoped that eventually such marriages will, in every
country, be under the ban of the law.—(G. F. L.)

Hering's binocular contrast. According to Burch, (*Practical Exercises
in Physiological Optics*, p. 86) "An ordinary stereoscope is very convenient for this purpose, a square of red glass being inserted on one
side of the central partition, and a square of blue glass on the other—

or a plain box divided down the middle with a pair of eyeholes at one end and the colored glasses at the other will do equally well, no lenses being required. A small, black wafer is fixed at the centre of each glass, with a white wafer close to the left side of the one on the right-hand glass, and another close to the right side of that on the left-hand glass. The two black wafers, being fixed binocularly, combine to form a single image, with the white wafers, each seen with a different eye against a different color, one on each side of it. If preferred, the white wafers may be one above and one below the black spot. The instrument may be directed to a sheet of white paper, or to a mirror reflecting the light of the sky. To bring out the full effect the light upon the white wafers must not be too bright. It should be reduced until the contrast colors show up strongly, orange against the blue glass and blue-green against the red. The point brought out by Hering is this: Helmholtz had said that contrast effects were judgments of the mind. Hering shows that if you look with both eyes at once, though the colors of the two fields may combine, as they do with many people, to produce the impression of purple, the two contrast colors will not combine to produce the complementary yellow-green unless they too are superposed, but will retain each its own hue. It is difficult to imagine the mind combining two impressions, and at the same time keeping separate the judgments they give rise to. Hering argues very properly that contrast phenomena are functions of the retina rather than of the brain." See, also, **Contrast**.

Hering's cyclops-eye. In physiological optics, this is an imaginary eye, supposed to be located midway between the two real eyes in the region of the root of the nose. See p. 3653, Vol. V, of this *Encyclopedia*.

Hering's experiment. THE DROP TEST. HERING'S FALL TEST. A delicate test of stereoscopic or at least of binocular vision in which the

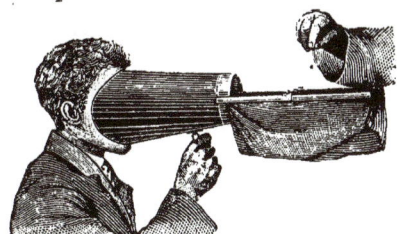

Hering's Drop Test of Binocular Vision.

perception of degrees of depth is tested by means of falling bodies, seen through a long tube. The patient looks with one eye through a long tube at a thread stretched vertically. Glass beads are then dropped in front of and behind the thread. If binocular vision is present the patient will correctly state whether the beads fell in front of or behind the thread; if blind in one eye he will make numerous mistakes. See the figure. See, also, Vol. V, p. 3829, of this *Encyclopedia.*

Hering's kymograph. A modification of the hollow spring instrument for recording wave-like oscillations of the pulse, muscle contractions, etc. The vibration of the levers connected with the writing style are limited by a connecting-rod dipped in a tube containing oil or vinegar, and the tube containing the sodic carbonate solution is connected with a syringe that regulates the amount of the fluid in the tube.

Hermodorus. An ancient Greek oculist, or Roman oculist with a Greek name, whose seal was found at Beaumont, Puy de Dôme, France. The seal bears an inscription in eight lines, as follows: *"Aulus Uritius. Hermodorus: Melinum Opobalsamum ad Aspritudines. Diasmyrnes lenementum Thurinum ad (Suppurationes). Crocodes ad Caligines."* Nothing else is known about this man.—(T. H. S.)

Hermofenil. This remedy, like fluorol, is used for washing out the sac in obstruction of the tear passages. It has been recommended especially by V. Landazabal. (*Archivos de Oftalmologia,* October, 1912) who has treated a number of cases of dacryocystitis by injection of 5 to 7 and 2 per cent. solutions respectively, after or without probing. The results were gratifying, and the author considers that success was obtained in many instances in which extirpation of the sac would otherwise have been necessary.

Hermonis collyrium. (L.) A collyrium containing long pepper, white pepper, cinnamon, costum, atramentum sutoris, nard, cassia, castor, gall-nut, myrrh, saffron, frankincense, lycium, ceruse, opium, aloes, calamine, acacia, antimony, and gum.

Hermon of Thasos. A classical patient, whose votive-tablet, placed in the temple of Asclepios at Epidaurus about 300 B. C., is still extant. The tablet reads: "Hermon of Thasos. This man was healed by the god [Asclepios] of his blindness, and, as he did not pay the fee into the sanctuary, the god made him blind once more. As, however, he came again, and once more slept in the temple, the god made him well."—(T. H. S.)

Hernia corneæ. (L.) An old term properly signifying a bulging forward of the membrane of Descemet through an ulcerative process in the anterior layers of the cornea; formerly and incorrectly used for keratocele.

Hernia iridis. (L.) Prolapse of the iris through a wound or perforating ulcer in the cornea or ciliary region. See **Hernia of the iris.**

Hernia oculi. (L.) An old term for exophthalmia.

Hernia of Descemet's membrane. In perforating ulcer of the cornea, just before the disease has penetrated the entire thickness of the membrane and when the ulcer has acquired great depth, there may be a projection of the membrane of Descemet, in the form of a transparent vesicle *(keratocele),* which fills the floor of the ulcer and may advance beyond the level of the cornea.

Hernia of orbital tissue. The fatty tissue of the orbit is normally held in place by the tarso-orbital fascia, orbicularis muscle, and skin. As a result of atrophy in elderly persons, or from trauma at any period of life, these tissues may become weakened and permit of protrusion of. the orbital fat between the orbicularis muscle and the skin. The hernia can be pushed backward into the orbit. If of sufficient size to cause deformity, the protruding tissue may be readily removed through an incision made parallel with the orbicularis fibres.—(J. M. B.)

Hernia of the eyelids. See Vol. VII, p. 5010 of this *Encyclopedia.*

Hernia of the iris. A prolapse of a portion of the iris after iridectomy, cataract extraction, corneal ulcer, trauma, etc. If the prolapse follows an accident, the surgeon may either attempt to replace the prolapsed portion or excise it. The former method, which is condemned because of the danger of infecting the eye, is accomplished by gently pushing the iris back into place with a clean spatula, after the conjunctiva has been cocainized and flushed with a solution of mercuric bichlorid or other antiseptic. After replacement a miotic is to be used three times a day for two or three days. Prolapse of the iris occurring after a cataract extraction should be treated by excision (iridectomy) when the condition is observed early. If it is noticed after firm adhesions have formed, it should not be interfered with. See **Cataract, Senile.**

Hernia of the vitreous. A term applied by Elschnig to a form of glaucoma in which a localized depression in the floor of the cupped papilla (extending below and beyond the lamina cribrosa) is lined with fibrous tissue and filled with firm vitreous. Oguchi *(Ophthal. Review,* p. 202, July, 1909) describes such a case and regards the tubular depression as due to the breaking down of one or more optic nerve-bundles.

However, E. Temple Smith *(Ophthalmoscope,* p. 269, May, 1914) gives quite a different definition of this term, and in describing his case of *intraocular hernia of the vitreous,* following a blow on the eye, reports that a gelatinous transparent mass, oscillating freely with the movements of the eye, was seen overhanging the upper part of the lens, and projecting into the anterior chamber. The free edge of the mass had a bright-red border, which was probably pigment derived from the blood in the chamber. The lens was *in situ,* and the fundus was very dimly seen through the cloudy lens, below the gelatinous body.

Roemer (*Text book of Ophthalmology,* Vol. VII, p. 330) corrobo rates Temple Smith's view of the significance of this expression. He says that with a Zeiss loupe one may distinguish something that looks like a clear, transparent drop that hangs down from above into the anterior chamber and quivers with every movement of the eye. It is not a subluxated lens; that organ is in its normal place and position; it is a large prolapse of the vitreous into the anterior chamber. A rupture of the zonule must evidently precede the occurrence of this complication, but it cannot be demonstrated, as the lens is normally fixed. The vitreous in the anterior chamber is the cause of increased tension and should be removed.

Herniaria alpestris. A plant species found in Europe, containing herniarin, saponin, and paronychin. The herb was formerly used in hernia, dropsy, bladder and kidney diseases, as well as in ophthalmia.

Hern's operation. For glaucoma. See p. 5487, Vol. VII, of this *Encyclopedia.*

Heroin. DIACETYLMORPHIN. This is a highly organized, white, crystalline, bitter, odorless powder, soluble in acidulated liquids, insoluble in cold water and oils. The *hydrochloride,* owing to its greater solubility in water, is commonly employed as an antispasmodic and sedative. Dose, 1/12 to 1/6 grain.

Heroin occasionally produces amblyopic symptoms. Solès (*Archivos de Ginecopatia Obstetric.,* No. 13, 1899) reports a case of a woman, suffering from asthma, who took 0.167 grm. of the powder. Four hours afterwards she suffered from general weakness, slowness of pulse, cramps in the legs, loss of vision and miosis. After three injections of caffein she recovered her sight. In another case reported by Dillingham (*Medical Record,* p. 664, 1890) the remedy was given for cough, in two doses of about 0.005 grm. Shortly afterwards the patient became comatose, with dilatation of the pupil.

Herophilus. A celebrated Greek anatomist, of about 300 B. C., the first to perform a dissection of the human cadaver, and the first to dissect the living human subject (condemned criminals), whose name has been perpetuated in the "torcular Herophili." He wrote a large number of works, chiefly on anatomical subjects, but of these only fragments survive in the writings of Celsus, Galen, Rufus, and Theophilus. Of chief importance to ophthalmologists was his *"Peri Ophthalmon."* He described distinctly the sclera, the choroid, the retina, and the vitreous humor.—(T. H. S.)

Herpes conjunctivæ. One of the synonyms of *conjunctivitis phlyctenulosa;* also used to indicate any herpetic disease of the conjunctiva. See p. 3025, Vol. IV, of this *Encyclopedia.*

Herpes corneæ. See Vol. V, p. 3372 of this *Encyclopedia.*

Herpes febrilis. See **Cornea, Herpes febrilis of the.**

Herpes frontalis. See **Herpes zoster ophthalmicus.**

Herpes iris. HERPES IRIS OF THE CONJUNCTIVA. This very rare disease has nothing to do with the *iris,* the name being employed in the usual dermatological sense to describe the disease as it affects the conjunctiva; a central, reddened or pigmented area surrounded by a ring of vesicles being found not only on that membrane but generally also on the surrounding skin, or on the buccal mucosa.

Hans Barkan (*Arch. Ophth.,* XLII, 236, May, 1913) reports one case and refers to the 20 others in the literature. The former was of the malignant type, with photophobia, violent ciliary and conjunctival injection, fibrinous exudate, and corneal ulceration. After the acute attack there was ankyloblepharon, symblepharon, corneal maculæ, with photophobia and secretion of mucus persisting a year after the initial attack.

Herpes of the eyelids. See p. 5010, Vol. VII, of this *Encyclopedia.*

Herpes ophthalmicus. Herpes zoster ophthalmicus.

Herpes of the iris. This name has been suggested by W. Gilbert (*Sammlung zwangloser Abhandlungen aus dem Gebiete der Augenheilkunde,* Vol. 9, No. 2, 1913) who observed in herpes corneæ febrilis and herpes zoster ophthalmicus a peculiar affection of the iris, which did not fit into the familiar inflammations of the anterior uveal tract. He asserts that this disease furnishes a well-defined clinical picture not due to a secondary spreading of a corneal process to the iris but to a genuine, primary, herpetic disease of the uveal tract. Within three years it occurred in 6 out of 40 very carefully examined cases of herpes of the cornea; in one out of four cases of herpes zoster; in one case of parenchymatous keratitis and in one case of vitiligo; altogether 9. All these affections belong together, being due to trophic or vasomotor disturbances of the fifth nerve, caused, as found by Head and Campbell in zoster, by an affection of the spinal ganglion, chiefly hemorrhagic inflammation. Herpes of the iris is characterized by initial neuralgic pain, circumscribed swelling of the iris, correspond-

ing to the eruptions of zoster on the skin, general or circumscribed
hyperemia of the iris, especially within the small circle, subsequent
hemorrhages, after which the pain subsides.

The prognosis is good if a hemorrhage occurs only once or twice,
but is impaired if the hemorrhages relapse more frequently or if a
large hypopyon sets in. Atrophy of the iris, occlusion and seclusion
of the pupil, and eventually secondary glaucoma may develop. The
treatment is the same as in herpetic affections and iritis.

In hemorrhages, mydriatics and miotics must be avoided, and
operative procedures postponed as long as possible.

The anatomical changes of an excised piece of iris corresponded
with those found by Sattler and Verhoeff in enucleated eyeballs of
patients with herpes zoster. From these Gilbert considers the
development of capillary nevi in consequence of irritation of the
nerves as the anatomical base of herpes of the iris.

The author also discusses in this connection the possible herpetic
character of certain cases of choroiditis, opacities of the vitreous, optic
neuritis and conjunctivitis complicating vitiligo and herpes zoster.
(Abstract in *Ophthalmology*, 1913.)

Herpes, Zonular. Herpes zoster ophthalmicus.

Herpes zoster ophthalmicus. HERPES OPTHALMICUS. HERPES FRONTALIS.
HERPETIC ULCER OF THE CORNEA. OCULAR SHINGLES. ZONULAR HERPES.
ZONA OPHTHALMICA. This affection is an acute, specific disease of the
nervous system characterized by an eruption of vesicles, upon inflamed
bases, over the area supplied by branches of the ophthalmic, or first
divison of the trigeminal nerve. The branches usually affected are
the supraorbital, supratrochlear, occasionally the lachrymal, and,
much less frequently, the nasal. The inflammation, which arises without any obvious peripheral or central cause, is located in either the
trunk of the nerve itself or in the Gasserian ganglion, or in both
nerve and ganglion.

It was pointed out by Jonathan Hutchinson, in his clinical report
on "Shingles Affecting the Forehead and Nose" (*Royal Lond. Oph.
Hosp. Reports*, Vol. 191, 1866), that "if the skin of the nose be extensively affected by herpes there is a special risk of the iris and cornea
also becoming inflamed." This association has since been confirmed
by many observers, indeed, it was at one time believed to be the invariable rule that when the skin of the nose was affected the ocular
structures also were sooner or later involved. Yet, in several cases
where vesicles have covered the side of the nose the eye itself has
wholly escaped. Hyberd found that in fifty-eight cases in which

the nose was affected, thirty-five showed eye changes while in eighteen cases the cornea and iris were normal.

This affection, it should be noted, has been known to ophthalmic surgeons as a distinct disease only since the latter half of the nineteenth century; it is, indeed, an uncommon disease, notwithstanding that it has been said to have shown a tendency to epidemic outbreaks, yet many practitioners have never seen a case. In twenty years of private practice, if I may be permitted to speak of my own experi-

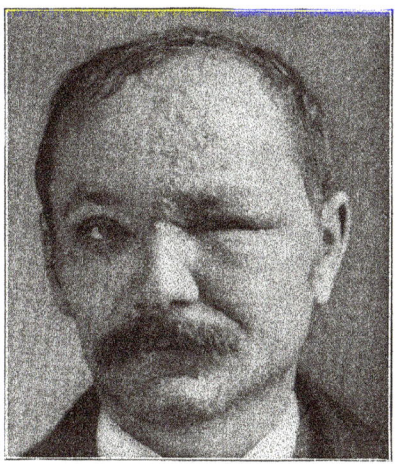

Herpes Zoster Ophthalmicus.

Showing distribution over brow, forehead and scalp. Reproduced from a photograph by the kindness of Dr. J. F. Schamberg.

ence, I have had the care of only four persons afflicted with it, and amongst 30,447 cases of all forms of diseases of the eye that came to the clinics of the Wills Hospital in the years of 1913 and 1914, only five were cases of zoster ophthalmicus (*Annals of Ophthalmology*, December, 1915). In Greenough's series of cases, intercostal herpes was fourteen times as frequent as the facial varieties; and in herpes of the face, out of a total of one hundred and sixty cases, only sixteen showed affection of the lids. Knowles' record of general herpes zoster, in 31,337 cases of diseases of the skin, seen in a period extending over nine years, shows how infrequent ophthalmic zoster is in dermatologic practice, for out of his total number of two hundred and eighty-six cases, only five occurred involving the supraorbital region, and only two of these showed affection of the cornea.

Zoster is a mysterious disease; we are still in doubt as to the cause of the neuritis, and equally uncertain whether it be central or peripheral in origin. Whatever the poison may be, the reactions of its manifestations are those of an acute specific infection, the clinical facts

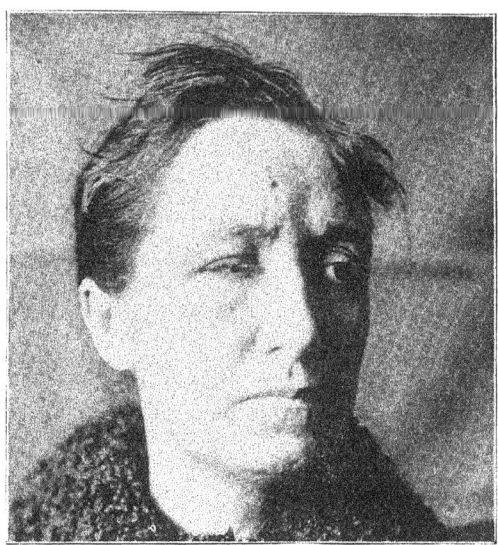

Herpes Zoster Ophthalmicus.

Showing distribution over brow, forehead and scalp. Reproduced from a photograph by the kindness of Dr. J. F. Schamberg.

of which are not militated against by another fact equally well-settled, that various kinds of nerve poisons may set up similar inflammations, if they do not actually produce the eruption of zoster.

A certain number of cases of zoster ophthalmicus seem to bear a distinct relation to, or association with, diseases of the general nervous system, for zoster has been noticed in the course of the general paralysis of the insane, and it frequently accompanies certain of the acute infectious diseases, notably pneumonia. Notwithstanding this comparative frequency, in the majority of cases the cause of its outbreak is not known. In some cases zoster has been seen to develop as the result of chilling of the body. Stieren was able in his cases to trace a history of exposure to cold or dampness in those who had become exhausted by unusual exertion and fatigue, in persons of sedentary habits. "Taking cold," however, is in itself a vague term, but since it has become possible to explore the sinuses of the skull adjacent to and communicating with the nasal passages, we have learned that many cases of "cold" are really expressions of inflammatory states within those sinuses. While there are no data at hand to justify such an assumption, yet the belief is entertained that time will show us that disease of the sinuses bear a close relation to outbursts of ophthalmic

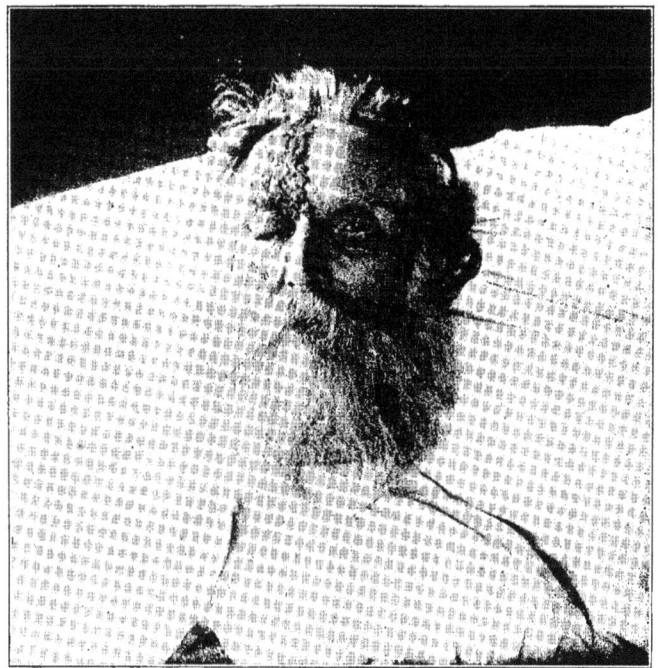

Herpes Zoster Ophthalmicus. (E. A. Clarke.)

herpes—if not as the basic cause, at least as a contributory. While it may be accepted as true that the exit of nerve branches from bony foramina renders them subject to the effects of exposure, and, as we shall see further on, that it is at these sites that we note painful neuralgias, both during the course of the disease and among the sequels of it, may it not be conceived that filaments of the nerves supplying the sinuses have been affected in their passage through the sinuses and that they thus transmit infections to the nerve branch?

In other cases it has been said to arise after injuries to the head, as by a blow on the cheek or eyelid; in others by poisoning by coal gas; in certain others after the toxic use of arsenic, which, however, according to Head, can be but a remote cause, only insofar as it renders the patient susceptible to attack. Severe mental emotion has appeared to be the exciting cause in a good many cases, yet there is scarcely any proof that emotion can produce it. Besnier, according to Crocker, relates the case of a student who, while studying a case of ophthalmic herpes, was himself seized, and permanent facial paralysis ensued! Other cases have preceded, accompanied or followed attacks of influenza, the consideration of which affection, however, can hardly be dissociated from the study of the acute inflammations of the nasal sinuses.

Early writers ascribed zoster to the effects of rheumatism, while later observers believed zoster to be dependent upon intestinal toxemia, to diabetes; and it has been observed during the course of nephritis. It can thus be seen that zoster ophthalmicus does not arise spontaneously in presumably perfectly healthy individuals, but rather it attacks those who have been weakened by some preëxisting disease. In my own examples, comprising six cases, no definite cause had been assigned in any case. Sattler regarded certain reported cases accompanied by pareses to be not true types of spontaneous zoster, but, on the contrary, believed them to be dependent upon lesions or growths about the base of the skull. This supposition strengthens my own belief that a study of the condition of the cranial cavities will throw a very strong light upon the origin of ophthalmic zoster. The value of a knowledge of the condition of the nasal sinuses as a safeguard for the maintenance of the good health is now fully appreciated.

The studies of Head and Campbell were carried on in county asylums, and the majority of their patients suffered from general paralysis. They were not able to decide whether the zoster was symptomatic, or whether the debilitated condition of such patients rendered them prone to attacks. In the best of circumstances, the physical condition of the inmates of county asylums is indeed bad, and it is not always possible to attend to the carious teeth or to prevent oral sepsis among such patients, two conditions from which infection can extend not only to the cranial cavities, but enter the general system as well.

While it has been said that sex does not have any special influence on general zoster, ophthalmic zoster occurs in both sexes with equal frequency; yet in Hutchinson's cases, males were more often attacked than females, for eleven were males and seven females. In my own observation of six cases, four occurred in men.

Ophthalmic zoster occurs at any age, but it is more commonly seen among the elderly in feeble health than among robust adults and young children; yet the young presenting no constitutional depression may be attacked. MacNab had a case in a boy of six; Rachmaninow also reports a case in a young child, and Knowles noted a case of corneal involvement in a girl of four. In Hutchinson's series the average age of eighteen cases was forty-seven years, while in the six cases of my own group, the average was fifty-two years.

There seems to be no special racial predilection to the incidence of ophthalmic herpes. All of my cases were in native-born Americans, of which the most disastrous occurred in a negro, a race seldom affected, as Knowles saw but twelve instances of general zoster in the negro.

Many attempts have been made to prove that zoster ophthalmicus occurs more frequently at one season of the year than at another, but results are conflicting. The probability of the idea that it is dependent upon atmospheric influences is favored, however, by the frequent occurrence of cases in groups.

As the trigeminal is the nerve in whose territory this affection occurs, the vesicles more frequently occupy the region of the distribution of the first or ophthalmic branch of that nerve. The eruption, therefore, is confined to the forehead, the anterior part of the scalp, the eyelids, and the side of the nose. It may be confined to only certain branches of the ophthalmic nerve, as shown in a case by MacNab, in which the vesicles were limited to the middle of the nose, from the tip to the level of the eyebrow above, and laterally the margins of the eruption projected out on the cheek.

It is a characteristic feature of the exanthem that it is almost always confined to one side of the face and head, and that the affection of the skin is sharply limited at the middle line. The disease is rarely bilateral; Hutchinson believed it never to be so. He found the right side affected in five cases and the left in nine. In all of his cases the tract supplied by the frontal nerve, that is, the forehead and front part of the scalp, were affected; in eight the side of the nose was inflamed, and in six of these the cornea and iris were involved. In none of his cases in which the frontal nerve alone was involved was the eye inflamed, whilst the eye suffered in all in which the naso-ciliary branch was implicated, but in none in which the nasal branch was not involved was the eye inflamed. This dictum cannot be taken as a law, however, because the globe was not always affected when the naso-ciliary branch was involved. In one of Hutchinson's cases there was zoster on the chest, and Knowles' list includes a case with eruption on the mucous surfaces of the lips as well as in the supraorbital region.

The vesicles, then, are found upon the upper lid, upon the fore-head as far as the scalp, and on the nose. When the district supplied by the second branch of the trigeminal is affected, the vesicles are situated upon the lower lid, over the region of the malar bone. Some-times the terminal expansions of both branches are affected simul-taneously; in the case of the negro in my series the lower lid was quite deeply pitted. It is extremely rare for the regions supplied by the second and third branches to be involved. Head saw a case of typical zoster ophthalmicus associated with an equally well marked eruption over the area of the second division (infraorbital) of the trigeminal. His table of four hundred and sixteen cases of zoster shows the tri-geminal to have been affected in all three branches on the right side, including the lids, cheek, upper lip, the mucous membrane of the cheek, the tongue and the tonsil.

The attack may be preceded by a prodromal stage of varying length, during which the temperature is raised and the patient has the sense of an impending illness; very much in the manner of the invasion by one of the acute infections. There is usually violent neuralgia, the pains being of either a darting or boring character, over the supra-orbital region, in the course of the trigeminal, or it is manifested by hemicrania and by pains in the scalp. When there is great soreness of the scalp the hair may fall out. The surface of these hyperalgesic areas may become reddened and be more or less edematous, and if the case is seen before the rash appears, it is sometimes possible to map out the area to be subsequently occupied by the eruption by means of these painful areas. In a few cases neuralgic symptoms may be en-tirely wanting. In some cases there may be a slight conjunctivitis for two or three days. These symptoms may endure with varying inten-sity for ten days, although it is most usual for them to exist for only a day or two. When the prodromal symptoms are severe they are followed on the third or fourth day by a sudden eruption of vesicles. The patient may become quite ill, especially when the extent of the eruption is wide and the evolution rapid, and, along with moderate fever and faintness, he may be seized with nausea and vomiting which persist until the eruption has fully appeared; but when the efflores-cence is complete the pain lessens and the general symptoms soon dis-appear. The temperature of the affected parts is decidedly increased, but commonly the sensibility is diminished. The manner of such severe attacks not unreasonably may be compared to that of an attack of pneumonia. The inflammation is marked by a sudden onset, but it shows no tendency to spread beyond what may be present at the first outburst; therefore, as much as is to be affected presents the signs at once. If the eye is involved at all, it will be affected at about the time of the appearance of the vesicles on the skin.

Among the ophthalmic lesions accompanying herpes zoster there may be swelling with, perhaps, vesication of the conjunctiva; the formation of vesicles on the cornea, which usually lead to ulceration and kerato-iritis, but in which hypopyon rarely develops. All of the ocular structures may be involved, although the external muscles, the conjunctiva and cornea are the parts most frequently affected. The eyelids during the active stage are nearly always congested and edematous; in mild cases there may be merely irritability and photophobia, with slight congestion, yet in more than half the cases lesions of the globe occur, although the deeper structures are only occasionally involved. Lachrymation with tenderness over the lachrymal gland may be observed, and, early in the disease, the adjacent glands sometimes enlarge and frequently are found to be tender.

The ocular complications do not, as a rule, set in until the eruption is at its height, or when it is already beginning to decline. They may be present, however, early in the attack, appearing primarily in the cornea at the same time as the vesicles on the skin, as was noted in Haab's case; indeed, ulceration of the cornea has been found within the first week. It may, however, happen, when there is much scabbing or an eczematous condition of the eyelids, that the conjunctiva becomes inflamed some days or weeks after the onset of the skin trouble.

Great edema of the lids and chemosis of the conjunctiva may be present when the supraorbital is densely affected, and one of the earliest signs, in cases in which the cornea becomes involved, may be an irritability of the conjunctiva for three or four days preceding the outburst of the vesicles.

Vesicles may be found on the conjunctiva, especially when the nasal branches of the nerve have been affected, and, after a day or so, the cornea itself may be invaded.

As has already been pointed out, the most serious and the most frequent of all the ocular manifestations is the eruption of vesicles on the surface of the cornea. Such an eruption is usually preceded by a period of insensitiveness of the cornea to touch. This quite pronounced and conspicuous symptom may be the only one observed; it may extend so far as to amount to the total abolition of the sensibility of the cornea. In other cases the corneal substance itself may be invaded, although when it does, the course of the invasion shows nothing characteristic of zona, but resembles the characteristics of herpes febrilis—with this difference, however, that the acute vesicular form is less often seen in zona than in herpes febrilis. In herpes ophthalmicus the vesicles are arranged in groups and speedily rupture, thus exposing minute ulcerations which form, enlarge, and become fused with one another, whereby, in a short time, a considerable area of the cornea may become denuded of its epithelium, and as the area expands the border of the denudation becomes crenated.

Usually the area remains shallow, yet it may penetrate deeper and become invaded by purulent infiltration, and, if perforation occurs, the iris prolapses with all the consequences following such a compli-cation. In other cases a typical dendritic ulcer forms, in which, in one or more directions from the minute ulcer, gray striæ extend, grow-ing longer and longer, throwing out lateral branches until finally the surface of the cornea breaks down, although such ulcers are commonly only superficial and never penetrate deeper unless they have become infected, in which case hypopyon usually results. Dendriform ulcers are extremely chronic and prone to relapse, and in the majority of cases of zoster they seem to arise more deeply than in the case of herpes febrilis.

Much more frequently, too, than in febrile herpes, the vesicles of zoster are accompanied by deep infiltration of the cornea, yet infil-tration may occur without ulceration; and in zoster herpes, too, is more likely to be complicated with iritis, which complications may not easily be observed because of the blepharospasm, the pain and the irritation which may hinder if they do not prevent a close examina-tion, whereby a single bleb on the cornea may be overlooked and the process not detected until serious damage has occurred. In some cases, as in the first of my series, the anesthesia may affect only cir-cumscribed areas, and, when it is easy to make a thorough examina-tion, small round dots may be detected, which dots are likely to be followed by ulcerations; or, more happily, they may disappear with-out breaking down. Haab believes such opaque spots are dependent upon anesthesia or disease of the trifacial. It is still open to question whether or not true interstitial changes can occur without there hav-ing been a loss of the superficial surface. Such cases as have been reported have been described as having been manifested at an ad-vanced stage of the cutaneous affection. Terson, however, has re-ported a case in which the corneal infiltration preceded the cutaneous eruption fully two weeks, in which, as the epithelium was not affected, complete recovery followed. Sometimes a regular keratitis profunda develops, when, as might be expected, it takes a longer time for the opacities to disappear, if, indeed, they ever disappear at all.

It has been noted frequently that the pupil becomes dilated and the iris immobile, failing to contract to light and accommodation;

and, quite early, the iris has become hyperemic, even though there may not have been serious involvement of the cornea. But the iris may be affected by a true infiltration of lymph, which binds the pupil by posterior synechiæ, and there may be a filling in of the pupillary space by a plastic exudation. Hutchinson believed that in all cases in which the eye was affected, paresis of the iris took place so that immobility of the pupil ensued. Such symptoms have been seen when the trochlear nerve has been affected; they are produced, perhaps, by the ophthalmic ganglion becoming disturbed through irritation from the ophthalmic nerve. So early an observer as Hebra noted that the mobility of the iris may be so much impaired as to simulate iritis. This would make the diagnosis particularly confusing when it occurs in those cases in which, along with the early symptoms, there has been hyperemia of the conjunctiva also.

It may be seen, therefore, that iritis does occur with keratitis, which is contrary to what is the case in febrile herpes. The iritis may be quite severe, and it may extend to the ciliary body and be accompanied by the presence of precipitates in the aqueous. In numerous cases iritis has not arisen until late; in such instances, without doubt, it has been dependent upon a general systemic toxemia rather than the herpetic pathogeny.

Diffuse retinal hemorrhages have been noted during attacks of zoster ophthalmicus, and retinal degeneration, too, has been said to follow an attack; yet such statements are not incontestable, because it is not quite clear how such effects can arise. So also is it likewise extremely difficult to say with certainty that retinitis, choroiditis, and optic neuritis with consequent atrophy, in given cases, were brought about by the effects of zoster, and were not present prior to the attack. Head stated that he examined every case of ophthalmic zoster that came under his notice, and that even in the most severe cases of the disease he had never seen changes in the retina or optic nerve.

The intraocular tension is not infrequently lowered while the inflammation is recent—indeed, it is commonly stated as characteristic that the intraocular pressure becomes decreased; yet in other cases, as in the first of my series, increase of tension has been observed to set in; while Bradburne reported a case of zoster which was ushered in by an attack of glaucoma, but in which the tension fell below normal later in the attack.

For many years it was a much debated question as to whether or not ophthalmic zoster is ever complicated by lesions of the oculomotor nerves, but in the past twenty years cases have been reported so frequently that we now know that it is, though rarely, accompanied or followed by paralysis of one or more of the ocular muscles. which paralysis may persist long after the cutaneous symptoms have disappeared. Of the one hundred and fifty-eight cases of ocular paralyses of various kinds associated with ophthalmic zoster, collected by Hunt, eighteen cases involved the third nerve, one the fourth, and five the sixth nerve. His results may be accepted as typical, and, therefore, it is accepted as true that the third nerve, in one or more of its branches, is the nerve most frequently affected, the next in order being the sixth, while the fourth is very exceptionally involved, although Traquair cites four cases and reports another under his own observation. Harlan described a case exciting paralysis of all the external muscles supplied by the third nerve, yet without myosis. Silcock had two cases of complete ophthalmoplegia, externa and interna. Paralytic symptoms may involve the whole third nerve or produce separate symptoms like ptosis or mydriasis, and there may be also distinct ptosis when the trochlear is affected.

It is an interesting fact that paralysis of the facial nerve, on the same side, may follow or accompany herpes in the distribution of the fifth nerve. Rare though this complication is, several carefully recorded cases prove its occurrence beyond question. These palsies have shown a slow but complete recovery, as a rule. The close proximity of the nuclei of origin of the fifth and seventh nerves in the floor of the fourth ventricle, suggests a method of extension of inflammation which would account for these curious and rare cases of oculomotor and facial paralyses.

Beauvois has reported a case of parlysis of the sixth nerve, which occurred in an aged woman. The prodromal symptoms had been quite severe and the paresis, a most rare affection, persisted for six months, fading at the patient's complete recovery. Galizowski tells of another case in a man of eighty-two years, who, after an attack of pneumonia, was seized with a very extensive eruption on the face which invaded the cornea. After a year the paresis disappeared, but Galizowski ascribed the paresis to the effects of the pneumococcic infection. Gasper cites a case of complete paralysis of the fourth nerve, together with total paralysis of the facial on the other side; and Galizowski reports a case of paralysis of several muscles of the eye innervated by different nerves. This case is interesting from an association of paresis of the sixth nerve and an internal ophthalmoplegia. Communications between the ophthalmic and the motor nerves have been described. Such combined affections are not difficult of explanation, for the sixth nerve passes quite close to the ophthalmic, and as the intrinsic musculature is innervated by the oculomotor through the intervention of the ciliary ganglion, which receives the sensory root from the nasal, a branch of the ophthalmic, the connection may readily be seen.

It may be well for us to recall the anatomic arrangement and distribution of the ophthalmic branch of the fifth or trifacial nerve. The trifacial, according to Leidy, resembles the spinal nerves in that it has a motor and a sensory root. The sensory or larger root is provided with a ganglion, the semilunar, or Gasserian ganglion, which the nerve enters on its upper border. From the anterior border are given off three nerves, the smallest of which is the ophthalmic, which proceeds forward through the sphenoidal foramen into the orbit. This nerve, together with the superior maxillary, the next in size, is purely sensory.

In its course from the cavernous sinus to the sphenoidal foramen the ophthalmic is in company with the third and fourth nerves. At the foramen it divides into three branches, the lachrymal, the frontal and the nasal nerves. After leaving the ganglion it gives off a small recurrent branch to the tentorium, and in its further course it is connected by filaments with the third, fourth and sixth nerves, and with the cavernous plexes of the sympathetic.

The lachrymal nerve runs along the outer part of the orbit above the external rectus muscle to the lachrymal gland and upper eyelid, to which it is distributed. The frontal nerve runs along the root of the orbit above the palpebral elevator and divides into the supratrochlear and the supraorbital nerves. The supratrochlear leaves the orbit external to the pulley of the trochlear muscle and ascends to the forehead close to the bone. It supplies the skin and conjunctiva of the upper eyelid and the skin of the forehead. The supraorbital, the main branch of the frontal, passes from the orbit through the supraorbital foramen and is distributed by two branches to the skin of the forehead and the upper part of the scalp. The nasal nerve enters the orbit in close association with the external rectus muscle and the third nerve. A branch re-enters the cranial cavity and is then distributed to the nasal cavity by the cribriform plate of the ethmoid. Its internal branch is distributed to the mucous membrane; the external branch also supplies the mucous membrane, but leaves the cavity between the nasal cartilage and the nasal bone to be distributed to the skin of the tip and wing of the nose. In its course the nasal nerve gives off a branch to the ophthalmic ganglion, a slender filament running on the outer side of the optic nerve; the large ciliary nerves, which pierce the sclerotic and supply the ciliary muscle and iris; and the infratrochlear nerve which leaves the orbit at the inner angle, and is distributed to the lachrymal sac and caruncle, the conjunctiva, the skin of the eyelids, and the root of the nose.

As has already been pointed out, the territory most frequently affected, to quote Hutchinson, is that of the supraorbital nerve, and next to it comes the supratrochlear. The frontal is often affected without the supratrochlear, but the latter never suffers alone. Both, too, are often affected without the other branches, but when this occurs the eye is not inflamed.

We have next to consider the lachrymal branch. This branch gives filaments to the lachrymal gland, to the conjunctiva, and lastly, to the skin of the upper eyelid. It is, therefore, not very easy to tell in any given case of ophthalmic shingles whether or not it is affected; and it is likewise difficult to tell whether or not the lachrymal gland also is inflamed, as both the conjunctiva and the upper eyelid receive branches from other sources than the lachrymal. In any instance, however, in which the eruption is unusually free on the upper eyelid, and there is great swelling and much conjunctival congestion, we may safely believe that the lachrymal nerve is concerned. The most important of the branches, so far as ophthalmic zoster is concerned, is the nasal nerve, or as it is better named, the oculo-nasal. This nerve, soon after leaving the main trunk, to repeat what has already been described, gives off the long root of the ciliary ganglion, from which the short ciliary nerves pass to the iris. It next gives off the long ciliary branches which run directly to the ciliary muscle and iris, and, subsequently dividing into two branches, under the names of infra-trohclear and external, supplies sensation to the middle and tip of the side of the nose. It follows, then, that to know whether or not the nasal nerve is concerned in an attack of ophthalmic shingles, we must look for vesicles on the side of the nose, especially near to its tip.

The pathology of herpes zoster is of great interest, because for many years it was the subject of conjecture only. Mehlis, in 1818, was the first to suggest that the eruption of herpes zoster follows the distribution of nerves, but it was not until 1861 that von Bärensprung declared it to be definitely of nervous origin. The first case examined postmortem was one occurring in a person who died of tuberculosis, in which von Bärensprung found lesions in the posterior ganglion.

Later observers had opportunities to make postmortem examinations, their findings extending and confirming von Bärensprung's contention. In 1871 Wyss reported a case of zoster of the whole first division of the trigeminal nerve. In this case death followed a few days after the appearance of the eruption, and the lesion was found confined to the locality of, and included, the Gasserian ganglion. In 1875, in a case of ophthalmic herpes, Sattler found an inflammatory lesion with hemorrhages destroying both the nerve cells and the fibers of the Gasserian ganglion. The ganglion was filled with round cells, the ganglion cells markedly destroyed, while the ophthalmic division of the nerve was degenerated.

In 1900 Head and Campbell exhaustively investigated the subject of herpes zoster and added twenty-one cases to the list of those already studied by pathologic investigation. Two of their cases showed involvement of the supraorbital; up to that time there had been but two other well reported autopsies on cases of zoster ophthalmicus, namely, by Wyss and by Sattler.

Head and Campbell's twenty-one cases bore the signs of all stages after the eruption, varying from a few days to one and a half years, and their findings may be accepted as authoritative, their work indeed monumental. In their studies changes in the ganglia of the posterior root, in the posterior nerve root, in the peripheral nerves and in the spinal cord were noted. The cases exhibiting disease in the area of the trigeminal were examined with special care, and as the lesions noted in them could not be interpreted except in the light cast by that obtained from the more general cases, a résumé of their findings will be given.

In the ganglion of the posterior root. In the stage of active eruption the ganglion was profoundly inflamed and the tissues invaded crowded with small round cells, masses of which were scattered in clumps around the periphery and in the center of the ganglion. These foci were occasionally found around extravasated blood. In other cases the center of the ganglion would be ploughed up by large hemorrhages. The hemorrhages and inflammations were found upon the dorsal aspect of the ganglion in the portion opposed to the anterior root.

The ganglion substance showed signs of destruction to a greater or less extent, but in the center of the hemorrhagic foci the cells were absolutely destroyed. In some cases the nuclei of the ganglion cells were swollen and void of nucleolus. The substance of the cell body was blurred and without structure. The extent to which these changes appeared varied in different cases, and such changes that were noted were not those commonly seen in degenerative diseases of the nervous system—there were no ganglion cells with extruded or eccentric nuclei with vacuolation or an absence of Nissl's particles. The contrast between the gross lesions in a case of fracture and another of malignant disease and the herpetic was most pronounced.

The sheath of the ganglion also exhibited changes; the vessels were engorged and showed extravasations, and in severe cases there was an invasion of small round cells. In others not so severe, the inflammation was noticed to have passed away, leaving no trace behind in the ganglion. But the greater the severity of the eruption and the greater the scarring, the more certainly permanent changes occurred in the root ganglion.

On the subsidence of the inflammation absorption began, the effusion undergoing retrogressive changes. Ultimately the inflammation became converted into fibrous tissues, the density of the scar depending upon the severity of the original inflammation; thus in certain instances the scar occupied one-sixth to one-half of the ganglion, in which area all the structures were destroyed. The sheath became thickened, dense and fibrous.

In the posterior nerve roots. The changes in the posterior nerve roots corresponded to the results that might have been expected from the lesions of the ganglion. They consisted of an acute degeneration followed by a greater or less amount of secondary sclerosis, according to the severity of the acute destruction. The anterior root was in all cases normal.

In the peripheral nerves. Marked secondary changes were produced in the fibers that enter the posterior root ganglion, depending, of course, upon the extent and severity of the disease. The degeneration seemed to have appeared and disappeared, and was replaced by sclerotic changes at the same periods after the initial lesion in the ganglion as in the case of the invasion in the posterior roots. Hemorrhage and inflammation occurred just as was noted in the ganglion. The degeneration could be traced back to the fine twigs which passed upwards to the skin to supply the area over which the eruption was distributed.

In the spinal cord. Such lesions of the ganglion as already described, as might be expected, were attended by acute degeneration of the root fibers in the posterior columns of the spinal cord. The degeneration appeared at about the period of the ninth or tenth day of the eruption. The products of degeneration were removed much more slowly than was the case of degeneration of the fibers in the posterior roots, but when the products were removed they left no perceptible sclerosis behind.

In zoster of the trigeminal hemorrhagic foci were found in the Gasserian ganglion, together with destruction of nerve cells in that portion corresponding to the first or ophthalmic division of the trigeminal, together with sclerosis of the root bundles, without there being, however, degeneration in any part of the central nervous system referable to the lesion in the Gasserian ganglion.

The lesions observed in the Gasserian ganglion were an exact reproduction of what took place in the posterior root ganglion of other areas, and just as the sheath of the spinal ganglia became implicated in the lesion, so did the pia of the Gasserian ganglion show signs of thickening and infiltration. Degeneration followed in the root of the fifth nerve and degenerated fibers could be traced to the pons and into the medulla, the products of degeneration being removed just as in the spinal cord. The investigators concluded, therefore, that zoster of the branches of the trigeminal is associated with a lesion in the Gasserian ganglion similar to that found in the posterior root ganglion in cases of zoster of the trunk and limbs, and that the lesion causes secondary degeneration in the sensory root of the Gasserian ganglion within its extra and intramedullary courses.

Accordingly, as the eruption of herpes zoster is caused by or is the outcome of an intense and concentrated inflammation of the posterior root ganglion of the nerve area involved, there is, to repeat, good evidence for believing that ophthalmic zoster is dependent upon definite lesions in the Gasserian ganglion, which ganglion is the homolog of a large number of posterior root ganglia, and, it follows, that such a lesion causes secondary degeneration in the sensory root of the Gasserian ganglion.

The Gasserian ganglion, according to Head and Campbell, may be considered as a triangle, from the inner angle of which the greater part of the central root fibers come off. The first or ophthalmic division of the trigeminal nerve enters the ganglion at the preaxial angle of the triangle, and the third or maxillary division enters at the postaxial angle and is connected with cells at the ganglion. The second division of the trigeminal is closely allied with the third division in nature and function, but the first, the ophthalmic division, is distinct.

We are accustomed to regard sensory nerves as conveying only afferent impulses, therefore, "it is difficult," according to Parsons, "to imagine how an inflammatory block in the course of the nerve can produce the pathologic changes in its distant terminations. It is a well established fact that the nerve fibers are under the trophic control of the posterior root ganglia, yet the trophic control of the tissues supplied by the fibers is not so readily explained. It is probable that the ends of the nerve are subjected to some abnormal irritation, whether by blood clot, pus or other agent, and such irritation can only make itself felt in the reverse direction to the normal by an efferent impulse or by the transmission of deleterious agents along the nerve." Whatever the bacterial or other agent may be it seems to have a specific attraction for the posterior root ganglion. In this connection, it is interesting to include Sunde's report of a case of herpes zoster frontalis complicating a fatal bronchopneumonia. At the autopsy the Gasserian ganglion on the side of the herpes was found to be enlarged by an acute inflammatory process. Sections of the ganglion on the side of the zoster showed a number of Gram positive cocci arranged after the manner of diplococci or in short chains. This case of Sunde's suggests the appropriateness of referring in this place to the report by Howard of a case of herpes facialis accompanying pneumonia, in which hemorrhagic lesions akin to those of true zoster were demonstrable in the Gasserian ganglion.

Notwithstanding the fact that the occurrence is not constant nor frequent, the association of herpes zoster with pneumonia may not be without significance. In seeking to explain the mystery of the origin of zona ophthalmicus, the thoughts arise that there may be some association between it and pneumococcal infection, and of the likelihood of a transference of pneumococcic virus from the nasal passages to the Gasserian ganglion, which lies not too remote to be subject to infection by such a route. It is singular, indeed, that whatever the infection may be and the mode of its entrance in zoster ophthalmicus, it should manifest a predilection for the Gasserian ganglion, and for that ganglion only, and that in only the rarest of cases it affects structures distantly removed from the functions of the ganglion or external to its associations. As the process does not arise through the vascular system, but rather through the nervous, to which it is confined, the possibility of a direct transmission of infective material to the ganglion by way of the peripheral nerve twigs spread out in the nasal mucous surfaces ought not to be overlooked. It may be that the solution of the problem lies hid within the nasal chamber and that a thorough study of the sinuses in a large number of cases may yield results fit to be associated with those already attained by Head and Campbell. The pneumococcus may be the true infecting agent, although its presence and activities await demonstration.

The changes in the skin, as outlined by Head, based upon his studies of sections through an unruptured vesicle of herpes zoster, show an unilocular cavity, the floor of which is formed of naked papillæ. These papillæ are infiltrated with masses of small round cells which stain deeply. The infiltration extends down to the terminations of the sweat glands and hair follicles, while here and there, in the deeper layers of the skin, too, are seen collections of small round cells apart from the hair follicles and sweat glands. The vesicle itself is split into incomplete cavities by septa extending from the roof to the floor. These septa are evidently the remains of incompletely raised epithelial layers that retain their attachment to the roof and to the floor of the vesicle.

The cavity of the vesicle is filled with fluid which coagulates under the influence of the hardening agent into a somewhat granular hyalin mass. Within this mass lie small round cells, which take the stain deeply, and broken down epithelial cells of all sizes and shapes which have lost their prickles. Restitution takes place under a scab, which consists of the contents of the vesicles, and in the covering of the base of the vesicles by an ingrowth of growing cells from the periphery.

Nerve twigs can be traced in the deep layers of the corium, the axis cylinders and the neurolemma of which show swollen and degen-crated sheaths, while larger branches show marked degenerative changes as early as ten days after the onset of the eruption.

Microscopic examination of sections of the skin revealed no signs of microorganisms, nor were there any in the serum contents of the vesicles; the vesicles, therefore, are undoubtedly sterile. It may be that the pathologic process of zoster is the same as that of ordinary inflammations, and that it is of toxic origin, the agent of which most certainly does not enter the system by way of the skin.

The vesicles begin to dry up and to form scabs about the fifth to the tenth day after their first appearance. At the end of six weeks, beyond some freshly healed scars, nothing is to be seen, and by the arrangement of the scars it is usually easy to recognize it in a patient who has suffered from the disease even years after its occurrence. Where the skin is thin, scars rarely result; whereas the thicker the skin, the greater the likelihood of scarring, because the papillæ are placed deeper. The marks remaining are distinctly characteristic of the disease, and resemble none other, unless they be the pits of smallpox. They extend in lines like the branching of the twigs of a tree, or map-like, with clear spaces between the lines. They are more like erosions etching their way over the surface of the skin but sharply limited from encroaching beyond the median line.

Generally, for several weeks after healing, the skin may continue to be tender and remain anesthetic for many months. In some cases there may be cutaneous anesthesia dolorosa, such as was complained of by a man under my own observation who could not wear a hat, so great was the pain. In others the skin feels stiff or parchment-like and the scars may become keloid. It is not only that the parts affected remain painful, but their sensation, too, may be impaired; thus the cornea may be left anesthetic, and, therefore, especially disposed to ulceration from the action of foreign bodies, etc. Patients sometimes continue to suffer pain for months or years after the disease has subsided. There is partial or complete anesthesia in the region of the skin affected, which may continue after the subsidence of the pain and inflammation.

As a sequel of the corneal involvement, nebulæ or troublesome phlyctenules may be left. The scars on the cornea are invariably extensive and dense, the surrounding portions remaining hazy. The haziness of the cornea may continue for a long time, perhaps because it has lost the sensitiveness which it never fully regains. This fact must render the cornea especially prone to subsequent inflammatory trouble from the entrance of dust or other foreign body. The globe may continue injected and more or less sensitive for many weeks. Even when there has been only an infiltration of the cornea, the globe may remain tender.

The paralyses may persist for weeks or months and then gradually fade; no permanent pareses so far have been reported.

The prognosis of ophthalmic zoster is less favorable than that of herpes febrilis, and, by the presence of complications affecting the globe, it is rendered essentially worse. The prognosis must be grave when iritis develops. The pain may persist for a long time, the affected eye continuing irritable and subject to an increase of tension; and, the older the patient, the more is this neuralgia to be dreaded the longer it persists. The severity of both the eye lesions and the skin eruption is likely to be greatest in patients of advanced age. Therefore, the exhaustion consequent upon the pain and loss of rest becomes of serious moment.

The course may be over in three weeks; in other cases it may last from three to five months. The severity of the eruptive process may vary widely; in certain cases there may be only a single bleb at the limbus, while in others the blebs may be so numerous that enucleation of the globe may be necessary. In conclusion, it may be accepted as a rule that when the eye is markedly affected the prognosis must be very guarded; vision may be wholly lost, owing to iritis or destruction of the cornea, or, in less grave cases, the eye may be left irritable and congested, or manifest increased tension long after the attack has subsided.

The disease is rarely, if at all, bilateral, and very rarely occurs twice in the same nerve area. It seldom relapses, although it has been known to occur three times in the same individual; when it does so recur, it is probable that it depends upon some chronic peripheral irritation.

Stress must be laid on the fact that herpes zoster ophthalmicus is the frequent subject of mistakes in diagnosis. The disease may be mistaken for erysipelas, from which it should be distinguished by the acute neuralgic pain and the formation of vesicles in the course of the set of nerves. The inflamed area is confined to one side of the face, showing no tendency to spread, in erysipelas, on the contrary, the eruption is not confined within such limits, and, moreover, the vesicles in erysipelas are large, while in zoster they are small and coalesce in patches on sites corresponding to the terminal distribution of the nerve. By the formation of cicatrices the vesicles of zoster are distinguished from those of herpes febrilis, in which the epidermis alone is detached by the fluid, so that the vesicle of herpes heals without leaving any trace of its previous existence. From simple herpes, zoster, it is to be distinguished by the more severe course, the irritative symptoms persisting after the rupture of the vesicles, and, when the cornea has been invaded by the parenchyma becoming deeply clouded at the spots where the vesicles were situated, and, to the other symptoms, iritis is often added.

The more abundant the eruption on the two sides of the face, the less likely it is to be true zoster. The eruption of herpes about the lips and nose or in the cheeks common in febrile states, or in the course of naso-pharyngitis, bears no relation to true zoster. This form of eruption is always bilateral, and the vesicles are noted for their recurrences, frequently returning with each cold in the nose. Zoster is rarely if ever bilateral; but as febrile herpes may be concurrent with zoster, an unusually wide distribution of herpetic vesicles may confuse its diagnosis, however. Febrile herpes is not accompanied nor preceded by the characteristic neuralgic pains of zoster.

When the rash appears it is well to dust it quickly with a powder consisting of oxid of zinc in rice starch. During the evolution of the vesicles an ointment of oxid of zinc and rice starch rubbed up in vaselin may prevent suppuration as well as promote the healing. Locally anodyne lotions are useful, as of lead-water and laudanum, when the globe is not affected; weak carbolic acid or belladonna. Ichthyol ointment, too, is valuable. Calamin lotions, if painted on early, have sometimes diminished the severity of the lesions. Arlt covered the side of the face with a mask of red celluloid and directed the patient to sit in the sun so as to get the therapeutic benefit of the red rays. In his experience, pain was relieved and healing followed without scars.

Internally, anodynes are nearly always required, as the severe pain must be mitigated by opiates and morphin hypodermatically. Quinin in full doses, iron, strychnin, arsenic, sodium salicylate, cod liver oil and a highly nutritious diet generally offer the best chance of combating the neuritis.

When ocular complications set in they should be managed on the general principles governing the treatment of conjunctivitis, keratitis, iritis, cyclitis, etc., from other causes. Carefully applied protective bandages, with which to seal the part from the air, may possibly ward off neuro-paralytic keratitis. For this reason it should be employed when anesthesia is the only symptom, and it is imperatively demanded when there is destruction of the corneal tissues. The use of galvanism has been recommended for the relief of persistent neuralgia. McNab has been gratified with his results of ionic medication, consisting of the introduction of sulphate of quinine by means of the positive pole over the whole area affected. Usually two applications to the skin area are sufficient, at an interval of from seven to ten days, using a current of one to one and one-half milliamperes per square inch of surface for fifteen or twenty minutes. He thus cured the neuralgic pains and the disturbance of local sensibility, as well as relieved the iritis.

The treatment of herpes zoster ophthalmicus is unsatisfactory; it is doubtful whether we can shorten the duration of the attack, and it is equally difficult to decide whether a rather shorter course than usual follows spontaneously, or can be due to the drug or other measures employed, for in many cases the evolution of the eruption is incomplete.

The above is a résumé of the accepted facts regarding zoster; for obvious reasons quotations have been given for the most part without acknowledgment to the bibliographic references obtained in a review of the literature of the subject. Those who desire lists of references are recommended to consult Hutchinson's papers, Wilbrand and Sänger's *"Neurolgie des Auges,"* Parson's *"Pathology of the Eye,"* the *Ophthalmic Year Books,* Head and Campbell, in *"Brain"* for 1900, and Head's article in *"*Allbutt's *System of Medicine.""*—(B. C.) See, also, Vol. V, p. 3374, of this *Encyclopedia.*

Herpetic ulcer of the cornea. See **Herpes zoster ophthalmicus.**

Herschel, Caroline Lucretia. (1750-1848), sister of Sir Frederick William Herschel. She lived in Hanover until 1772, when she went to England to live with her brother at Bath. When William turned astronomer she became his constant helper, and on his being appointed private astronomer to King George the Third she acted as his assistant. While discharging her duties in this position she discovered several comets; and several remarkable nebulæ and clusters of stars included in William's catalogues were described from her original observations. In 1798 she published at the expense of the Royal Society, *A Catalogue of Stars taken from Mr. Flamsteed's Observations,* which contained five hundred and sixty-one stars omitted in the British catalogue. In 1828 the Astronomical Society conferred on her their gold medal. See her *Memoir and Correspondence,* edited by Mrs. Herschel (1876).—*(Standard Encyclopedia.)*

Herschelian rays. Invisible, infra red heat rays of the spectrum.

Herschelian telescope. A direct front-view reflector.

Herschel, Sir John Frederick William (1792-1871), the only son of Sir William Herschel, was born in Slough, England, and educated at Eton and St. John's, Cambridge, where, in 1813, he was senior wrangler and first Smith's prize-man. His first publication was *A Collection of Examples of the Application of the Calculus of Finite Differences.* (1820). In 1822 he applied himself especially to astronomy and for a time he worked with Sir James South in re-examining the nebulæ and clusters of stars described in his father's catalogs. The results of the examination were given in 1833 to the Royal Society in the form of a catalogue of stars in order of their right ascension. His treatises on Sound and on the Theory of Light appeared in the *Encyclopedia Metropolitana* (1830-31); his treatise on Astronomy (1831) and the *"Preliminary Discourse on the Study of Natural Philosophy"* in Lardner's *Cyclopedia;* not to mention his papers in the *Transactions of the Astronomical Society.* In January, 1834, Herschel arrived at the Cape of Good Hope, with the intention of completing the survey of the sidereal heavens, by examining the southern hemisphere as he had done the northern. Here he established his observatory at Feldhausen, six miles from Table Bay; in four years working all the time at his own expense he completed his observations; in 1847 he published a volume of *Astronomical Observations made at the Cape; being the Completion of a Telescopic Survey of the Whole Surface of the Visible Heavens commenced in 1825.*

On his return to England honors were showered on him—he was made D. C. L. of Oxford and on Queen Victoria's coronation a baronet. He was president of the Astronomical Society and in 1849 became master of the Mint. His articles on Meteorology, Physical Geography and the Telescope, contributed to the *Encyclopedia Britannica,* were published separately; and his *Popular Lectures on Scientific Subjects* (new Ed. 1880) and *Collected Addresses* are well known works. Herschel was also a distinguished chemist, and attained important results in photography independent of Fox Talbot. His researches on the undulatory theory of light were very valuable. He had also a profound interest in poetry and made translations from Schiller and from the *Iliad*. He was buried in Westminster Abbey near Sir Isaac Newton. See Agnes M. Clerke, *The Herschels and Modern Astronomy* (1896).—*(Standard Encyclopedia.)*

Herschel's double prism. This small instrument, like the Risley double prism, is used for determining not only the strabismic angle in a squinting eye but the degree of convergence. The Zeiss catalogue gives the following description of it—in combination with the Landolt graduation: In a frame provided with a handle are two prisms having two similar refracting angles and coupled in such a manner that, as one is made to revolve, the other rotates at the same rate but in the opposite direction. This produces a continuously variable prismatic deflection in one direction, the pencil of rays being deflected in a plane at right angles to the handle. The prisms are rotated by means of a milled ring which bears the graduations, motion being imparted to it by the thumb or index finger of the hand holding the instrument. On the opposite side to the graduated face the instrument has a revolving vulcanite cup which fits snugly the rim of the orbital cavity so as to give the instrument an immovable position in front of the eye. The cup is so arranged that it will accommodate a green glass or a Maddox cylinder, the object of the former being to mask the dispersion at large angles of deviation.

The milled ring carries in front two graduations. Of these the upper one, which is read by the upper index, shows the deviation in degrees produced by the two prisms. The zero point of the scale is marked by the nickel-plated screw. The zero point serves also to indicate the position of the base. This is always situated at right angles to the handle and always on the side of the zero point of the upper scale, as indicated by the nickel-plated screw.

If, for example, the deviation in any given case be found to be 5° a prism of 5° may be prescribed for either eye, since the angle is about twice as great as the angle of deviation.

The lower scale, as devised by Landolt, reads the deviation in terms of metre-radians. Since these depend upon the magnitude of the basal line the scale is so arranged that the metre-radians can be read off for various basal lines. At the bottom edge will be found the metre-radian for a basal line of 58 mm., the first ring reads the values for 60 mm., the second ring for 62 mm., the third ring for 64 mm., and the inner edge those for 67 mm. Readings are taken by the long index. If, for example, with a basal line of 58 mm. the reading shows a deficiency of 3 metre-radians it will be 2.9 metre-radians for a basal line of 60 mm., 2.8 metre-radians for 62 mm., 2.7 metre-radians for 64 mm., and 2.5 metre-radians for a basal line of 67 mm.

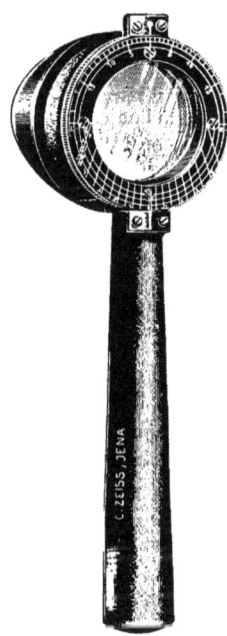

Herschel's Double Rotary Prism.

The symbols —L and —R indicate the nature of the deviation of the squinting eye, they show accordingly whether the strabismus is divergent or convergent.

When the prisms are held in front of the right eye and the images brought to coincidence when a reading is taken on the side bearing the symbol —R this shows that the squint is divergent and in this case the base occupies a nasal position. If a reading be taken for the right eye on the side bearing the symbol —L the squint is convergent and the base of the correcting prism occupies accordingly a temporal position. The symbol —L corresponds therefore to +R and, conversely, —R corresponds to +L.

When using the prisms in front of the trial frame it is best to remove the vulcanite eye cup.

Herschel, Sir William (1738-1822), was born at Hanover, the son of a band-master and was educated as a professional musician. In 1757 he established himself in England, becoming a teacher of music in the town of Leeds, whence he went to Halifax as organist, and subsequently (1766) in the same capacity to Bath. Here he would seem to have first turned his attention to astronomy. Wanting a superior telescope and unable to afford to buy a good reflector he made one for himself—a Newtonian of five foot focal length—and with this applied himself to study the heavens. In 1781 he made his first discovery, a new planet, which he at first took for a comet. The result of his discovery was his appointment to be private astronomer to George III. He then went to live at Slough near Windsor, where, assisted by his sister Caroline, he continued his researches. Herschel married a Mrs. Mary Pitt, and left one son. He was knighted by George III. He greatly added to our knowledge of the solar system; he discovered Uranus (called by him Georgium Sidus) and what he took for its six satellites and two satellites of Saturn. Besides this he detected the rotation of Saturn's ring, the period of rotation of Saturn itself and that of Venus; the existence of the motions of binary stars, the first revelation of systems beside our own. His catalogue of double stars, nebulæ, etc., and tables of the comparative brightness of stars and his researches in regard to light and heat would have in themselves entitled him to the first rank as an astronomer and natural philosopher. He erected a famous monster telescope of forty feet in length. It was begun in 1785 and finished in 1789, in which year he by means of it detected the sixth satellite of Saturn. See Herschel's *Life and Works* by E. S. Holden (1881) and *William Herschel and his Work*, by J. Sime (1900).—*(Standard Encyclopedia.)*

Herse-curette conjonctivale. (F.) Conjunctival rake-curet.

Hertel's exophthalmometer. See Vol. VII, p. 4597 of this *Encyclopedia;* as well as the captions **Exophthalmometer** and **Exophthalmos.**

Herter's test. This is one of several well-known tests for simulated blindness (q. v.) with the plane mirror.

Hertzell's electric perimeter. See **Perimeter**; as well as **Perimetry.**

Hertzell's ophthalmo-diaphanoscope. See p. 3948, Vol. V, of this *Encyclopedia.*

Hertz, Heinrich Rudolf. This distinguished scientist was born at Hamburg, Germany, in 1857, and studied at Berlin. In 1880 he became assistant to Helmholtz, in 1885 was called to the technical school at Karlsruhe and in 1889 succeeded Clausius as Professor at Bonn. He greatly advanced the science of electricity, was the continuator of the work of Faraday and Clerk-Maxwell and was a singularly ingenious experimenter. He demonstrated the existence of electromagnetic waves of comparatively slow frequency. "Hertzian" waves are propagated through space, and can be reflected, refracted and polarized like light. Wireless telegraphy is the practical development of his discoveries. Three volumes of his collected works appeared in 1894 and have been translated into English by D. E. Jones (1893-99). Hertz's untimely death occurred in 1894.

Hervorrufung. (G.) Development.

Herz. (G.) The heart.

Herzensthätigkeit. (G.) The action of the heart.

Herzgifte. (G.) Cardiac poisons.

Herzklemme. (G.) Stenosis of the aortic, mitral, tricuspid, or pulmonary aperture.

Herzschall. (G.) The sound of the heart.

Hess, Wilhelm. A well-known German ophthalmologist. Born at Giessen, June 23, 1831, he was a student at Giessen, Wurzburg, Heidelberg, Vienna, and Prague. In 1853 he began to study ophthalmology under Albrecht von Graefe, whose close personal friendship he enjoyed. In 1857 he settled for practice in Mainz. He possessed remarkable executive, as well as operative, ability. He was one of the founders of the (Heidelberg) *Ophthalmologische Gesellschaft* and was for a long time its permanent secretary. He was a man of impressive appearance and charming personality. He died in 1905.—(T. H. S.)

Heterobaphia. (L.) That state of a body in which its surface shows two or more colors.

Heterochromia, Ocular. ANISOIRIDOCHROMIA. CHROMHETEROPIA. HETEROPHTHALMOS. HETEROCHROMIA IRIDIUM. ANISOCHROMIA.

In this condition the irides are of different colors. The difference may involve the entire surface, or in one iris a half or a sector is of a different color from the remainder. The sector may remain blue while the rest of it is brown; or patches of brown may be scattered about in a blue iris forming what is termed a "piebald iris."

The color of the iris is always proportionate to the pigmentation of the rest of the body, and as a rule blondes will have a light and brunettes a dark-hued iris; the dark races therefore, always have a dark iris.

Pigment is deposited in the epithelial layers of the iris very early in fetal life, and does not make its appearance in the mesoblastic elements until after birth. At first the stroma is thin and contains but little pigment, so that the posterior pigment layer is seen through it,

but as age advances, the stroma becomes thicker, and, if the pigmentation does not increase, the iris simply becomes of a light blue or gray.
Blue eyes accordingly show the normal pigmentation of the retinal
epithelium, the stroma being deficient in pigment; if, however, there
is an increase in the pigment as well as the stroma, the iris becomes
of a brown color. The color of the iris depends, therefore, upon the
pigmentation of the stroma as well as upon its structure and density;
accordingly, most children are born with a deep-blue or grayish iris,
but the color changes in the first years of life.

Irregularities in the disposition of pigment in the iris may occur,
in some cases only temporarily, while in others they persist throughout
life. Accordingly, the transformation of a blue iris into a brown
is occasionally confined to a portion of the membrane, so that a
brownish sector is seen in an otherwise light-colored iris. Moreover,
though the occurrence is rare, the iris of one eye may be blue and
that of the other brown. The sectoring is usually confined to one eye,
but, rarely it may be seen in both eyes, when it is spoken of as bilateral
heterochromia, or dicorus.

The cause of heterochromia is not known. It has been noted in
some cases that the parents have been of different complexions, one
fair with blue eyes, the other dark.

It has been observed in certain cases that heterochromia has had
other anomalies or defects of structure associated with it, and that
such individuals have been preternaturally subject to cataract, the
cataract developing in the lighter eye. It is probable that these were
not true cases of congenital heterochromia, but were dependent upon
disturbances of nutrition, because, in addition to the clouding of the
lens, evidences of a chronic cyclitis were manifested by the deposition
of minute granules in the aqueous humor; the cataracts were, therefore, complicate. The differences in color in such cases may be slight,
one iris being of a somewhat lighter blue or gray than the other, the
lighter showing pronounced degenerative changes while the other remains normal, although Butler, in 1912, reported a case in which the
changes took place in the dark eye. This acquired form of heterochromia has been seen at as early an age as 8 years. It has been suggested by Bistis that paralysis of the sympathetic may occupy an
important place in the discussion of the etiology of acquired
heterochromia.

Heterochromia, therefore, appears in two forms: as a simple anatomic anomaly, and, as a symptom of a definite and rare disease of
the ciliary body, called heterochromic cyclitis.—(B. C.)

[That heterochromia iridis is not infrequently associated with, or is often due to, *paralysis of the sympathetic* has been maintained by a number of observers. M. S. Mayou (*Ophthalmic Review,* June, 1910) reported two such cases occurring in young children.

J. Bistis (*Archives d'Ophtalm.,* Sept., 1912) reports a similar case, but in a woman aged 38, and believes that trophic disturbances, as evidenced by the presence of cyclitis, etc., must be held to be responsible for the change in color in the acquired form, just as much as they are the cause in the congenital form, and that the origin of the trophic disturbances is to be found in disease of the cervical sympathetic. He suggests that heterochromia might well be added to the cardinal symptoms of Horner's syndrome,. and says that the fact of it not being constant in all such cases is no argument against a sympathetic paralysis.

Galezowski communicated to the Société française d'Ophtalmologie several examples of heterochromia with signs of paralysis of the sympathetic, such as inequality of the pupils and narrowing of the palpebral fissure. In one of these cases there were indications of excitation of the sympathetic on the opposite side, viz., dilatation of the pupil, widening of the palpebral fissure and proptosis.

The most elaborate argument in favor of the frequent connection between paralysis of the sympathetic and heterochromia is stated by Scalinci (*Archivio di Ottalmologia,* Feb., 1915). He adopts the classification .of de Vries, who suggests the occurrence of four varieties of heterochromia: (a) the congenital; (b) congenital plus chronic iridocyclitis; (c) the depigmented iris, such as is not infrequently met with in glaucoma; and (d) that occurring as a true iridocyclitis, particularly in myopic eyes. Another might be added in which, apart from any obvious cyclitis, this want of symmetry develops during adult life, with or without signs of cyclitis. In Scalinci's opinion it would be best to keep the name heterochromia for the instances in which there has not been any obvious pathological process in the eye, such as rise of tension or iridocyclitis.

Altogether Scalinci concludes that the condition known as heterochromia would be better named aniso-iridochromia; it may be primary or secondary; if primary, it may be congenital or ·acquired. He further contends that primary heterochromia, in either form, is a complex disturbance of the eye; the deficiency of pigment in the iris stroma (and elsewhere) is caused by a lesion of the cervical sympathetic. Insidious inflammation of the ciliary body, coming on in such an eye either in virtue of diminished resistance on its part, or on account of the loss of pigment, does not exist in these cases in the true sense of the word. The appearances presented (depigmentation, presence of precipitates on the posterior surface of the cornea, etc.) can be accounted for by the existence of a lesion of the cervical sympathetic of a paralytic nature. The loss of pigmentation on the one hand and the presence of precipitates in Descemet's membrane on the other are to be looked upon not in the light of cause and effect, but rather as two manifestations of the same lesion of the sympathetic. The cataract which occurs, and which has been regarded by some as induced by cyclitis and trophic lesions of the lens, is by Scalinci looked upon rather as due to changed physio-chemical relations with the circulating nutritive fluids, or perhaps to biological alterations in the contents of the nutrient fluid itself, to the passage into the blood of substances alien to the normal intra-ocular contents, this escape being due to vasomotor paralysis.] See also **Congenital anomalies**.

Heterochromous iris. An iris in which part is of one color and part of another.

Heterocrania. (L.) Headache on one side only.

Heterogenesia. (L.) The development of parts that are abnormal as to situation.

Heteroglaucia. (L.) A term adopted by Wallroth, to describe the anomalous production of greenish or glaucous spots.

Heteroglaucous. Having one eye blue and the other black or gray.

Heterograft. A transplant, generally of skin, from one individual to another.

Heteroinfection. Infection of the organism with a poison not generated within itself.

Heterolateral. Occurring on the opposite side.

Heterologous. Not homologous; of opposed sides or kinds, as for instance the injection of horse's serum into the human body.

Heteronymous. Opposed or opposite; not homonymous. Applied in *diplopia* to crossed double images, such as are seen when there is a relative divergence of the eyes.

Heteronymous images. Double ocular images apparently displaced from one another in the contrary sense to the displacement of the eyes in which they are produced.

Heterophoralgia. Eye-strain or ocular pain caused by heterophoria.

Heterophoria. HETEROPHORIA IN GENERAL. Insufficiency and imbalance of the extrinsic ocular muscles will be considered not only under the caption **Muscles, Ocular**, but under the several headings into which the nomenclature of Stevens divides the subject; so that it will not be pursued to any length here. This nomenclature has been generally accepted and is as follows:

Orthophoria. Perfect or mathematical binocular balance.

Heterophoria. Imperfect binocular balance. Heterophoria naturally presents many varieties, to-wit:

Esophoria. A latent tendency of the visual axes to swing inward.

Exophoria. A latent tendency of the visual axes to swing outward.

Hyperphoria. A latent tendency of one visual axis to deviate above that of the other.

Hypophoria. A latent tendency of one visual axis to deviate below that of the other.

Combinations of the above are:

Hyperesophoria. A latent tendency of one visual axis to deviate upward and inward.

Hyperexophoria. A latent tendency of one visual axis to deviate upward and outward.

Hypoesophoria. A latent tendency of one visual axis to deviate downward and inward.

Hypoexophoria. A latent tendency of one visual axis to deviate downward and outward.

To these have been added

Anaphoria. A latent tendency of both visual axes to deviate above the horizontal plane of the head.

Kataphoria. A latent tendency of both visual axes to deviate below the horizontal plane of the head.

Cyclophoria. An insufficiency or overaction of the obliques; seen principally in connection with oblique astigmatism.

The *diagnosis of and tests for heterophoria* are discussed under **Examination of the eye,** as well as under **Muscles, Ocular,** and the minor captions referred to in this section.

Heterophorometer. An instrument for the detection of heterophoria. See **Examination of the eye.**

Heterophthalmia. (L.) An old term for a difference, either of color, position, or size, between the two eyes; also a term proposed by Coulomb (*Annales d'Oculistique,* Aug., 1912), instead of the French word "borgne," to denote a one-eyed person.

Heterophthalmos. An incorrect term for heterochromia.

Heteroplasty. Plastic surgery by the transplantation of portions from another organism, especially one of a different species. See **Enucleation,** and **Cornea, Transplantation of the.**

Heteropoda. Pelagic gasteropods, in which the "foot" has become a swimming organ. In association with their active life on the surface of the ocean must be noted not only the locomotor foot but the protective transparency, the highly developed nervous system and sensory structures, eyes, ears and smelling organ. See **Comparative ophthalmology.**

Heteroptics.   Perverted uses of the eyes; false vision.

Heteroscopy.   Any visual defect.   Deuteroscopy.

Heterotopia.   (L.)   An anomaly of situation; misplacement of an organ; the occurrence of a particular tissue in an abnormal situation according to Haeckel, in evolution, the appearance of an organ in an abnormal position or its development from a part different from that in which it develops in members of the same division.

Heterotropia.   Another name for that form of strabismus, or squint, in which there is decided deviation of the visual axes of non-paralytic origin.   This subject will be fully treated under **Muscles, Ocular.** Here it may be said that to this class of muscular anomalies the term comitant strabismus is given, because of the distinguishing feature that the angle of deviation remains the same whether the eyeballs are turned in the direction of the squint or in the opposite direction; or, in other words, that the affected eye follows its fellow fully in all its movements.

The terms *convergent* (in), *divergent* (out), *sursumvergent* (up), and *deorsumvergent* (down) strabismus are used to distinguish them according to the direction assumed by the deviating eye.

The following nomenclature has been given by Stevens to the condition of equilibrium and to the various deviations therefrom:

Orthophoria, the condition in which muscular equilibrium is maintained with the minimum of nervous effort.

Heterotropia, a deviation of the visual lines from parallelism in such a manner that they cannot habitually be united at the same point of fixation.

The class of heterophorias includes:

Esotropia, a deviation of the visual lines inward.

Exotropia, a deviation of the visual lines outward.

Hypertropia, a deviation of one visual line above the other.   (The term is a relative one and must be prefixed by the designating word *right* or *left*.)

Intermediate deviations are termed *hyperesotropia* (right or left) and *hyperexotropia* (right or left).

Variations of the equilibrium, which may or may not be consistent with parallelism of the visual lines, but in which, with the least innervation of the eye-muscles, the visual lines would tend below or above the most favorable plane for the minimum effort, are termed, respectively, *cataphoria* and *anaphoria*.

A rotary tendency, due to insufficiency of the oblique muscles, has been described by Savage and has received the name *cyclophoria.*

Aside from the above characteristic symptom, which alone would serve to distinguish this form of squint from the paralytic variety, there is usually absence of diplopia, equality of the primary and secondary deviations, and amblyopia of the deviating eye by which to differentiate them.

Deviations of the visual axis may have their origin in anomalies of refraction, structure, and insertion of the ocular muscles, and in the development of the orbits, in innervational disturbance, and as the result of congenital and acquired monocular amblyopia (opacities of the media and diseases of the fundus).—(J. M. B.)

See, also, p. 3297, Vol. V; as well as p. 4052, Vol. VI, of this *Encyclopedia.*

Hetol. SODIC CINNAMATE. SODIUM CINNAMYLATE. $NaC_9H_7O_2$. This is a white, crystalline powder readily soluble in water. It is mostly employed in eye diseases by sub-conjunctival injection, the eye being first cocainized. Half a gram of à 1 per cent. solution is at first injected every other day and then daily. More or less pain is the result, followed by a feeling of comfort. A number of observers have testified to its value in interstitial keratitis, corneal ulcer, herpes ophthalmicus, episcleritis and in the various forms of uveitis.

Both Pflueger and Cohn observed much benefit from the use of this remedy in parenchymatous keratitis. The latter used it in the form of collyrium—a one per cent. solution—to which he added the same quantity of cocain to minimize the pain. He believed that it exerted a favorable effect on the disease both in its acute and chronic phases.

Cohn (*Woch. f. Ther. u. Hyg. des Auges,* June 19, 1913) also reports success with hetol in three cases of iritis. Two were undoubtedly of a tuberculous nature, the third probably tuberculous.

Following 3 per cent. cocain he instilled 2 to 5 per cent. hetol and 1 per cent. novocain dissolved in normal salt solution, this procedure being repeated every other day, and the number of drops gradually increased.

Heubacillus. (G.) Bacillus of hay fever.

Heuermann, Georg. A celebrated Copenhagen surgeon, who devoted much attention to ophthalmology. Born at Oldesloe, Holstein, in 1723,* he studied for a time at the Copenhagen University, and, in 1749, received from that institution his medical degree. In 1750 he

---

* According to Hirschberg, but the ''*Biographisches Lexikon der Aerzte*'' says in 1722.

became prosector at the University, and eight years later "physician and chief surgeon to the mobilized army." He was appointed professor of surgery at the Copenhagen University in 1763, but did not begin to lecture till three years later. In 1768 he died. His medical writings are as follows: 1. *De Linguâ Humanâ*. (Diss., 1749.) 2. *Physiologie*. (In four parts; Copenhagen and Leipsic, 1751-55. According to Hirschberg, more than 200 pages of this work are devoted to the eye.) 3. *Abhandlung der Vornehmsten Chirurgischen Operationen am Menschlichen Körper*. (3 parts; Copenhagen, 1754-57. Especially rich in the surgery of the eye.) 4. *Vermischte Bemerkungen und Untersuchungen der Ausübenden Arzneiwissenschaft*. (2 parts; Copenhagen; 1765, 67.)—(T. H. S.)

Heufieber. (G.) Hay fever.

Heurteloup's leech. See p. 633, Vol. I, of this *Encyclopedia*.

Heurtin, Marie. An interesting account of the education of this deaf, blind and dumb girl is given by S. H. Brown (*Ophthalmic Record*, p. 586, 1910). The dramatic features of the case engaged the attention of the French Academy of Sciences and one of its sessions was devoted entirely to it.

The story as narrated by those familiar with the facts relates how on March 1st, 1895, Heurtin, a caskmaker, with his wife and ten-year-old child, Marie, after traversing the polygon of the Arsenal at Poictiers, reached the Convent of de Larney, supported and managed by the Sisters of Wisdom. This was the beginning of a new epoch in the life of the child. When she was ten years old she presented none of the characteristics of a girl of that age and was repulsive in every particular. She was deaf, dumb, and blind from the time of her birth, and the nystagmus of which she was the subject made her appearance especially startling. Being out of all communication with those about her, she was deprived of all the ordinary training of mind and her traits were more or less animal in character. The uncertainty of where she was stepping compelled her to crawl for the most part, and when she did assume the erect posture she had a peculiar dragging gait. Added to these outward deflections was the possession of an ungovernable temper.

The parents of the poor child sought admission for Marie to the various institutions only to be met with disappointment from time to time. The blind asylums refused her because she was deaf; the deaf because she was mute; and the mute because she was blind and deaf. Those institutions that had taken her were unable to do anything with her on account of her ferocious temper, and she was returned after a short stay to her parents. But at last, upon the advice of the Curé of Nantes, they sought in despair the aid of the Sisterhood at the Convent of de Larney, after a tramp of two hundred miles. The Mother Superior was much impressed by the history of the child as told by the father and by the dire distress of the parents, and accepted the child as an inmate, although she was the first of the kind they had ever encountered. The work of the institution had to do entirely with the deaf and dumb.

The handling of such a case was naturally perplexing. For the first few months she was allowed her own way for purposes of observation and her bestial tendencies were marked. Her temper manifested itself in pseudo-convulsions and strange noises. Day and night having no significance to her at this time, she would get out of bed at night and crawl indefinite distances guided by the floor and the walls. The latter she distinguished by the plaster, which she scraped off in her wanderings. Anything portable with which she came in contact she straightway destroyed. These maniacal outbursts were at times witnessed by outsiders, and the report became current that they were superinduced by cruel treatment on the part of the Sisters.

This naturally led to investigation and the public were surprised to learn that instead of torturing an inmate one of the pious Sisterhood, Sister Sainte Marguerite, was making it her special life work to educate the apparently hopeless deaf, dumb and blind imbecile. This pious woman with wonderful patience set about her task and watched every detail of the child's natural tendencies without interruption, for an indefinite period. Gluttony being the most pronounced of the child's traits, she determined to make the entering wedge through this channel. She learned that Marie was especially fond of eggs, and while feeding her one day she withdrew the egg after it had already been in the girl's possession and made the symbol of egg in the youngster's hand.

The wrath of the child knew no bounds, but she failed to obtain it again and other food was given to her instead. For several successive days a similar experiment was made and at last the light dawned upon the feeble mind that she was expected to make the sign suggested to her if she were to get the egg. From this beginning Sister Sainte Marguerite exerted her infinite ingenuity until the child had mastered the alphabet of the blind. With this means of communication with the surrounding world established, the Sister was able to teach this stunted brain the elements of ethics, morality, and religion, and slowly but surely the ferocious animal-like temper dwindled and the intellect flourished. She eventually learned to manipulate a sewing machine in addition to accumulating quite a fund of intellectual knowledge.

Her teacher, Sister Sainte Marguerite, was complimented by the French Academy and by the President of the French Republic. Marie Heurtin is now (1910) 25 years of age, and while she cannot see, she has six different means of conversing and is capable of engaging in a conversation of considerable range. She is able to knit, sew, make chairs and baskets, and draw upon the blackboard, all of which accomplishments she owes to the devotion of the Sister. This remarkable case suggests an obvious course in all similar instances.

Heusinger, Johann Christian Friedrich Karl. A celebrated German natural historian and physician, who devoted some attention to ophthalmology. Born at Farnroda Feb. 28, 1792, he received his medical degree at Jena in 1812, and, after a year of further study at Göttingen, became a military physician in active service in the Prussian army. Returning to civil life, he became an assistant to von Himly at Göttingen, then professor at Jena, then at Würzburg, and, finally at Marburg, where he spent the remainder of his days. In 1876 he was ennobled, and on the 5th of May, 1883, he died, aged 91.

Heusinger's chief ophthalmologic writing is "Untersuchung der Augen eines Amaurotischen" (*Rust's Mag. f. d. Ges. Heilk.*, Bd. I).— (T. H. S.)

Hewson, Adinell. A famous American surgeon, of some importance in

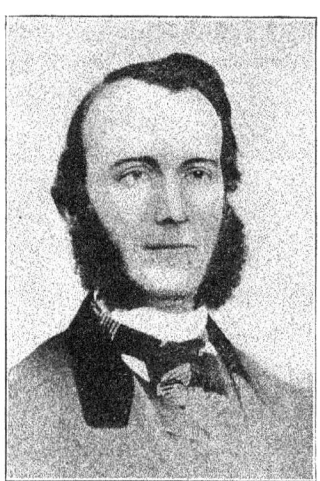

Adinell Hewson.

ophthalmology. Born Nov. 22, 1820, eighth son of Professor Thomas T. Hewson, of Philadelphia, he received the degree of A. B. at the

University of Pennsylvania in 1848, and that of M. **D.** at the Jefferson Medical College in 1850. For a time he studied at the Rotunda Hospital, Dublin. Returning to Philadelphia in 1851, he practised there for the remainder of his life. He was for several years surgeon to the Wills Eye Hospital, and wrote the following papers of ophthalmologic interest: "On the Prominence of the Eyeball with Sinking of the Caruncle and Semilunar Folds Following the Ordinary Operations for Strabismus" (*N. Am. Surg. Review,* Phila., 1858); "On Localized Galvanism as a Remedy for the Photophobia of Strumous Ophthalmia" (*Am. Jour. of Med. Sciences,* Phila., 1860). He also edited, with numerous excellent notes, William Mackenzie's *"Practical Treatise on Diseases of the Eye"* (1855).

Dr. Hewson married, in 1854, Rachel Macomb Wetherill, daughter of Dr. William Wetherill, of Philadelphia, by whom he had three sons and three daughters. He died Sept. 11, 1889.—(T. H. S.)

Hexagon. A figure enclosed by six straight lines.

Hexagonal pigment-cells of the retina. See **Histology of the eye.**

Hexahedron. A solid figure having six faces.

Hexamethylene-tetramin. UROTROPIN. FORMIN. AMINOFORM. CYSTAMIN. CYSTOGEN. This abundantly named agent is a white, crystalline powder sublimable and soluble in water. It is much used in cystic and renal diseases in doses of 8 to 25 grains (0.5—1.5 grm.).

Major Kirkpatrick (*Indian Medical Gazette,* June, 1915) has treated several cases of hypopyon keratitis with urotropin given in doses of fifteen grains thrice daily, and is quite sure that the drug has hastened the cure of the disease. Its use has been combined with atropin locally. Paracentesis, in addition, has been required in some cases. Major Miller, the chemical analyst, of Madras, found the drug in the tears of a patient with a septic ulcer of the cornea who was under urotropin treatment.

The treatment was first tried in a case of acute infection following cataract extraction. The corneal wound was much infiltrated, the anterior chamber was half full of pus, and the pupil blocked by exudate. Fifteen grains of urotropin were given every four hours, cyanide of mercury was injected under the conjunctiva, and atropin and conjunctival irrigations were used. The case cleared up in a very striking manner, and in four weeks' time, the eye had vision 6/36 when corrected.

A case of gonorrheal ophthalmia in an adult is also related, in which the administration of urotropin three times a day was combined with the "usual treatment." There was rapid improvement.

Henry Gradle (*Illinois Med. Journ.,* Nov., 1913) has found it of decided value in several ophthalmic cases, and believes its chief clinical importance lies in its use as a prophylactic against infection. He says:. "During the past two years I have had the local surgeon at one of the wire mills give large doses to every man immediately upon suffering a perforating injury of the eyeball. During this period of time, I have not had a single case of panophthalmitis develop where my instructions have been followed, and only one case of endophthalmitis septica. During the two years preceding, approximately three cases out of every ten lost the eye because of a panophthalmitis developing within the first forty-eight hours. This may be mere coincidence, but I believe that I am justified in attributing the results to the free and early use of hexamethylamin. Every case of intraocular operation is given hexamethylamin for at least two days preceding and for four days following operation. Here, too, my results have shown a remarkable freedom from infection."

Hexangular. Having six angles.

Hexen-Hasel. (G.) Witch hazel.

Heyfelder, Johann Ferdinand. A famous ophthalmologist of Petrograd, Russia. Born at Küstrin, Germany, Jan. 19, 1798, he studied medicine at Berlin, Jena, Würzburg, Tübingen and Breslau. At the last named institution he received his degree in 1820, presenting as dissertation "De Prosopalgia Fothergilli." After a year or more spent in travel, he settled in Trier, where he became a very successful practitioner. In 1831 he was sent to Berlin to investigate a terrible epidemic of cholera raging there. The result was a work entitled *"Beobachtungen über die Cholera Asiatica"* (Bonn, 1832). With a similar purpose he went to Paris in 1832, and again the result was a book, *"Die Cholera in Frankreich"* (Bonn, 1832). In 1841 he became professor of surgery and ophthalmology and director of the Surgical Clinic at the University of Erlangen. Here he was known as a daring operator, a careful and critical editor, and a brilliant teacher. Dissentions arising, however, between himself and his colleague, he resigned his position as professor, and joined the Russian army. In his capacity of army surgeon, he was present at the bombardment of Sveaborg. At the close of the war, he settled in Petrograd. Here he resided for fifteen years, honored, and admired by all. He died, June 21, 1869. To the industry of Hirschberg we owe the following bibliography: 1. Das Chirurgische und Augenkranken-Clinicum der Universität Erlangen von 1. Oktober 1841 bis zum 30. September 1842 von Prof. Heyfelder (*Heidelberger Med. Annalen*, 1842). 2. Das Chirurgische und Augenkranken-Clinicum zu Erlangen von 1. Oktober 1842 bis zum 30 September 1843, von Dr. Heyfelder (Erlangen,

1843). 3. Das Chirurische und Augenkranken-Clinicum der Universität Erlangen, vom 1 Oktober 1843 bis zum 30 September 1844, von Dr. Heyfelder (Berlin, 1845). 4. Sur l'Influence de la Commotion sur l'Oeil. Par le Dr. Heyfelder, etc.. Traduit de l'Allemand, sur le Manuscrit de l'Auteur, par le Dr. Ph. van Meerbeck d'Anvers. (*Annal. d'Ocul*, xiii, S. 145-157, 1845.) 5. Mikroskopische Untersuchungen über die Krankhaften Geschwülste (*Heidelberger Klin. Annalen*, 1845). 6. Anatomische Untersuchung eines Auges mit Koloboma Iridis. (Ammon's Z., III, 467, 1833.)—(T. H. S.)

Heyfelder, Oscar. Son of Johann Ferdinand Heyfelder (q. v.). Born at Trier, Apr. 7, 1828, he studied at the Universities of Heidelberg and Erlangen, at the latter institution receiving his degree in 1851. For a number of years he was chief of the surgical and ophthalmological clinic at Erlangen. He died June 1, 1890.—(T. H. S.)

Heyl, Albert Gallatin. A distinguished American ophthalmologist. Born at Philadelphia, Oct. 2, 1847, he studied in both the academic and the medical departments of the University of Pennsylvania, receiving his professional degree in 1870. After a period of special study in Vienna, London, and Heidelberg, he returned to Philadelphia, and, for the remainder of his life, practised ophthalmology exclusively. He is said to have been a brilliant operator.

Among his more important writings are: 1. A Case of Uremic Amblyopia. (*Am. Jour. of the Med. Sc.*, 1874.) 2. A Case of Hypemia following Lens Discision. (*Phila. Med. Times*, 1875.) 3. Coloboma of the Crystalline Lens. (*Int. Oph. Cong.*, N. Y., Sept., 1876.) 4. Metastatic Tenonitis in Diphtheria.. (*Med. Jour.*, 1880.) 5. Remarks on Lipemia Retinalis Occurring in a Case of Diabetes Mellitus.: (*Phila. Med. Times*, 1880.) 6. Thermometric Observations in a Case of Traumatic Diphtheria of the Orbit. (*Phila. Med. Times*, 1882.)ı 7. Acute Glaucoma Induced by Duboisin. (*Am. Jour.*, 1882.)—(T. H. S.)

Heymann, Friedrich Moritz. A celebrated Dresden ophthalmologist. Born at Schneeberg, in Saxony, May 24, 1828, he received the degree of Doctor in Medicine at Leipsic in 1850, and pursued the study of ophthalmology at Prague, Vienna, Paris and London. In 1851 he settled in Dresden as ophthalmologist, and eight years later was placed in charge of the Division for Eye-Patients at the Deaconness Institution. He was a very skilful operator, and a clear and forceful writer. He died of suppurative meningitis Oct. 21, 1870, at the early age of 43.

Heymann's ophthalmologic writings are as follows: 1. Exposer l'Influence Respective des Divers Nerfs sur le Mouvement de l'Iris.

(Awarded a gold medal by the Belgian Academy of Medicine at Brussels.) 2. Ueber die Beziehungen der Erkrankungen der Verschiedenen Gebilde des Auges zur Sogenannten Amaurose. (*Prager Vierteljahrschrift,* XIII.) 3. Zur Sclerotico-Chorioiditis Posterior. (Graefe's *Archiv,* II.) 4. Ueber Amaurose bei Bright'scher Krankheit und Fettdegeneration der Netzhaut. (*Ibid.,* II, 2.) 5. Frische Netzhauthämorrhagien. (*Ibid.,* VIII.) 6. Ueber Glaucom in Aphakischen Augen. (*Klin. Monatbl. für Augenheilk.,* V.) 7. Ein Fall von Netzhautgliom mit Zahlreichen Metastasen. (v. Graefe's *Archiv,* XV.) 8. Krankheiten der Orbita. (v. Graefe's *Archiv,* VII.) 9. Die Autoskopie des Auges und eine neue Methode derselben. (1863.) 10. Ueber Künstliche Beleuchtung. (*Prager Vierteljahrschr.,* C.)—(T. H. S.)

Hey, William. A celebrated surgeon of Leeds, England, who devoted some attention to ophthalmology, especially to comparative ophthalmology. Born at Leeds, Sept. 3, 1736, the grandson of a well-known surgeon, he lost the sight of his right eye in early childhood as the result of a wound made by a penknife. He studied at Leeds and in London, returning to Leeds as a general practitioner of medicine. He founded the Leeds General Hospital, in which institution he practised with much success for more than forty-five years.[*] He became a Fellow of the Royal Society, and died Mar. 23, 1819.

Hey's only strictly ophthalmologic writing was "A Description of the Eye of the Seal" (*Memoirs of the Philos. Soc.,* 1790). However, in his *"Practical Observations on Surgery"* (London, 1803) he treats in a general way of a number of eye diseases.—(T. H. S.)

Hieracion. In ancient Greco-Roman times, regarded as an ophthalmic remedy. See **Hawkweed.**

Hieracis collyrium. A collyrium containing myrrh, ammoniacum, thymiamatis and ærugo rosæ.

Hiéranose. (F.) Epilepsy, i. e., the sacred disease.

High frequency currents. See **Electricity in ophthalmology.**

High lights. Those parts of the photographic picture which are brighter than the rest.

Highmore, Antrum of. The ocular symptoms arising from diseases of the maxillary sinus and their treatment has been fully discussed under **Cavities, Neighboring,** especially on p. 1879 and following pages.

---

[*]According to the usually accurate Hirschberg (*Englands Augenärzte,* pp. 394 and 395) Hey was only a mediocre operator (als Augen-Operateur nur mittelmässig) while, eighteen lines later, the same William Hey is declared to have been "an excellent operator" (ein trefflicher Operateur)!

Highmore, Nathaniel. A celebrated English anatomist, who discovered the accessory nasal sinus which bears his name today. Because of the important pathological relations which this large, but imperfectly drained, cavity bears, directly and indirectly, to the eye, its discoverer should be remembered by ophthalmologists.

Highmore was born Feb. 6, 1613, at Fordingbridge, England. He received his medical degree at Oxford in 1642, and at once proceeded to the practise of medicine and surgery at Sherborne, in Dorsetshire. In this little place he continued to practise for the remainder of his days, becoming celebrated not only as an anatomist, but also as a general practitioner of both medicine and surgery. He died Mar. 21, 1685.

His most important works are: *"Disquisitio Corporis Humani Anatomica"* (Hague, 1651) and *"The History of Generation, Examining the Opinions of Divers Authors and chiefly of Sir K. Digby, and Concerning the Cure of Wounds by Sir Gilbert Talbot's Sympathetic Powder"* (London, 1651).—(T. H. S.)

High-power objective. Objectives of high magnifying power and short focal length.

Hildreth, Joseph Sullivan. This early American ophthalmologist was born at Cohassett, Norfolk County, Massachusetts, May 1st, 1832. Nothing concerning his family is known other than the suggestion that it was the same as that of Richard Hildreth, the historian. He went to Chicago from Paris, France, where he was superintendent of Desmarres' Eye and Ear Institute, under its famous founder. He also studied two years in Berlin under Virchow. In June, 1862, he married Mary Elizabeth, daughter of the Hon. Jacob M. Howard, then a member of the United States Senate from Michigan. The records of the war department show that he was appointed surgeon of United States Volunteers in 1863, stationed at Chicago, and honorably mustered out of the service, December 10, 1865. In the summer of 1863, the Chicago City Hospital was occupied by the United States military authorities, and in July, 1865, surgeon J. S. Hildreth took charge. The scope of treatment was limited to diseases of the eye and ear, and the hospital was termed the Desmarres Eye and Ear Hospital. Its location was at the corner of 18th and Arnold streets; capacity, 130 patients, and it boasted forty attendants. In 1866 it became the Cook County Hospital, and Dr. Hildreth became a consultant on its medical staff. Dr. Hildreth was a pioneer in ophthalmology, the first professor of ophthalmology and otology in the Chicago Medical College, and held that position at the time of his death. His practice at that time was very large and lucrative. He contributed papers on ophthalmology to the Chicago and Illinois state

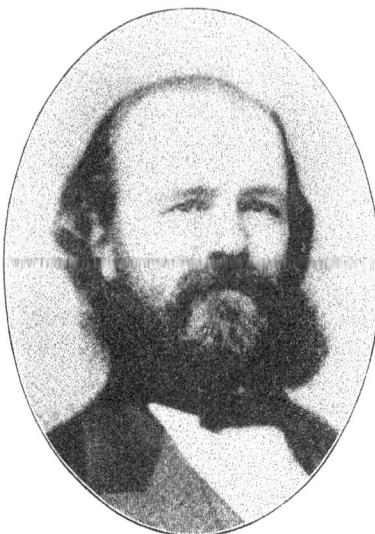

Joseph Sullivan Hildreth.

medical societies. His death came very suddenly, July 22nd, 1870.—
[From photograph and data collected for the Society of Medical
History of Chicago, by F. D. DuSouchet.]

Hilliard, Walter. A well-known ophthalmologist and oto-laryngol-
ogist of Denver, Colorado. Born Jan. 17, 1845, at Oxford, N. C., son
of Jeremy and Amelié King Toole Hilliard, he received his medical
degree at Tulane University, New Orleans, in 1869, and, for twenty-
six years, practised at Denver as a specialist in diseases of the eye,
ear, nose and throat. He was twice married: first to Victoria Houghton, of Shreveport, Louisiana, and, some years later, to Jessie Benton
Davis, of Cincinnati, Ohio. He had three children: Julia, wife of
Dr. E. K. Macomber, Amsterdam, N. Y., a son, Dr. Houghton Hilliard,
of Manilla, and another daughter, Dorothea Martina. Dr. Hilliard
died of cirrhosis of the liver at Denver, June 17, 1915, aged 70.

Dr. Hilliard was a man of high ideals and of great public spirit.
He was very helpful to the younger men in his profession. A Demo-
crat till recent years, he then became a staunch Republican. He was
very religious, but, withal, broad-minded and tolerant. He was a
member of the Episcopal Church. He had decided views on all
religious matters, for example, he could not tolerate fine church buildings, paid choirs, and the like, and would not ask grace at meals, for
fear the procedure might become perfunctory from frequent repeti-
tion. He was very charitable, and gave away large sums without

ostentation. Perhaps his highest praise is sounded by an ophthalmologic brother who was very well acquainted with him: "He was the gentlest man I ever knew."—(T. H. S.)

Hillmer. A Prussian quack, who flourished about the middle of the 18th century. He was a very rough and careless operator, who boxed his patients' jaws, even while the point of his cataract-needle lay within their eyes. It is said that, immediately after a cataract operation, he would not infrequently permit the patient to walk to his own home, and would even advise him to drive, or else to ride about on horseback. Hilmer, as might have been expected, had but few successes. He worked, or, rather, blundered and plundered, chiefly in Paris, Lyons, Dijon, Montpellier, Madrid, Lisbon, and numerous towns and cities in Germany.

His exact life dates are unknown. He was, however, at Lyons in June, 1749, and in the *Courrier, d'Avignon* for Aug. 17, 1756, we read as follows: "Doctor and Professor Hillmer, adviser to his majesty, the King of Prussia, arrived in this city the third of this month, coming from Lisbon *via* Madrid. From the fifth until now, he has not discontinued his operations, and the success which they have had have merited for him the eulogies of many physicians and surgeons, and of numerous persons of distinction who have been eye witnesses to the cure of several blind persons, one of whom had been blind from birth. The success of these operations has justified the high idea which had been formed of the talents of Dr. Hillmer, for the patients who were cured during the first days go about and do as they like without the assistance of guides, as if they had never been deprived of vision.

"M. Hillmer will return in a short time to the Court of Berlin."— (T. H. S.)

Hilon. (F.) Hernia of the iris through the perforated cornea.

Himly, Carl. A famous German ophthalmologist, re-discoverer of artificial mydriasis for use in ophthalmology, co-founder (with Adam Schmidt) of the first ophthalmologic journal, and one of the earliest teachers of ophthalmology as a specialty. Born at Braunschweig, April 30, 1772, he studied both there and at Göttingen. In 1795 he became professor in the Medico-Chirurgical Klinik at Braunschweig, a position which he resigned in 1801 in order to accept the chair of internal medicine at Jena. In 1803 he removed to Göttingen, in order to become Director of the Academic Hospital in that city. In the same year he began to give instruction in a course devoted exclusively to ophthalmology. Himly at the same time, founded, together with Adam Schmidt, the first ophthalmologic periodical, *Die Ophthalmologische Bibliothek*. This journal became defunct in 1807, but, in

1816, was revived by Himly alone, under the slightly altered title, *Bibliothek für Ophthalmologie.* This journal, like its predecessor, was short-lived, passing away in 1819.

Himly has been said to have been the first to make use of artificial mydriasis in ophthalmology. This, however, is a mistake. The first was undoubtedly Reimarus, of Hamburg, and the second, Loder, of Jena. Himly was only a slow third.

Himly's chief ophthalmologic writings are as follows: 1. *Ophthal-mologische Beobachtungen und Untersuchungen* (Bremen, 1801). 2. *Einleitung in die Augenheilkunde.* (Jena, 1806.) 3. *Die Krankheiten und Missbildungen des Menschlichen Auges und deren Heilung.* (2 vols., Berlin, 1842-43; edited and much improved and enlarged by the author's son, E. A. W. Himly.) The subject of this sketch was drowned in the Leine Mar. 22, 1837.—(T. H. S.)

Hindu ophthalmology. The native Hindu ophthalmology is very ancient and alike remarkable for two important and reciprocal facts. (1) It never did contribute, even in the slightest degree, to the ophthalmology of ancient Greece. (2) It never received the slightest contribution from any foreign source, Greek, Roman, Assyrian, or any other. Hindu ophthalmology, in other words, is strictly *sui generis.* To a certain extent it flourishes today in India, side by side, as one may say, with the modern ophthalmology of Europe and America.

At just what date East Indian ophthalmology was born we have no means of knowing. Its records appear, however, in the Sanscrit medical Shastras, and, almost exclusively, in the works of Charaka (q. v.) who was first and foremost a physician, and of Susruta (q. v.), who, first and foremost, was a surgeon. Both these men are declared to have flourished, according to some authorities as early as 1000 B. C., according, however, to others, as late as 1000 A. D. The really probable date for both is about the beginning of the Christian era.

The following codification, or abridgment, of the ancient Hindu ophthalmology (the beginnings of which date back to centuries, one might almost say to millenaries, before the time of the two great commentators, Charaka and Susruta) is taken, with only the slightest editing, from Wise's *"Commentary on the Hindu System of Medicine"* (Calcutta, 1845). This excellent compilation would, in fact, seem to be of the highest possible authority on its subject:

ORDER IV.

Diseases of the Eyes, (Akírogah).

It is related that *Janaka,* rájá of Mithilá or Tirhoot, did not perform the usual ceremonies and prayers to the sun, for which he was afflicted with the diseases of the eye. By abstinence and humiliation before the sun, however, he was cured of the disease; and since then, by proper offerings he obtained the favor of, and was instructed by, *Surya* concerning these diseases. He afterwards wrote a *Shástra* on the subject, called *Salaka Tantra,* which is stated to be "in profundity like the ocean."

There are 76 diseases of the eye. Of these 10 are air diseases, 10 bile, 13 phlegm, 25 are produced by the derangement of the three humors, 16 by blood, while 2 are external diseases. These diseases are again subdivided into 9 of the joinings of the eye, 21 of the eyelids, 11 of the white part of the eye, 4 of the black part, 17 of the eye in general, 12 diseases of the true organs of vision (Dristí), and two external diseases from injuries.

1. *Description of the Eye.* After a description of the size of the eye, the organ is stated to be formed by a combination of all the elements. Thus, the flesh is produced by the earth, the blood by the fire, the black part from the air, the white part from the water, while the different canals for the tears are produced by ether, or sky. The black part extends over one-third of the eye, the pupil comprising about one-seventh of the black part. The tunics are the two eyelids, and those of the globe of the eye. The first surrounds the vitreous humor (Tezajla, or glistening water), the second is covered with flesh, the third with fat, and the fourth with bone. They distinguish five circles, the eyelashes, eyelids, the white sclerotic coat, the iris, and the pupil. There are five joinings, the eyelashes with the eyelids, the eyelids and white of the eye (sclerotic), the white with the transparent cornea, and this with the pupil, and the caruncula lachrymalis. The humors are carried into the eye by the vessels, and produce many diseases.

The causes of these diseases are bathing when the body is very hot, intensely regarding minute objects, or those at a great distance, or sleeping at irregular periods, frequent crying, grief, anger, external injuries, excessive venery, constipated or sour articles of food, or a kind of pea *(Máskalái).* Irregularities of seasons produce them, retaining the tears in the eye, smoke and dust, profuse vomiting, or the sudden stoppage of vomiting. These causes, with derangements of air, bile and phlegm or blood, produce diseases of the eye. The deranged humors are conveyed into the eye by the vessels, and produce the different diseases in the different parts of the eye. The general symptoms of diseases of the eye are changes from its natural color, pain, redness, a discharge of tears, and a burning sensation in the eye as though there was an external body in it. The eyelids feel painful, as if thorns were under them, and there is intolerance of light.

2. *Inflammation.* There are four varieties of inflammation of the eye, produced by derangement in the air, bile, phlegm, and blood. The ten diseases of the air are characterized by severe pain in the eye, which remains immovable, a feeling of sand in the eye, which is dry, while the patient feels an inclination to rub the organ. The patient complains of headache, and the tears are cold.

Bile produces inflammation of the eye, which is characterized by burning and the discharge of blood and pus. Cold applications are grateful. The eye seems to be covered with a haze, feels hot, and presents a yellow color. There is likewise a discharge of warm tears.

Cough produces inflammation characterized by the fact that hot applications are grateful. The eye feels heavy, swelled, itchy, and cold. There is also a copious discharge of tears, of an oily nature.

Blood produces inflammation characterized by discharge of a copper color. The eye is red, the small vessels of the eye being turgid. Before this turgidity appears, the peculiar symptoms of bile are present. When this inflammation is neglected, or improperly treated, it produces one of the four varieties of severe ophthalmia *(Adimanta).* This aggravated form presents the following symptoms: severe pain, as if the eyes were torn; throbbing, which extends to half the head, and is characterized by the foregoing symptoms of each variety. When this is produced by phlegm, it will destroy the eye in seven days; if the blood is diseased it will destroy the organ in five days; if air, in six days; and if bile, in one day. In the acute stage of this ophthalmia the pain is severe, as if a foreign body were in the eye. There are redness and swelling, and a copious discharge of tears. When the disease is merely chronic, the pain is less, with itchiness in the part, the discharge of tears is slight, and the eyelids can be opened, and the globe appears healthy. When the inflammation produced by air is neglected, the accessions recur at intervals, and produce pain of different kinds. The eye swells, suppurates, and is red like a wild fig. It suppurates without swelling, when the other symptoms are the same. The eye in such cases is very painful, and the disease is incurable.

Another form of the disease is named *Bátaparjiya,* in which the air is deranged, and the eyebrow and eye are painful, so that the person winks, and brings the eyelid forcibly together.

Suskákipáka. When the eyelids are dry, and suppurate, the eye is very painful, the sight is troubled, and the patient cannot shut the eyelids.

Anutáyabáta. When the air of the neck and head, ears, cheeks, or vessels of the back of the neck are deranged, as well as that in other situations, the eyebrow and eye are very painful.

In *Amládhasita,* the eye is of a green color with a red circumference, from the color of the blood in the part. It extends over the eye, which is hot, swelled, and tears continually flow. This disease is produced by sour articles of food.

Sirotpáta. This is accompanied by more or less pain in the eye, which becomes red. When neglected, this form is called *Siráharsa,* when the discharge is of a copper color, and the person cannot see. These are the general diseases of the eye.

2. *The Diseases of the Black Part of the Eye.*

Ulcers of the cornea, (Bruna-sukra). In this disease the black part appears spotted; the discharge is very hot, and if the trouble is not near the pupil and there is only one spot, which is without pain and any discharge, it may sometimes be cured.

When the ulcer is of long standing, extensive, and deep-seated, it is difficult to cure. When it is depressed in the middle and its margin is elevated, it will destroy vision. When both coats (cornea and iris) are destroyed by a long standing ulcer, with a red margin, the condition is incurable.

Abruna-sukra. When the inflammation is in the black part of the eye with a burning sensation, it is very white, like the moon, and is curable. If it be of long standing, white, large, and deep-seated, it will be cured with difficulty.

Pákátiya, or opacity of the cornea following inflammation.

Ajakáyáta, small tumors, like the litter of goats, slightly red. These protrude through the cornea, from which proceeds a bloody discharge mixed with pus.

The *Dristi* (crystalline lens) is the principal part of the organ of vision. It is like the form of a pea *(masurí),* and is produced by a mixture of the essential parts of the five elements. It resembles the firefly, and it is largely supplied with the eternal fire *(Abaytazi).* It is covered by the external tunic of the eye, and has externally an opening (pupil?). By cold it is kept in a healthy state. The diseases of this part of the eye are very tedious in their cure.

3. *Diseases of the Membranes of the Eye.*

When the first tunic *(Pratarnapatala)* is deranged, the vision is indistinct. When the second tunic is affected, the sight is very imperfect, and the person sees an appearance of motes, mosquitoes, hairs, and nets. In other cases the appearances are in the form of a circle like spectres, rays, and is as if everything were indistinct and immersed in water, or like rain, clouds, and darkness. The person cannot distinguish distance, so that near objects seem at a distance.

When the third membrane is deranged, he can neither see above nor below; large objects appear covered, and he cannot distinguish the features of a person placed before him. Such a person has often double vision.

Linganása. In this form the whole crystalline lens *(Dristí)* is affected, and, if not very deep, the person can see the moon, star, and lightning. When the *air* is much increased, the patient sees every object red; and when the *bile* is affected, he can see the sun, the rainbow, and lightning. In other cases everything appears black, variegated, and like the feather of a peacock. When affected by *phlegm,* every object appears as if covered with oil and white. When the three humors are deranged, everything appears spotted as of a mixture of different colors. When the *blood* is deranged, every object appears red and dark. In *Linganása* the color is made of six different tints.

When the eye is affected with deranged *bile,* the condition is called *Pittabidagdha dristí.* It is characterized by yellowness, the images appearing yellow. If it affects the third membrane, the patient cannot see during the day, but can see at night.

When the *phlegm* is affected, the condition is called *Sleshmabidagdha dristí.* This is characterized by a white appearance, and by everything seen seeming white. When deranged in the three membranes of the eye, it is called *Nyctalopia,* or night-blindness. The patient can see during the day. Grief, fever, vexation, severe diseases of the head, cause this disease of the eye, in which every object appears enveloped in smoke; hence the disease is called *Samadarsher.* In other cases the person cannot see small objects during the day, but sees everything at night. This is called *Rasajáta.*

When air, bile, and phlegm are deranged, and produce a change in the iris like the mungoose eye (which is very red) everything appears of a mottled appearance during the day. The condition is named *Nakulándha.*

Gambiraká. When the *air* is deranged, it produces the disease in which the pupil of the eye is contracted, and it diminishes the size of the eye, and is accompanied with great pain.

Linganása is of two kinds. The first is called *Sanimita* and the second *Animita:* the first is produced by inflammation of the eye, and the second by the sight of holy sages, by regarding a kind of large snake *(Maharaza)*, or luminous objects by which vision is destroyed. The eye in this disease does not lose its natural appearance.

Abigáta hatadristí is produced by accidents or injuries to the eye, by which the person cannot see; the organ becomes red like coral, and severe pain is felt as if a person were tearing the eye out.

4. *Diseases of the White Part of the Eye.*

Prastáríjarma. In this disease there is a thin red or dark-colored membrane covering the white part of the eye.

Suklárma. The enlargements in this disease are white and soft. The affection advances slowly.

Raktárma is characterized by fleshy growths of a red color.

Adimánsarma (Pterygium) is a liver-colored thickening of the white part of the eye. It is stationary. Another form is thick, fleshy, and of a white color.

Stárjarma is a fleshy swelling of the white of the eye.

Sukti is the name when there are many small spots of a green flesh color.

Arjana is the name of a condition in which there is a red spot.

Pistaka is a round white elevation of the white of the eye, resembling a drop of water.

Jála. The white part in this case is like a net-work, with hard small vessels of a red color.

Sirája, is a disease in which, in the white of the eye, appear white pimples surrounded by enlarged vessels.

Balásaka is a silvery, copper-colored spot, surrounded by vessels.

5. *Diseases of the Joinings of the Eyes:—of the Eyeball, Cornea and Sclerotica, Eyelids, Eyelashes, etc.*

These diseases are nine in number. The parts sometimes swell, suppurate and are painful; the disease is called *Puyalisa*. In these cases blood and thick pus are discharged. In another form there is much swelling, but no suppuration; itching, but no pain. The condition is called *Upanáha*.

When air, bile, and phlegm are deranged at the joints, and the passage of the tears are discharged over the eyelids in the form of tears, the condition is called *Netranári* (fistula lachrymalis), of which there are four varieties, according to the nature of their discharges. When pus alone is discharged, the disease is called *Parsásarba*. When phlegm is alone diseased, and the joint suppurates without pain, the discharge is of a white color, thick, and shining like oil: the trouble is then called *Sleshmásrába*. Diseased blood sometimes produces this disease, and when there is a hot discharge mixed with much blood, the name is *Raktasrába*. When bile is diseased, the discharge has a yellow color, and the affection is called *Pittasrába*.

When small pimples appear at the joints of the eye, of a red color, they burn and are painful. They are called *Parbaniká*. Sometimes they occur at the juncture of the cornea and sclerotica, and are accompanied by the same symptoms as the last. They are of a red color, and are called *Alaghi*.

Krimágranti. Sometimes worms are produced at the juncture of the eyelids, and eyelashes. They produce much itching; and sometimes they form between the eyelid and the white part of the eye. They are of different colors and forms, and destroy the eye.

Diseases of the Eyelids.

There are twenty-one diseases of the eyelids. In this class of diseases, air, bile, and phlegm may be diseased in a combined or in a separate form. In other cases these derangements affect the vessels of the eye, and the blood and flesh, etc., may separately, or when combined, produce diseases of the eyelids.

Atsangani are small eruptions on the external part of the lower eyelids. They are produced by diseases of the blood, and often open internally.

Kanbiká are swellings at the borders of the upper eyelid. When they break, pus and blood are evacuated. They are like small castor oil seeds.

Another form of swelling is of the color of blood; of the size of a mustard seed, hard, and itchy; water, pus, and blood are evacuated from them. When painful they are called *Pataki*. When numerous clusters of small eruptions are rough, elevated, and situated on the inner side of the lid, they are called *Bartasarkará*. In another form they are small, like melon seeds; cause little pain, are situated in the eyelids, are rough to the feel, and are called *Arsabarta* or *Bartársi*. When like the new shining germ of a plant, the eyelids are long, hard, rough, indolent and irregular, and the patient cannot open the lid, the disease is called *Saskúrsa*, or dry hemorrhoidal tumors of the eyelids.[*]

Another kind are very hot, painful, and of a copper color. They are soft, and small. They are called *Angannanámika*.

---

[*] This sentence, though much involved, the present writer [T. H. S.] has not attempted to edit, because he is not quite certain of its meaning.

Sometimes the eyelids are covered with small eruptions, and all the small swellings have the same appearance and color, and are stationary. They are called *Bahalabarta*.

Another form of swelling is when the lids are swollen, itchy, and painful, the lids being tied over the eye, and not completely covering the globe. The diseases is called *Bartabanda*.

When the internal part of the eyelid is spongy, hot, painful, of a copper color, and changes quickly to a red color, it is called *Klistahbarta*.

If in this disease bile is deranged and affects the blood, much dirty matter is discharged called *Bartahkardama*.

When there is both external and internal swelling of the lids, together with burning and itching and a dark yellow discharge, it is called *Sábabarta*.

When the upper lid is externally swollen, is of a red color, and much matter is discharged from its inner surface, the condition is called *Prákninabarta*.

When the eyelids are shut, and cannot be opened without being previously soaked in water, on account of the secretion, the disease is called *Akhnabarta*.

When the joints of the eyelids become immovable and everted, the trouble is called *Bátahattabarta* (Entropium).

When a pendulous swelling forms on the inside of the eyelid without pain, and is caused by blood, it is named *Arbuda*.

When the vessels which move the eyelids are deranged, they produce winking, or a continual movement of the eyes. This is called *Nimassa*.

When the small fleshy excrescences, situated in the eyelids, are red, soft and painful, and grow again when removed by the knife, they are produced by diseased blood, and are called *Sunitársa*. Another form of tumor on the eyelids is like a plum, hard, soft and moist. It does not suppurate, but becomes large and knotted. It is called *Lagannah*.

When air, bile and phlegm are deranged, the swelling appearing above the eyelid, it breaks, and blood, water and pus are discharged through many openings. The pain is so severe as to resemble that of poison, and is called *Bishabarta*. In other cases these derangements contract the eyelids so that the person cannot see distinctly. This disease is called *Kuncharna*.

When air is deranged, the eyelashes are turned inwards, and inflame the eye, and the person is always rubbing them. It is called *Pakakapat* (entropion), and is a difficult disease to cure.

Bile, when deranged in the eye, produces falling of the eyelashes; when the eyelids are itchy and hot, the disease is called *Pakaksáta*.

Treatment of the diseases of the eye. Eleven of these diseases are cured by excision of the diseased part; nine by scarifications; five by incisions; fifteen by punctures; twelve by the use of different instruments; seven are cured with difficulty; and fifteen diseases are incurable. The two general diseases of the eyes are considered incurable.

In treating ophthalmia *(Abisanda)*, the patient is to have his body anointed, and fomented according to custom; and in both *Adimanta* and *Adisanda* venesection is to be employed, followed by oleaginous glysters and purgatives. Cooling washes, and the vapor of certain medicines, with errhines, are to be applied to the diseased eye. It is then to be covered with a yellow-colored cloth. Warm fomentations, and boiled hot flesh is to be applied to the eye, with poultices made of milk and rice. The patient should drink milk boiled with the decoction of those plants which cure diseased air. Goat's milk, boiled with the decoction of the root and leaves of the castor oil shrub is to be applied to the eye while warm.

When the ophthalmia is produced by derangement of the bile, bloodletting, purgatives, and the applications recommended in other inflammations are to be used. In other cases ghee and goat's milk are to be prepared with the following medicines. Take of

> *Gundrá* (Cyperus pertenuis),
> *Sháli,*
> *Shaibala* (Vallisneria octandra),
> *Loclobido,*
> *Dárbi* (Zanthorrizon),
> *Elá* (Cardamoms),
> *Udpoloh,*
> *Rodhra,*
> *Mustaka* (Cyperus rotundus),

and the leaves of the water-lily and other cooling medicines. Ghee is to be used as an external application. The other parts of the antibilious treatment is to be followed; and gold rubbed in the milk of a woman, and mixed with honey, may also be applied. Liquorice root, mixed with woman's milk or sugar and water; or a piece of cloth made of the wild silk is to be first moistened with water, and then applied to the eye.

When ophthalmia is produced by phlegm, blood-letting, fomentations, errhines, and colleria,* with the application of vapor, are to be

* The spelling of Dr. Wise, I have, in general, preserved.—(T. H. S.)

used. Different gargles, and irritants for the discharge of mucus from the nose are recommended. The colleria, etc., are to be prepared with medicines which cure phlegm. The patient should eat of such substances as do not increase phlegm, the ghee should be prepared with bitter plants. This should be repeated daily. The fomentations should be prepared with the decoctions of

Bálá (Hibiscus tortuosus),

Suntí (Dry ginger),

Debdáru (Erythroxylon sideroxcylloides),

Kushta (Costus speciosus).

The vapor of these medicines is to be applied to the eye. At other times various medicines are formed into a mixture, and applied externally to the eye: such as myrobalan, *haridrá,* (turmerick), *maduka,* (liquorice), *anjana,* and antimony. These medicines are dried in the sun, and when the mixture is to be used, moisten it and apply it upon the eyelids.

When blood produces diseases of the eye, use general and local bleeding, strong and frequent purgatives, errhines, cold applications, and apply a mixture of different medicines upon the eyelids. If there is much pain use soothing fomentations, leeches, and the usual treatment for bile. The juice of *nimba* leaves, mixed with iron and copper, is also recommended. The juice of sugar-cane, honey, sugar, woman's milk, *darbia,* and *maduka,* (liquorice), are to be applied externally, with the juice of the pomegranate. Water and sugar, rock-salt, and whey are also used as external applications.

Besides the seventy-six diseases, which are common both to children and to the adult, there is another which is peculiar to the former. This is called *Kukunáka,* or purulent ophthalmia. It is caused by the bad milk of the mother, and also by the derangement of phlegm, air, bile, or blood, singly or collectively. It affects the eyelids. The symptoms are continual rubbing of the eye, as well as of the nose and forehead; great intolerance of light, and a copious discharge.

In the *treatment* bleeding is first recommended with scarifications of the eyelids. Then, stimulating substances, mixed with honey, in order to discharge the bad humors. With this the usual medicines recommended for the mother and child, for purifying the humors and improving health are to be given; such as emetics. A decoction of the young leaves of *jumbu* (rose apple), *ámra* (mangoe), datree mulica, and myrobalan trees, are also recommended. The eyes are to be washed with this, as well as with other astringent medicines. The following mixture is also recommended. Take of:

Nipálaja (red sulph. of arsenic), *maricha* (black pepper), burnt *kunch* (a shell), *rasánjana* (sulph. of antimony), and *saindhaba* (rock-salt), with jagary and honey. These medicines are mixed with the honey and treacle, and applied to the eye with a probe.

There are many peculiarities in the diseases of the eyes that cannot be described in a book; but by these general precepts an intelligent person will be able to vary his treatment according to the circumstance of each particular case.

The diseases of the eye in which the use of instruments is required are:

> *Utsinjiní,*
> *Bahalabárta,*
> *Hurdamabárta,*
> *Shábabárta,*
> *Bandabasta,*
> *Klistabárta,*
> *Pataka,*
> *Kambíkíni,* and
> *Bátasarkárá.*

Scarifications. Before undergoing this operation the patient should take an emetic and a purgative. He should be placed in a closed cool room without much light, the eyelids separated by the thumb and forefinger of the left hand. Moisten the eye with a piece of soft cloth which has been dipped in warm water; and with the point of a knife on the rough leaf, as of the wild fig-tree, etc., the scarifications are to be made. Continue the application of the warm water as a fomentation; after which the following mixture is recommended. Take of

> *Manageh* (Red sulphurate of arsenic),
> *Káses* (Sulphurate of iron),
> *Baso* (long and black pepper and dry ginger), and
> *Saindhaba* (Rock-salt).

Mix with honey, and apply a small portion with the probe to the inside of the eyelid. This is to evacuate more completely the bad humors. After these have been discharged, the medicine is to be removed by bathing the eye with warm water. Ghee is to be applied to the eye. These applications are to be used, with the exception of the scarifications, every third day.

The effect of these scarifications on the inside of the eyelids is to stop the morbid discharge, and to diminish the swelling and itching as the eyelid becomes smooth. Such results prove that the eyelid has been properly scarified. If not performed well, the following are the symptoms: The redness, swelling, and discharge continue, and the symptoms of the disease are not removed. The eyelid becomes black, heavy, and is moved with difficulty. There is much itching and irritation in the eyelids; and sometimes it produces suppuration of the eye.

The nine diseases in which scarifications are to be used, are:

Bortábabandá,
Clestabártang,
Bálabártang,
Pataki,
Sáhabarta,
Cardamaburta,
Cambikini,
Súkárá, and
Utsanjani.

The characteristic symptoms of these diseases of the eyelids are mentioned above.

Incision of the eye should be employed in

Bishagrenti. In this disease fomentations are first to be used; when matter forms, open the abscess, and then apply powdered rock-salt with the sulphate of zinc *(kásis),* long-pepper, red sulphurate of arsenic with honey, and then a bandage.

In *Lágana* divide the parts and then apply the powder of *Ráchanás* (supposed to be the concrete bile of the cow), saltpetre, sulphate of copper, and honey. In other cases the actual cautery must be applied. Treatment of *Unjánámeká* (styr), consists of fomenting the abscess, and then applying the sulphurate of antimony with honey.

For the cure of *Bishagrenta,* first foment, open the part, and then apply the powder of the three kinds of *matabah, tuto* (sulphate of copper), *kásis* (sulphate of iron), and rock-salt. These medicines irritate, and increase the secretion of tears, and clear the organ. Later, use astringent applications.

In *Upanáha* cut off the diseased part, and then apply fomentations and a mixture of long-pepper, rock-salt, and honey.

Excision. In *Udemánsarniá* (pterygium), excision is to be used. First mix ghee with the patient's food; then apply stimulating powder to the part, followed by fomentations. The eye is then to be rubbed with the finger, and, when the eyelids are somewhat loosened, apply a hook, and draw the fleshy growth slightly outwards. Then pass a needle under the diseased growth; tie it, and then separate the diseased part from the cornea and sclerotica with a round formed knife. Then apply fomentations and a bandage.

The only diseases in which excision is employed, are:

Sírâjâla,

Sorbanícá,

Ursa,

Sarskársa Urbada, tumors.

In *Pakakapat* (intropeon). In this distressing disease it is recommended that from the inner to the outer canthus of the eye a portion of the skin be removed, about three lines in breadth, in the lower third of the upper eyelid. This operation is particularly described by Susruta, who states the kind of room which should be used as an operating room, that in which the patient is to be placed, his diet, etc. After the operation apply honey and ghee to the wound, which should be brought together by hair sutures. These are removed on union taking place. If this operation is not successful, destroy the roots of the hair by the actual or potential cauteries.

Amaurosis (*timra* or darkness). The patient is first to get oleaginous purgatives prepared with old ghee which has been kept for some time in an iron vessel. The ghee is also recommended to be prepared from amphibious animals. It is to be rubbed up with water and applied to the eye; different preparations of antimony are likewise recommended, such as antimony, honey, sugar, red sulphurate of arsenic, mixed together, and applied to the eye. Different colleria, fomentations, errhines and other external applications are also to be used. These preparations of antimony with other stimulants are to be used. Bleeding is not recommended, but errhines are highly extolled. Various other remedies, with nutritive diet, are recommended, as barley with much ghee, the juice of myrobalan, and the flesh of wild animals and birds.

Cataract (linganása). In treatment of this and other diseases the patient should first take ghee, as it is supposed to cure the diseases of *air*, which are supposed to derange the other humors. The weather should neither be very hot nor very cold in which the operation is to be performed. The eyelids are to be kept properly separated by an expert assistant; the patient is then to be directed to look to his nose, and a knife with a point shaped like a grain of barley is to be held between the fore and middle fingers, and thumb of the right hand if the left eye is to be operated on, and in the left hand, if the right eye. The knife is then to be carried forward near the junction of the sclerotica with the cornea, neither high nor low in the eye (near the transverse axis), and pass it on until water escapes. Then introduce a probe with a hook at its extremity, which is to detach and remove the cataract. When the person sees well, immediately after the operation, it has been properly done, particularly when the pupil appears clear like the other eye. After the operation apply the milk of a woman to the eye, with fomentations. Then cover the eye with a bandage. For ten days after the operation the patient must remain perfectly quiet in a dark room. During this time his food should be light.

In the treatment of the following diseases of the eye, the knife is not to be used:

Sukákipáka,
Kaphabidagdhadristí,
Pittabidagdhadristí,
Sakra,
Urjana,
Pishtaka,
Amlakí,
Akílnabarta,
Damadarsí,
Suktí,
Príkelnabarta,
Balásabasta.

In external injuries, and their consequences, the following diseases are cured by bleeding:

Sîrágála,
Siráharsa,
Nainapáka,
Pabanunátah,
Pueálása.

Also in acute and purulent ophthalmia.—(T. H. S.)

Hintere Augenkammer. Posterior chamber of the eye.

Hintere Brennweite. (G.) Posterior focal distance.

Hinterer Kapselstar. (G.) Posterior polar cataract.

Hintergrund. (G.) The background (of the eye).

Hinunterziehender Augenmuskel. (G.) The inferior rectus muscle of the eye.

Hipparchus. The first systematic astronomer on record was born at Nicaea, in Bithynia and flourished between 160 and 125 B. C. The only authority we have regarding his researches is the *Syntaxis* of Ptolemy; from it we learn that Hipparchus discovered the precession of the equinoxes and the eccentricity of the sun's path, invented the planisphere, and drew up a catalogue of ten hundred and eighty stars.

Hippel's (von) disease. ANGIOMATOSIS RETINÆ. This extremely rare disease—only about thirty cases have so far been reported—was first intelligently described by von Hippel in 1904. Seven years subsequently this writer (Graefe's *Archiv fuer Ophthal.*, Vol. 79, Part 2, 1911) was able to examine anatomically the eye that formed the basis of his first paper. He found an angiomatosis of the retina with secondary disease of the retinal vessels, obliteration of the nervous retinal elements, proliferation of the glia and extensive subretinal hemorrhages with subsequent organization.

The ophthalmoscopic diagnosis is usually easy, being dependent principally upon the presence of reddish, spherical formations, the enormous dilatation, tortuosity and uniform color of one or more arteries and their collateral veins.

The disease is distinctly chronic; the prognosis as regards vision is absolutely unfavorable, blindness and secondary glaucoma being the ultimate results. Enucleation is indicated only when pain supervenes, and it will probably never be possible to obtain a specimen showing the incipient stages of the disease.

Of the cases subsequently described, Moore's (*Oph. Year-Book*, p. 234, 1912) patient was a woman of 20, who had only noticed impairment of vision for two weeks shortly after having quinsy. But both eyes were affected with characteristic lesions. See the illustration.

In the account given by Bane (*Annals of Ophthalm.*, p. 399, April, 1913) the right upper temporal vein and artery were both tortuous and three times the normal diameter. Up and out three and one-half disc diameters from the disc was a rounded tumor two disc diameters across, and having a sharp edge except at the upper outer side, where the edge was feathery. The mass was in intimate relation with the main upper temporal vessels. On a branch vessel to its upper outer side were two much smaller tumors. The artery, as it left the disc and for a disc diameter beyond, was narrow and intermittently beaded. The vein disappeared as it reached the disc. Some distance below and slightly to the outer side of the main tumor, were some fine whitish deposits. The left upper temporal artery and vein were irregularly enlarged. The artery became normal for one and one-half disc diameters after it had gone a disc diameter from the disc, and then became beaded and enlarged for some distance. The vein was constricted as it left the disc, then dilated to double normal caliber, and then gradually fell away to normal caliber.

Ginsberg and Spiro (*Archiv f. Ophthalmologie*, Band LXXXVIII, Heft 1, 1913) observed the development of a case of angiomatosis retinæ from its very beginning, and were able to follow the progress

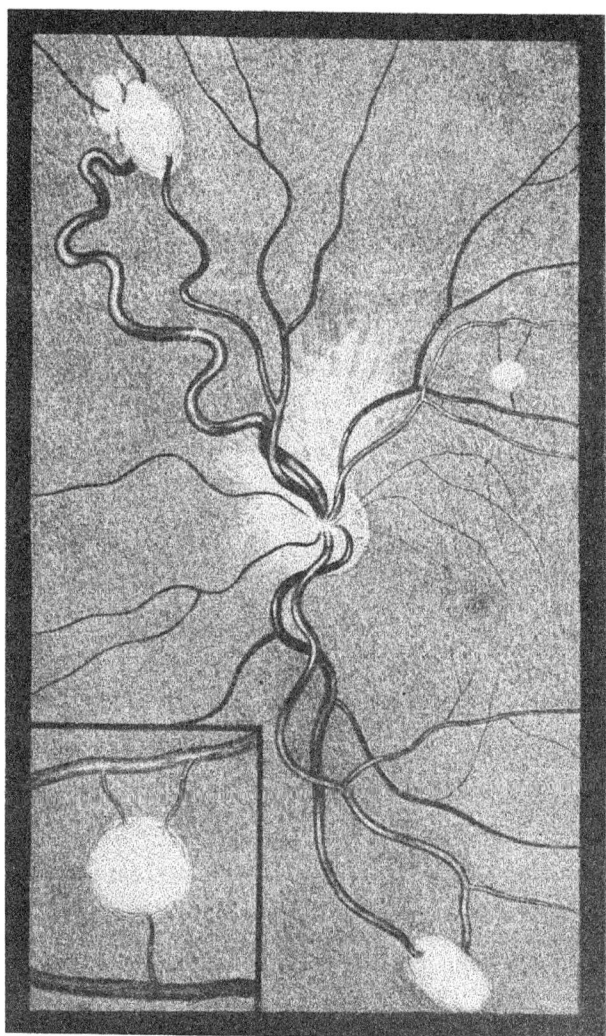

Angiomatosis of the Retina.

Left eye. Lower left corner shows middle tumor with connected artery and vein, enlarged. (Moore.)

of the case for seven years, and finally examined microscopically the affected globe, which they enucleated on account of glaucoma. They are of opinion that there is a new formation of tissue in the retina which is to be regarded as tumor formation, and two different tissues take part to a varying extent, in the formation of this tumor, namely, the neuroglia and the blood-vessels. In other words, the process is a true angio-gliomatosis. They have found in some parts of their specimen a pure gliomatosis and in others a mixture of the two. The gliosis is of a different nature to the glioma retinæ of infancy. It is only locally malignant just as the gliomata of the brain are. It is conceivable, upon this explanation, that one or other of these tumor elements may alone be present, or that the second may be so poorly represented as to be negligible, in which case one would obtain tumors of widely varying appearance, but still essentially of the same nature.

The case of Darier (*La Clinique Ophtalmol.*, Dec. 10, 1913) was first published in 1890 but not recognized as one of angiomatosis retinæ until after the publication of von Hippel's description.

Probably the best bibliography on this subject is given by Vossius (*Sammlung Zwangl. Abhandl.*, p. 32, Vol. 9, No. 1, 1913), who in the same monograph also describes fully two cases of his own.

Hippiatrie. (F.) Veterinary medicine.

Hippocrates. The father of medicine, and, therefore, of ophthalmology. Inasmuch as the works and personality of Hippocrates will be treated at length under the heading **Ophthalmology, History of,** the reader is referred to that rubric.

Hippocratism. The doctrine that was taught by Hippocrates of imitating nature in the treatment of disease by studying the spontaneous efforts toward recovery and the crises that occur in the course of many diseases.

Hippomane mancinella. The manchineel-tree, the celebrated poison tree of Central America, is generally found near the sea-shore. It is one of the sources of caoutchouc. Its juice is very acrid and poisonous, and is used as an arrow-poison. It has caused blindness by the hands coming in contact with the eyes after handling the plant. It is used externally to remove fungous growths, especially those of syphilis, and the leaves yield an extract used in skin diseases, including leprosy.—(Foster.)

Hippuryltropin. One of numerous feeble mydriatics belonging to the tropin series.

Hippus. PUPILLARY ATHETOSIS. An old term for a rapid alternate contraction and dilatation of the pupil, independent of light and the accommodation. It was also confounded with nictation.

This extremely rare symptom is defined by Bach as rhythmic contractions and dilations of the pupils occupying on an average from 1 to 3 seconds, which are generally unassociated with variations in illumination. Rarely is the phenomenon unilateral. The pupillary excursions are about equal in the two eyes, and measure from 2 to 3 mm. Bach states that hippus has no diagnostic value, and its cause is not known.

Knies says that it is observed in recovering paralysis of the motor oculi and is then associated with nystagmus. It is much rarer as an independent condition, and is then found almost always in diseases—such as tabes, multiple sclerosis, etc.—in which there are numerous lesions in the region of the nuclei of the ocular muscles. Hippus has also been noted in neurasthenia, hysteria, epilepsy and brain tumor.

Fromaget (*Arch. d'Ophtal.*, Apr., 1906) reports a case: A laundress, 38 years of age, in good health and without hereditary taint, applied for treatment of a slight blepharospasm of the right eye which was otherwise normal. There was almost complete ophthalmoplegia—extreme divergence and partial ptosis of the left eye. The pupil of this eye, examined in full light, appeared to be of the same size as the other—about two mm., but in testing the reflex by raising the eyelid, after a few seconds of exclusion, and exposing the eye to a bright light, the pupil dilated slowly, instead of contracting. When it reached the maximum of dilatation the pupil maintained it for three or four seconds and then slowly contracted for eight or ten seconds and maintained the maximum of contraction for ten seconds. Then the sphincter yielded and the pupil returned slowly to the state of dilatation, the action lasting about 30 seconds. After three seconds of arrest, the phenomenon was repeated, so that every minute the pupil changed its form, with equal rests at the maximum of dilatation and of contraction.

The author thinks that the symptoms point to a nuclear lesion, probably of encephalitic origin, and that the phenomenon called hippus is a myosis which occurs in a rhythmic manner, in an iris in a state of mydriasis. The sphincter of the iris, under the influence of a central excitation, contracts slowly, during some seconds, the maximum contraction persists about ten seconds and then, the excitation failing, the sphincter relaxes slowly to reproduce the mydriasis.

These contractions, occurring slowly in a muscle incompletely paralyzed, resemble what occurs in other muscular territories and that have been studied by Hammond, Charcot and others under the name of athetosis.

It is probable that in the case under consideration the nucleus of the oculo-motor of the left side had been in great part destroyed, but that, in association with the destruction, there are irritative phenomena which cause this rhythmic spasm of the sphincter. See, also, **Pupil**.

Hird's hand-perimeter. The perimeter devised by R. Beatson Hird (*British Medical Journal*, Sept. 14, 1912) is a modification of a pre-existing hand perimeter. It is simple in structure, with no mechanism to get out of order. The handle is detachable, and the whole can be carried in an ordinary handbag. It is light, so that any patient can easily hold it in position. There is a rotating half arc enabling the field to be mapped out rapidly, the dial registering the part of the field that is being tested. The face-rest is made of vulcanite for the purpose of being cleansed, and the fixation object is a white spot 10 mm. in diameter, so that it can be seen by presbyopes. The field is tested by white and colored squares mounted on black handles which are carried along the arc. A book of 100 charts is provided. The fields can be mapped out accurately and quickly for white and colors, and with it the fields of a patient in bed can be taken if desired.

Hire, P. de la (1640-1718). A distinguished French ophthalmologist, who, in 1709, repeated the submersion experiment of Jean Méry on the eye of the cat, and first furnished the correct solution of the most important question raised by that experiment. Méry's experiment (1704) was this: He submerged a cat under water, and then beheld in all its glory the animal's *fundus oculi*—the entrance of the optic nerve, the vessels and all the various hues of the brilliant choroid coat. Méry's explanation of his own experiment, however, was very erroneous. He believed that the reason why the fundus could be observed in the submerged, but not in the unsubmerged, eye, was that the water "evened over" the various tiny "inequalities" which must exist on its anterior corneal surface. De la Hire, two years later, came forward with the correct explanation. He made it entirely clear that the reason why the fundus of the submerged eye could be perceived was that the water did away with all the corneal refraction of the light, so that all the light-rays leaving a given point upon the fundus, emerge from the eye not as a parallel, but as a strongly divergent, pencil. He also observed incidentally that all the disturbing light-reflexes which appear on the cornea *in aero* are done away with by submersion.—(T. H. S.)

Hirn. (G.) Cerebrum; brain.

Hirnanhang. (G.) Pineal gland.

Hirnbeinhaut. (G.) The pericranium.

Hirnbläschen. (G.) Cerebral vesicle.

Hirnëntwickelung. (G.) Development of the brain.

Hirnfuss. (G.) Base of the brain.

Hirngeschwülst. (G.) Brain tumor.

Hirnhaut. (G.) A membrane of the brain. Meninges.

Hirnhautentzündung. (G.) Meningitis.

Hirnlos. (G.) Anencephalous.

Hirnrinde. (G.) The external portion of the cerebral hemispheres.

Hirnschale. (G.) Cranium.

Hirnseuche. (G.) Cerebro-spinal meningitis.

Hirnsichel. (G.) The falciform process of the dura.

Hirnwassersucht. (G.) Hydrocephalus.

Hirsch, August. A celebrated German hygienist and historian of ophthalmology. Born at Danzig, Oct. 4, 1817, he studied at Leipsic and Berlin, at the latter institution receiving his medical degree in 1843. His dissertation was ''De Laryngostasi Exsudativa Vulgo Croup Vocata.'' He settled for a time at Elbing, later removing to Danzig. Here he wrote *''Ueber die Geographische Verbreitung von Malaria Fieber und Lungenschwindsucht und den Räumlichen Antagonismus dieser Krankheiten''* (1848), as well as a number of other articles. In 1863 he became professor of Medicine at Berlin, to which city he then removed. In 1873 Pettenkofer and he secured the appointment by the Government of the ''Cholera Commission for the German Empire.'' He himself, as a member of this commission, investigated the cholera in West Prussia and Posen. The result of this investigation was *''Das Auftreten und der Verlauf der Cholera in den preussischen Provinzen Posen und Preussen,* May-Sept., 1873'' (Berlin, 1874; 2d ed., 1875). In 1874 he attended the International Cholera-Conference at Vienna, as a delegate from the German government. In 1879 he investigated the pestilence in Russia, and wrote upon this subject *''Mittheilungen über die Pest-Epidemie im Winter 1878-79 in dem russischen Provinz, Astrachan''* (Berlin, 1880). One of the most important of all his writings was the *''Handbuch der Historisch-Geographischen Pathologie''* (2 vols., Erlangen, 1859 to '64; 2d ed. 1881 to '86; English trans. by the New Sydenham Society, 1883).

His most important ophthalmologic writing was the well known *''Geschichte der Augenheilkunde''* (Leipsic, 1877), which formed the seventh volume of the first edition of the Graefe-Saemisch *Handbuch der Gesamten Augenheilkunde.* This monumental work was of vast importance in its day, but has now been wholly superseded by the voluminous *''Geschichte''* of Hirschberg. Of almost equal importance, however, in the history of ophthalmology, are the *''Geschichte d. Medicinische Wissenschaft in Deutschland"* (Munich and Leipsic, 1893) and the *"Biographisches Lexikon der Hervorragenden Aerzte Aller Zeiten und Völker"* (Vienna and Leipsic, 1886), of which he was chief editor. Professor Hirsch died Jan. 28, 1894.—(T. H. S.)

Hirschberg, Magnet of. See p. 4252, Vol. VI, of this *Encyclopedia.*

Hirschler, Ignaz. For many years this surgeon was the only ophthalmologist in Hungary. Born at Pressburg, Hungary, 1823, he received his medical degree at the University of Vienna, and for a time was the assistant of von Rosas. In 1847-48 he studied ophthalmology under Desmarres at Paris. In 1849 he settled as ophthalmologist at Budapest, where he practised until shortly before his death, which occurred Nov. 10, 1891.—(T. H. S.)

Hirudo medicinalis. The medicinal leech, an aquatic species found throughout Europe, but especially in the northern parts. It has an olive-green back, with 6 dorsal stripes interrupted with black spots, and a belly yellowish-green or spotted with black, and 86 teeth. See **Leech;** as well as p. 2544, Vol. IV, of this *Encyclopedia.*

Hirundo rustica. (L.) A species of leech, the young of which were formerly used in France for the relief of angina, ophthalmia, epilepsy, etc.

Hispiditas. (L.) An old term for irregularity of the eyelashes.

Histogenesis. (L.) The origin and development of the tissues. While all the tissues originate from an ovum, it is common to attribute their direct origin to the epiblast, hypoblast, or mesoblast.

Histology of the eye. The minute structure of the normal tissues of the human eye.

Although this section is not here illustrated references are from time to time made to explanatory cuts and plates under various captions of the *Encyclopedia.*

THE EYELIDS.

The eyelids are the movable curtains situated in front of the eyeball, to cover and protect it. The free margins are flattened and are surmounted by eyelashes from the external canthus to a point about 5 mm. from the inner canthus. Internal to this the lid margins are rounded and devoid of eyelashes, and form the upper and lower boundaries of a triangular space—the lacus lacrimalis—in which is the caruncula lacrimalis. See the colored and other illustrations of this subject on pp. 408*a—d,* inclusive, Vol. I, of this *Encyclopedia.*

The very thin skin covering the lids is but loosely attached to its bed by a lax, non-fatty connective tissue. The skin of the lids has the usual structure. It contains small sweat-glands, and the follicles of small hairs, and at the edge of the eyelid the large hair follicles from which the eyelashes grow. The subcutaneous tissue is loose and devoid of fat and in it are found the fibres of the orbicularis muscle. A small separate bundle of the orbicularis which occupies the margin of the lids behind the eyelashes, is called the *muscle of Riolan.*

In each lid there exists a dense framework of condensed fibrous tissue which gives the lid its consistence and shape. In front of these tarsal plates are fibres of the orbicularis palpebrarum muscle and the integument, while imbedded in its posterior surface is a row of long sebaceous glands (the Meibomian glands), the ducts of which open at the edge of the eyelid. The superior tarsal plate is larger than the inferior, and at the extremities of the two are found the external and internal tarsal ligaments.

The *Meibomian glands* are elongated sebaceous glands with numerous lateral offshoots. They are embedded in the tarsal plates, and filled with cubical epithelium. Between the eyelashes and the muscle of Riolan are found two or three rows of modified sweat-glands, termed the *glands of Moll.*

There are two voluntary muscles found in the lids, namely, the *orbicularis palpebrarum* and the *levator palpebræ superioris.* The former is a flat, expanded cutaneous muscle, which surrounds the palpebral fissure in the form of a circle. It is divided into two parts, an internal and an external. The levator palpebræ superioris arises at the bottom of the orbit and runs forward on the superior rectus. It is attached in three portions, to the deep surface of the skin, to the superior tarsal plate, and to the fornix conjunctivæ. The fibres of Mueller's muscle run from between the striated fibres of the levator to the upper margin of the tarsus.

The eyelid may be readily divided into two parts. The skin, cilia, and fibres of the orbicularis forming the anterior part, while the posterior is made up of the tarsus, with the Meibomian glands, and the palpebral conjunctiva.

THE CONJUNCTIVA.

The conjunctiva is a mucous membrane which covers the posterior surface of the lids and is reflected over the anterior surface of the eyeball. In the cornea it is represented by the anterior layer of epithelium. The conjunctiva, which forms a sac open anteriorly, is divided into three parts, according to its position: 1. The conjunctiva bulbi; 2. The conjunctiva palpebrarum; 3. The conjunctiva fornicis.

Histologically it is divided into two layers: (1) the epithelium; (2) the mucosa.

The bulbar conjunctiva is that part which coats the anterior surface of the eyeball. Slightly altered in character it is continued over the cornea. This gives rise to a division of the bulbar conjunctiva into two parts, the conjunctiva sclerae and corneae. See the figures on p. 354, Vol. I, of this *Encyclopedia.*

The *conjunctiva sclerae* is connected with the sclera by connective tissue (the episcleral tissue) so loosely that movement from side to side is very free. At the periphery of the cornea the scleral conjunctiva is very thin and elastic. It is covered with laminated pavement epithelium and contains no glands. It forms at the inner angle of the eye a crescentic duplication, the plica semilunaris, which represents the remnant of the palpebral tertia of animals. The *caruncle,* a small island of skin lying to the inner side of the semilunar fold, is a small reddish prominence, its surface is covered with minute hairs and it contains sebaceous follicles and glands like Krause's.

The *conjunctiva palpebrarum* is immovably adherent to the subjacent tarsus. It contains small glands called Krause's which resemble the lachrymal in structure and which are found along the convex border of the tarsus. The conjunctiva fornicis is a very lax portion of the conjunctiva. This character renders movement of the eye very free, while its abundant blood supply renders it peculiarly liable to great swelling when inflamed.

The epithelium in the different parts of the conjunctiva varies. The conjunctiva of the lids is covered with a laminated cylindrical form. There are, in fact, two layers of epithelium—a superficial cylindrical and a deep flattened. The superficial cells are cylindrical with oval nuclei which lie towards the base of the cell, while the deep cells are flat with oval, horizontal nuclei.

The *bulbar conjunctiva* is covered with laminated pavement epithelium, the best example of which is found at the limbus. As in the cornea one may distinguish three layers. The superficial consists of flat cells with horizontal oval nuclei; the middle, of many layers of polygonal cells, while the basal layer is formed by a single layer of small cylindrical or cubical cells.

Goblet cells are found in the epithelium of the normal conjunctiva in varying numbers. They were described by Stieda in 1867. They are large, round, or oval cells, which are found at different depths, in different sizes, and which have a definite opening on the surface. These cells contain mucin. The flattened nucleus forms a crescent at the base.

The mucosa of the conjunctiva is divided into two parts, (1) the adenoid layer, lying directly under the epithelium, and (2) the fibroid layer. The former is absent in the new-born until about the third month. It varies in thickness from 40 microns in the palpebral to 50 to 70 in the fornix and 15 to 27 in the bulbar (Villard). Among its fine fibres one finds lymphocytes in all its parts. During inflammation their number is greatly increased. The fibrous, which is thicker than the adenoid layer, contains thicker meshes and many elastic fibres. It is thin over the tarsus with which it is continuous. The chief arteries, veins, lymphatics and nerves are found in the fibrous layer, though the adenoid is also well supplied.

The palpebral conjunctiva contains true large acino-tubular glands called Krause's. They are serous glands and are found beneath the fornix and the edge of the tarsus, especially towards the nasal side. They are much more common in the upper than in the lower lid, there being, according to Krause, 42 in the upper and 6 to 8 in the lower. The acini unite to form a large duct which opens on to the fornix.

There are also gland-like depressions which occur in the basement membrane. They are of varying depths and are lined with cylindrical epithelium. Fine tubular glands also occur in the conjunctiva under normal and pathological conditions. They are called *Henle's glands*.

THE CORNEA.

The cornea forms about the anterior sixth of the outer tunic of the eyeball. Apart from the indistinctness of the marginal portions, the cornea everywhere has a uniform transparency. It is thinner at the centre than at the periphery. The cornea proper consists of five layers from before backwards: Epithelium; Bowman's membrane; Substantia propria; Descemet's membrane; Endothelium.

See the figures on pp. 367-371, Vol. I, of this *Encyclopedia*.

The *epithelium* over the greater part of the cornea has a uniform thickness of 37 to 58 μ, and in the regularity of its anterior surface probably surpasses the epithelium of all other parts of the body. It is the stratified pavement variety with five to six layers of cells. The superficial cells are flattened, with oval nuclei. While the cells of the second layer are of about equal size in all their dimensions, a beginning flattening is apparent in the third layer. The second layer consists of polyhedral elements with convex anterior surfaces and concave posterior ones, the edges between these concave surfaces are more or less drawn out into the shape of wings. The long axis of the nucleus is parallel to the surface of the cornea, and the protoplasm is of darker color than that of the basal cells.

The cells of the deepest layer are cylindrical. Each cell turns an absolutely flat surface towards Bowman's membrane, and a rounded end (head) to the surrounding cell layer. The nucleus is slightly oval and lies with its long axis at right angles to the surface of the cornea.

The cells are united by means of cell bridges. The intercellular spaces are plainest between the basal cells, towards the surface they gradually disappear.

Leucocytes are quite often found in the system of spaces, characterized by heavy staining, constricted or fragmented nuclei, and under normal conditions are only to be found between the bases of the first cells just in front of Bowman's membrane.

Bowman's membrane, while it does not extend over the entire cornea. has a uniform thickness of 10 to 16 microns. Embryologically it is shown to be part of the substantia propria and is to be looked upon as a superficial, modified layer of the stroma. The posterior surface does not show so sharp a contour as the anterior. It is not possible to detach Bowman's membrane from the stroma. It differs from the other lamellæ in having no corneal corpuscles, and, by ordinary stains, appears structureless. It consists of fine connective tissue fibres.

Bowman's membrane is a thin, homogeneous structure, chiefly connected with the corneal lamellæ lying beneath it. It may be said to represent the uppermost layer of the stroma of the cornea which has become homogeneous and destitute of cells. It is separated from the epithelium by a sharply-defined border.

The *substantia propria* is composed of a ground substance and cells. The ground substance in its ultimate constitution consists of fine fibrillæ of connective tissue united by a cement substance into flat bundles. The individual elementary lamella consists of fine, straight, connective tissue fibrillæ strictly parallel to one another. The direction of the fibrillæ varies from lamella to lamella. There are about sixty lamellæ which run parallel to the surface and cross at right angles in alternate layers.

The bundles are bound together by ground substance. "By means of injection under very low pressure, a network of anastomosing stellate spaces between the lamellæ is obtained. These are v. Recklinghausen's canals. If mercury is used and the pressure is greater, tubular passages running at right angles to one another in the different layers are injected (Bowman's corneal tubes)."—(Parsons.)

Between the lamellæ are found the cells of the stroma, which are of two kinds: (1) The fixed corpuscles of the cornea, and (2) the motile corpuscles.

The first are cells with a large nucleus, a protoplasmic cell body, the numerous branched processes of which are connected with the processes of adjoining cells, so that in this way there is formed a system of connected protoplasmic bodies. They are flat, stellate cells, with long ramifying processes, which anastomose with those of the other cells. They lie between the lamellæ and are surrounded by lymph spaces, which also communicate along the processes with those of the neighboring cells. The cytoplasm is clear except near the nucleus where it is granular.

The second variety, the motile corpuscles of the cornea, the wandering cells of v. Recklinghausen, are migratory leucocytes which are derived from the peripheral blood vessels and move about in the system of lymph passages.

Descemet's membrane is a homogeneous elastic lamina which forms the posterior boundary of the cornea. It is 5-7 mm. thick in the middle portion. In staining reaction it is distinctly different from the corneal stroma, and is very resistant alike to chemical agents and pathological processes.

The posterior epithelial layer or endothelium of the cornea consists in a single layer of flattened cells which are rich in protoplasm with the nucleus completely embedded in it. This endothelium extends over nearly the entire inner surface of the Descemet membrane.

The cornea is traversed by a network of nerve fibrils, which are not demonstrated by the ordinary stains. For this the gold chloride, Dogiel methylene blue method, or Gregi method, is necessary. The nerves retain their medullary sheath for 1 to 2 mm., and form a plexus near the anterior surface of the substantia propria.

Blood vessels are entirely absent from the stroma of the cornea proper. At the periphery there are a series of minute loops from which the cornea receives nourishment.

THE SCLEROTIC.

The sclera, together with the cornea, forms the supporting envelope of the eye. It is the firm, opaque membrane which forms about five-sixths of the outer tunic. It is thinner in the child than in the adult, is thickest in the posterior segment and gradually diminishes anteriorly, being thinnest at the equator. The outer surface of the sclerotic coat is covered by a layer of endothelium and is in contact with the capsule of Tenon. The endothelial covering is reflected over all the vessels, nerves and muscles of this space. The intervening space is called "the supra-scleral lymphatic space."

The deep surface is of a brownish color. It is loosely attached to the choroid except at the entrance of the optic nerve and in the region of the sulcus sclerae. The entrance of the nerve is funnel-shaped and situated 1 mm. below and 3 mm. to the nasal side of the posterior pole of the eyeball. The fibrous sheath of the nerve and the outer part of the sclera blend, while the nerve bundles pass through a series of openings. This portion is called the lamina cribrosa sclerae. There are also openings around the entrance of the nerve for the passage of the ciliary nerves and short ciliary arteries.

The inner surface of the sclerotic is lined by flattened endothelial cells, and between the sclera and the choroid there is an extensive lymph space, the spatium perichoroideale. In this space are found ciliary nerves and arteries and a meshwork of fine, pigmented connective tissue and lamina fusca. This loosely attaches the sclera to the choroid. See the figures on pp. 373 and 374 of this *Encyclopedia.*

At the junction of the cornea and sclerotic the fibrous tissue of the latter passes continuously into that of the cornea and here in the deeper part is a circular canal, the canal of Schlemm. This communicates internally with the anterior chamber of the eye and externally with the veins of the sclera. The sclerotic coat consists of bundles of fine fibrillae of connective tissue which have a meridional course. Between these we find equatorial and oblique bundles. They form several layers which have spaces between them. These spaces are filled with cells, the sclerae corpuscles. With the white fibrous tissue there are a large number of fine elastic fibres, which run as wavy fibrils in the same direction as the white fibres. They are more numerous in the outer than inner layers and more posteriorly than anteriorly. They form a ring around Schlemm's canal and the optic nerve and are plentiful in the lamina cribrosa. They are well demonstrated by the resorcin-fuchsin method.

Pigmented cells are also found, plentiful in the lamina fusca, in smaller numbers, also, near the optic nerve and corneo-scleral junction. Occasionally patches of pigment occur (melanosis sclerae— Hirschberg). They are usually found associated with abnormally dark pigmentation of other parts of the eye or body.

The sclera receives its blood supply from the short posterior ciliary and anterior ciliary arteries. "Branches of the posterior ciliary arteries anastomose with branches of the central retinal vessels and form an anastomotic ring situated in the sclerotic around the optic nerve. This is important as being an indirect anastomosis between the choroidal and retinal circulations.''—(Parsons.)

The veins open into the venæ vorticosæ and anterior ciliary veins.

The nerve supply is derived from the ciliary nerves which pass through the fibrous bundles.

The canal of Schlemm. At the bottom of the scleral furrow there are found one or more lumina, which have a closed endothelial covering, and which are usually considerably larger and more prominent than the spaces of the meshwork of the iris angle. These lumina form the so called Schlemm's canal.

''The endothelial lining has the same appearance as in other vessels, and forms an extremely thin membrane with nuclei projecting inward. Aside from the endothelium, Schlemm's canal has no real wall, at least none such as one finds in other vessels of the same size; It seems to be simply entrenched in the adjoining tissue. On the other hand, it is not correct to say that the endothelium lies immediately upon the sclera, for a loose tissue, poor in fibres but rich in cells, is interposed between the two, as a rule; one sees this layer best in sections stained with Von Giesen; the tissue is then sharply set off from the deep red of the sclera by its yellow color.'' In prepared specimens the lumin of the canal is empty or contains only a few red blood cells. Schlemm's canal occupies only about the posterior half of the scleral furrow, the rest of the depression is filled out by the meshwork of the iris angle. This consists of a three-sided prismatic band, the anterior edge of which is extremely sharp, and unites with Descemet's membrane, and the posterior lamellæ of the cornea. Behind, it unites with the scleral roll, the anterior surface of the ciliary body, and with the root of the iris. Its outer surface borders upon the corneal and scleral tissue, in front, and upon the inner wall of Schlemm's canal, or the loose tissue surrounding it further back; its inner surface is free and turned toward the chamber space.

THE IRIS.

The middle tunic of the eye, consisting of iris, ciliary body and choroid, is called the uveal tract, or uvea.

The iris forms a circular plate, the outer margin of which is called the ciliary, the inner, the pupillary border. These two parts are separated by a zig-zag line. The two zones, ciliary and pupillary, vary in structure and sometimes in their color. According to Salzmann (Brown) the cellular meshwork of the iris is made up of vessels which run in a radial direction from the ciliary to the pupillary border, a thick adventitia which encloses them, and a loose meshwork of branched and fragmented cells which surround and fill the interspaces between the vessels. See pp. 383 and 387, Vol. I, of this *Encyclopedia*.

It is necessary to have sections in the three main directions for an accurate understanding of the histology of the iris.

1. The *medional* or *radial section,* perpendicular to the surface of the iris, shows an irregular limitation in front. The various crypts are recognized as interruptions of the most anterior layer of the tissue, the contraction furrows as sharp angular indentations of this layer. From this border the sphincter pupillæ is seen stretching out into the stroma of the iris, the firm connective tissue which supports it from behind and unites it with the posterior surface of the iris.

2. The section at right angles to the radius may be called the *transverse section.* The farther one goes from this point the more oblique are the elements encountered and the less clear the picture. In general this section shows a smoother course along the anterior border of the iris.

3. The *surface section* presents apparently the least instructive picture, partly because the individual layers of the iris are much too lacking in evenness for the section not to vary into the cells of the next higher or lower layer.

From in front backwards the iris may be histologically divided into: 1. Anterior limiting layer; 2. Endothelium; 3. Anterior border layer; 4. Posterior limiting membrane; 5. Retinal pigment layer.

The anterior limiting layer is a specially dense layer of cells which forms the anterior surface of the iris. The layer of endothelium is a continuation of the endothelium of Descemet's membrane and covers the entire surface of the iris as far as the pupillary margin. This endothelial layer is very hard to demonstrate histologically. It is deficient at those spots which correspond to iris crypts.

The anterior border layer, which has to do with the color of the iris, is modified iris stroma which differs in its intensity. It is made up of cells, chromatophores, between which are collagenous fibrillæ and nerve endings. The cells have usually one or two processes, which are often arranged in little bundles. Between the cells is a thick plexus which in the middle portion is uniformly developed in all directions.

The anterior border varies in thickness in different parts and fails entirely at the entrances of the crypts, while it is thickest on the pupillary border and ciliary zones.

The anterior border through its pigment and density gives the color to the iris. There are two kinds of pigment, the stroma pigment which lies in the branched cells, and the pigment found in the epithelial cells. Pigment always abounds in the latter while the amount in the stroma varies considerably.

The vessel layer, the main mass of the iris, contains numerous blood vessels and nerve plexuses in a delicate stroma which is an extremely delicate tissue containing pigmented and non-pigmented stroma cells, clump cells and wandering cells. The blood vessels enter the periphery and converge towards the pupil. Near the latter the small arteries form an anastomosis from which a capillary network passes towards the pupil. The arteries possess a thin muscularis and a weak intima.

In a similar way the nerves of the iris pass through the periphery and form a plexus in front of the larger vessels. The chromatophores are formed chiefly about the vessels and nerves.

Apart from a few fibres in the periphery elastic fibres are not found in the iris.

The vessel layer undergoes a special modification in the pupillary zone of the iris by the interposition of the muscular band which contracts the pupil, the *sphincter pupillæ*. This is a flat band of smooth muscular fibres which lies close to the posterior surface of the iris.

The *posterior limiting membrane* (Bruch's membrane) consists of fibres extending in a radial direction from the periphery to the pupillary border and which form the *dilator pupillæ*. This muscle, the fibres of which are of a peculiar character, is made up of two layers, according to Salzmann (Brown): (1) A non-nucleated membranous layer in front and (2) a layer of nucleated pigmented spindle cells.

The *dilator pupillæ* extends along the posterior surface of the vessel layer of the iris from the ciliary border of the sphincter pupillæ almost to the root of the iris in an absolutely uniform development.

The layer of pigment epithelium coats the posterior surface of the iris extending to the pupillary margin where it is seen as a black rim. Its cells are densely filled with dark-brown pigment granules, and consist of two layers of epithelial cells which merge into one another at the pupillary border.

THE CILIARY BODY.

The ciliary body forms a girdle of 5 to 6 mm. in width and is divided into two parts—the anterior zone, bearing the ciliary processes, is called the *corona ciliaris*, while posterior to this is the *orbicularis ciliaris*, which is smooth and of a uniform black color. The corona ciliaris is much more uniformly developed throughout its entire circumference than is the orbicularis ciliaris.

The meridional white striation so strikingly seen, even on macroscopical examination, is due to the summits of the ciliary processes. They give the name to the zone and number about 20 in the entire circumference. The interspaces between the processes carry numerous similar projections. See the figures on pp. 386 and 408e, Vol. I, of this *Encyclopedia*.

The whole system of elevations and projections is succeeded in front by a circular ridge which juts forth about opposite the border of the lens. At its posterior border the ciliary body is not any thicker than the peripheral parts of the choroidea; where the ciliary muscle begins, however, some 3 mm. behind the anterior border, the thickness of the ciliary body gradually increases and attains a maximum of 0.8 mm. at its very anterior border. With this maximal thickness the ciliary body ceases as such, as a rule, and thereby acquires a three-sided prismatic form. An outer surface is turned towards the sclera, an inner towards the vitreous, and a narrow anterior surface is turned toward the centre of the cornea or the pupil. The inner and anterior surfaces unite in a rounded ridge, projecting in the direction of the border of the lens; this is called the *inner ledge*.

The insertion of the iris root into the anterior surface lies in the neighborhood of this ledge.

If the ciliary process is examined from without inwards one comes first upon the *ciliary muscle*. In its outer layers the bundles have an almost fine meridional direction—the meridional portion. Forward the thickness of this portion gradually increases up to one-third of the maximum of the entire muscle. At the very fore part it again thins and ends at the scleral wall.

The *radial portion* succeeds the meridional inwards. In this the structure of the framework is most pronounced and the section therefore shows an irregular net-form marking. Many of the bundles appear to end blindly. The interstices of the framework are filled out by a pretty dense connective tissue, which carries the blood vessels and the especially numerous nerve branches, and in heavily pigmented eyes also a few scattered chromatophores. The radial portion attains its greatest thickness in the neighborhood of the inner ledge of the ciliary body.

Here lies the circular portion of the ciliary muscle, the so-called *Mueller's muscle*. It is characterized by a circular course of the bundles and therefore appears as a group of cross sections in the meridional section. The blood vessels peculiar to the ciliary muscle lie throughout in its interstitial tissue and are small in calibre.

Beyond the root of the iris and in front of the circular portion of the muscle, or in it, one encounters in all meridional sections the cross section of an artery, the *circulus arteriosis major*. Large veins are not found in the ciliary muscle.

The *ciliary nerves* branch before entering the ciliary muscle, forming first a wide-meshed plexus and then, continuing to branch, pass on through the muscle. The nerves to the ciliary muscle itself, as well as those to the neighboring parts, are given off from this plexus.

2. The *vessel layer of the ciliary body* is a direct continuation of the vessel layer of the choroid. The larger elevations of the ciliary body, such as the ciliary processes, are due to local thickenings of this layer. In its histology the vessel layer of the ciliary body agrees with that of the choroid. An exception is that the chromatophores are less numerous and may be entirely absent in the front in many eyes. See the illustration on p. 405, Vol. I, of this *Encyclopedia*.

3. The *elastic lamella* is a continuation of the lamella of the same name in the lamina vitrea of the choroid. It is seen with all stains, as a fine, very sharp, straight line in case the section goes perpendicular to the surface, for this lamella courses absolutely smooth over the orbicularis ciliaris.

4. The *interlamellar connective tissue* is a continuation of the delicate layer of collagenous fibrillæ found by Wolfrum, between the two layers of the glass membrane of the choroid. It is thick enough in the ciliary body to be demonstrated by ordinary stains, and here and there contains elongated nuclei. It has no blood vessels.

5. The *cuticular lamellæ,* which covers the whole uveal portion of the ciliary body as far as the neighborhood of the iris root, is a continuation of the corresponding membrane of the choroid. It is very thin. Three varieties of the reticulum, with respect to height of ridges and width of meshes, can be made out, according to Salzmann (Brown).

(a) The larger meshes are rounded or polygonal, and have a width of 40 to 50 mu. and a depth of as much as 40 mu.

(b) The smaller meshes have only about one-half or one-third the diameter of the large meshes.

(c) Among these appear ridges characterized by special thickness, height and striation.

6. The *pigment epithelium* of the ciliary body is a direct continuation from the choroid and consists of a single layer of pigmented epithelial cells. The pigment consists of large, dark, round granules.

The form of the cells changes in various parts of the ciliary body; being short and cylindrical where the inner surface is smooth. The union between the individual pigment epithelial cells is possibly no more firm than it is in the territory of the choroid. The outer surface of the pigment epithelium everywhere forms a perfect mould of the inner surface of the cuticular lamella.

7. The *ciliary epithelium* consists of a simple, smooth layer of cells, aside from several folds, in the anterior part of the orbicularis.

The protoplasm of these cells is in general free from pigment which is found in the ciliary epithelium anteriorly in the neighborhood of the iris root.

The form of the cells varies from that of circular to a cube, and in general their height increases from behind forward. The inner ends of the cells show a form varying much with the direction of the cells.

8. The *membrana limitans interna ciliaris* is a structureless layer on the inner surface of the ciliary epithelium. It is plainly differentiated from the protoplasm of the ciliary epithelial cells by its staining reaction and homogeneous structure. It is probably best looked upon as a cuticular formation of the ciliary epithelium and corresponds in its position to the membrana limitans interna retinæ.

THE CHOROID.

The choroid is between the retina and sclera and reaches as far forward as the ora serrata of the retina. In many animals it is black in color, in the human it is dark-brown. It is a soft, thin membrane possessing a certain degree of elasticity. It is pierced posteriorly by the optic nerve and at this point is firmly adherent to the scleral coat. The inner, smooth surface is next to the pigmented layer of the retina.

The choroid consists of blood vessels and branched pigment cells embedded in a loose connective tissue. It is made up of five principal layers which from without in are: 1. The surface choroid; 2. The layer of large vessels, or Haller's layer; 3. The layer of medium sized vessels, or Sattler's layer; 4. The layer of capillaries, or membrane of Ruysch; 5. The lamina vitrea, or membrane of Bruch.

See the illustrations on pp. 408f and 410 of this *Encyclopedia*.

1. The *lamina suprachoroidea* consists of a series of fine, non-vascular lamellæ, each containing a delicate net work of elastic fibres, among which are stellate, pigmented and ameboid cells.

It is without vessels. The long posterior ciliary arteries come through the perichoroideal space, but they do not give off any branches here.

The *perichoroideal space* lies between the inner surface of the sclera and the outer surface of the uvea. It is limited anteriorly by the insertion of the ciliary bundle into the scleral roll, while behind it ceases some distance in front of the nerve.

This whole space·is traversed by delicate lamellæ which go from the uvea to the sclera. They fuse together here and there and contain large round openings. In this way the suprachoroideal space is not divided into smaller communicating ones.

"Each suprachoroideal lamella has an *endothelial coat* as a basis. This is an entirely transparent, structureless, extremely fine membrane, with only here and there an oval, or somewhat irregular, very flat nucleus, and one to two fine nucleoli. This membrane is supported by a rich plexus of elastic fibres. These fibres stain in the usual way, notably heavier than those of the sclera, but always much more delicately than those of ordinary connective tissue. They are straight, or weakly bowed; for the most part they form a plexus, i. e., the fibres cross in various directions, and the angular branchings and insertions here and there seem to form a reticulum. No particular direction predominates; only at the margins of openings in the lamellæ do the fibres press together and form a sort of ring."—Salzmann (Brown).

In the suprachoroidea one finds branched, flat cells with oval or irregular nuclei, which have in their bodies and processes fine brown pigment. In the outer layers of the suprachoroidea these cells are plump, with short, broad processes, while in the inner layers the processes are slender and longer.

Chromatophores are found through the whole uveal tract. With certain properties common to all they vary, however, in form and pigment contents. The melanin is seen as fine, round granules, both in the cell body and processes.

Wandering cells are also found in varying numbers and are characterized by the density with which the nucleus stains and their frequently granular protoplasmic seam.

The suprachoroidea is without vessels. The space is traversed by the ciliary nerves and the two long posterior ciliary arteries, and by an irregular network of pigmented connective tissue which attaches the choroid to the sclera. The ciliary nerves give off numerous small branches, which again break up into finer plexuses. These are found in the inner layers of the suprachoroidea.

2. *The layer of large vessels (Haller)* forms the main mass of the choroid. This layer may be subdivided into two parts of larger and

smaller vessels. In the layer of larger vessels the arteries predominate, while in the layer of smaller vessels, the veins.

The interspace one finds filled out with choroidal stroma which changes in its make-up from without inwards, especially as regards the chromatophores. In the internal layers there are many endothelial membranes, and flat chromatophores. As one goes inward, however, the dimensions of the chromatophores increase; the endothelium becomes less prominent.

Through the choroidal stroma one finds numerous nerve fibres, the last branches of the ganglionated plexus which begins in the suprachoroidea. They are found usually in company with the arteries.

3. The *layer of medium-sized vessels,* or Sattler's layer, consists, as its name implies, of medium-sized vessels lying in an elastic network, with a few pigmented cells. It has an endothelial covering on its outer side as well as endothelial cells on the inside. The veins have no muscular tissue. They are enclosed in an adventitia which is separated from the internal endothelium by a perivascular lymph space. This communicates with the intercapillary spaces of the chorio-capillaris. The perivascular lymph spaces are said not to communicate with those present between the planes of the supporting connective tissue.

4. The *chorio-capillaris, or membrane of Ruysch,* is composed essentially of small capillaries which form an exceedingly close network embedded in a finely-granular or almost homogeneous tissue. This is the characteristic layer of the choroid.

The network of the capillary layer is especially thick in the posterior part of the choroid, while toward the periphery the meshes of the capillary net continually become wider and longer. The chorio-capillary does not extend forwards into the ciliary body, and has no pigmented cells.

The capillaries consist of simple endothelial tubes strewn with oval nuclei. In the interspace one finds a homogeneous non-nucleated stroma.

5. The *lamina vitrea,* or membrane of Bruch, is a transparent and nearly structureless layer which coats the inner surface of the choroid. It stains feebly with elastic tissue stains. In cross section it appears highly refractile, with a stroma present only in the interspaces of the capillary net. It is made up of two lamellæ, the outer, darker and finely granular; the inner, straight and uniform except in old age. The membrane, especially its outer lamella, becomes thicker.

The outer or elastic lamella bears a clear network first described by Sattler. Smirnow later demonstrated a dense plexus of finest elastic fibres in this network by the orcein stain. The Sattler network corresponds to the larger bundles of this elastic mesh only, and Smirnow called it the *stratum elasticum supracapillare*. As stated, this is united with the elastic fibres of the capillary interstices, and to a certain extent closes off the whole elastic system of the capillary layer inward. In general the lamella has no measureable thickness; by itself it appears only as a contour on cross section, and moreover the elastic fibre stain only makes this contour sharper, not broader. In the region of the optic nerve entrances alone, the elastic lamella is thicker and to the same extent that the glass membrane in general is thickened. Its fibrillæ come out more plainly and take on a more and more circular curve.—Salzmann (Brown).

Upon the inner surface of the choroid is found the pigment epithelium which lies upon the lamina vitrea, and gives the choroid the dark-brown color. It is made up of a single layer of protoplasmic hexagonal cells. The cell bodies are uniformly filled with pigment, while the round nucleus is free from it. From this the entire layer acquires a dark-brown color.

The ciliary nerves enter the sclera near the posterior pole and form in the choroid a dense plexus in which numerous ganglion cells are intercalated. The choroid seems to be devoid of sensory nerves.

THE RETINA.

The retina is a thin, transparent, inelastic membrane with a smooth inner surface, attached to neighboring structures only at the optic nerve and the anterior end, the *ora serrata*. It is thickest at the border of the optic nerve and thins out toward the periphery except on the temporal side. Here one finds the fovea centralis, which is a funnel-shaped depression, the centre of which is 3.5 mm. away from the border of the *foramen opticum choroideæ*.

In this region the retinal wall on the nasal side is somewhat higher than on the temporal. Another prominent point in the retina is the head of the nerve, or the *papilla nervi optici*, which occupies the posterior pole of the eye and is distinguished by its faint yellow color.

Histologically the retina consists of nine layers. From within outward they are: 1. Membrana limitans interna; 2. Nerve fibre layer; 3. Ganglion cell layer; 4. Inner plexiform layer; 5. Inner nuclear layer; 6. Outer plexiform layer; 7. Outer nuclear layer; 8. Membrana limitans externa; 9. Layer of rods and cones.

See the figures on pp. 390 and 391, Vol. I, of this *Encyclopedia*.

The membrane limitans interna is formed of the united bases of the fibres of Mueller, which are long stiff cells passing through several of the retinal layers. At the outer nuclear layer they branch and expand into a sort of honey-comb tissue which serves to support the fibres and nuclei of the rod and cone elements.

At the bases of the rods and cones this sustentacular tissue ceases, being here bounded by a distinct margin, the *external limiting membrane*. Each of Mueller's fibres as it passes through the inner nuclear layer has a nucleated enlargement, indicating the cell nature of the fibre. The *internal limiting membrane* lies between the retina and the vitreous. It is 1 to 2 mu. thick and continues uninterrupted and unchanged over the fovea centralis.

The *layer of nerve fibres* is formed by the expansion of the optic nerve after it has passed through the coats of the eye. The thickness decreases towards the periphery where this and the ganglion cell layer run together. Unlike the rest of the retina the nerve fibre layer shows an exquisite fibrous structure.

Besides the nerve fibres, and Mueller's supporting fibres, it contains neuroglia, which consists of cells and fibres. The cells having a long, densely-staining nucleus, with the axis directed parallel to the course of the nerve fibres and a small amount of protoplasm which varies in form. The nerve fibre layer also contains the larger retinal vessels which are embedded in this and the next layer.

The *ganglion cell layer* is composed of nerve cells of a varying size, somewhat like the cells of Purkinje of the cerebellum. These are multipolar and have numerous protoplasmic processes, which broaden out in the inner plexiform layer and are for the most part provided with axis cylinders going over into nerve fibres of the adjoining layer. The protoplasm contains the so-called Nissl granules which are of varying size and form.

Neuroglia cells are also found here. They have a flat body with smaller and more densely-stained nuclei than the ganglion cells.

The *inner plexiform layer* is comparatively thick and maintains the same thickness in all parts of the retina. It possesses a finely reticular appearance and permits secondary or sub-layers to be recognized. A few nuclei are scattered through it and it is traversed by the processes of the nerve cells and of the inner granules, by Mueller's, and fibres from the optic nerve layer.

The *inner nuclear layer* is mainly composed of bipolar nerve cells containing large nuclei. The inner nuclei, which make up the layer, are placed closely together. The layer consists almost wholly of cell nuclei with the mantles of protoplasm from which processes of varying number and direction go off.

According to Greeff the following elements can be distinguished in the inner nuclear layer: 1. The *horizontal cells* include (a) the *outer* horizontal cells. These are small flat cells whose processes broaden out in a direction parallel to the surface and end in the outer plexiform layer. They lie in the outer portion of the inner nuclear layer. (b) The *inner* horizontal cells are larger than the former and likewise broaden out in a direction parallel to the surface; their end branches mount up toward the outer plexiform layer. Some of these have a descending (proximal or inward directed) process as well,

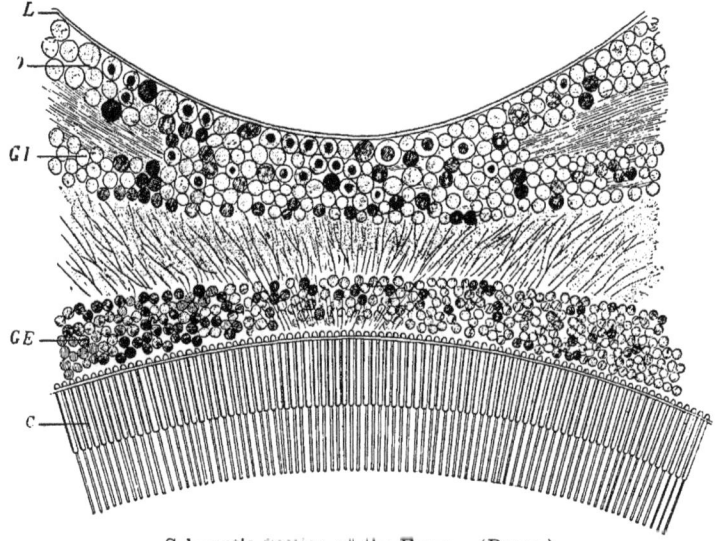

Schematic Section of the Fovea. (Panas.)

L, Membrana limitans interna; C, modified cones.

ending in the inner plexiform layer. They lie at a plane farther inward than do the outer horizontal cells.

2. The *tripolar cells*. According to their union these are divided into: (a) The *rod bipolars:* each of these has a basket of ascending (distal or outward) processes and by means of these is in contact with the ends of the rod fibres. The descending (proximal) process is a single fibre coursing through the inner plexiform layer and invests a cell of the ganglion cell layer by means of its less thick branches. (b) The *cone bipolars* lie very close to the outer plexiform layer, their ascending (distal) processes broaden out parallel to the surface of the retina and come in contact with the proximal ends of the cone fibres. The descending (proximal) process ends in the inner plexiform layer with branches parallel to the surface. Some of these cells

are characterized by specially numerous ascending processes (giant bipolars, Greeff).

3. The *amacrin cells* form a continuous layer in the innermost portion of the inner nuclear layer. Their pear-shaped body measures 10. to 13.7 mu. and gives off a single process inward. One finds: (a) Stratified amacrin cells: these have only one process ending in the inner plexiform layer with a superficially parallel branching. (b) Disseminated amacrin cells: the process branches many times and ends in all parts of the inner plexiform layer. (c) Association amacrin cells: these protoplasmic processes (dendrites) end in the first sub layer of the inner plexiform layer, the axis cylinder process curves parallel to the surface for a long stretch on the border between the inner nuclear layer and the inner plexiform layer and breaks up into numerous branches. These cells also come in contact with the centrifugal fibres.

4. The nuclei of Mueller's supporting fibres.—Salzmann (Brown).

The *outer plexiform layer* is thin and consists of a densely interwoven reticulum of fibrous elements arranged principally in two directions, perpendicular and parallel to the surface of the retina. Two well-separated portions can be made out, an outer thicker, and an inner thinner, which shows the fine reticular (plexiform) structure in a typical way.

The *outer nuclear layer* consists mainly of thickly-placed, rounded, or weakly-oval structures in which a thin, protoplasmic mantle and a densely-staining nucleus can be made out. The nucleus forms so large a portion of the outer nuclear element that the whole layer seems to be made up solely of nuclei. Two kinds of nuclei can be distinguished, one is smaller, more rounded, and more densely-stained, the other larger, plainly-oval and weakly-stained. The first form makes up the main bulk of the layer.

The *membrana limitans externa* is an extremely delicate, sieve-like, perforated membrane, visible as a fine, continuous or streaked line only, in absolutely perpendicular sections. The holes correspond exactly to the elements of the rod and cone layer in number and position, as they serve for the exit of the fibres going out from these elements.

The *layers of rods and cones* has two divisions, an outer, less densely-stained, and an inner, more densely-stained; the border between the two portions lies about half way between the ends of the pigment processes and the membrana limitans externa.

The *layer of rods and cones* has two divisions, an outer, less densely-cylindrical structures, with a length corresponding to the thickness of the entire layer,—the rods, each of which is provided with a some-what longer, slenderer, highly refractile *outer member,* and a shorter, thicker, finely granular *inner member.* The *cones* are flask-form struc-tures which also possess a thinner *outer* and a thicker *inner* member.

The outer member is narrowed conically toward the apex, the inner bags out. The form and dimensions of the cones, however, vary a great deal with their location. The longest and slenderest cones are found in the centre of the fovea, where they appear more like rods than cones. As regards their finer structure the rods and cones are very similar. The cones contain no visual purple.

THE CRYSTALLINE LENS.

See, in illustration of this section, pp. 378-383, Vol I, of this *En-cyclopedia.*

The lens is a laminated, fibrous body inclosed by a transparent elastic capsule, which lies between the iris and vitreous. With the zonula it divides the eye into an anterior and posterior section. It is a transparent and nearly colorless lenticular structure, whose an-terior surface is less curved than the posterior. The lens is kept in position by the suspensory ligament, or zonula ciliaris, which unites it with the ciliary body, and the ligamentum hyaloideocapsulare with the vitreous body.

The posterior surface of the lens is imbedded in the fossa patellaris of the vitreous. Histologically the lens is divided into three parts, the lens capsule, the lens epithelium, and the lens substance. The lens capsule forms the external envelope of the lens and is a structure-less, highly-refracting, firm, elastic membrane, which is very resist-ant to pathological influences. This homogeneous membrane is thicker upon the anterior than superior surface of the lens. The anterior capsule also differs from the posterior by having a single layer of cubical epithelial cells, the epithelium of the lens. The lens epi-thelium extends beneath the lens capsule over the whole anterior surface up to the equator.

The cells in the neighborhood of the anterior pole are not regular, and may take on a more or less stellate form. There may be spaces between the cells. Towards the periphery the cells become more of a cylindrical form. At the epithelial border the cells are arranged in meridional rows.

The lens fibres are long, flat bands, with finely serrated edges and in transverse section appear prismatic. Between the fibres is a cement substance which holds the fibres together. The fibres begin and end upon the anterior and posterior surfaces of the lens along lines which radiate from the anterior and posterior poles.

The lens substance may be divided into two parts, the cortex, which consists of the outer layers of the lens substance, and which is soft and without color, and the nucleus which consists of the harder, deeper layers, and is of a yellow color.

The lamellæ of the lens are made up of lens fibres. These are compressed, prismatic, band-like cells of considerable length. The lens fibre averages about 10 mm. in width in the region of the equator and about 2 mm. in thickness. On cross section the lens fibre has the appearance of an elongated, six-sided figure, with two long and two short sides. The relations between breadth, thickness and form on cross section change in the depth of the lens substance.

The zonula ciliaris consists of delicate homogeneous fibres which originate from the inner surface of the ciliary body. Leaving the apices of the ciliary processes the fibres of the zonula ciliaris pass over to the edge of the lens. The fibres change as they approach the lens, where they are broken up in the lens capsule, part going to the equator, part in front, and a part behind. The Canal of Petit is the name given to the triangular space, on cross section, between the fibres of the zonula and the equator of the lens.

THE VITREOUS.

The vitreous is a completely transparent, colorless mass of jelly-like consistence, which fills the posterior cavity of the eye. In front it has a depression, the fossa patellaris, in which the lens rests. It is fixed to the patella and to the inner surface of the retina, especially at the *ora serrata*. Salzmann suggests this point should be called, *the base of the vitreous*. In the fetal eye the vitreous is traversed by a canal which runs from the optic papilla forward to the posterior pole of the lens. In this canal runs the hyaloid artery. In the developed eye Cloquet's canal serves as a lymph channel. See the figures on pp. 365, 366, Vol. I, of this *Encyclopedia*.

The vitreous consists of a clear liquid substance enclosed in a transparent reticulum. It exceeds all the other refracting media of the eye except the aqueous. The framework consists of fine granular fibrils. The cells, which are round or star-shaped, are very sparse and are found chiefly in the peripheral parts. According to Salzmann the whole framework of the vitreous goes out from the base of the vitreous. Out of the somewhat complicated fibrillation of this portion a thicker layer is first separated off and this extends along the inner surface of the retina backwards as the *posterior border layer*.

That portion of the fibrillation of the base of the vitreous which does not enter the posterior border layer, radiates into the interior of the vitreous, broadening out like a fan, and forms the loose, often shreddy, *body of the vitreous* along with the branches of the border layers.

About the middle of the orbicularis ciliaris, a thickening of the framework of the vitreous again appears. It separates the vitreous from the posterior chamber and from the lens and is therefore called, the *anterior border layer*.

The framework of the vitreous consists of delicate fibrillæ, which are exceedingly fine and extremely soft.

Many fixed cells, blood vessels and nerve fibres, are entirely absent in the fully formed vitreous. Many cells, called *subhyaloid cells*, are found on the outer surface of the posterior border and at the vitreous base. These are isolated cells with simple or fragmented nuclei and a granular protoplasm.

THE OPTIC NERVE.

The optic nerve is divided into three parts: (1) The intracranial portion, which extends from the chiasm to the optic foramen; (2) The orbital portion, from the optic foramen to the eyeball, and (3) The intra-ocular portion, which is found within the sclera.

The intra-cranial, short portion of the optic nerve is flattened and enveloped only by the pial sheath. The optic nerve leaves the orbit through the optic foramen, which contains the ophthalmic artery besides. The optic nerve within the canal is lightly enclosed by bony walls and is particularly disposed to pathological changes.

The orbital portion consists of the trunk of the nerve and the sheaths. The trunk consists of nerve fibres and connective tissue. The nerve fibres vary greatly in size, are very numerous, and have between them neuroglia tissue which acts as a supporting and insulating substance. The nerve fibres are the same sort as are found in the white substance of the brain and spinal cord, and have an axis cylinder and medullary sheath, without a sheath of Schwann.

See the illustrations of this subject on p. 395, 396, and 397, Vol. I, of this *Encyclopedia*.

The fibres vary in size and the finer ones are looked upon as the actual visual fibres. The variation in their size in cross section is due to nodular swellings. Between the bundles of nerve fibres lie the supporting connecting tissue, in the form of thick, or thin, septa which traverse the whole nerve.

The blood vessels pass from the pial sheath into the optic nerve. The central artery is a branch of the ophthalmic. Both the artery and vein enter the optic nerve at a distance of 10 to 20 mm. behind the eyeball.

The three sheaths of the optic nerve originate from the three enveloping membranes of the brain and are called the pial, arachnoid and dural. From the pial, or inner, pass the bands of connective tissue, which form the septa to the interior of the nerve.

The intraocular portion of the optic nerve may be subdivided into a retinal, choroidal and scleral portion. "When one follows the nerve fibre layer in a centripetal direction in a meridional section one sees the nerve bundles curve over the choroidal foramen in bows into the line of the optic nerve axis. Since the nerve fibre layer, and with it the entire thickness of the retina, increases in thickness toward the optic nerve, this transition area bulges a little toward the interior of the eye (papillæ nervi optici). The prominence is, however, insignificant, and scarcely deserves the name papilla, especially since what one designates as such in ophthalmology has nothing whatever to do with the prominence."

In the middle of the papilla there is a depression, due to bowing apart of the nerve fibres. This varies considerably in form and size. The retinal portion of the optic nerve really forms only a ring; the blood vessels in this part of the optic nerve lie wholly superficial, that is, they are not covered by nerve fibres, but possess a thin glial covering on the vitreous side. An actual limitans interna does not exist in the region of the physiologic excavation. The layer of the retina ganglion cells—the rod and cone layer—ends at the border of the optic nerve, the inner earlier than the outer layers, corresponding to the bow-form course of the nerve fibres.

The pigment epithelium reaches up to the intermediary tissue at the optic nerve, but does not extend as far as does the glass membrane of the choroid, which is the only one—of retina or choroid—which reaches up to the optic nerve. The whole of the glass membrane of the choroid forms the inner opening of the optic nerve canal. The wall of the canal is formed by a white, or whitish-colored, fibrous tissue which is plainly set off from the choroidal layers.

The optic nerve canal shelters the choroidal and scleral portions of the non-medullated section of the optic nerve. In the entire non-medullated section of the optic nerve the individual nerve fibre bundles remain strictly separated from one another.

The framework is weakly developed in the retinal portion and at the level of the inner opening of the optic nerve canal; it thickens, however, in the choroidal portion as the optic nerve canal widens and the nerve bundles spread apart. The trabeculum of the choroidal portion is therefore called the *lamina choroidalis* by many, while the lamina cribrosa is given the name *lamina scleralis*. As a whole the lamina cribrosa shows a certain concavity inward; its thickness can be placed at 0.2 to 0.3 mm.

The histology of the non-medullated section of the optic nerve agrees most closely with the nerve fibre layer of the retina. Its various non-medullated fibres are arranged in plainly separated bundles; immeasurably fine glial fibres support the nerve fibres and interlace with them.

THE LACHRYMAL APPARATUS.

This subject is illustrated by the figures on pp. 350 and 351, Vol I, of this *Encyclopedia*.

The lachyrmal apparatus consists of: The lachyrmal gland; The lachrymal canals; The lachrymal sac; The nasal duct.

The lachrymal (an acinous) gland, with short-branched gland tubules, is divided into two parts, known as the superior and inferior lachrymal glands. The superior occupies the fossa lacrimalis in the inner aspect of the external angular process of the frontal bone, and is fixed to the periosteum by fibrous bands. Its inferior surface is in contact with the levator palpebræ superioris and external recti muscles, which intervene between it and the globe. The inferior is much smaller and consists of one or two lobules, and is known as the accessory lachrymal gland.

The lachrymal is a compound racemose gland resembling in structure the serous salivary glands, such as the parotid. *The lachrymal sac* and *nasal duct* together form a passage by which the tears are conveyed from the lachrymal canals to the nose. The upper, expanded portion of this passage is called the lachrymal sac. It lies in a groove formed by the lachrymal bone and the nasal process of the superior maxillary. Above, it has a rounded, blind end, while below it narrows into the nasal duct. The nasal duct is lined with mucous membrane, which is thrown into inconstant folds, several of which have been described as valves. The epithelium is columnar and in part ciliated.

In this section free use has been made of E. V. L. Brown's translation of Salzmann's well-known work on the *Anatomy and Histology of the Eye*. The text-books of Fuchs, Greeff and Parsons have also been frequently consulted. See, also, especially for illustrations, **Anatomy of the eye; Development of the eye; Comparative ophthalmology;** as well as **Eyelids; Iris** and similar minor captions.—(S. H. M.)

Histomarmarygae. (Obs.) Dazzling subjective appearances before the eyes, as of lines or fibres.

Histopin. This proprietary remedy is praised by Kayser (*Woch. f. Ther. u. Hygiene des Auges,* 10 April, 1913) who has found it very useful as a local application in blepharitis and hordeolum.

History of ophthalmology. See **Ophthalmology, History of.** See, also, **Periodic ophthalmic literature; Literature, Ophthalmic,** as well as **Galen;** and other minor captions.

Hitzschlag. (G.) Sunstroke.

Hives of the lid. See **Urticaria of the lid,** also p. 5010, Vol. VII, of this *Encyclopedia.*

Hjort, Johan Storm Aubert. A well-known Norwegian surgeon, who devoted much attention to ophthalmology. Born at Christiania, Norway, April 10, 1835, the son of Jens Johan Hjort, a prominent general surgeon, he received his medical degree at Christiania. In 1864 he accompanied the Danish army on a military expedition and spent the year 1865 in travel. In 1873 he was made Professor of Medicine at the University of Christiania, and Chief Physician to the Surgical Division of the Royal Hospital. He wrote a large number of journal articles on ophthalmologic subjects: keratitis, glaucoma, the visual purple, coloboma of the iris, etc. He died in 1905, aged 70.—(T. H. S.)

Hocken, Edward Octavius. An ophthalmologist of Exeter, England, whose life-dates are unknown. A pupil of Barnes and de la Garde, he was surgeon to the West of England Eye Infirmary from 1836 to 1839.

His writings are as follows: 1. *A treatise on Amaurosis.* (London, 1840.) 2. Injuries of the Eye. (*Lancet,* XXXVIII, p. 282, 1840.) 3. Classification of Ulcers of the Cornea. (*Lancet,* XXXVIII, p. 934, 1840.) 4. Amaurosis from Hysteria. (*Edin. Med. Jour.,* 1842, pp. 49-69.) 5. Hyperaemial Amaurosis. (*Edin. Med. Jour.,* 1842, pp. 324-355.) 6. Essays on Diseases of the Eye. (*Lancet,* XLV, 678, 721, 1847.)—(T. H. S.)

Hock, Jakob. A well-known ophthalmologist of Vienna. Born at Prague, Oct. 31, 1831, he received his medical degree at Vienna in 1861, and then, for a time, pursued the study of ophthalmology under Ed. Jaeger. In 1866 he settled in Vienna for the practice of ophthalmology, and was almost immediately successful. In 1872 he qualified as privat docent at the University, and seven years later established a private eye infirmary. He was also ophthalmic surgeon at the Rothschild Hospital and at the Blinden Institut auf der Hohen Warte.

Among his more important writings are: 1. *Ueber Scheinbare*

Myopie (Vienna, 1872). 2. *Ueber Syphilitische Augenkrankenheiten* (Vienna, 1876). 3. *Ueber die Function der Längsfäsern des Ciliarmuskel* (Vienna, 1878). 4. *Propaedeutik zum Studium der Augenheilkunde* (Vienna, 1887). He died Feb. 2, 1890, after a long and painful illness.—(T. H. S.)

Hoden. (G.) Testes.

Hodge's mixture. See **Silver iodide.**

Hodgson, Joseph. A well-known surgeon of Birmingham, England, who devoted considerable attention to diseases of the eye. Born of indigent parents at Penrith, Cumberland, in 1788, he proceeded to London at a very early age, and there began to study medicine at St. Bartholomew's. Pagel relates that, on a very eventful evening, Hodgson lost at cards twenty pounds out of a hundred which had been presented to him by an uncle. Seeing the error of his ways, he afterwards became a most diligent student and highly moral man. In 1811 he won the Jacksonian prize by his "Essay on Diseases of the Arteries and Veins," which was in 1815 published in London in book form. Later, it was published at Hanover in German (1817), at Paris in French (1819), and at Milan in Italian (1823).

At first Hodgson practised in Chelsea, then at Cheapside. In 1818, however, he settled in his native city, as surgeon to the Birmingham General Hospital and the Birmingham Eye Infirmary. In the former institution he was active for thirty years, in the latter for a short time only. He seems to have written nothing on the eye, although he devoted much attention to ophthalmic diseases in his practice.

Because of failing health, including the blindness of one eye, Hodgson retired in 1848 from active work of every kind, and removed to London, where he lived in retirement. He never ceased, however, to take an interest in the progress of ophthalmology. He died Feb. 7, 1869, aged 81.—(T. H. S.)

Hoeve's (van der) symptom. Enlargement of the blind spot and central scotoma in sinus diseases. Ruebel (*Klin. Monatsbl. f. Augenh.*, August, 1912) reports four cases in which the visual fields were carefully studied in relationship to the nasal condition. His observations lead him to the conclusion that van der Hoeve's symptom is not constantly present in affections of the sinuses behind the nose, but that it has real worth as a diagnostic aid.

Hof. (G.) Area; areola; halo.

Hofmann, Moritz. A celebrated German anatomist, surgeon and botanist, chiefly remembered as the discoverer of the pancreatic duct, and of some (slight) ophthalmologic importance, because of his "*Diss. de Lacrymis*" (Altdorf, 1662). Born in Mark, Brandenburg, Sept. 20,

1622, he studied at Altdorf, Padua, and again at Altdorf, where, in 1645, he received the degree of Doctor in Medicine. Settling in Altdorf, he there became, in 1648, Professor Extraordinary for Anatomy and Surgery and, in the following year, Full Professor of Medicine. In 1653 he was given also the chair of Botany. He died April 20, 1698.—(T. H. S.)

Hog. The ashes of the thigh of a hog, specially of the wild hog, was a favorite remedy in ancient Greco-Roman times, for *lippitudo sicca*. The eyes were also sometimes fumigated with burning lard, and the marrow was used as an ointment in affections of the lids.—(T. H. S.)

Hogg, Jabez. A well-known ophthalmologist of London, England. Born in 1817, he studied at Charing-Cross Hospital, London, and became a member of the Royal College of Surgeons of England in 1850. He was, for a long time, Consulting Surgeon to the Royal Westminster Ophthalmic Hospital, Surgeon to the Bloomsbury Eye Hospital, and to the Royal Masonic Institution.

His chief ophthalmologic writings are: 1. *A Manual of Ophthalmoscopic Surgery* (1863). 2. *A Parasitic or Germ Theory of Disease: the Skin, the Eye, and Other Affections* (1878). 3. *Cure of Cataract and Other Eye Affections* (1878). He also wrote a book on the Microscope, very popular in its day. He died in London, April 23, 1899, aged 82.—(T. H. S.)

Hogg's test. This important and valuable test for the detection of ocular malingering is by some authorities ascribed to Z. Laurence. See Vol. II, p. 1181, of this *Encyclopedia*.

Hog gum. See **Tragacanth.**

Hog's bean. The same as "broad" bean. *Faba vulgaris*. Bean meal, mixed with honey, was once employed as a poultice for "black eyes," or, mixed with frankincense, roses and the white of egg, for hypochyma (cataract.)—(T. H. S.)

Hog's bread. The same as "sow's bread." *Cyclamen europœum*. In ancient Greco-Roman times, the juice of this plant was used for cataract and for affections vaguely known as "weakness of the sight."— (T. H. S.)

Hog's fennel. *Peucedanum officinale*. Used, according to Pliny and Dioscorides, for hypochyma (cataract), caligo, and epihora.— (T. H. S.)

Hogue-California trial frame. See p. 4733, Vol. VI, of this *Encyclopedia*.

Hohläugig. (G.) Hollow-eyed.

Höhle. (G.) Antrum; cavity; crypt; sinus.

Höhle des kleinen Hirns. (G.) Fourth ventricle.

Hohlmeissel. (G.) Concave chisel.

Hohlnadel. (G.) Hypodermic (or hollow) needle.

Hohlspiegel. (G.) Concave mirror.

Hoin, Jean Jacques Louis. A celebrated French surgeon, of considerable importance in ophthalmology. Born at Dijon, April 10, 1722, he became surgical externe at the Dijon Grande Hôpital and a Fellow of the Dijon Academy. He contributed much to our knowledge of after-cataract, of the structure of the crystalline lens, and of cataractine pathology. He died in 1772.

His chief ophthalmologic writings are: 1. Lettres Concernant quelques Observations sur Diverses Espèces de Cataractes. (*Mercure de France*, August, 1759.) 2. Seconde Lettre à M. Daviel sur la Cataracte Radiée, la Convexité du Chaton du Crystallin, etc. (*Ibid.* March, 1760.) 3. Essai Historique sur les Différentes Opinions Concernant la Nature de la Cataracte. (*Ibid.* Dec., 1764.) 4. Observ. sur l'Extirpation de l'Oeil. (*Mém. de l'Acad. Royale de Chir.*, T. III.)— (T. H. S.)

Holder, Sponge. One of the simplest forms of this useful device for

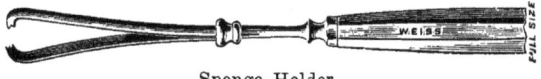

Sponge Holder.

holding sponges of gauze and cotton for ophthalmic purposes is depicted in the text.

Hole at the macula. HOLE IN THE RETINA. CHOROIDAL CRATER. · As the result, generally of injury but occasionally of other causes, a peculiar ophthalmoscopic picture is sometimes found at the macula. It consists of a circular red disc or ''hole,'' which is from one-third to one-half the diameter of the papilla, through which the uncovered choroid is visible. Its depth, according to Ogilvie, is about one-half millimetre. Unlike choroidal diseases, in this condition alterations in the pigment epithelium and choroid are absent. The condition is permanent. Vision is not greatly disturbed unless a detachment of the retina coexists. A central scotoma may be present. The condition does not admit of treatment.—(J. M. B.)

As A. C. Sautter (*vide infra*) points out, it was Knapp (1869) and Noyes (1871) who first called attention to this anomaly of the fundus, but it was not until after Kuhnt's and Haab's studies in 1900 that references to macular hole became fairly numerous. While the majority of the cases reported followed a concussion injury of the eye, in a considerable number of cases traumatism could be positively excluded, the affection being then observed in association with various pathologic conditions of the eye, e. g., ulcerative keratitis, uveitis, albuminuric retinitis, retinitis pigmentosa, senile changes and retinal vascular disease. A nontraumatic example is reported by de Schweinitz in 1904, and in one of Zentmayer's cases reported in 1909. The lesion has also been observed to follow post-operative iridocyclitis.

No case has been studied ophthalmoscopically and then examined microscopically, if we exclude two rather atypical cases; one published by Parsons, of amaurotic family idiocy, and the other by Kipp and Alt, in which a true tear of the retina, complicated with a rupture of the optic-nerve, occurred.

Cases of traumatic rupture of the retina differ clinically and anatomically from the typical macular hole, and both Coats and Fuchs emphasize the importance of differentiating between these two affections.

Pathologic studies have been made by Fuchs, Coats, v. Hippel, Murakami, Pagenstecher and others of eyes which would have presented the typical picture of macular hole had ophthalmoscopic examination been possible, these investigations included eyes with and without a previous history of traumatism. Histologic examination in these cases showed a cystic degeneration of the retinal layers, the formation of a hole at the macula resulting from rupture of the cyst walls.

Coats attributes this degeneration to an edema of the retina at the posterior pole; he believes a completely typical picture of macular hole necessitates a defect of all the retinal layers, but that the appearance of a hole may follow involvement of the inner layers alone.

Fuchs believes that the pathology is probably the same in most instances, whether due to traumatism, vascular or toxic changes. There may be a primary fluid exudation, followed by a secondary pressure atrophy (albuminuric retinitis, neuritis), or a primary tissue atrophy followed by cavity formation (senile changes). In traumatic cases he considers edema probably the primary causative factor, although he concedes that a contusion might result in serious molecular changes, followed by death and absorption of the cells, without the occurrence of extravasations or lacunar degeneration.

Twietmeyer (*Practical Medicine Series*, Eye, p. 134, 1909) reported two cases, caused by contusions of the eyeball through blunt objects. The macular region was at first opaque, the veins engorged and tortuous. In from about 10 days to 3 weeks a round hole, half the size of the optic disc, had formed at the macula, the depth of which was of a marked lower level than the surrounding retina. It was red and was covered with white dots, and surrounded by a diffuse grayish opacity, gradually passing into normal retina. In the second case this opacity showed also a great number of shining, yellowish crystals. Subjectively a central scotoma corresponded to the seat of the affection.

R. Foster Moore (*Ophthal. Review*, p. 94, March, 1910) has described the fundus appearances in a male, aged 24, who had been struck in the left eye with a piece of wood. By ophthalmoscopic examination both eyes showed symmetrical changes at the macula, occupying an area about 1⅓ the size of the disc. In the right eye there was a circular, hazy, edematous area well-defined and slightly raised at the edges with some small exudates on the surface. The left eye showed an affection of a similar nature, but here there was the appearance of bright-red holes with shelving edges, and many whitish areas of all sizes scattered about in this region.

Zeeman (Graefe's *Archiv fuer Ophthal.*, Vol. LXXX, Part 2, 1911) published the histologic findings in a case of hole formation at the fovea centralis. He believes that a perifoveal retinal zone exists, which is especially susceptible to injurious agents; this susceptibility is the result of special vascularization; the predisposition to cyst formation in the region of the fovea and ora serrata is an expression of this relatively deficient vascularization; the most pronounced cyst formation occurs in the temporal half of the ora serrata, because of the greater distance here from the efferent central vessels; perifoveal lesions induced or favored by insufficient blood supply may lead to hole formation; true hole formation at the fovea results either from a union of cystoid spaces or from rupture consequent to cicatricial contraction from the immediate vicinity.

Harrison Butler (*Zeit. f. Aug.*, 26, p. 128, 1912) described the ophthalmoscopic condition in a woman, aged 28, with high myopia.

At the posterior pole of the right eye was a fusiform excavation (in its horizontal meridian) a little larger than the disc; the vertical meridian equaled two-thirds of the horizontal. It had a light-green color and contained three dark-green foci. Excepting a small staphyloma posticum, the fundus was normal. The left eye presented another aspect which explained the condition of the right fundus. From the disc, scars in the form of yellowish long stripes extended laterally over the posterior pole. At the macula there was also a small green hole, and a large hemorrhage veiled the whole posterior pole. The green color was undoubtedly due to changed coloring matter of the blood. See, also, **Green spot about the macula.**

In the case reported by E. M. Blake (*Ophthalmic Record*, December, 1912) the patient, a man aged 52 years, had been struck in the left eye with a baseball. Two days later there was seen in the region of the macula lutea a sharply-defined, bright-red area of about one-third the diameter of the disc. The edges of the spot were slightly wavy, and in the depths of the red area were three small white dots, probably sclera. Vision = fingers at fifteen feet; field of vision normal, except for a scotoma corresponding to the lesion.

Three cases are reported by Purtscher (*Klin. Monatsbl. f. Augenheilk.*, January, 1913), in which after trauma defects were found at the macula. One case, which was seen within a few hours after the injury, showed no central scotoma, but the macular region showed a commotio retinæ. A few days later, when the commotio had disappeared, a macular deficiency with scotoma was found. The findings lend evidence to Fuchs' opinion, that these holes are the result of tissue destruction, perhaps by absorption, and not the sequela of tearing of the tissues.

In the case described by A. C. Clapp (*Ophthalmic Record,* Feb., 1913) a colored man, æt. 35, had been struck by piece of wood over the right eye two years before. The ophthalmoscope showed on the right side a large oval excavation about one-third the size of the nerve head, situated a little below the macula and inward towards the nerve. The long diameter of the oval extended upward and outward and downward and inward. The excavation seemed to be at least one millimeter deep with very precipitous sides, but no line of pigment at its margin. The retina surrounding it was yellowish in color and seemed to have a predominance of the fibrous element; the floor was mottled in appearance, but no vessel could be made out. Around the periphery of the fundus there was a marked punctate condition of the retina. The left eye showed a similar excavation, although not quite so large and being slightly above the nerve level and position of macula. The long diameter also extended upward and outward, and downward and inward. No definite macula could be made out in either eye. In the periphery of the left eye there was marked pigmentation, seemingly in the retina, as the retinal vessels were covered in places. The retinal vessels were very tortuous in the periphery, almost suggesting a detachment. There were cholesterin crystals in the left vitreous, with some deposits in the retina.

The diagnosis of hole at the macula was in this instance based upon its position being at or very close to the macula, on its shape, either perfectly round or slightly oval and on the appearance of the surrounding retina having a yellowish or grayish appearance. The bottom of the excavation was dark-red and mottled in appearance, which distinguished it from an atypical macular coloboma in which there was also absence of the choroid.

In his later paper on this subject Alt (*Amer. Jour. of Ophthal.*, Vol. XXX, No. 4, April, 1913) reported a case following an injury from explosion of a dynamite cap. The eye was enucleated two weeks after the accident and on section there was found a localized swelling of the macular region, due to edema of this part of the retina.

The edema having caused an amount of pressure and consequent destruction of the tissue elements which they could no longer withstand, had finally suddenly burst through an opening into the inner layers and the inner limiting membrane, and the current of the liberated fluid had drawn nuclei and fibers in its course inward towards the vitreous chamber. That the hole is not clean-cut, as it appears in older cases, is, of course, perfectly natural, as the partly destroyed parts have not yet been shed and absorbed, nor has there been time for the formation of the scar tissue.

Just outside of the macula the retina assumes its normal appearance; even the rods and cones show no pronounced pathologic changes. This is the case in the direction of the optic papilla, as well as in the direction toward the periphery of the retina.

It seems from this specimen, which evidently represents a very early stage of the formation of a hole in the fovea centralis, that a high degree of hyperemia of the choroid may, with the aid of some mechanical or chemical influence, lead to a localized edema in the macula lutea and its nearest surroundings, which, if it persists long enough, may lead to a rupture of the inner layers and the inner limiting membrane, and thus may cause the formation of a hole. It may seem doubtful that such a process alone would account for as large a macular hole as others and the writer have found, but there is nothing to prevent a small hole in the fovea centralis from growing into a larger one.

A. C. Sautter (*Annals of Ophthalm.*, July, 1913) reports and depicts a case following a blow on the left eye. The disc is vertical oval, with well-defined margins, and is distinctly atrophic in appearance, the temporal half being slightly excavated and the lamina almost entirely exposed. The nasal half of the nerve is of a pale-rose tint. The arteries appear slightly reduced in size, but the veins are of normal caliber. A macular arterial branch shows in its proximal portion an envelope of connective tissue. Crossing the temporal edge of the disc are two extremely slender vessels, barely discernible, the lower one running obliquely downward and apparently joining a branch of the inferior temporal vein. Encircling the nerve head, but particularly extensive above and to the temporal side, is an irregularly outlined pigmented patch of old retino-chloroiditis about three and one-half times the area of the disc. (See the figure.)

In the macular region, separated from this patch by a stippled, moderately pigmented zone of retinal tissue, is a sharply-circum-scribed, somewhat depressed, dark-red disc, pyriform in shape, with the rounded extremity situated temporally. This area is on a level with and just a little below that of the optic disc, the long axis of the

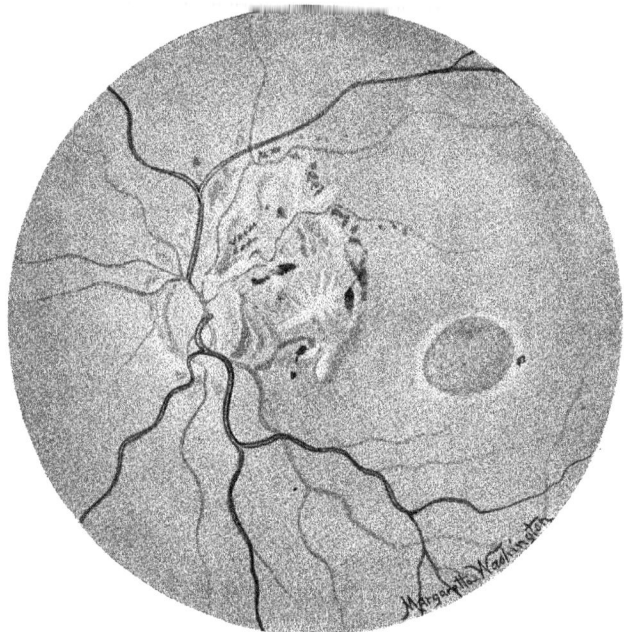

Hole at the Macula.   (Sautter.)

oval being directed slightly down and in. In its widest part it is rather wider than the nerve head, but in length it does not quite equal that of the disc. This area has a more or less mottled appearance, contains some pigment and yellowish deposits, but no visible choroidal vessels. It is surrounded by a broad, grayish-white ring, with an inner shelving margin, especially well-marked temporally, the nasal half of the ring being broader, with its inner edge sloping more gradually towards the excavation. Within this opaque band are a number of brilliant white specks and some spots of pigment. The adjoining retina exhibits many shifting reflexes. At the lower temporal border of the encircling gray zone there is a larger pigment clump, which aids materially in the demonstration of parallactic deviation, the refractive difference between the base of the excavation and the surrounding retinal tissue being about one diopter.

Among the more recently published cases of macular hole not associated with trauma is that of Deutschmann (*Beiträge Zur Augenheilk.*, 87, 1914), who draws attention to somewhat similar cases published by Kuhnt, by Noll (in whose case the condition was complicated by the presence of retinitis pigmentosa) by Roll and by Bradburne. His own case is as follows: a young man of 21 came in 1911 for glasses. Vision after correction of the compound myopic astigmatism was 5/12 in the right eye and 5/10 in the left. Jaeger 3 was read fluently. Ophthalmoscopically the optic discs and retinal vessels appeared normal, but at each macula there was a round, sharply-defined red spot one-fourth the size of the optic disc. No pathological pigment anywhere in the fundus. The parents were nearly related to each other. In good light the fields were found to be almost normal, very slightly contracted upwards in each eye for white, color fields normal, and no color scotoma. In dim light, on the other hand, a decided contraction of the fields was found, and an indefinite paracentral scotoma, relative for colors, was found above the fixation point. The patient admitted that his vision was not at all good in subdued light.

Hole in the disc. Crater-like cavities in the optic nerve-head are exceedingly rare. Not more than twenty-five authentic cases have been reported to date. The first one seems to have been published by Wiethe (*Archiv f. Augenheilkunde*, Vol. IX, 1878). Excellent vision is generally retained and other fundus lesions are almost uniformly absent.

The condition appears to be twice as common in females as in males, the position of the hole is, as a rule, in the outer half of the disc, and never above the horizontal meridian, the depth would seem to vary greatly, and in one case two holes were present.

Reiss and Stephenson have described the hole as being covered in anteriorly by a fine tenuous pellicle which it is extremely difficult to see.

A good example of these defects is furnished by R. R. James (*Ophthalmic Review*, Feb., p. 38, 1913), in which case, by the way, the sight was affected and the macular region was found to be pathologic. A child, aged 6, was brought for squint. On examining the fundus (see the accompanying figure) the disc "is seen to be a little paler than usual, but not enlarged, the vessels emerge from the centre and take a usual course; the temporal edge shows the physiological rim of pigment."

Just below the horizontal meridian of the disc on the temporal side is seen the hole which reaches at one spot up to the pigmented edge, and has steep upper, lower, and outer edges, while the inner edge is more sloping. It is obviously a deep hole from the parallax obtained by moving the lens. The reflex from it is of a slatey-blue color.

The macular changes appeared to be quite superficial; the central part was of a dull-yellow color, while there was a massing of fine pigment around the edge.

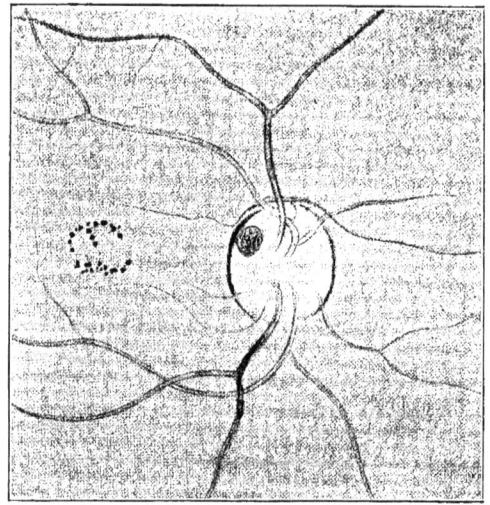

Hole in the Disc.　(R. R. James.)

Examination by the direct method was difficult on account of the child's age, and the presence of his squint; repeated attempts did not allow more than a rough guess at the depth of the hole. See, also, **Cavernæ, Schnabel's**; as well as p. 2937, Vol. IV, of this *Encyclopedia.*

Hole in the iris. Actual holes through the whole thickness of the iris are, apart from traumatisms, excessively rare. In most instances they are congenital (polycoria) or are due to circumscribed atrophy of the iridic tissues. An account of one such instance is furnished by Polte, for which see p. 2854, Vol. IV, of this *Encyclopedia.* See, also, **Polycoria.**

Höllenstein. (G.) Lunar caustic; nitrate of silver.

Hollow prism. A glass device with parallel faces, filled with fluid prism.

Hollow-root. BIRTH-WORT. This plant was frequently employed in Greco-Roman antiquity as a remedy for what was vaguely called ''weakness of the sight.''—(T. H. S.)

Holman, James. A celebrated blind traveller and writer. Born at Exeter, England, Oct. 15, 1786, he entered the navy at a very early age, and, soon afterward (in 1807), was made lieutenant. At the age of twenty-five he lost his sight completely.

Resigning from the navy, he entered the University of Edinburgh with the intention of devoting himself to literature. His health failing, he left the University, and being possessed of a roving turn of mind, decided to devote his life to travelling. In his thirty-third year, alone and absolutely blind, and before the days of railroads and steam vessels, he set out on those wanderings that have formed the subjects of a number of well known and delightful volumes.

The first of his journeys included France, Italy, Savoy, Switzerland, Germany, and the Netherlands. The results of the trip appeared in a book entitled *''The Narrative of a Journey Undertaken in the years 1819, 1820, and 1821.''* The volume went through five editions in thirteen years, and procured for its able author a fellowship in the Royal Society.

On returning from the first of his tours, Holman was made a Royal Knight of Windsor, and given an abode at Travers College, but, possessed of the true roving instinct, he set out in 1822 on a journey round the world. He proceeded at first to St. Petersburg, intending to traverse the whole of the Russian Empire and then to return to England. When, however, he had gone five thousand miles, he was stopped by a Russian officer and sent back. The order had come from the czar, who seemed to suspect that Holman was a spy, who merely pretended to be blind. The result of the trip was a volume entitled *''Travels through Russia and Siberia''* (London, 1825).

He again attempted to circumnavigate the globe, and this time was successful. Throughout the journey, he persuaded his fellow passengers, whenever he could, and one after another, to write down memoranda for him; or, in default of such assistance, he used the nocturnograph himself. Most of his notes he also committed to memory.

Holman was a keen observer, and had the strongest kind of relish for adventure and for traits of human nature. He was also brave, cheerful and serene. His favorite lines were the following from ''Othello'':

"When remedies are passed, the griefs are ended,
By seeing the worst which late on hopes depended,
To mourn a mischief that is passed and gone
Is the next way to draw new mischief on.
What cannot be preserved, when fortune takes,
Patience her injury a mockery makes.
The robbed who smiles steals something from the thief,
He robs himself who spends a bootless grief."

Holman died at his lodgings in John Street, Trinity Square, in London, July 29, 1857.—(T. H. S.)

Holmes, Edward Lorenzo. A famous Chicago ophthalmologist. Born at Dedham, Mass., in 1828, he received the degree of Bachelor of Arts

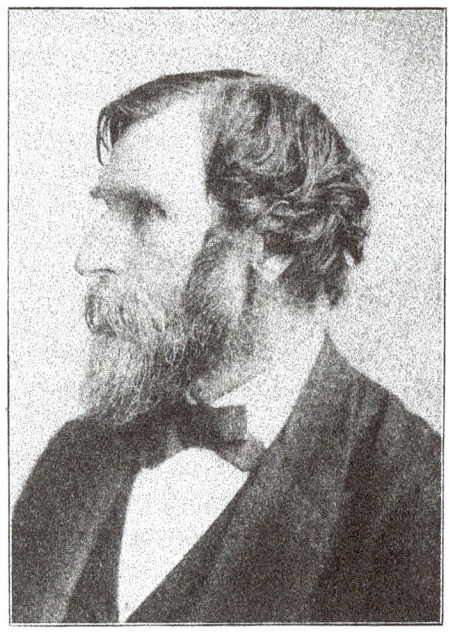

Edward Lorenzo Holmes.

from Harvard University in 1849. For a time he taught in the Latin School at Roxbury. In 1854 he received his medical degree at Harvard, and spent the following year as interne in the Massachusetts General Hospital, making a specialty of ophthalmology and otology. For further study in these subjects he proceeded to Europe, where he remained for a year and a half.

.Returning to America, he settled in Chicago, where he was almost immediately successful. Hardly a medical movement occurred in the State of Illinois in which, up to the time of Dr. Holmes's death, he had not a guiding hand. In 1858 he founded the Illinois Eye and Ear Infirmary at Adams and Peoria streets. In 1884 he was one of the founders of the Presbyterian Hospital. He was a trustee of Lake Forest University, a director in the Central Free Dispensary, a life member of the Illinois State Medical Society, and an honorary member of the Ophthalmological and Otological Societies.

In 1860 he was appointed lecturer on ophthalmology and otology in the Rush Medical College. In 1867 he received the full professorship, a position which he filled with distinguished ability until his resignation in 1898—31 years. He was President of the school from 1890-98.

For a time he was editor of the *Chicago Medical Journal*. His contributions to ophthalmology and otology, both in that publication and in others, are numerous and valuable.

Dr. Holmes married, in 1862, Miss Paula Wieser, of Vienna. Of the union were born five children: Mrs. E. A. Gray, Mrs. R. H. M. Dawbarn, Miss Jeanette R. Holmes, E. L. Holmes and R. W. Holmes.

Dr. Holmes was a man of impressive appearance: tall, slender, long-bearded; very sober and dignified. As to manner he was, in fact, somewhat ministerial. He was an active worker in the Unitarian church, had a host of friends, and exerted a world of influence. He died Feb. 12, 1900, of pneumonia.—(T. H. S.)

Holmgren, Alaric Frithiof. A celebrated Swedish physiologist, of considerable importance in ophthalmology. He was born at Asen, Sweden, October 22, 1831, and began the study of medicine at Upsala in 1850. His medical progress seems to have been considerably interrupted; for, between 1850 and 1861, he became, successively, a teacher of the natural sciences at a school in Norrköping, a cholera physician, an assistant physician in a hydropathic institute at Söderköping, etc.

In 1861 he received his medical degree at Upsala. He was at once appointed adjunct professor of theoretical and practical medicine in his alma mater. The next year, however, he received a commission to continue his education in experimental physiology in foreign countries, and, upon returning, to found a physiologic laboratory at Upsala. In accordance with this commission he studied from 1862-64 with Brücke, Ludwig, and du Bois-Reymond. In 1864 he returned to Upsala and organized the physiologic laboratory above referred to— the first of its kind in Sweden. In the same year he was appointed to the full professorship of physiology in Upsala University.

In 1869 he studied for a time with Helmholtz.

. Among his articles, the following are of special ophthalmologic interest: 1. Die Farbenblindheit in ihren Beziehungen zu den Eisenbahnen und der Marine (Leipsic, 1878). 2. Metod att Objectivera Effekten af Ljnsintryck på Retina. 3. Om Retinaströmunen. 4. Om Färgblindheit och den Young-Helmholtz'ske Färgteorien. 5. Om Förster's Perimeter och Färgsinnets Topografi.

The Holmgren test for color-blindness, known all over the world, is fully described in the non-historic portions of this *Encyclopedia*.

Holmgren died Aug. 14, 1897, at Upsala, of heart disease.— (T. H. S.)

Holmgren's chromatoskiameter. See p. 2205, Vol. III, of this *Encyclopedia*.

Holmgren's wool test. See **Color sense and color blindness;** also **Examination of the eye,** as well as **Examination of the eyes of soldiers, sailors, etc.**

Holocain. HOLOCAIN HYDROCHLORIDE. AMIDIN. PARADIETHOXYETHENYL-DIPHENYLAMIN. This derivative of phenacetin is a colorless, odorless, neutral crystalline powder, having a slightly bitter taste. It is soluble in 40 parts of water.

It is four times as anesthetic as cocain; it is non-toxic and does not affect the cornea, pupil or ciliary body. However, its instillations produce more hyperemia of the conjunctiva and more local irritation than cocain. On account of its irritant quality it is best used in conjunction with cocain. The fullest anesthetic effects can be had from the instillation, every two minutes for ten minutes, of a single drop of the following mixture: Cocain. hydrochlor., gr. j.; Holocain. hydrochlor., gr. ¼; Aquæ dest., fld. ℥jj. To be freshly prepared.

The patient should keep the anesthetized eye closed before and after the operation for which it is instilled.

On boiling in glass vessels the aqueous solution becomes turbid owing to a separation of a small quantity of the free base by alkali derived from the glass. It should form a clear, colorless solution in water, neutral or faintly alkaline, yielding precipitates on addition of silver nitrate or ammonia. The base obtained by precipitation with ammonia and crystallized from alcohol forms colorless needles which melt at 121 degree C. (249 degrees F.). Incinerated on platinum it leaves no residue.

It is incompatible with alkalies and the usual alkaloidal reagents. Glass vessels should be avoided in preparing and preserving the solution, porcelain being used instead.

R. L. Randolph has seen many cases of foreign body in the corneæ of railroad men from the shops. Generally the foreign substance is either a particle of rust or a minute piece of emery. When the patient is first observed the foreign body has generally been picked at and an infected ulcer is present. When every trace of the extraneous substance has been removed Randolph finds this collyrium most soothing and antiseptic: Holocain., gr. ss; Sod. chlor., gr. iii; Aquæ dest., ʒii. A small quantity is given, for healing usually takes place in from 24 to 48 hours.

Holometer. An instrument for measuring angles in any directions; a pantometer.

Holophotal. Reflecting or refracting without perceptible loss.

Holophote. An optical system by which practically all the light from a radiant is projected.

Holophotometer. An instrument for measuring the total light emitted by a radiant in every direction.

Holostemma adakodien. This and several other plants of the same genus, found in the Deccan, tropical Himalaya, Pegu and Burmah, are used in the East for various diseases of the eye. The pulverized root when applied to the eyes is said to cure "amblyopia." Combined with other medicines, it is also used as an ointment in "ophthalmia."

Holosteric. Composed of solid matter throughout.

Holthouse, Carsten. A well-known London surgeon, of considerable importance in ophthalmology. Born in London, Oct. 2, 1810, he studied first under a Yorkshire surgeon, then at St. Bartholemew's Hospital, and, in 1834, in Paris. In 1836 he settled as surgeon in London, where he resided and practised until his death. From 1840 till 1870 he was Instructor in Anatomy, Physiology, and Surgery at the Aldersgate Medical School and at the Medical School of Westminster Hospital.

Holthouse's ophthalmologic writings are as follows: 1. Six Lectures on the Pathology of Strabismus, and its Treatment by Operation, etc. (London, 1854.) 2. On Squinting, Paralytic Affections of the Eye and Certain Forms of Impaired Vision. (London, 1858.)—(T. H. S.)

Holth's operation in glaucoma. In addition to iridencleisis antiglaucomatosa known as *Holth's operation,* that operator has also devised a *scleral punch operation* for the relief of glaucoma, the instruments for which, as well as a diagram showing the steps of the procedure itself, are depicted on pp. 5524, 5525 and 5526, Vol. VII of this *Encyclopedia.* Harrison Butler (*Ophthalmoscope,* June, 1914) has slightly modified this punch method, which he describes as follows: The usual Elliot flap is cut and reflected down to the limbus with squint scissors, and the cornea is split with a small scalpel as far as was usual in the older Elliot operation, to bring the opening close to the cornea, but not necessarily into it. The flap is held down with fine forceps which have no teeth, and the point of the knife is entered at a spot 1.5 mm. from the limbus. The flap is replaced over the knife by the assistant, and the instrument is pushed forward till its point is seen in the anterior chamber. The point of the keratome may catch in the iris and produce a slight iridodialysis. This, Butler thinks, is an advantage, because it helps to clear the iridic angle, which is desirable in glaucoma. The patient must then look down while the punch is inserted slowly and the scleral disc punched out. It must be noted that the cutting blade is underhung, so that the lower (female) blade must be passed in further than may appear to be necessary. A D-shaped orifice results, which should just include a portion of the cornea. If any iris prolapse, it should be seized and excised,. Otherwise, if an iridectomy be desired, the iris should be withdrawn with Liebreich's (Matthieu's) forceps. The flap is finally replaced and held in place with a suture. The eyes are covered with a double pad for forty-eight hours, and then inspected. If there be any undue injection, atropine is instilled. After forty-eight hours, the eyes are left open, using a large shade to exclude glare.

Holth's plate. This test for central scotomata is fully described on p.

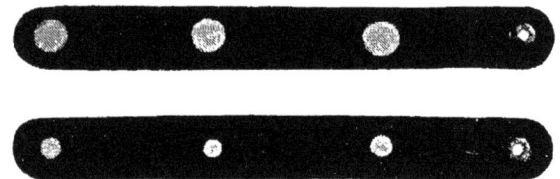

Holth's Ebonite Plate for Testing Central Color Perception.

2419, Vol. IV, of this *Encyclopedia,* which should be studied in conjunction with the (adjoining) figure in this volume.

Holzbock. (G.) IXODES RICINUS. This form of tick pierces the skin of man and animals and occasionally attacks the eyelids, showing the point of partial entrance of the body by a little vescicle. It can be removed by the application of strong salt solution, care being observed to remove the sting, otherwise a severe dermatitis will be set up.

Holzgeist. (G.) Methyl alcohol.

Homalometopus. (L.) A term suggested by Lissauer for a skull having a frontal angle between 130.5° to 141°.

Homalopisthocranius. Lissauer's term for a skull in which the angle formed by lines joining the external occipital protuberance and the occipital point with the highest point of the skull is between 140° and 154°.

Homaluranus. Lissauer's term for a skull in which the angle formed by lines joining the occipital point and the bregma with the highest point of the skull is between 147.5° and 163.5°.

Homans, John. A well-known general practitioner of Boston, Mass., who paid considerable attention to ophthalmology. Born in Boston Nov. 26, 1836, he received the degree of Bachelor of Arts at Harvard University in 1858, and his medical degree from the same institution in 1862. Serving for a time in the Civil War as assistant surgeon, he settled for practice in Boston and was very successful. He devoted much attention to ophthalmology, but at no time wholly relinquished general practice. He was president of the Massachusetts Eye and Ear Infirmary, and a member of numerous medical societies, both general and special. He died in Boston, May 4, 1902.—(T. H. S.)

Homatropin. OXYTOLUOLTROPINE. $C_{10}H_{21}NO_3$. The hydrobromide (or hydrobromate) is the commonest salt of this alkaloid, although the hydrochloride and sulphate form, like it, regular, white crystals. The first named seems best adapted for clinical purposes. It is soluble in 10 parts of water, the solution being permanent. The alkaloid forms regular, limpid crystals. It is slightly poisonous and dilates the pupil and paralyzes the ciliary muscle almost as energetically as atropin.

This mydriatic agent is chemically a mandelic ether of tropin. It was discovered by Ladenburg, of Kiel, and its clinical value in ophthalmology lies in its use as a cycloplegic substitute for atropia and scopolamin, since the fullest paresis of accommodation produced by it passes off in twenty-four hours. In the experiments which the Editor, in 1890, originally made with this agent he found that the best results are obtained from discs of homatropin (alkaloid) and cocain (alkaloid), containing gr. 1-50 each. One of these is placed, from the tip of a moistened camel's-hair brush, on the eyeball three or four mm. from the superior limbus (while the patient looks down and the upper lid is raised by drawing the eyebrow upward) every twenty minutes for an hour. These three disks, the eye meantime being left closed, set up very little irritation and produce the most complete cycloplegia in an hour and a half after the introduction of the first disk. If the pupils are not normal on the next day a drop of a half per cent. solution of eserin sulphate in castor oil will soon contract them.

The aqueous solution, commonly employed in the form of the hydrobromide, is used in about 2 per cent. strength as a mydriatic and (sometimes) in greater strength as a cycloplegic; a drop of 1-500 strength instilled into the conjunctival sac every five minutes, five times, will produce a maximum dilatation of the pupil in three-quarters of an hour, returning to normal in 14 to 18 hours. Other soluble salts of homatropin also used in ocular therapy in the same dosage are the sulphate, salicylate and methylbromide.

Cocain increases the effect of this drug and is used for that purpose in solution just as in gelatin discs.

An effective formula is: Homatropin. hydrobrom., Cocain. hydro-brom. aut hydrochlor., āā gr. iv; Aquæ dest. fld. ℥iv.

The patient should keep the eyes closed one-half the time until the examination. It must be remembered that homatropin and its salts are very expensive agents and should be prescribed with due regard to economy.

According to Jackson, strong solutions (4 to 5 per cent.) induce a burning sensation in the conjunctiva of five minutes duration without causing marked hyperemia. On the other hand, even weaker solutions may, after 3 to 10 minutes, induce a marked congestion of the vascular zone about the cornea; also of the vessels of the sclera, the same as after the instillation of atropin. After instillations of large doses of homatropin, its bitter taste becomes perceptible, but not the dryness of the pharynx which follows the use of atropin.

Batten (*Ophth. Rev.*, January, 1908) finds that the chief difference between homatropin bromide and homatropin methyl bromide, in 1 and 2 per cent. solutions, is the shorter duration of the mydriatic effect of the latter—about one-half to one-third as long.

A highly neurotic woman was examined by S. H. Brown (*Annals of Ophthalm.*, April, 1906) for an error of refraction. Two drops of a 2 per cent. sol. homatropin were used to suspend the accommodation. The patient fainted before the examination was completed, then became delirious and incoherent. This condition continued for twenty-four hours.

One of the advantages from using in the form of gelatin discs such agents as are required to be applied to the conjunctival sac, is the freedom from toxic symptoms. After many years' use of homatropin and cocain discs the Editor has never seen a single example of poisoning from them.

In LeFevre's (*Oph. Record*, June, 1908) case three instillations, one grain to forty-eight minims in two hours and a half, were followed half an hour later by light-headedness and faucial dryness. Thickness of the voice and delirium, with hallucinations of the sight, and apparently of hearing, were present. There was pronounced muscular prostration and incoordination. Recovery was complete in 6 hours.

Harris (*Oph. Record*, Sept., 1908) reports the case of a woman aged 35, of unstable nervous system, in whom four instillations of 2 per cent. solution in each eye, were followed by dryness of the throat, flushed face, hallucinations of sight and hearing, muscular prostration and incoordination. She recovered in 9 hours.

Hömen's sign. ROSENBACH'S SIGN. In exophthalmic goitre, trembling of the upper lid when the eyes are gently closed. It disappears when the eyes are opened, and it is seen occasionally in healthy subjects.

Homeopathy in ophthalmology. [The following essay is contributed at the request of the Editor, by a well known and representative homeopathic ophthalmologist, for the purpose of presenting an authoritative statement of the subject.]

There is little doubt but that Hofrat Samuel Hahnemann (1755-1843), M. D., Erlangen, 1779, was, like Hippocrates and Pasteur, an epoch-maker in medicine. Hippocrates laid the foundation for the scientific study of diseases; Hahnemann initiated the scientific study of drug action. Pasteur revolutionized the practice of surgery; Hahnemann revolutionized the practice of internal medicine. He demonstrated that drugs produce in the healthy body diseases like natural diseases except that they cease when the drug is stopped.

Hahnemann was not the first to declare that likes may be cured with likes (Hippocrates enunciated this), nor was he the first to try the effects of drugs upon the healthy—Stoerck did this in 1760, and Haller was the first to suggest that if we wish to know the action of drugs they should be tested upon the healthy. But to Hahnemann is due the credit of creating and building up a therapeutic system of cure by similars based upon drug provings on the healthy. He alone possessed the requisite medical, chemical and literary knowledge, the scientific insight and thoroughness, the perseverance and the intellect to grasp the subject in mass and detail that were necessary for the development of what had been but a vague idea in the minds of others.

A master of ancient literature and of ten languages (besides a smattering of Chaldaic), Hahnemann was a prominent physician and chemist, well-known beyond the borders of his own country for his masterly translations and discoveries in chemistry; he possessed distinguished friends of high position in the medical profession and among the reigning nobility. Ahead of his times, disgusted with the errors, uncertainties, confusion and failures of medicine, he gave up practice shortly after his marriage and supported his family by translating; later, he resumed practice when he advanced far enough to do so homeopathically.

In 1790, while translating Cullen's *Materia Medica,* he was led to experiment upon himself with Peruvian bark, to study its effects upon a person in health, and discovered that it could produce the same phenomena, symptoms, as those of ague, which disease it had a reputation for curing. This led to testing other drugs upon himself and upon many (healthy) friends; he verified his observations by ransacking the materia medica for recorded experiments, and the whole history of poisoning. Six years were thus spent, when he published in Hufeland's *Journal der praktischen Arzneykunde und Wundarzneykunst,* Vol. II, parts 3 and 4, 1796, his Essay on a New Principle for Discovering the Curative Powers of Drugs.*

Hahnemann demonstrated that all cases of constitutional disease which are curable with medicine will be cured by the administration of that which has the power to cause similar symptoms in the healthy body. While he was emphatic that theory and explanation are secondary in importance to observed facts, he submitted a vitalistic explanation of how the homeopathic remedy cures. Facts speak for themselves; their explanations will necessarily change with our conceptions of pathology.

Observing that nature at times cures by the advent of a stronger *similar* disease, Hahnemann asserted that homeopathy is the natural way to cure: that the drug disease if similar in its manifestations (symptoms) carries off the patient's disease with it as it passes off; hence the name homeopathy, *omoios,* like or similar, and *pathos.* disease or affection. Hahnemann perceived that we can have actual knowledge only of phenomena (facts); that we can recognize disease only by its phenomena (its symptoms, subjective and objective), that hence the essential similarity between a diseased condition and its remedy is its symptom-similarity. Therefore he formulated his method of practice *Similia similibus curantur,* "let likes be treated with likes." (*Transactions American Institute of Homeopathy,* 1899, p. 99.)

This phrase formulated the means by which one may select the curative remedy; it expresses the relation, symptom-similarity, between two series of observed facts: (a) the facts of disease—all that we can ascertain about the sick patient, and (b) the facts of the remedy—all the subjective and objective symptoms that the remedy *has been found to cause* in the healthy body. *This therapeutic law of cure is a scientific expression of relationship between the science of*

---

* *Organon of Rational Healing;* first published in 1810. The fifth edition appeared in 1833; this has been translated 15 times (21 editions) into French, English, Russian, Spanish, Italian, Hungarian and Swedish.

pathology on the one hand and the science of pharmacology on the other; it is unaffected by advances in knowledge of either of these sciences, except that thereby it may be applied more exactly. Its application is an art. "Homeopathy is a method of therapeutics, as multiplying numbers is a method of mathematics. Therapeutics explains the limitations of homeopathy." (*Jour. of Am. Institute of Homeopathy,* March, 1913, p. 836.)

Hahnemann stated that every reasonable physician will first remove removable causes, that local mechanical conditions are to be treated surgically, that in dangerous emergencies antipathic and hygienic palliatives are permissible and useful.*

Other therapeutic axioms are: 1. Homeopathy is a therapeutic law of cure through symptom-similarity, applicable to medically curable constitutional diseases with or without secondary lesions, and formulated *similia similibus curantur* (let likes be treated with likes) with the understanding that the similarity here meant is symptom-similarity.

2. It is a scientific expression of relationship between the science of pathology (all ascertainable phenomena of the patient) on the one hand and the science of pharmacology (the ascertained pathogenetic effects—subjective and objective—of the remedy) on the other hand.

3. It is a system of medicine limited (strictly speaking) to medicinal therapeutics but extending throughout the practice of medicine and surgery wherever and whenever internal medication is applicable; based upon cure by symptom-similarity and upon individualization of patient, case and remedy, it involves the single remedy, small dose, potentization, provings (tests upon the healthy), verifications and a complete organization of societies, colleges, hospitals, etc., books and periodicals peculiar to but not necessarily limited to itself.

A medicine is a homeopathic prescription only when it is selected, and because it is selected, upon the homeopathic principle. The second tenet of homeopathy is the single remedy; this is a corollary of the first.

The scientific way to study drug action is to "prove" it by administering one drug at a time to the healthy body, with due precautions that the symptoms observed are properly attributable to the drug. It is well to supplement this with larger, lethal, doses to animals for

---

* For a simple exposition of the teachings of the Organon, see Dr. Samuel Lilienthal's "*Catechism of Samuel Hahnemann's Organon*" in the *California Homoeopath,* March, April, May and June, 1889, which appears in the *Homoeopathic World* (London), June and July, 1889, as "The Essence of Samuel Hahnemann's Organon."

the study of structural changes.*   The proper study of the pathogenetic effects of a drug requires a large number of provings upon
numerous people, both males and females, by administering it in
various doses.   The same drug affects different parts of the body in
different individuals; when a symptom occurs in two or more provers,
or is repeated in one prover each time and only when the drug is
taken, it carries more weight because it is then more certainly attributable to the drug.

The third tenet of homeopathy is the small, the "minimum" dose.
Hahnemann found by experience that a patient is particularly sensitive to the remedy which is homeopathic to his or her condition at
the time, that too large a dose will aggravate the disease and may
even precipitate death.   Hence he gradually diminished his doses,
but never went to such extremes as did some of his followers.   He
wrote (Organon, sect. 278, 279, 280) : "Pure experiments and observation alone can solve the question of the dose.   The doses are to be
reduced so far that they will merely produce an almost imperceptible
homeopathic aggravation, a slight intensification of the symptoms,
immediately after having been taken."   Some, if not most, of the
older "high potency" physicians adopted the extreme dose because
they found it more successful after having tried "allopathic," empiric,
crude and low potency prescribing.

The Homeopathic Pharmacopeia of the United States (in harmony
with the British Homeopathic Pharmacopeia) has a uniform drug
strength for tinctures—1/10 drug power, referred to the dry crude
drug making allowance for the plant moisture (they are made always
when possible from the fresh green specimen).

Insoluble drugs are ground for an hour or more in individual
clean mortars with nine parts by weight (usually 10 and 90 grains)
of finely powdered milk-sugar until the largest drug particles do not
exceed 1/100 inch in diameter; this makes the first decimal trituration, Ix.   To one part (10 grs.) by weight of this, in a fresh mortar,
are added nine parts by weight (90 grains) of milk-sugar and triturated until the largest drug particles are not more than 1/2000",
except in case of drugs with which experiment has demonstrated the
impossibility of attaining this degree of fineness, this is the second
decimal trituration, IIx.   Subsequent triturations are made in the
same way, the largest drug particles of the IIIx should not be more
than 1/4000" in diameter if possible; in and after the fourth the

---

* The best exposition of this is the Test Drug-Proving of the American
Homeopathic Ophthalmological, Otological and Laryngological Society. A Re-
proving of Belladonna, by Howard P. Bellows, M. D.   665 pages.   Boston, 1906.

grinding should be continued until each 100 grains has received as much trituration as that drug required to make its IIx.

Dilutions of soluble drugs are to be made by adding nine cubic centimeters of water, alcohol or water and alcohol, to one cubic centimeter of the next lower attenuation and shaking hard at least ten times until thoroughly mixed; this is best done in vials of four or more dram capacity and each downward shake should be suddenly arrested. These attenuations are, respectively, tincture, 2x, etc., "dilution;" both dilutions and triturations are also spoken of as "potencies" or "attenuations."

Insoluble substances were first triturated to VIx, one grain of this was dissolved in 50 minims of distilled water and 50 minims of alcohol added thereto, then "succussed," shaken as above, at least ten forcible shakes with each dilution.

Hahnemann, and his súccessors for many years, made the potencies on the centesimal scale: one part to 99. Each attenuation on this scale contains as much of the original substance as would be indicated by a fraction with a numerator of 1 and for denominator 1 followed by twice as many ciphers as there have been steps in the trituration or dilution. These preparations are written I, II, III, etc., or 1, 2, 3, etc.; they are also indicated with a c instead of an x, but this is not necessary—it is not found in the literature until within the last few years. The American Institute of Homeopathy voted that the centesimal scale is to be understood unless the decimal is expressly indicated. As an instance of the difference: the third decimal contains 1/1000 of the original drug, while there is but 1/1,000,000 in the third centesimal. Only 2970 c.c., less than three liters, of alcohol will suffice to run up the 30th centesimal dilution from the tincture, and 5400 grains of milk-sugar will suffice to make the 60th decimal trituration.

After awhile Hahnemann observed that the non-venereal chronic diseases, even after having been repeatedly and successfully removed by the then known homeopathic remedies, continually reappeared in a more or less modified form and with a yearly increase of disagreeable symptoms. "This proved to me," Hahnemann writes (*"Chronic Diseases,"* 1828) "the fact that the phenomena which appeared to constitute the ostensible disease should not be regarded as the whole boundaries of the disease—otherwise the disease would have been completely and permanently cured, which was not the case—but that this ostensible disease was a mere fragment of a much more deeply seated primitive evil." For ten years he studied this problem, and concluded that chronic diseases are due to one of three chronic "miasms" (what we now term dyscrasia): psora, syphilis and sycosis.

Then he proved drugs that would reach the root of the trouble: "antipsorics," like sulphur, calcarea, etc., and "antisycotics" of which thuja is the representative.

By the psora miasm Hahnemann meant that dyscrasia wherein the sarcoptes scabiei thrives; we all know that one individual is contaminated by the touch of a person or article carrying the itch insect while another escapes as if he or she were repugnant to the insect. (The same is true as to fleas, etc.) Today Korndoerfer (*New England Med. Gaz.,* p. 170, Apr., 1913) offers *lowered immunity from hypothyroidism* as the modern explanation of Hahnemann's much discussed and misunderstood "psora miasm;" he shows the identity of their symptoms.

Hahnemann taught the dual action of drugs (which the dominant school is only now beginning to realize). By this is meant not reaction but that opposite effects follow the administration of small as against large doses, both pathogenetically and therapeutically. The size of the dose must be left to the judgment of the prescriber because it has been found impossible to formulate definite rules for it. Some have said "Give the smallest ("minimum") dose that will cure." The writer feels that much harm would have been avoided if it had been put "Do not give so large a dose as to impede the cure or do any harm." Constantine Hering advised that "the more accurately the remedy is selected, the closer and fuller its similarity, the higher should be the potency. The late Dr. Henry M. Dearborn taught and practiced: "in chronic diseases lower the attenuation, increase the dose, until some effect be noticed, either aggravation or amelioration, then give smaller doses, higher attenuations, or stop the remedy, as improvement progresses. This of course when one is satisfied that the right remedy has been selected." A minute medicinal aggravation is evidence that the right medicine is being administered.

The dose will vary according to whether we wish a chemic, mechanic or dynamic effect, also with the drug and with the susceptibility of the patient. The patient should be cured *"tuto, cito et jucundo."* The small dose obviates disturbing the stomach and does not upset the patient or set up a drug condition which is later to be combatted; and when it acts it is usually more prompt and more thorough. Dilution and trituration increase the points of contact and thus more than compensate for lessened quantity of drug.

Broadly speaking, the homeopathic prescription is based upon the drug's secondary symptoms and the dominant school administers a remedy for its primary—immediate—effect. For example, belladonna in a large dose is a mydriatic; mydriasis, when not due to belladonna, is one of the important indications for the administration homeopathically of belladonna, and is best met with a smaller dose than would dilate the pupil if administered internally.

Verifications—cures of symptoms under the homeopathic law—form an essential part of homeopathic literature, provided they are properly reported. Every clinical report should be so clear and full that the reader or hearer will agree with the reporter in the diagnosis and will concede that the cure or relief claimed is properly attributable to the remedy (or treatment, whatever that was) and to nothing else. Care should be taken to mention all adjuvant treatment and other change in environment, the duration of the symptoms or disease and also the promptness and permanence of the relief. It would be well to indicate the symptoms which led to the selection of the remedy.

The fundamental principle of homeopathic practice is individualization; individualization of patient, of case and of remedy. It is the patient who is sick and is to be restored to health, not the disease which is to be combatted and cured. Diagnosis is necessary for intelligent therapeutics, but the symptoms of most importance in making the diagnosis are not the most important ones in selecting the remedy. This is because the generic symptoms, while classifying disease, are not particular enough to characterize the individual case of illness. For this, reliance must be placed upon the peculiar symptoms—peculiar to the patient and to the attack; they may be unexplainable and apparently trifling. Among these are the modalities—conditions of aggravation and amelioration, of time, locality, etc. Mental symptoms are very valuable and, as a class, subjective are more important for prescribing than are objective symptoms. So-called physiological prescribing points out a class of remedies but fails to indicate which one to select.

There are varying degrees of similarity; the more complete the similarity the more satisfactory will be the cure. While the most brilliant homeopathic cures have been constitutional, the principal is often applicable in apparently local troubles with but few symptoms. A remedy is often selected, with gratifying result, upon only three or four "characteristic" symptoms.

Even after the lapse of a hundred years our provings are yet incomplete; they should be brought up to date with the use of modern instruments of precision and examinations by experts. This will be done, ultimately. In practice the provings have been supplemented by "clinical symptoms," symptoms which according to careful observers have repeatedly disappeared after the administration of a given remedy. These have crept into the materia medica and repertories, indicated by °, so that practically our only "pure" materia medica is found in Hahnemann's *Reine Arzneimittellehre*, Allen's *Encyclopedia*, and his *Handbook*, in the *Cyclopedia of Drug Pathogenesy*, and scattered through medical literature in provings and poisonings.

In the *Cyclopedia of Drug Pathogenesy* are recorded drug effects consecutively as they occurred; but this arrangement is not convenient for reference, hence Hahnemann arranged the symptoms of his *Materia Medica* according to an anatomical schema. The objection to this, particularly for study, is that each proving is scattered in pieces —the sequence of symptoms is lost.

The best books for studying the homeopathic materia medica are Farrington's *Lecture on Clinical Materia Medica*, Kent's *Lectures on Materia Medica*, and Richard Hughes' *Parmacodynamics*. Some object to this last work because it teaches organotherapy and pathological drug action rather than true homeopathy. The classical work on homeopathy applied to ophthalmology is "*Ophthalmic Diseases and Therapeutics*" by Arthur B. Norton, M. D., 3d edition, 1902.

See, also, *Homeopathic Therapeutics in Ophthalmology*, 1916, by John L. Moffat, New York.

As an example of the application of the foregoing principles in ophthalmic homeopathic practice, the curative remedy for a given case of iritis will be found not by depending upon the diagnostic symptoms— belladonna, bryonia, mercurius, spigelia, and each of more than twenty other drugs will cause these—but that one must be selected which has the characteristic, individualizing, symptoms presented by the individual patient; sometimes it is a remedy that has never been known to cause or cure iritis.

If the patient is rheumatic, irritable, constipated, aggravated by heat and motion and is worse in the morning, has soreness in, around and particularly behind the eyeball, with sticking pains on motion in the eyes—bryonia will cure.

But the mercurius patient presents an entirely different picture: He is worse at night after going to bed and in damp weather, the eyes are particularly sensitive to the light of the fire, gas, candle, etc., he has night sweats, nocturnal pains in different portions of the body, bad breath, metallic taste in the mouth, the tongue is flabby and indented, there may be a diarrhea; all or most of these symptoms in addition to those of iritis proper. While spigelia, classed as a neuralgic remedy has repeatedly made brilliant cures of iritis when indicated by the totality of its symptoms, characterized usually by neuralgic pains radiating from the eye through the temples, face and head.

Homeopathy is not organotherapy, yet some remedies do undoubtedly manifest a selective affinity, so to speak, for certain tissues or organs: e. g. belladonna, duboisia, gelsemium, mercurius corrosivus, phosphorus, cause congestion and inflammation of the ocular fundus even when introduced into the stomach or some other part of the system remote from the eye; the choice among these must be determined by the patient's drug picture—it may be indicated by three or four characteristics.

It is impossible to memorize the homeopathic materia medica, nor all the symptoms of any one of the leading remedies; recourse must be had to the assistance of repertories which must be followed by verification in the materia medica. It is because of this difficulty that the majority of physicians, oculists, etc., who believe in homeopathy find themselves unable to apply it regularly in the stress of their daily work and the demands of other phases of medical study. With persistent study, however, and experience one can become so familiar with the characteristics of such remedies as prove successful in his hands that he can recognize them in his patients as one will pick out a familiar face in the crowd. As a matter of fact, very many so-called homeopathic prescriptions are but empirical; e. g. bryonia given in iritis because it has a reputation for that disease might be a stumbled-upon cure—empiricism, but it would be more scientific, more certain, and the doctor would have learned more, if it had been chosen on account of its symptom-similarity.

The official definition of the homeopathic physician is: "One who *adds to* his knowledge of medicine a special knowledge of homeopathic therapeutics and observes the law of similia. All that pertains to the great field of medicine is his by tradition, by inheritance, by right." Krauss *(loco cit.)* suggests: "A homeopathic physician is a medical practitioner who *consciously* practices homeopathy when homeopathy is indicated."

From the foregoing it may readily be seen that a physician is a homeopathic specialist or exclusivist, just as one may devote special or exclusive attention to electricity.

Homeopathy is applicable in ophthalmology, just as it is wherever any other medicinal therapeusis is called for. The eye as a living part of a living body is influenced by the patient's constitution and by disturbances in other parts of the system.

A committee of the American Homeopathic Ophthalmological, Otological and Laryngological Society reported *(Journal of Ophthalm. Ot. and Laryng.,* p. 4, Jan., 1913) upon the facilities in this country and Europe for special education in diseases of the eye, ear, nose and throat, and concluded that "there is great need of a higher and more uniform standard of special training in this country." It found that "the New York Ophthalmic Hospital is the only institution in the country having an organized course covering the field of ophthalmology, otology, rhinology and laryngology as they should be covered." Adding, "The plan of this college comes nearer, we believe, to meeting the demands for modern instruction in these specialties than perhaps any other in the world."—(J. L. M.)

Homer. The greatest poet of all time, who is sometimes said to have been blind. Hence, he is often called "The Blind Old Bard of Chian's Strand," "Blind Melesigenes," etc. He is supposed to have flourished about 1000 B. C. The fact, however, seems to be that Homer is a mythical person, though the ancient Greeks undoubtedly believed in his actual, historical existence, and, in fact, never questioned it. The so-called *"Works of Homer,"* were probably the product of various early tribes, or, rather, of the bards of those tribes. Eight Greek biographies of "Homer" have come down to our day, all untrustworthy. One of these is plainly by Plutarch, while another is ascribed, though falsely, to Herodotus.

The more important Homeric writings are the *Iliad, The Odyssey, Hymns, Battle of the Frogs and Mice, Jests,* and *Margites.* These are too well known in the world of letters generally to require the slightest discussion in this work.—(T. H. S.)

Homoarecolin. ARECAIDINETHYL ESTER. A colorless liquid, soluble in water and alcohol; less toxic than arecoline but possessing similar miotic powers.

Homobaric. Of uniform weight.

Homocentric. Concentric; having the same center.

Homocentric rays. In *optics,* rays that emanate from one and the same point on the optic axis.

Homochromous. Of the same color. In botany, having the male flowers, when present, ligulate and of the same color as those of the disc.

Homochronous inheritance. HOMOCHRONISM. A term introduced by Haeckel to define inheritance of a character in an offspring at an age corresponding to that at which the character appeared in the parent.

Homococain. ETHYL-BENZOYL-COCAINE. COCA-ETHYLINE. This crystalline substance, a by-product in the manufacture of cocain by synthesis, forms salts which have an anesthetic action, but much weaker than that of cocain.

Homœopathy. See **Homeopathy.**

Homofocal. Confocal; having the same focus.

Homogeneous immersion system. A system of lenses in which the layer of air between the cover-glass and the objective is replaced by a liquid (generally oil of cedar) whose refractive index is equal to that of the cover-glass and the front lens of the objective.

Homogeneous light. Light of only one wave-length, therefore, of one color, mono-chromatic light.

Homogeneous medium. A medium having throughout the same composition and the same density.

Homoiopathia. (L.) A similarity of morbid conditions.

Homolateral. IPSOLATERAL. Occurring on the same or the corresponding side.

Homologous. HOMOLOGIC. Having the same relative position or proportion.

Homolographic. Exhibiting true relative areas.

Homonymous. Coming under the same general designation (thus the two external recti muscles are homonymous); also, occurring on or within the same lateral half of the body, *homonymous diplopia* or *hemianopia,* for example.

Homonymous diplopia. See p. 4006, Vol. VI, of this *Encyclopedia.*

Homonymous hemianopsia. See **Hemiopia.**

Homonymous images. Double ocular images apparently displaced from one another in the same sense as the displacement of the eyes in which they are produced.

Homopathy. Homeopathy, or homoeopathy.

Homorenon. ETHYLAMINOACETOBRENZCATECHIN HYDROCHLORIDE. ETHY-LAMINOKETONE. This agent is a derivative of suprarenin synthetic. It is a stable product, appearing as a small crystalline substance, very soluble in water.

A 4 to 5 per cent. solution corresponds in efficiency to a 1 to 1,000 solution of suprarenin synthetic, or the product obtained from the adrenal gland. It is more easily employed than suprarenin synthetic, as the quantity needed for making solutions can be accurately weighed, and solutions therefore extemporaneously made.

Homotopic inheritance. A term attributed to Haeckel, the inheritance of acquired character.

Honey. Honey, in Greco-Roman times, was thought to have a "purifying" action on the eye—i. e., to remove from that organ all and every noxious humor that might perchance be pent within it. Honey was deemed especially useful, therefore, in ulcers of the cornea.

Beeswax, on the other hand, was merely employed as a menstruum in the preparation of ophthalmic ointments.—(T. H. S.)

Honeycomb choroiditis. A synonym of Doyne's or familial choroiditis. See **Familial eye affections.**

Honig. (G.) Honey.

Hood. A device by means of which a lens is protected from extraneous light.

Hookah. NARGILEH. The water tobacco-pipe of the Arabs, Turks, Persians, Hindus and other orientals. It consists of a bowl for the tobacco, a water bottle and a long flexible tube ending in the mouthpiece. The smoke passing through the water, is cooled, cleansed and deprived of a portion of its nicotine and other poisonous agents before being drawn through the mouth. By some authorities it is believed that hookah (or nargileh) smoking is less likely to produce toxic amblyopia than is the common pipe.

Hooke, Robert. One of the most ingenious of experimental philosophers. He was born, the son of a minister, at Freshwater, in the Isle of Wight, July 18, 1635. In 1658 he entered the University of Oxford. Becoming assistant to Boyle, he rendered a great amount of service to that brilliant investigator in connection with his invention of the air-pump. In 1662 Hooke was appointed "Experimenter" to the Royal Society, and, in 1678, its Secretary. He is chiefly to be remembered by ophthalmologists as the first to measure (not to discover— on that head, see **Euclid**) "the minimum visual angle." The passage in which this great discovery is recorded is found in Birch's *"History of the Royal Society"* (1757, III, p. 120) and runs as follows: "If a graduated ruler be held at such a distance from the eye that the interval between any given division-mark and the next appears under a smaller angle than one minute, then the sharpest eye can no longer discriminate the two marks from one another." On this great discovery is based a very large proportion of the daily work of every practising ophthalmologist.

Hooke also invented the clock spring, the watch spring, and probably (the point is much disputed) the reflecting telescope.

He died of overwork at London, Mar. 3, 1703.—(T. H. S.)

Hooke's experiment. HOOKE'S LAW. See **Hooke, Robert.**

Hookfront. One of the names given to "grab" fronts. See p. 4921, Vol. VI, of this *Encyclopedia.*

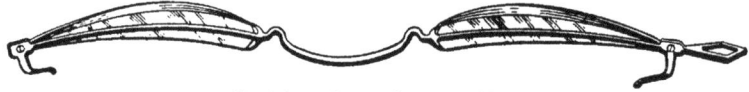

Hookfront Binocular Magnifier.

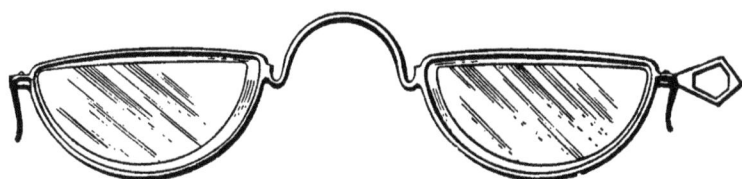

Hookfront Binocular Magnifier.

Hooks. This class of instruments may be subdivided under the heads of *strabismus* or tendon hooks, *capsule* hooks, *iris* hooks, both sharp and blunt, *fixation* hooks. Models of each class are shown in the illustrations.

The blade of R. H. Elliott's instrument (*Trans. Oph. Soc. United Kingdom*, p. 219, 1909) is 5 cm. long. The large curve of the blade has been moulded on the antero-posterior curvature of an average eye, and corresponds to a little less than half its circumference. The extremity of the hook is bent back 4 mm. in the smaller curve, the opening of which has been so graduated that it will admit and hold firmly an optic nerve.

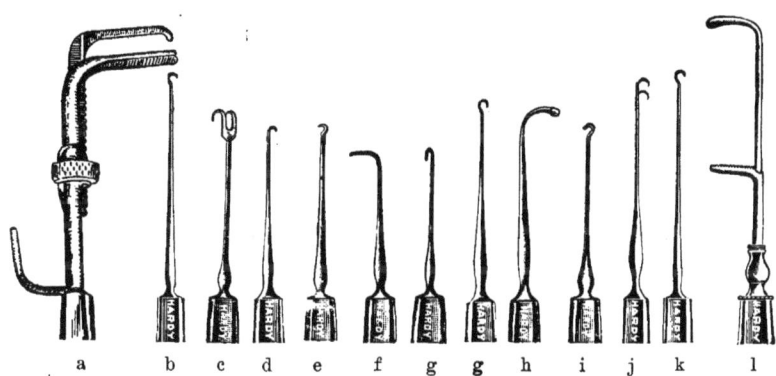

a   b   c   d   e   f   g   g   h   i   j   k   l

Hooks. a. Double Hook for Use in Advancement Operation, b. Jaeger's (sharp iris), c. Double fixation, d. Beard's (extraction), e. Blunt iris, f. Stevens' (squint), g. Tyrrell's (blunt iris), h. Graefe's (squint), i. Sharp iris, j. Weber's (double), k. Himly's (blunt iris), l. de Wecker's (double).

H. Knapp's (*Trans. Am. Oph. Soc.*, p. 107, 1873) is quite small, grooved and roughened on its concave side and made of flexible silver, so that its curve may be changed to suit the case.

Other hooks for various purposes figure in the text. Their purpose is more fully set forth under such appropriate captions as **Muscles, Ocular; After-cataract; Enucleation** and **Iridectomy.**

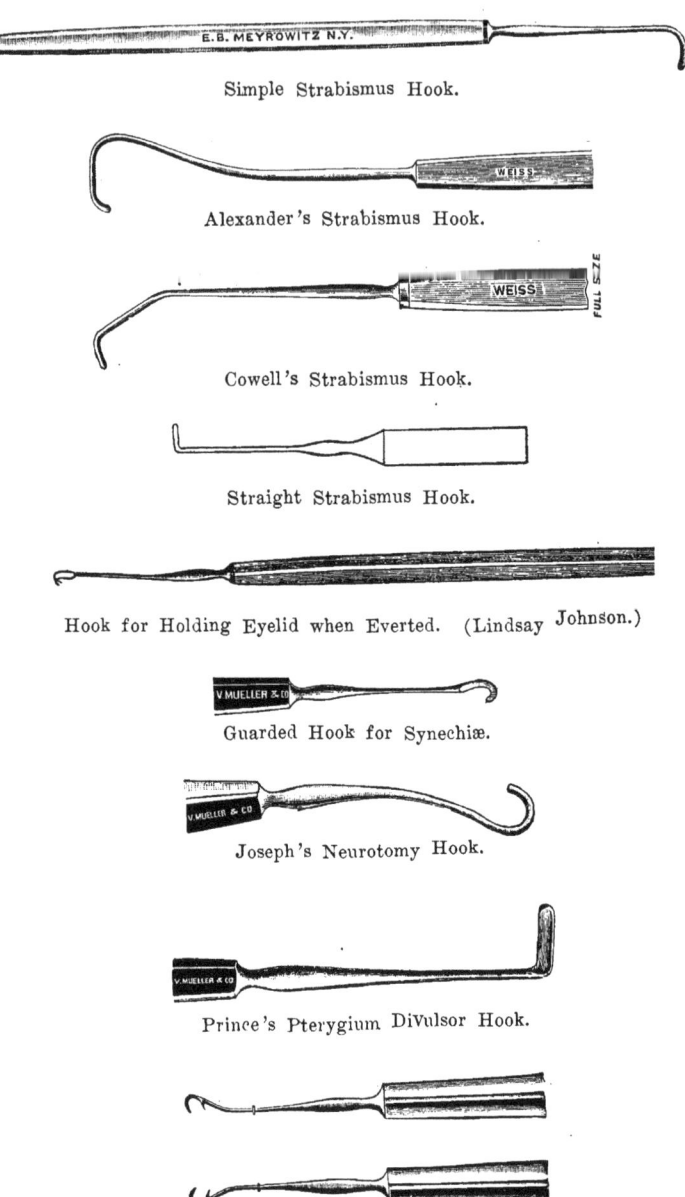

Simple Strabismus Hook.

Alexander's Strabismus Hook.

Cowell's Strabismus Hook.

Straight Strabismus Hook.

Hook for Holding Eyelid when Everted.   (Lindsay Johnson.)

Guarded Hook for Synechiæ.

Joseph's Neurotomy Hook.

Prince's Pterygium Divulsor Hook.

Weber's (Double) Right and Left Cataract Extraction Hooks.

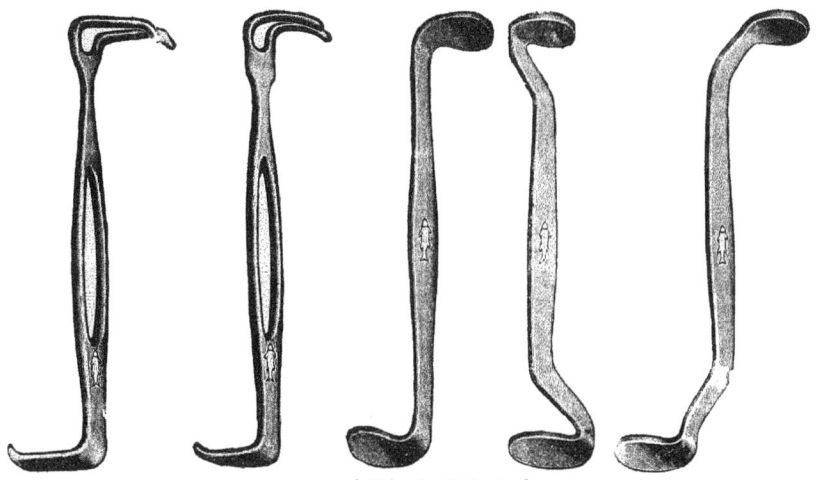

Axenfeld's Orbital Hooks.

Hookworm disease. The parasite *Ankylostoma duodenale* or *Necator Americanus* is the cause of this disease which, also known as miners' anemia, mountain or tunnel anemia, is now a terrible scourge, especially of the south states. Known to other countries for years, it was discovered to be common among the poor whites and southern negroes by Dr. Charles Wardell Stiles, chief of the Division of Zoology of the United States Public Health and Marine Hospital Service (1896). The hookworm, a parasite about one-fourth of an inch long and the thinness of a pin, thrives in moist and sandy soil and gains access to the human body through the soles of the feet, causing a "ground itch" or "foot itch," and passes into the intestines. They there attach themselves to the mucous membrane and cause hemorrhage, produce anemia, heart weakness, indigestion, emaciation, and perverted taste (shown in clay or dirt eating). The disease is commonest in Virginia, North and South Carolina, Georgia and Florida, where it attacks not only the poor but the well-to-do. Dr. Stiles concluded that the eggs of the hookworm were found in about sixty-eight per cent. of the farms of the south and that about twenty per cent. of the people of the south were affected. In Georgia alone it had ruined the constitutions of over two hundred thousand people and caused the deaths of many young children. He recommended a treatment consisting of Epsom salts following a dose of thymol and avoidance of any fat or oil. As the parasite comes out in human excrement, this must be dealt with in a sanitary manner. Lands were to be treated with blazing oils and burnt over with straw, and all the people were to wear shoes. In 1909 John **D**. Rockefeller gave one million of dollars for aiding measures of extermination and a Rockefeller Hookworm Commission met in January, 1910.—*(Standard Encyclopedia)*.

J. W. Jervey *(Jour. Am. Med. Assocn.*, p. 151, July 11, 1914) has fully studied the eye symptoms in (fifty-three cases of) hookworm disease. He concludes that hookworm disease produces eye lesions only indirectly, by way of the anemia which results from it, and that none of the eye lesions occurring with the disease are sufficiently distinctive or characteristic to be of diagnostic value. In discussion of this paper Calhoun held to his previously expressed opinion that the more serious ocular changes are directly due to a toxin rather than merely to the secondary anemia.

See, also, p. 487, Vol. I, of this *Encyclopedia.*

Hooper, Robert. A famous London physician, medical lexicographer, and natural historian, who devoted considerable attention to ophthalmology. Born at London, he studied at Pembroke College, Oxford, and in 1805 received the degree of Doctor of Medicine at St. Andrews. Settling in London, he became physician to the Marylebone Infirmary, where he was very successful as well as in his private practice. He died May 6, 1835.

Hooper is chiefly remembered for *"Hooper's Medical Dictionary"* and *"The Physician's Vade Mecum."* His only ophthalmologic writing was *"A Diagram of the Human Eye; with Observations"* (1804). —(T. H. S.)

Hopfen. (G.) Hops.

Hopkins, Woolsey. A promising ophthalmologist of New York City, who died at the age of thirty-two. Born at Alexandria, Va., in 1868, he received his professional degree from the College of P. and S. of the City of New York in 1890. He was assistant surgeon to the Manhattan Eye and Ear Hospital, and a member of the American Laryngological, Rhinological, and Otological Society. He practised ophthalmology and oto-laryngology in New York City for several years, and died in 1900.—(T. H. S.)

Horama. (L.) In medicine, that which is observed.

Horamagraph. An instrument for studying the field of vision. This term was suggested by Matthew A. Adams, of Maidstone, Kent, England.

Horasis. (L.) A seeing or observing.

Horaticus. (L.) Capable of seeing.

Hordeolum. STYE. HORDEOLUM ZEISSIANUM. This form of infection is a small furuncle that develops in the anterior margin of the free border of the lid among the eyelashes, from infection of one or more of the glands of Zeiss.

It is usually a painful affair, and may cause considerable swelling of the lid. If it does not yield to abortive treatment (hot applications and antiseptic lotions) it should be incised with a very sharp, narrow scalpel at the place where it seems to be pointing, the incision being parallel to the lid border. The subcutaneous injection of a drop of 1 per cent. cocain solution into the tissues for anesthetic purposes may be made, but this is usually as painful as the incision. The part is better anesthetized with a spray of ethyl chlorid, with proper precautions for the protection of the eyeball.

Occasionally one or more of the Meibomian glands become acutely infected, producing a condition known as *hordeolum internum*, or acute chalazion.

By everting the lid, a yellowish spot, corresponding to the infected glands, may be seen shining through the conjunctiva. If this lies near the lid border, an attempt may be made to express the contents through the orifices of the duct by pressure of the lid between the finger and the thumb nail.

If the case is of any severity, an incision into the little abscess should be made from the conjunctival side, at right angles to the lid border, and therefore in line with the Meibomian glands.—(W. H. W.)

Hordeolum, External. The ordinary form of stye; one produced by suppuration of one of Zeiss's glands.

Hordeolum hydatidosum. (Obsolete.) A supposed hydatid form of hordeolum.

Höring, Carl Friedrich von. A German ophthalmologist, son of Friedrich, and nephew of Gottlob Friedrich Höring. The dates of his birth and death cannot now be ascertained. He was born at Schwaigern, Neckarkreise, Württemberg, Germany. He studied at Tübingen, Würzburg, Prague, Vienna, and Berlin, and received his medical degree in 1845. Settling in Ludwigsburg, he began to devote his attention exclusively to ophthalmology. He founded in 1859 a Private Eye Infirmary, which was very successful. He was pensioned in 1882.

He wrote: 1. Mittheilungen aus der Augenheilkunde für den Prakt. Arzt, von Hofrath Dr. v. Höring. (Stuttgart, 1877.) 2. Bericht über die 25jähr. Wirksamkeit der Privat-Augenheilanstalt zu Ludwigsburg von Hofrath Dr. v. Höring. (Stuttgart, 1885.)— (T. H. S.)

Höring, Friedrich von. A well-known German ophthalmologist, brother of Gottlob Friedrich, and father of Carl Friedrich, Höring. The subject of this sketch was born Sept. 24, 1792, at Willsbach, near Weinsberg, Germany, the son of a surgeon who was well-known locally. He studied with an uncle for five years, then, for a very brief period, with Friedrich Jaeger. In 1812 he became assistant to Köllreuter in Stuttgart. He then for a time was a student at Tübingen University, at which institution he received his degree in 1817. He next proceeded to Vienna, where he made a specialty of ophthalmology and became assistant to Friedrich Jaeger and to Beer. He then for a time resided in Württemberg, but in 1823 removed to Neuenstadt, where he practised surgery and ophthalmology and remained for eleven years. He afterwards removed to Ludwigsburg, where he became a celebrated operator. He died Dec. 10, 1867, having practised medicine almost fifty years.

He wrote: 1. Verunglückter Versuch, eine Kropfgeschwulst durch Unterbindung der Art. Thyr. Super. zu Heilen (*Rust's Magazin*, 1820). 2. Über Myotomia Ocularis. (*Württem. Correspondenzbl.*, 1841.)—(T. H. S.)

Höring, Gottlob Friedrich. A well-known German ophthalmologist, brother of Friedrich, and uncle of Carl Friedrich, Höring. The subject of this sketch was born in 1813 at Willsbach, near Weinsberg, Germany, and in 1838 received his medical degree at the University of Tübingen. His dissertation on this occasion was entitled ''Über die Wirkungen des Broms'' [Bromine], and was crowned by the faculty. From 1830 to 1840 he studied with his uncles in Vienna. In 1841 he settled in Heilbronn, where, in 1844, he died.

He wrote: 1. Recherches sur le Siège et la Nature de la Cataracte. (*Ann. d'Ocul.* VIII, 1842-3.) 2. Über den Sitz und die Natur des Grauen Stars. (Heilbronn, 1844.) 3. Cysticercus de la Conjunctive. (*Ann. d'Ocul.* II, 1839.) 4. Über die Dislaceratio Capsulæ. (*Württemberger Corr.*, 1841.) 5. De l'Emploi de l'Appareil de Rotation Electro-Magnetique dans les Maladies de l'Oeil. (*Ann. d'Ocul.*, XVI, 1846.) 6. Iritis Syph. (*Anal. d'Ocul.*, XXX, 1854.) *—(T. H. S.)

Horizon. The line separating the visible from the invisible part of, the earth from a single point of view.

In *craniometry*, a line that extends around the skull, touching the lower border of the orbital cavities and passing through the auricular points.

In *astronomy* the circular line formed by the apparent meeting of the earth and sky is called the *sensible* horizon. The *rational* horizon is the circle formed by a plane passing through the center of the earth, parallel to the sensible horizon, and produced to meet the heav-

---

* For all material contained in this sketch I am indebted to Professor Julius Hirschberg, who, in turn, acknowledges his obligations to Sleich.

ens. The *artificial* horizon is a small trough containing quicksilver, the surface of which affords a reflection of the celestial bodies. The *dip of the horizon* is the angle through which the sea-horizon appears depressed in consequence of the elevation of the spectator.

Horizon glass. The half-silvered glass plane of a sextant.

Horizon of a globe. The horizontal ring in which a terrestrial globe is usually mounted.

Horizontal exclusion. Suppression of a double image in the horizontal direction.

Horizontal hemianopsia. See **Hemiopia.**

Hormones. One of the most important advances in physiology in the last few years has been the discovery of hormones by Starling and Bayliss of University College, London, England. The term hormone means chemical messenger. By a series of ingeniously contrived experiments observers have proved that the stimulus to secretion of the pancreas is carried to the gland by the blood stream, the active substance, or ''chemical messenger,'' as they called it, being a substance elaborated in the intestinal mucous membrane under the influence of the dilute acid of the gastric secretion. Prior to this, it was believed that pancreatic secretion occurred as the result of nervous influence, the secretion being a reflex act initiated by stimulation of the acid. Starling and Bayliss's researches disprove this view. To this chemical messenger they give the name of secretin, and its importance lies in the fact that it is only one of a large number of similar chemical messengers (hormones) which, traveling by way of the blood stream from one organ to another, bring about a stimulation of the functions of the organs concerned. On the whole, these hormones correspond to the substances hitherto spoken of as internal secretions. The few hormones which have been isolated possess all the characteristics of well-defined chemical compounds, e. g., the hormone of medulla of the suprarenal gland is the well-known substance adrenalin. Much has already been learned regarding the hormones of the thyroid, pituitary body, para-thyroid gland and ovaries. A further knowledge of the bearing of the hormones theory upon the generative organs of the female is likely to largely add to our knowledge of the interrelationship of the various ductless glands. From a practical standpoint, the further study and development of this interesting theory is sure to yield many valuable results and it is anticipated that many diseases of obscure origin may later be explainable by the hormone theory. A full account of hormones is given by Starling in the *Journal of Surgery, Gynecology and Obstetrics* (1909).— *(Standard Encyclopedia.)*

Horn, Corneal. CICATRIX HORN. This rare and curious condition is almost invariably a papilloma of the cornea which has undergone dense epithelial changes. Bowman first described it as a "warty condition" of the cornea. More recently Baas reported a corneal horn which consisted of a papilloma covered by horny epithelium. Lawson (*Trans. Oph. Soc. U. K.*, Vol. XX, 1900) has also described a

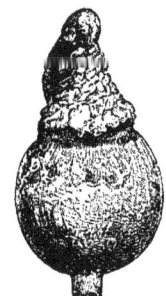

Corneal Horn.   (Parsons.)

case of "cicatrix horn" which grew directly from the cornea. It was conical in shape, five-eighths of an inch in length, and an inch and a half round the base. It grew from an anterior staphyloma, and consisted of an outer layer of fibrillated material, staining badly, and an inner layer occupying three-quarters of the section, composed of small, round, nucleated cells. It can hardly be doubted that this was no true new growth, but merely a mass of granulation tissue which was unusually exuberant. Projecting between the lids, the surface became dry, and the detritus was not cast off by movements of the lids, etc., owing to the marasmic condition of the patient.

Horn, Cutaneous. See p. 3524, Vol. V, of this *Encyclopedia.*

Horner, Johann Friedrich. Discoverer of the disease known as herpes corneæ, as well as, according to some, the introducer of antiseptics into our special field of work. He was born at Zurich, March 27, 1831, and in 1854 received his medical degree at the university in that place. For a time he was assistant to Albrecht von Graefe, and, for three or four months, he studied in Paris with Desmarres.

In 1856 he was docent in ophthalmology at his alma mater, and, in 1862, full professor.

He was a cautious and able diagnostician, a very successful operator and a copious and interesting speaker. He died of apoplexy Dec. 20, 1886.

Horner was a man of medium height, with full gray beard and

prominent eyes—in a general way, of "rugged mold." He was a great and untiring clinician. From 8 a. m. till noon he worked in the hospital, and, after a hasty lunch, took up his private practice, which occupied him until night. He was then too much exhausted for literary labor. In fact, he had an abhorrence for every sort and kind of writing. Thus, a former student of his has written to the present writer: "In connection with the fact that he had long been at work on an article on diseases of the eyes of children for Gerhardt's '*Handbuch*'—an article which he never finished—he continually referred to himself as 'ein fauler Esel.'" Neither was he much of a laboratorian; his strength lying, in fact, in the twofold capacity of diagnostician and operator. He always, in consequence, had at his heels a chain of American students (rare enough in Zurich in those days) and this addendum of admirers used to be jokingly referred to by the other professors as the "tractus opticus."

Despite his disinclination for literary labors, however, Horner did manage to perform considerable literary work. His more important writings are as follows: 1. Zur Retinalerkrankung bei Morbus Brightii. (*Klin. Monatsbl. für Augenheilkunde*, 1863.) 2. Ein Fall von Periostitis Orbitae und Perineuritis Nervi Optici. *(Ibid.)* 3. Tumor Retinæ. *(Ibid.)* 4. Fremde Körper in der Iris. *(Ibid.)* 5. Carcinom der Dura Mater: Metastase der Mm. Recti; Exophthalmus. (*Ibid.* 1864.) 6. Colobom des Augenlids mit Zahlreichen Dermoid geschwülsten. *(Ibid.)* 7. Eine Kleine Epidemie von Diphtherit. Conjunctivæ. (*Ibid.* 1869.) 8. Zur Behandlung des Keratoconus. *(Ibid.)* 9. Ueber eine form von Ptosis. *(Ibid.)* 10. Tumoren in der Umgebung des Auges. (*Ibid.* 1871.) 11. Ueber Herpes Corneæ. *(Ibid.)* 12. Refractionsänderungen. (*Ibid.* 1873.) 13. Zwei Fälle von Trigeminuslähnung mit Secund. Augenaffectionen. (*Correspondenzbl. für Schweizer Aerzte*, 1873.) 14. Desinfic. Behandl. Einiger Hornhauterkrankungen. (*Zehender's Klin. Monatsbl.*, 1874.) 15. Ueber den Anatom. Befund bei Entzündl. Kapselcataract. *(Ibid.)* 16. Keratitis Mycotica. *(Ibid.)* 17. Ueber die Entstehung und Beschaffenheit des Pterygiums. (*Correspondenzbl. für Schweizer Aerzte*, 1875.) 18. Ueber Strabismus Converg. bei Myopie. (*Ibid.* 1876.) 19. Indicationen und Contraindicat. von Atropin und Calabar. (*Ibid.* 1877.) 20. Ueber Intoxicationsamblyopien. (*Ibid.* 1878.) 21. Ueber die Verbreitungswege der Sympathischen Entzündung. (*Ibid.* 1879.) 22. Die Krankheiten des Auges im Kindesalter. (*Gerhardt's Handb. f. Kinderkrankhh.*, Tübingen, 1880.) 23. De la Myopie Congénitale. (*Revue Méd. de la Suisse Romande*, Genève, 1881.) 24. Die Antisepsis bei Augenoperationen. (*Internat.*

Med. Congress, Lond., 1881.) 25. Ueber Brillen, aus Alter und Neuer Zeit. (*Neujahrsbl. zum Besten des Waisenhauses in Zürich,* 1885.)—(T. H. S.)

Horner, William Edmonds. A celebrated American physician, discoverer (in 1822) of "Horner's muscle," *i. e.,* the *tensor tarsi,* and the first to explain in a satisfactory manner the passage of the tears from the conjunctival sac to the nose. Born of English extraction at Warrenton, Fauquier County, Va., June 3, 1793, he received the

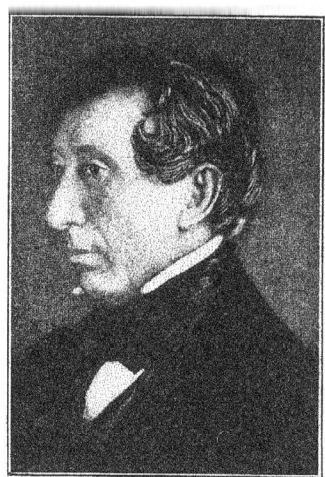

William Edmonds Horner.

degree of Doctor in Medicine at Philadelphia in 1814. For a time he was a surgeon's mate in the U. S. Army, but in 1816 settled in Philadelphia. There he became prosector, in 1819 adjunct professor, and in 1831 titular professor, of anatomy, in the University of Pennsylvania. In 1847 he founded St. Joseph's Hospital. For a time he studied in Europe. Returning to Philadelphia, he practised there until his death, Jan. 23, 1853.

Horner's only writings on the eye are those which deal with the muscle discovered by him. These, which are three in number, are here subjoined, in accordance with our plan to reproduce, so far as possible, all the briefer classics in ophthalmology.

The first of the articles appeared in *"The London Medical Repository,"* Vol. XVIII, No. 103, July 1, 1822, at p. 32, and its title and text were as follows:

A Description of a Muscle connected with the Eye, lately discovered *by* W. E. HORNER, M. D., one of the Professors of Anatomy in Philadelphia.*

"I have lately had occasion, in a dissection of the human eye, to observe a part of its muscular apparatus, which I believe not to be generally known to Anatomists, judging from the reports of my professional brethren in this country, and from a reference to the more approved authorities among the systematic writers, as Soemmering, Albinus, Caldani, who has quoted from the first, Bichat, Sabatier, &c., of the continent of Europe; and Munro and Bell, of Great Britain.

"The part alluded to is a small oblong muscle, found on the posterior part of the lachrymal ducts. It arises from the os unguis near its junction with the os planum, and passing forwards and outwards, terminates at the internal commissure of the eyelids, near the puncta lachrymalia. As it approaches the eyelids, it splits into two parts; one is inserted into the upper lid, and the other into the lower; the superior fibres of the first-named part, or the upper, being blended, in some measure, with the orbicularis muscle, but the lower having fully a distinct and well-marked insertion. The muscle is about half an inch long, and one-fourth of an inch wide, its upper and lower margins being well defined. I have also had occasion to make some new remarks on a tendinous structure enveloping the lachrymal ducts, and the position of these ducts, by which the curvature of the internal commissure of the eyelids is kept up, and which would prevent any deformity of the lids, even if the tendon of the orbicularis were cut through in the operation for fistula lachrymalis. The origin of the muscle is at least half an inch posterior to the orbicularis tendon, at its attachment to the nasal process, and it lies on the tendinous matter including the ducts. To get a view of this muscle, cut through the eyelids, and separate them from the ball, except at the internal canthus; then turn the lids over on the nose; remove the valvula semilunaris and the tunica conjunctiva in the neighborhood, with the fatty matter, and you will be sensible of the arrangement described.

---

* Mr. Shaw favoured us with this communication, which was contained in a letter from Professor Horner to him. We have placed it among the *Original Communications*, because its author wished to have it announced in a British journal, previously to its appearance in a future volume of Transactions of the Philosophical Society of Philadelphia.

Mr. Shaw has also favoured us with the following opinion respecting its originality, in which we entirely concur: "I think that the muscle described by Professor Horner is the same which has been already depicted in Rosenmuller's plates; but the description given here is so different and so much better that I have no hesitation in admitting Professor Horner's claim to the merit of having discovered it, without having derived any assistance from the labours of other Anatomists." [Footnote accompanying original article.]

Its use is to draw in the puncta, and to keep the edges of the eyelid properly adjusted to the ball, &c.

"Philadelphia, 6th April, 1822."

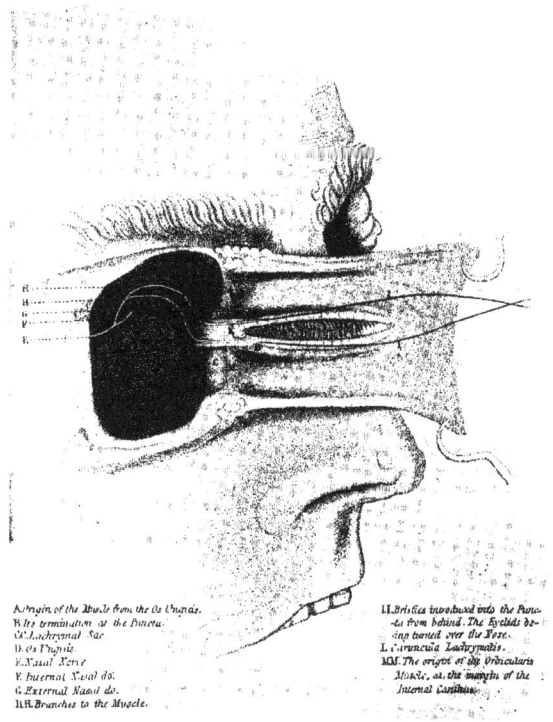

A.Origin of the Muscle from the Os Unguis.
B.Its termination at the Puncta.
C.Lachrymal Sac.
D.Os Unguis.
E.Nasal Nerve.
F. Internal Nasal do.
G.External Nasal do.
H.H.Branches to the Muscle.

I.I.Bristles introduced into the Puncta from behind. The Eyelids being turned over the Nose.
L.Caruncula Lachrymalis.
MM.The origin of the Orbicularis Muscle, at the margin of the Internal Canthus.

Horner's Muscle.

The second of Horner's articles proceeds much farther into detail. We venture to believe, moreover, that it possesses a very decided value, even now, as an anatomical and physiological treatise respecting the parts involved. It is found in *"The Philadelphia Medical Journal,"* Vol. VIII (1824), pp. 70 ff., and runs as follows:

Description of a Small Muscle at the Internal Commissure of the Eyelids. By W. E. Horner, M. D., Adjunct Professor of Anatomy in the University of Pennsylvania.

"During the winter of 1821 and 1822, while engaged in the dissections connected with the Course on Anatomy, and having at that time under my hands several sheep's eyes, intended to illustrate some points in the structure of the human eye—it occurred to me, that the known apparatus for conducting the tears from the surface of the eye to the nose, was insufficient to account for all the phenomena of this function. The desideratum was, to ascertain the causes of the constant application of the puncta lachrymalia to the surface of the eye, in the several conditions of extreme corpulency, emaciation, sleeping and watching. My mind had been previously prepared for the inquiry, by observing in an elderly acquaintance, a continual running over of the tears at the internal corner of the eye, apparently owing to the internal commissure being so loose, that the puncta were in some measure averted from the balls of the eyes. I had also observed, that in a sudden fit of fainting, which had come on the late Professor Wistar during his last illness, and while he was sitting upright, the lower lids of his eyes had fallen from their balls, so as to leave a very conspicuous interval between them. Impressed with these facts, and actuated by the impulse of the occasion, I first sought for a new apparatus in the orbits of the sheep's heads before me, and not being satisfied with what I saw in them, in a minute afterwards I laid open the orbit of a human subject, and forthwith had the pleasure of finding a small muscle, which from its position and connexions, seemed well adapted to supply the defect in the known mechanism of the lachrymal passages. This first dissection has been so frequently and invariably confirmed by my own observations, by those of my associates, among whom I name the very distinguished and indefatigable anatomist, the late Dr. Lawrance, and by the observations of very learned and skilful anatomists in Europe, that though from the beginning I had no doubt of the accuracy of my own perceptions, additional weight will accrue from such testimony.

"The muscle alluded to, lies on the posterior face of the lachrymal ducts and sac. It is oblong, being in the adult about three lines broad and six lines long. It arises from the posterior superior part of the os unguis, just in advance of the vertical suture between the os planum and the os unguis. Running forwards for three lines it bifurcates. One bifurcation is inserted along the superior lachrymal duct, and terminates at its punctum or near it. The other bifurcation is inserted along the lower lachrymal duct, and terminates at its punctum also, or near it. The base of the caruncula lachrymalis is placed in the bifurcation. The superior and inferior margins of the muscle touch the corresponding fibres of the orbicularis palpebrarum, where this latter is connected with the margin of the internal canthus of the orbit—but they may be very readily distinguished from the orbicularis, by their running straight forwards. The nasal face of this muscle adheres very closely to that portion of the lachrymal sac which it covers, and also to the lachrymal ducts. The lachrymal sac rises about a line above its superior margin, and is seen in the orbit to extend four lines beneath its inferior margin. The orbital face of the muscle is covered by a lamina of cellular membrane, and between this lamina and the ball of the eye are placed the valvula semilunaris, and a considerable quantity of adipose matter. The bifurcated extremities of the muscle as following the course of the ducts are consequently covered by the tunica conjunctiva. If the muscle be examined with the eyelids in situ, it will be seen forming a curve, the concavity of which is orbital, and the convexity nasal. The most satisfactory view of it may be got by making a dissection corresponding with the plate, and the distinction between it and the orbicularis palpebrarum, will be manifested, by the body of this muscle arising at least three lines behind any acknowledged origin of the orbicularis, and in such a way, that the attentive observer will scarcely confound the two into one. The superior fork, however, of the muscle, has a few of its fibres blended with the ciliaris.

"A compend of the foregoing description was published two years ago, which having attracted the attention of the Italian anatomists, a very interesting observation has been superadded by the learned Dr. Joseph Trasmondi, Professor of Practical Anatomy in the Hospital of Consolation at Rome. This gentleman, on seeing the account of the muscle in the *Medical Observer* of Naples for June, 1823, immediately verified its existence in a female subject of seventy years. Having further satisfied himself by repeated dissections, he proceeded to investigate the nerves of the muscle, and in a pamphlet, which I have had the honour of receiving from him, he gives the following account of his researches. 'We have found in fact by dint of patient and repeated observations, that two nerves coming from the external nasal branch, derived from the ophthalmic nerve of the trigemini or fifth pair, supply the muscle of Horner.'*

" 'It is known that the ophthalmic nerve gives off, first, the branch to the lachrymal gland—secondly, the frontal branch—thirdly, the nasal branch. It is also known that this last is subdivided, first, into the internal nasal branch, to be introduced through the anterior and internal orbitar foramen, and to be thence diffused in the cavity of the nose—secondly, into the external nasal branch, which until now

---

* This gentleman has by mistake called me Hermer in his pamphlets, published in the Italian language, and for the translation of which, I am indebted to the politeness of Dr. Jno. Bell of this city. [Horner.]

was, by many, and among others by Bichat, thought to be the only continuation of the nasal branch, prolonged into the internal parietes of the orbit. This writer, in giving a description of the above mentioned branch, says that it is a continuation of the principal branch, and is prolonged into the internal parietes of the orbit—but that having arrived near and under the trochlea, it anastomoses with a filament of the frontal branch, and thence goes out from the orbit and is divided into several branches. The external of which are distributed, first, to the superior palpebra, where they meet the filaments of the frontal branch—secondly, to the inferior palpebra, where they are united to the suborbital filaments, and some of the facial—thirdly, to the lachrymal sac. The internal filaments are then spread, first, on the dorsum of the nose, where they sometimes anastomose with the subcutaneous filaments of the internal nasal branch, which pass from the anterior to the exterior of the nose—secondly, on the pyramidalis—thirdly, on the skin. If this most learned anatomist had had the slightest idea of the muscle of Horner, he would certainly have made more diligent researches, nor would the nerves belonging to this muscle have escaped his powerful mind.

" 'It is now therefore evident from the ascertained facts, that the continuation of the external nasal branch, is not single, but that about six lines distant from the first division, there is a second one forming two ramifications. These are distributed to the cellular membrane, one under, and the other near the trochlearis muscle. From this point the upper one, after having anastomosed with a filament of the frontal branch, and after having given off all those small ramifications to the palpebræ, the dorsum of the nose, &c., turns away. Thence the inferior nerve, also taking its turn, they continue their course, during which they separate from each other, and are implanted into the muscle of Horner, to which they adhere by means of a cellular structure, and pass on to its extremities, and to the puncta lachrymalia, in such a manner that the ramification which had passed under the trochlea goes to the superior extremity, and the other to the inferior one.'

"The existence of this muscle being fully established by observations which every anatomist can readily verify, it will be extremely useful to ascertain its agency on the motion of the eyelids, and its influence in conducting, or in assisting to conduct, the tears from the ball of the eye to the nose. It appears to me clear, from its origin and insertion, that its contraction in a moderate degree will tend to apply the puncta lachrymalia to the ball of the eye, and is therefore so far efficient in regulating the lachrymal passages, by keeping the

puncta immersed in the tears that accumulate at the internal commissure of the eyelids. When the muscle contracts very forcibly,
which it can be made to do by the action of volition in certain individuals, and of which I have seen two cases, one in a student of medi-
cine.and the other in a lady, it draws the eyelids towards the nose,
and buries the puncta and the internal commissure under the fold of
skin which is formed at the same time on the internal canthus of the
orbit. I am indebted to Dr. Physick for a further suggestion in
regard to its uses. He thinks that in cases of extreme emaciation,
where the adipose matter around the ball of the eye is more or less
absorbed, causing thereby the eye to sink deeper into the orbit, and
consequently to retire somewhat from the lids, the effect of this muscle
is to draw the eyelids backwards and to keep them applied on the
ball.

"Mr. Trasmondi has added so much to my own views of the subject,
that I have great pleasure in quoting freely from his pamphlet. He
says, that 'we now understand how the lachrymal canals, being covered with moving fibres, may by a series of actions elongate—turn
their extremities towards the eye—dilate—receive the tears—and then
constrict and shorten themselves, so as to deposit them in the lachrymal
sac.' He also thinks that the compression exercised on the lachrymal
sac by the body of the muscle, may afterwards drive the tears into the
nose.

"The utility of this muscle being supplied by filaments from the
ophthalmic nerve, Mr. Trasmondi thinks is thus manifested. A sympathetic connection is thereby established between the lachrymal gland,
the pituitary membrane, and the muscle. In proof of which, if a
stimulus increase the secretion of the lachrymal gland, the action of
the new muscle is augmented, by which the puncta, the canals, and
the sac, quickly receive the separated fluid, and transmit it to the
nasal duct. Or if any stimulus affect the pituitary membrane, similar
phenomena occur in the rapid secretion and absorption of the tears.

"Mr. Trasmondi, in his reflections on this subject, has thought it
useful to inquire why the tears, having reached the lachrymal sac,
remain there for some time before they are expelled. His conclusions
are, that it depends upon the column of atmospheric air which is
introduced through the naris into the lower part of the ductus ad
nasum, and thus supports the column of tears above, according to a
principle well known to the natural philosopher. That air is admitted
into the lachrymal sac, under the common circumstances of respiration, he thinks is proved by its issuing through the fistulous opening
on the face, when one affected with fistula lachrymalis blows his nose.

The disproportion between the cubic contents of the canals and the ductus ad nasum is so much in favour of the latter, that the principle is greatly assisted by the mechanism of the parts. Wherefore the tears, passing by small drops from the canals to the sac, will be sustained there till they are accumulated in sufficient abundance: they will then, assisted by the muscle of Horner, press down the column of air and be discharged into the nose.

"In the ignorance of this muscle, anatomists have contrived many theories to account for the passing of the tears into the nose. M. Jourdan asserts that in a healthy state of the sac there is never an accumulation of tears in it, in consequence of the sac opening freely into the nose, by which the tears descend as fast into the nasal fossa as they are secreted. He considers it, therefore, perfectly unnecessary to admit of the existence of muscular fibres in the lachrymal sac, particularly as the most scrupulous dissection has not enabled him to find them. But if any fibres of the obicularis are attached to the external coat of the lachrymal sac, from their being in front they would rather have a tendency to separate the anterior from the posterior part of the sac, than to obliterate its cavity, or to squeeze out its contents. It therefore results, that no other impulsive force than the tonicity of the parts determining the course of the tears, they descend by their own weight, and by adhering to the internal coat of the lachrymal sac. M. Jourdan, in another place, reasoning on this, after positively denying again the existence of muscular fibres on the sac, says: But how does it happen that the tears flowing into the lachrymal sac (whose sides are of a very unyielding nature), continue to descend into it even when it is full, instead of running over on the cheek, and particularly as the lachrymal canals having but a small diameter, push the tears with but little force? This question is easily resolved by referring to the established laws of hydraulics. For in fact a liquid discharged into any cavity, by a pipe of a certain diameter, acts with the same force upon all the points of this cavity, whose diameters are equal to that of the pipe, in such manner that the force of impulsion is repeated or multiplied just the number of times that the surface of the cavity exceeds the diameter of the pipe. The tears, therefore, continue to flow from the canals into the sac, dilating it considerably at the same time.

"Sabatier's mode of accounting for the passing of the tears into the nose is, that when they arrive near the puncta, they are easily introduced into them—but he is not certain whether this is done by the contraction of the orbicularis muscle, or whether the canals, whose extreme smallness allows us to consider them as capillary tubes, pump up the tears by a kind of absorption.

"M. Boyer thinks that the lachrymal passages resemble a syphon, the sac being the long leg and the lachrymal ducts the short one, and that the tears are thus drawn from the surface of the eye. This theory might, perhaps, answer better if the body were always erect, for then we should have on our minds the idea of the long leg being constantly vertical, and of the preponderance of the fluid in it. But as we sometimes lie down, in which case, notwithstanding the principle of the syphon is destroyed, the tears do not overflow, it is therefore clear that M. Boyer is wrong.

"M. Bichat says that the entire passage of the tears from the globe of the eye to the nasal cavity is effected through the influence of the vital properties, and not by that of the mechanism of inert fluids in syphons, as J. L. Petit and many others after him have asserted, in comparing the lachrymal canals, the sac and the duct to a syphon, the long branch of which is represented by the latter. He believes, on the contrary, that the absorption of the tears, which continual winking favors very much, occurs chiefly at the moment when the eyelids approach each other, and by turning their margins backwards, the puncta are applied to the surface of the eye. This seems to be still more confirmed by the overflowing of the tears when we keep the eyelids open for some minutes. M. Bichat also thinks it well ascertained that the tears continue in the lachrymal sac a certain time before they flow into the nose.

"M. Portal, after asserting that no muscular fibres are to be found in the lachrymal passages, advances the same opinion with Bichat, in those words. The absorption of the tears occurring only as the effect of a certain sensibility in the lymphatic vessels and ducts destined to this use, it is not to be doubted that if they lose this sensibility, as occurs in certain paralytic affections, the passage of the tears will be diminished, interrupted and suppressed—as the absorption of the tears would be embarrassed, or would not proceed in a convenient manner if this sensibility should become too great. Wherefore it may be established as a rule, that if tonic lotions are occasionally indicated, the reverse also happens where relaxing and demulcent washes, anodynes, and preparations of opium are far better.

"The English anatomists do not seem to have studied this point so fully as the Continental—several of them (among whom is named with some surprise Mr. Pott) do not allude to it. Mr. Charles Bell, whose book is more read in this country, than the systems of any of his countrymen, introduces in a general way the opinions already advanced, but does not put much confidence in them. He has, indeed, approached much nearer to the true principle of the passing of the tears into the nose (though he has not exactly hit upon the appropriate apparatus), by asserting that the connexions of the orbicularis muscle over the sac, is of a nature to accelerate the passage of the tears, and even perfectly to compress the sac.

"Richter, the celebrated anatomist and surgeon, not succeeding in finding a muscular apparatus, still felt the importance of its existence. Not having his book to refer to, Mr. Trasmondi's pamphlet furnishes the appropriate quotations. 'The puncta lachrymalia have doubtless the power of contracting and of closing themselves, and it is very evident that the puncta, as well as the lachrymal canals, when the palpebræ are closed, contract and become shorter, which cannot take place without muscular fibres.' Again, 'without muscular powers the lachrymal sac cannot transmit the tears accumulated in it on to the nose, consequently the lachrymal sac is without doubt furnished with muscular fibres.'

"It appears to me that none of the opinions here introduced, will account for all the phenomena attending the course of the tears into the nose. It is much more probable, that the act is accomplished through the influence of the muscle which I have attempted.to describe, aided by the elasticity of the sac. The attachment of the muscle to the posterior face of the lachrymal sac is such, that it draws the posterior parietes of the sac away from the anterior parietes, and dilates the sac, thus tending to form a vacuum, particularly as the nasal face of the sac is fastened to the bony fossa and cannot move. This dilatation is aided by the cylindrical curve of the muscle, whose concavity is orbital, and which curve is brought into a straight line by the contraction of the muscle itself. Now if the diminished diameter of the lower part of the ductus ad nasum with the presence of mucus in it, present a greater impediment to the introduction of air into the lachrymal sac from below, than to the entrance of tears from above, through the lachrymal ducts—it is clear that while the vacuum is thus formed in the sac by the muscle, the puncta lachrymalia, being bathed continually in the tears collected at the internal commissure of the eyelids, will rapidly transmit the tears to fill up this vacuum. But when the muscle ceases to act, the elasticity of the lachrymal sac will drive the tears into the nose, as the mechanism of the passages is such, that it allows a fluid to pass more readily from the eye to the nose, than from the nose to the eye.

"If this explanation of the functions of the muscle be correct, it will enable us to understand why, in perfect obstructions of the ductus ad nasum, the sac fills itself to distension, and on being emptied through the puncta by pressure, it will fill itself again. It also suggests the probability of some cases of epiphora, depending only on an atony* of this muscle, and consequently to be removed by such remedies as strengthen it. It is scarcely necessary to say that these cases are indicated by an overflowing of the tears, where there is no proof by examination of the passages being obstructed. And that such cases do occur, the writings of surgeons much experienced in the treatment of fistula lachrymalis will sufficiently attest, notwithstanding the very general assertion of the systematic authors, that the foundation of this disease is always laid by a stricture in the ductus ad nasum.''

Like all discoveries of importance, that of Horner's little muscle was declared by many writers to be no discovery whatever. But Horner was more than a match for all opponents, and, as his answer to Flajani is an excellent summary not only of the arguments upholding his own priority, but also of the history of the matters involved, we here repeat it *in extenso*, from the *''Philadelphia Medical Journal,''* Vol. IX, 1824, p. 98 ff., as follows:

An Inquiry into the Discovery of the Tensor Tarsi Muscle, being an answer to the objections of Signior Gaetano Flajani, of Rome. By W. E. Horner, M. D., Adjunct Professor of Anatomy in the University of Pennsylvania.

''In the fifteenth number of the Journal was presented an account of the circumstances under which my attention was first called to this muscle. It was also demonstrated, that several of the standard anatomical works of modern times gave no account of it, and that though some of their authors, in their speculations on the manner in which the tears pass from the eye to the nose, felt the necessity of a muscular apparatus, they confess their inability to find it. The annunciation of this muscle, which was made near two years ago, in the European journals, has attracted the attention of the Italian anatomists particularly. By Signior Trasmondi it is unquestionably admitted as an original observation with myself—by Signior Flajani, the latter is as decidedly controverted. An allusion to this discussion in the July number of the very excellent Quarterly Journal of Mr. Anderson, London, and the expression of an expectation on the

---

* Mr. Trasmondi has taken a different view of the actions of this muscle, but also believes that a paralysis of it will produce epiphora—a case of which kind then under his care he cites. [Horner.]

part of the editor, that an answer would be given by myself, have induced me to make the following remarks.

"Contested points, in regard to priority of anatomical discovery, seldom obtain, or even deserve, much attention from the profession. They are founded too much upon self-love, upon the one side, and, frequently, critical and personal intolerance upon the other, to be carried on with a proper regard to the patience of the public, and to the importance of presenting private and subordinate matters in their most accessible shape. Wishing, therefore, to occupy as little time and space as possible, I shall confine myself to leading points in vindicating my own pretènsions, as to the original observation of the tensor tarsi muscle.

"It will not be denied that the standard anatomists of France, considering as such Winslow, Sabatier, Bichat, Boyer, Marjolin, Maygrier, Cloquet, Demours, make no mention of this muscle. That Mangetus and Soemmering, occupying a similar rank among the Germans, are equally silent. That Antonius and Caldini, having the same position in Italy, and who are the publishers of the most splendid collection of anatomical tables that have yet appeared, are equally silent. That in Holland, Albinus, whose name is forever associated with the muscles of the human body, was unacquainted with this. That in Great Britain, Cheselden, the Monros, the Bells, Innes, Fyfe, Shaw, Green, Hooper, the author of the *London Dissector,* are also silent. That in America, Wistar has overlooked it. From all which, it must be generally conceded, a charge of ignorance, or of inadvertence, as to the labours of their predecessors and contemporaries, against such diligent and successful anatomists, is inadmissible. Under these circumstances, I shall endeavour to refute the authority of some very indefinite accounts of the muscular structure, bordering on the lachrymal sac, which have been considered by Signior Flajani as militating against my own claims, and to show why so little attention has been bestowed on the former by these eminent authors.

"For the sake of greater perspicuity, I shall quote from my description of the muscle given in number fifteen, page 71, of this Journal. The tensor tarsi muscle 'lies on the posterior face of the lachrymal ducts and sac. It is oblong; being in the adult about three lines broad and six long. It arises from the posterior superior part of the os unguis, just in advance of the vertical suture, between the os planum and the os unguis. Running forward for three lines, it bifurcates. One bifurcation is inserted along the superior lachrymal duct, and terminates at its punctum, or near it. The other bifurcation is inserted along the lower lachrymal duct, and terminates at its

punctum also, or near it. The base of the caruncula lachrymalis is
placed in the bifurcation.'

"Signior Flajani asserts that this muscle was described by Haller,
Schobinger, Duverney, Rosenmuller, and Signior Alexander Flajani.
We find in Vol. I, page 234, of Haller's *Disputationes Chirurgiæ*, the
following paragraph: 'The same sac has about its *exterior* and *anterior* part, a small peculiar muscle arising by its own fibres around
the os planum, and extending itself over the above mentioned parts
of this sac, which muscle **D**. Duverney, a zealous anatomist and surgeon of the Royal Garden of Paris, public demonstrator of anatomy
and of operative surgery, the cousin german of the very celebrated
man just spoken of (Dom. Duverney), my most beloved preceptor,
first found, and frequently demonstrated to me in various subjects.'

"It is very evident, from this extract, that Schobinger gives the
merit of this observation to Duverney, and that Haller has been in no
wise connected with it, except in publishing the thesis of Schobinger.
It will also be seen, that in the essential points of situation on the
sac, of origin, and of insertion, the tensor tarsi muscle is a very different one from Schobinger's. The latter is on the anterior and exterior
part of the sac, and is inserted into the same—whereas, the tensor
tarsi is on the posterior surface, and is inserted along the lachrymal
ducts to the puncta.

"Rejecting then, as inadmissibly incongruous, the description of
Schobinger, let us take up that of his master Duverney. 'The little
muscle of the eyelids. This muscle takes its origin from the interior
of the orbit, and goes to spread itself out, and to be confounded with
the orbicularis, at the middle tendon of the great angle.' Again, in
a second work he says, 'Of the muscles of the eyes. The orbicularis
being detached and turned over the nose, one may, by removing the
fat, find a little muscle which takes its origin from the interior part
of the os planum, and comes to be inserted into the internal part of
the middle tendon opposite the insertion of the orbicularis. I believe
that it is not described. It may serve to direct the entrance of the
tears into the lachrymal sac.'

"The discordance between this description and mine, must also be
extremely obvious. Duverney's muscle arises from the os planum,
and is inserted into the tendon of the orbicularis—the tensor tarsi, on
the contrary, comes from the unguis, and is inserted along the lachrymal ducts. Besides the all important difference in origin and
insertion, Duverney's figure is essentially different. He has furnished
a plate of the muscle, in which it is represented as triangular, with
its base adhering to the orbicularis, near its tendon, and with an

acute angle, whereby it is inserted into the interior of the orbit, apparently, at the lower anterior corner of the os planum, without there being an indication of the slightest connection with the lachrymal sac. The muscle, in fact, looks like a mere appendage of the orbicularis, the fibres of which do not even change their direction, and are removed considerably from the course of the lachrymal ducts and puncta. For the accuracy of this statement I appeal confidently to the plate of Duverney, and only demand a comparison between it and my own. The tensor tarsi muscle, on the contrary, is oblong, its fibres parallel, its quadrilateral base is behind, fixed on the lachrymal sac, and its anterior termination bifurcated, so as to suit the situation of the lachrymal ducts, an insertion strikingly contrasted with one into the tendon of the orbicularis, which is much in advance of the ducts. Duverney's description, therefore, must also be rejected as inconsistent with my own.

''The next pretension is that of Rosenmuller, in the year 1805, and of Signior Alexander Flajani, in 1810. As the latter, according to his own admission, has repeated the description of the former, we will consider him as presenting a full state of the case, and in the following words: 'The most interesting part of this figure is the muscle of the lachrymal sac, which arises from the os unguis, and surrounds the internal side of the lachrymal sac, and terminates in that part of it, by which it is united with the tarsi.'

''The unsuitableness of this description to the tensor tarsi muscle, is very obvious. Flajani describes a muscle surrounding the internal side of the lachrymal sac (that next the nose), whereas the tensor tarsi lies on the side next the orbit, to which it belongs. This muscle, also, terminates in that part of the sac which unites with the tarsi— whereas the characteristic of mine is to embrace the lachrymal ducts, and to extend to the puncta lachrymalia. Rosenmuller is very far from providing for the latter arrangement—the only intimation of any resemblance to it is expressed in these words: 'Dice il Signior Rosenmuller di aver osservato alle volte estendersi alcune fibrille di questo muscolo fino ai canaletti lagrimale.' So that Rosenmuller's muscle, far from having the anterior bifurcation, with its fibres embracing the ducts to the puncta, has only *sometimes a few fibres reaching as far as the lachrymal canals*, which implies their stopping very short of the puncta lachrymalia.

''Signior Gaetano Flajani, in opposing my claims by those of Duverney and Rosenmuller, has abandoned their descriptions, which should have been his text, and very ingeniously adopts one derived from my communication, thereby virtually coming over to my side, but, as he seems to think, sustaining his own. He says, 'it is (the tensor tarsi) a fasciculus of parallel fibres, placed in the internal side of the orbit, of a quadrilateral figure, and bifurcated in advance, derives its origin from behind by very short tendinous fibres from the os unguis, at about the distance of one line from its aethmoidal edge—the superior margin is contiguous to that portion of the orbicularis which inserts itself into the internal orbital process of the os frontis. When it has arrived anteriorly at the point of junction of the lachrymal ducts, it adheres there closely, and then divides into two portions, which embrace the said ducts.'

"I will now leave it to the good sense of the profession whether my learned opponent, in adopting this description in place of adhering to his own text, has not changed his colours, and become the advocate of my own claims.

"Having thus pointed out the insufficiency of the preceding descriptions the next object of inquiry is, to what do Duverney and Rosenmuller allude when they speak of a muscle at the internal canthus of the eye, and whether there is any other part of the structure to which their descriptions are equally applicable, as to the tensor tarsi muscle. Haller, when speaking of the orbicularis muscle, says 'a portion of it, brought from the superior to the inferior place, is continued within its tendon, then beyond the same and beyond the lachrymal sac.'

"Duverney's plate and description suit this process, occasionally growing from the orbicularis, much better than they do the tensor tarsi.

"Haller moreover says, concerning the inferior oblique muscle of the eye, that he has seen some of its fibres manifestly inserted into the lachrymal sac, 'cujas aliquas fibras vidi sacco manifesto inseri.' Soemmering also reports, that sometimes the inferior oblique muscle arises from the lachrymal sac. Now, as the locality of all these muscles is at the internal canthus of the eye, it is, to say the least, quite as probable from the descriptions of Schobinger, Duverney, and Rosenmuller, that they have been attracted by the orbicularis, and by the inferior oblique, as by the tensor tarsi; for their description, I repeat, it is by no means an adequate one of the latter, in regard to the very essential points of origin, of insertion, of form, of attachments, of situation, and of the course of the fibres. In regard to Schobinger or Duverney, Haller gives no importance to their muscular fibres in conducting the tears. He omits his own anatomical observation, as well as theirs, saying, 'unquestionably the tears enter the puncta lachrymalia, are carried into the lachrymal sac, and moreover reach the nose by their own weight.' But if any doubt remain after this, as to Haller's real views on the subject, it must be dispelled by his saying unequivocally, 'a muscle is by some ascribed to this sac, but it is not yet sufficiently ascertained.'—*Physiology*, article 507. Edinburgh translation.

"I have now extended this discussion probably as far as the occasion requires, and feel well assured that the proof of Duverney and of Rosenmuller, having anticipated my description, is very defective. Let this be as it may, the more important point is established of there being a muscle at the internal canthus of the eye, hitherto excluded from classical works on anatomy, but henceforth likely to be regularly registered, and appreciated for its influence in conducting the tears from the eye to the nose, and for its probably determining certain cases of fistula lachrymalis.

"In regard to Signior Trasmondi being the discoverer of the nerves which supply it, he has unquestionably substantiated his pretensions in the discussions between M. Flajani and himself. The particulars are out of my province at present, but for them I refer to his pamphlet, entitled 'Risposta del Dottore Giuseppe Trasmondi Professore D'Anatomia pratica nel Ven. Ospedale della Consolazione al Signior Professore Gaetano Flajani intorno la scoperta Del Muscolo D'Hermer (Horner) e de nuovi due nervi dell' occhio umano. Roma, 1823.' "— (T. H. S.)

Horner, Muscle of. TENSOR TARSI. See p. 353, Vol. I, also p. 6009, Vol. VIII, of this *Encyclopedia*.

Horner, Syndrome of. J. F. Horner was the first (1869) to notice and report that occasionally the pressure of the enlarged thyroid gland (bringing about a paresis of the corresponding cervical sympathetic) produces on the side of the enlargement or of the greater enlargement, a slight enophthalmos with marked ptosis and pupillary contraction. It is sometimes noticed, also, that the pupillary reaction is less marked on the affected side and that the visual acuity is less. Dufour (*Révue Médicale de la Suisse Romande*, July 20, 1910) reports an example of this syndrome.

Horner teeth. A term sometimes applied to barred or scrofulous teeth.

Hornhaut. (G.) Cornea.

Hornhautblätter. (G.) An old term for cloudiness or opacity of the cornea.

Hornhautfalz. (G.) The margin of the cornea.

Hornhautgeschwür. (G.) A corneal ulcer.

Hornhautkörperchen. (G.) Corneal corpuscles.

Hornhautkrümmung. (G.) Corneal curve.

Hornhäutlein. (G.) Cornea.

Hornhautnagel. (G.) An opaque thickening of the cornea.

Hornhautnaht. (G.) Corneal suture.

Hornahautnarbe. (G.) Opacity or scar of the cornea.

Hornhautrand. (G.) The margin of the cornea.

Hornhautscheitel. (G.) Corneal vertex.

Hornhauttrübung. (G.) Opacity of the cornea.

Hornhautverdunkelung. (G.) Opacity of the cornea.

Hornhautvorfall. (G.) Staphyloma of the cornea.

Horn-trefoil. *Lotus sativus.* The juice of lote, mixed with honey, was, according to Dioscorides, of use in corneal affections.—(T. H. S.)

Horopter. The sum of all the points seen singly by the two retinæ while the fixation-point remains stationary. According to Mueller, a circle passing through the center of rotation of each eye and through the apex of the point of fixation of the visual lines. Noyes defines it as a line representing the curve along which both eyes can join in sight. See **Muscles, Ocular**; also **Physiological optics.**

Horrocks, Jeremiah (1619-1641). This scientist was an astronomer of remarkable genius, generally known as the first observer of the transit of Venus, an account of which phenomenon he has given in a Latin treatise entitled *Venus in Sole visa.* Newton, in the *Principia,* bears honorable testimony to the value of Horrocks's astronomical work, especially commending his lunar theory as the most ingenious yet brought forward. Hevelius printed the *Venus in Sole visa,* which first appeared in Germany; a translation of this work, with a memoir by Whatton, appeared at London in 1859. In 1678 Horrocks's fragmentary works were published under the auspices of the Royal Society, being edited by Wallis, with the title *Jeremiæ Horroccii Opera Posthuma.—(Standard Encyclopedia.)*

Horse-eye bean. See **Cali.**

Horse-tail. SHAVE GRASS. *Equisetum arvense.* This plant was, in ancient Greco-Roman times, tied around the neck for epiphora.—(T. H. S.)

Horst's eyewater. COLLYRIUM ASTRINGENS LUTEUM. According to the Austrian pharmacopeia this collyrium, recommended by Fuchs, especially in chronic catarrh of the conjunctiva, and frequently prescribed abroad, is made in the following manner: Take of ammonium chloride, 50 centigrammes and zinc sulphate, 125 centigrammes. Dissolve them in 200 grammes of distilled water and add a solution of 40 centigrammes of camphor in 20 grammes of dilute alcohol and 100 centigrammes of saffron. Digest for 24 hours with frequent agitation and filter. This collyrium is generally mixed with an equal quantity of water for use in conjunctival catarrh.

Hospitals, Ophthalmic. This section should be read in conjunction with such captions as **Illumination; Electromagnet; Anesthesia; Operation** rubrics; and other headings that are directly and obviously related to the equipment and administration of ophthalmic hospitals, their public wards and their private rooms.

Although ophthalmic hospitals * do not differ materially from those built for the care of general surgical cases, yet there are many details of the former that call for separate treatment.

So far as the comfort and well-being of the patients, as well as the absolute necessity for surgical cleanliness in the wards and operating rooms are concerned, these details are much the same.

One of the first essentials is the protection of the patient against fire by the construction of fireproof buildings. The wards should be built so that an abundance of fresh, clean air and sunlight are admitted to them without exposing the patients to unnecessary drafts and the glare of the sun's rays.

The question of *ventilation* is of the greatest importance and, without doubt, natural ventilation through open windows is the best. According to Ochsner and Sturm (*Organization, Construction and Management of Hospitals,* Cleveland Press, Chicago), "Transoms should be provided in the windows which, when open, will throw the entering air upward so that the entering cool air will mingle with the warm air of the upper room before descending to the floor; drafts will be reduced and inflowing air will be tempered before the breather is reached. The benefits of such a method of ventilation are important and large, provided the inflow of air is free and that harmful drafts and chilling effects are eliminated."

Ventilators may be inserted under the sash of the windows, some of which have an automatic device for the control of air by means of a swinging shutter. They may be built into the masonry work of the building, preferably in panels under the window, so that the air entering is brought directly in contact with the heating surface of the radiator and the chill taken off. The inlets for the air should be between beds. In all forms of natural ventilation it will, of course, be necessary to have some outlet for the air in the room in order to create the circulation necessary for ventilation. The doors should be provided with transoms and the corridor could thus be made a large and voluminous vent duct. Adequate means should be provided at

---

* The text and illustrations for this section have been largely drawn from the writer's article in a *System of Ophthalmic Operations.*

the opening of each corridor for carrying off the air which comes through the transoms. This can be done by means of ducts built through the wall above the windows, thereby creating a draft through the corridor.

Unfortunately, owing to the severity of the climate in many sections of the country, it becomes too cold for the air supply of the hospital to come directly from the outside through the open windows or through ventilating flues in the walls. It is then necessary to force air into the wards and rooms by means of revolving fans and other mechanical means.

Ochsner (*Jour. A. M. A.*, Nov. 2, 1902) advises that, in this contingency, "It should first be washed by passing through strands of oakum or other similar material suspended in the horizontal portion of the air shaft, a small amount of water being permitted to trickle over these strands constantly, then it should pass through a long shaft, extending preferably through the entire length of the building. This shaft should contain coils heated with steam or water. The outside of the shaft should be covered with some material which prevents the radiation of heat in order to economize fuel. Taking the air from a tower some distance above the roof of a high building, it is nearly free from micro-organisms; this can be freed from particles of dust and dirt and introduced into the hospital clean and heated to the desired temperature. The foul air can be carried out of the rooms and wards through flues opening near the floor."

The floors should be constructed of hardwood and covered by some material which can be easily cleaned and is impermeable to moisture; or, still better, made of tile or concrete.

The monolithic type of floor, when properly laid, has proven very satisfactory. All floors and angles of the walls should have cone bases as a matter of cleanliness.

The walls should be covered with enamel paint which can be thoroughly washed and scrubbed when necessary.

All articles of furniture, decoration, etc., should be of simple construction and made of non-porous material that can be easily and thoroughly cleaned. Wooden furniture is undesirable on account of its porosity, but if used it should be heavily coated with absolutely smooth enameled paint so that dirt that adheres to it can be readily washed off. Chairs, tables and beds should be made preferably of metal, either polished or covered with white enamel paint. The tops of tables should be of metal, glass or glazed earthenware. No cumbersome furniture should be given space in a ward. All draperies, pictures and other articles of adornment should be excluded, since they collect dust and are difficult to keep clean.

The furniture of each room should consist of a bed, chair and bedside stand. The bed should be single, made of iron about 26 inches

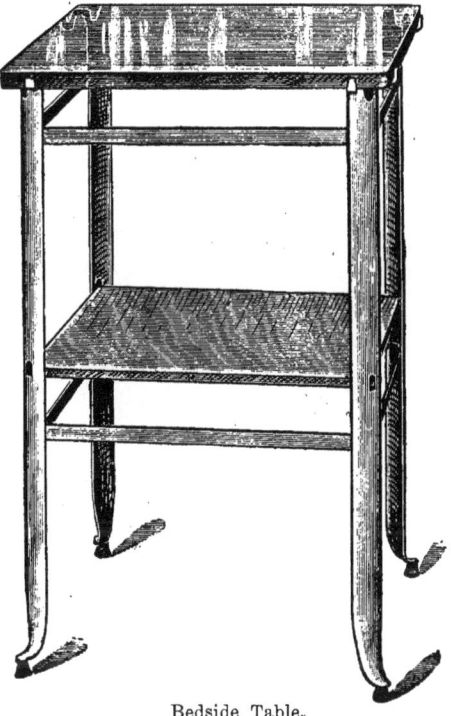

Bedside Table.

high, painted with white enamel. It should be on castors and easily movable and made with a low, movable head-piece so that operations, dressings and examinations may be readily made.

The springs should be woven wire and the mattress should be filled with horsehair. Each bed should be surrounded with sufficient space for proper ventilation, to give room for a chair and table and to allow ready access for the passage, on all sides, of the surgeon, nurse or other attendants.

The Manhattan Eye Hospital, of New York, uses an ordinary 3 by 6½-foot iron bed with woven wire springs. The two end pieces are of the same height and project enough above the mattress to keep the pillows from sliding off. In private rooms the beds have high head-pieces which can be lifted off when desired.

Chairs should be made of iron and enameled white. The legs should have rubber tips so they will not slip and can be moved with as little noise as possible.

A table or stand placed at the head of the bed should be made of

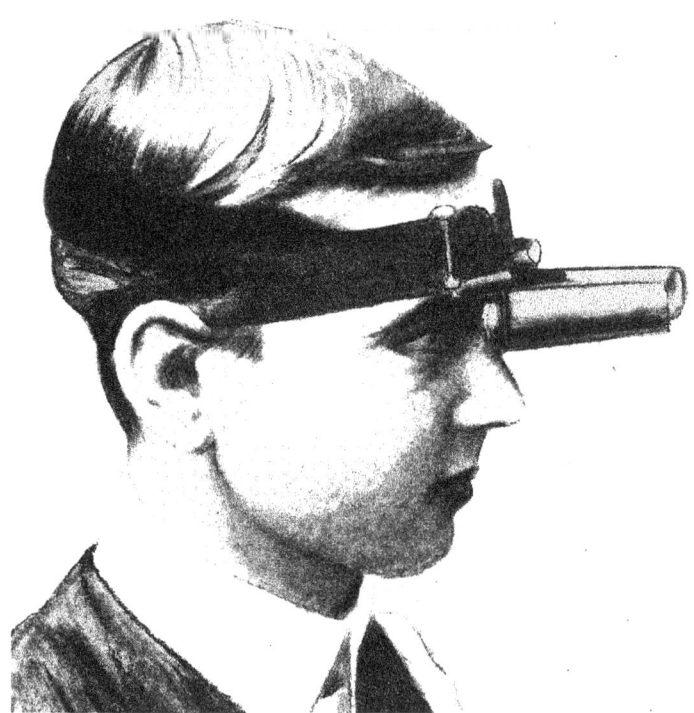

Portable Corneal Microscope for Hospital Practice.

steel, white enameled and mounted on rubber tips. The top is best made of polished glass with a rail around three sides to prevent articles from sliding off. It may be provided with shelves of the same material and a drawer.

Each ward should be provided with a stationary cabinet constructed preferably of steel and enameled, with glass doors and sides, in which may be kept drugs of various sorts, such as atropin, eserin, etc., and various kinds of sterilized dressings, eye-shades, instruments, appli-

cators and various appliances used for purposes of the ordinary examinations and dressings necessary in eye surgery.

The *wards or rooms in ophthalmic hospitals* should not be too exten-

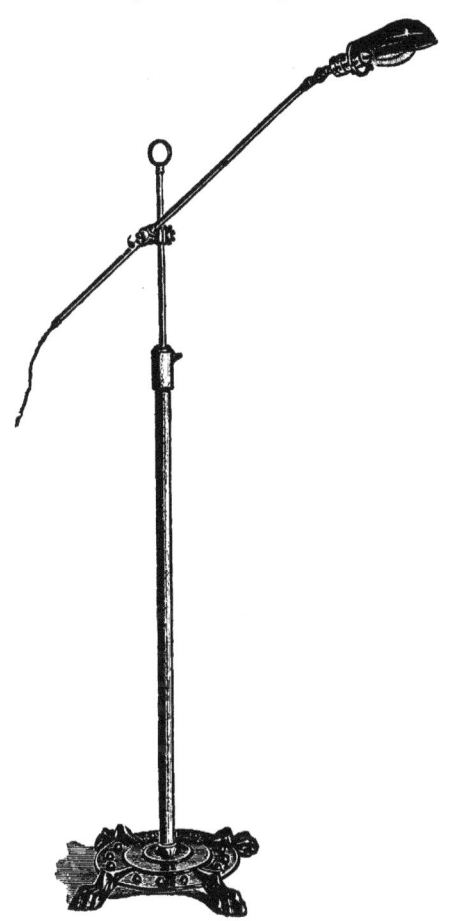

Adjustable Reflector on Stand for Operations and Examinations.

sive. In the Manhattan Eye, Ear and Throat Hospital they contain
from ten to twelve beds; the walls of the rooms are painted dark.
There is a large sitting room which can be made quite dark and so
arranged that patients can walk about in it for exercise.

The room containing one bed is for those who are so financially
situated that they are able to pay for their privacy, but does not

differ materially in furnishings from the larger ward which contains more beds.   Where possible, no ward should contain more than ten beds.

Ward furnishings.   The main point to be considered and insisted upon is simplicity in design and furnishing.   The contents of an ophthalmic ward or room should consist only of articles that are absolutely needed for the comfort and well-being of the patient and those appliances that are most needed in the proper care of the case.

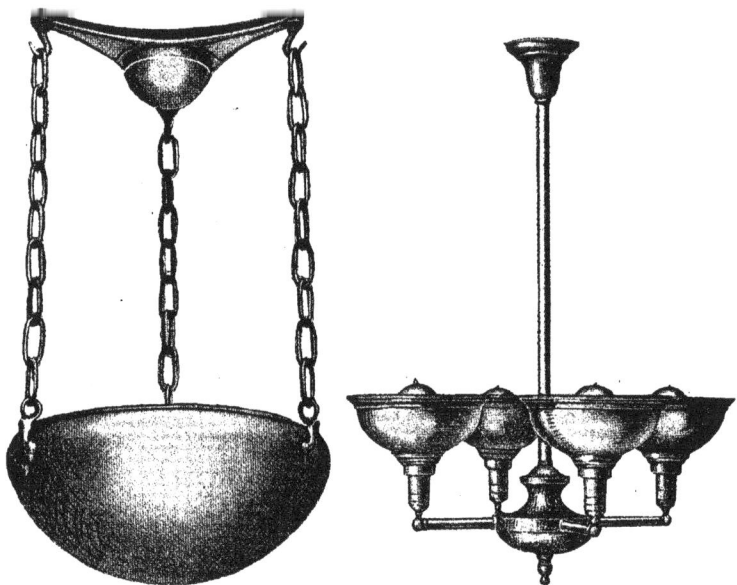

Convenient Electric Fixture for In-   Multiple Electric Lamp Fixture for
direct Lighting of Rooms.   Indirect (Ceiling) Illumination.

Ward and room lighting.   To a ward devoted to the care of general surgical and medical cases it is desirable to admit much outside light; the ophthalmic ward, from the nature of the cases under treatment, should not be brilliantly illuminated.

The light should be sufficiently subdued, although it is not necessary that the room be darkened; in fact, a darkened room under ordinary circumstances is apt to be depressing to the patients.   The windows should be shaded by blinds of a dark hue, and they should be adjustable and capable of being lowered to any desired height.

The wards should be lighted sufficiently to enable the nurses and attendants to go about their duties without undue effort.   There should be no streaks or flickerings of light and the surroundings should be so arranged that all reflection is avoided. The walls and ceilings should be painted a light cream or straw color, or a very light buff.

Artificial illumination should be by means of the incandescent electric light so shaded that the rays of light are reflected only from the ceiling.

Lamps for ward dressing. Where increased illumination is required for purposes of examination of the eye, the application of dressings,

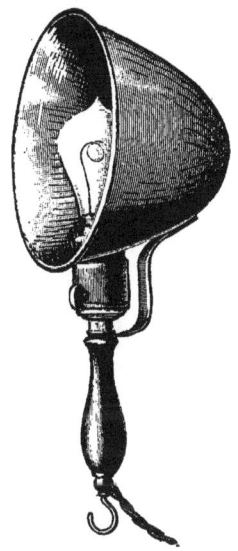

Electric Hand Lamp with Shade for use in Wards or Private Rooms for Operations, Examinations and Dressings.

etc., one of the many forms of electric lamps in the market will be found useful. Plugs should be placed in the wall at the head of each bed, to which an attachment can be made for an incandescent electric light. This may be a hand lamp attached to a cord running from this plug mounted on a flexible arm, easily movable, with a frosted bulb and so shaded that the light is not only not reflected into the examiner's eyes, but shines directly on the eye under examination.

In addition there should be a *portable dressing tray or ward carriage* which can be carried or wheeled from bed to bed by the nurse, on which are placed those solutions, ointments, instruments, dressings, etc., that are required at each visit of the surgeon in administering to the wants of each particular patient in the ward.

An irrigator stand on wheels which can be moved to any portion of the ward will also be found useful in dressing ophthalmic cases.

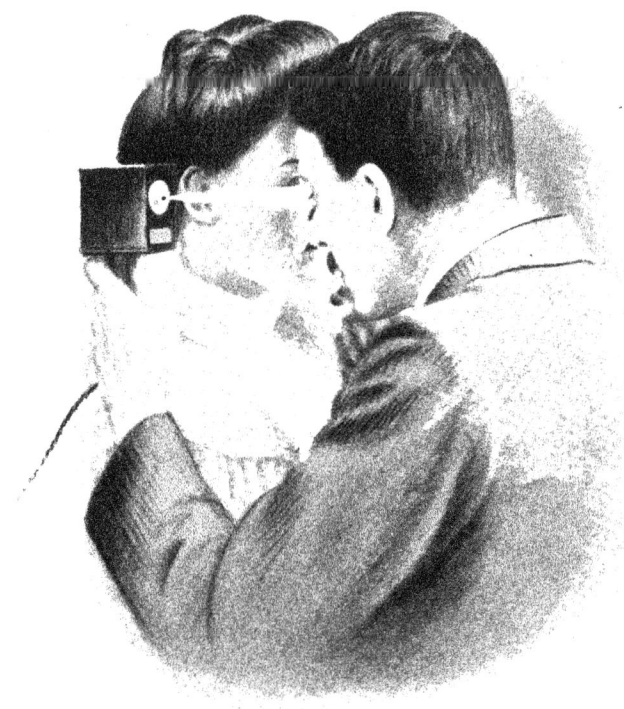

Ophthalmoscopic Lamp for Ward Practice.   (Gradon.)

The bottles containing the solutions should be adjustable in height and supplied with irrigator tube, stop cock and tip.   It may be used, also, as a dressing stand, to avoid a multiplication of ward furniture.

Wards for major ophthalmic operations.   Operative cases, especially those upon whom cataract extraction has been performed, should be kept, when possible, in a ward by themselves, hence it is desirable to have small wards so that cases can be more easily classified.   All contagious cases, such as purulent ophthalmia and trachoma, should, under all circumstances, have separate accommodations. The ultimate success of an operation may depend upon the separation of this class of cases. A separate ward should be provided for children, not only for hygienic reasons, but for purposes of quiet. Children are apt to be noisy. In addition, the children's ward may be so situated that it gets more sunlight. Separate sitting rooms should be provided for those patients who are recovering from operations and are able to be up and about. The surroundings should be cheerful and, when possible, corridors for exercise and sun parlors should be provided.

Careful attention should be paid to the regulation of the temperature of the wards. Whatever system of heating is used, it should be regulated by such appliances as will automatically control the temperature and so guard against excessive heat and dryness of the atmosphere. The air should be kept moist and fresh, without drafts and without sudden changes in its temperature.

OPERATING ROOMS AND THEIR FURNISHINGS.

The ideal operating room should be at the top of the building and contain at least a single, large window with a northern exposure. Although these advantages are highly to be desired in a general sur-

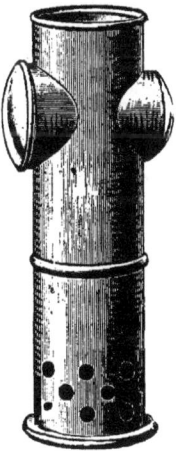

Priestley Smith's Lamp for Ward Use.

gical operating room where plenty of good daylight is required for operations, it is of secondary importance where ophthalmic operations are to be performed. In this class of operations a darkened room illuminated by artificial light is sometimes preferable to the natural illumination. In any case, no matter from what point of the compass the room receives its light, or how good the natural illumination is, means should be provided so that the field of operation may easily be illuminated by artificial means. Electricity is, on the whole, the best illuminant, the current being controlled from a switch on a side wall. The light rays may be concentrated by means of a reflector containing a number of electric lights placed above the table and attached to an adjustable arm swung to any angle.

The Nernst or similar lamps operating in a tube provided with lenses and affixed to an adjustable standard form very useful illuminants.

Fresh air should be provided without necessitating the opening of doors and windows, thereby creating unnecessary drafts or lowering the temperature of the room. The system of ventilation should be so arranged that the overheated, stale air is quickly given exit from the room by means of a flue in the ceiling operated by a fan. The floors, walls and ceiling should be constructed of such material as will stand the wear and tear of use without chipping, cracking or showing roughness of surface. They should be capable of being scrubbed with soap and water and made thoroughly aseptic without injury. There should be no projecting surfaces and all corners and angles should be rounded to admit of absolute cleanliness. Probably the best, although most expensive, covering for floors, walls and ceiling is glass. It is impervious to water, oil and acids. It comes in large pieces, allowing of very few joints. It is white in appearance and very easily kept clean. Terrazzo flake mosaic and tiling laid in cement have proven very satisfactory as to wear and cleanliness for flooring, and are much less expensive than glass. A wainscot of marble, glass or cement may be carried to any desired height and the walls and ceiling covered with a thick coat of enamel paint.

It should be possible to darken the room when necessary by outside shades which may be raised and lowered as desired.

There should be at least two operating rooms, one which is used exclusively for clean eye operations and the other in which only septic cases are operated upon.

Operating rooms should be so constructed that the highest possible degree of surgical cleanliness can be obtained. The doors and doorframes should be metal clad, without panels and perfectly plain. The window frames and sash should be all metal, or metal clad.

All windows and skylights should be of ground glass, especially if they are exposed to the sun's rays.

The fixtures and furniture of the room should be perfectly plain and made of metal, glass, marble and porcelain, so as to admit of thorough sterilization. There should be no built-in cases and all cases should have sloping tops so as to prevent the accumulation of dust and dirt.

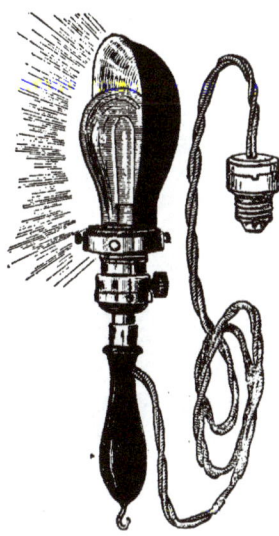

Hood Lamp for Use in the Operating Room.

The operating room should contain nothing in the way of furniture, except that which is actually needed for the work to be performed. Special rooms should be provided for the sterilizing apparatus, for anesthesia and for instruments, and a preparation room for the surgeon and assistants. These should all open into the operating room where possible, or be in close proximity.

Private ophthalmic hospitals. C. R. Holmes, whose private ophthalmic hospital is of recent date, has the floor in his operating room built of white three-inch hexagonal tiles with six-inch baseboard of the same material, with no angles. Under the operating table electric wires for light and cautery come through the floor and are protected from water by white marble. He recommends that the walls be covered to the ceiling with white tile or marble, although to a height of six feet is sufficient, in which case the wall above should be painted with smooth white enamel paint. No guards or shelves should be above the tiling.

On account of the variability of the daylight he does practically all of his operations with the aid of electric light and darkens the room by outside shades.

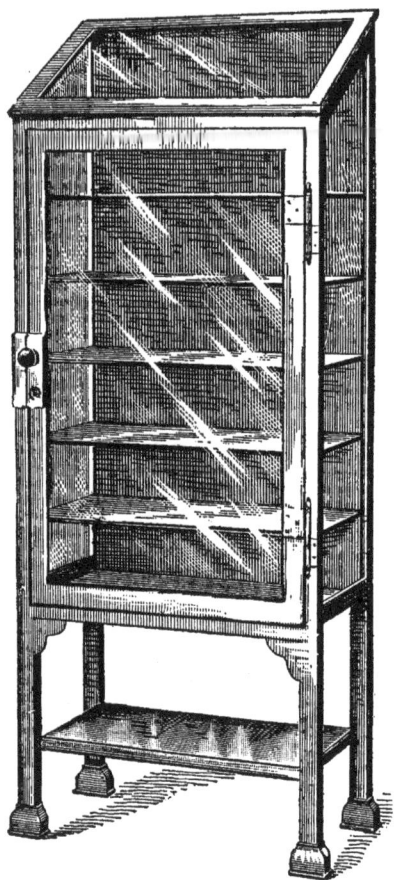

Instrument Cabinet for Ophthalmic Operating Room.   It has a Slanting Glass Top.

He always operates for cataract and does iridectomies with the patient in bed and in his own room or ward.   The bed should be substantial and made of such height as suits the operator, the head and foot-piece of equal height.   That the patient may lie firmly in bed he uses a board, 24 inches wide and the width of the bed, slipped under the wire springs and held in position by two iron fingers and two sliding bolts catching on the frame of the bed. This board is placed under the patient's hips and after operation is quietly dropped down by slipping the two bolts back. This device prevents all spring motion of the mattress.

Arnold Knapp does not advise an amphitheater in the operating room, as not more than six visitors are able to see what is going on. Railings answer every purpose to keep back the spectators. He performs all operations on a specially designed operating chair which is moved into the room in which the patient is operated upon. He claims that the chair has this advantage, that often during an opera-

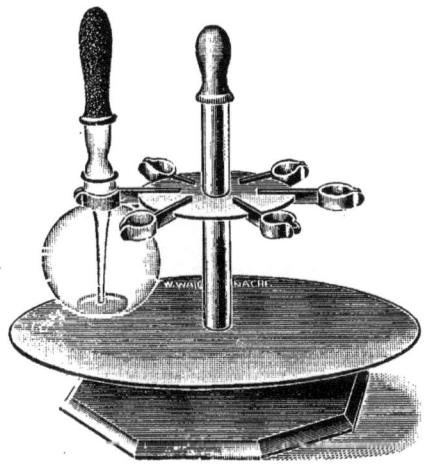

Revolving Treatment Stand for Ophthalmic Ward Uses.

tion the light has to be changed and then the chair can be more easily moved, and as it can be taken to the patient's room without difficulty there is a minimum disturbance of the patient.

Frank Todd has two operating rooms in his hospital, one for clean and one for septic cases. The operating room is tiled and besides the side light he has a large, slanting, opaque glass skylight which extends level with the operating table. He prefers a south exposure as it gives sufficient light in the darkest days, although it has the disadvantage of being too warm in summer. This is not a serious objection as eye operations are of short duration. To shut off too much light he uses a curtain on the outside which can be rolled over the glass.

All cataract cases are operated upon in the operating room in a specially constructed bed which has a low foot-board and large, rubber-tired wheels so arranged that the bed may be raised or lowered. There is no specially constructed amphitheater in the operating room, but there is a place under the skylight which is raised about a foot from the floor, where from six to a dozen may witness an operation.

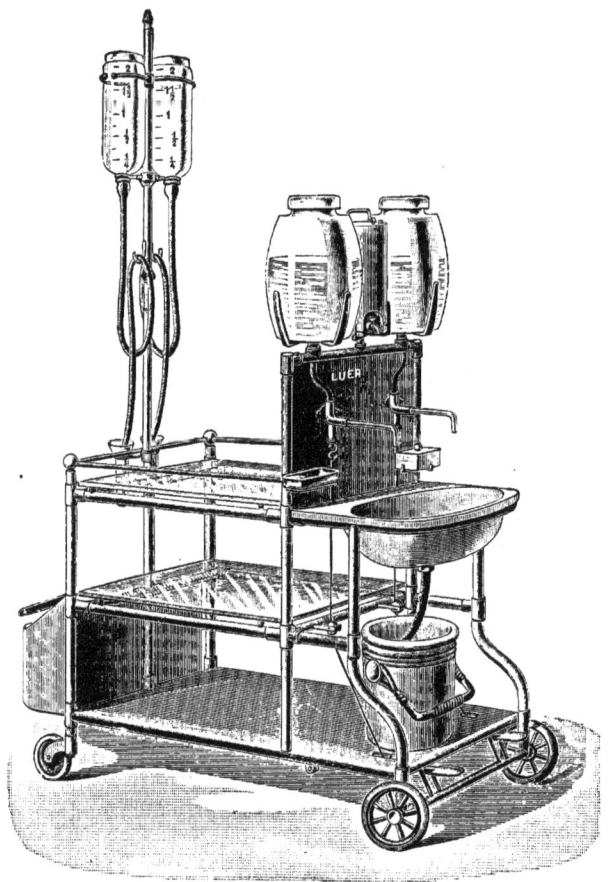

Washstand Wagon for Ophthalmic Rooms and Ward Use.

Contact of the spectators with the table is prevented by a nickel-plated railing.

Derrick T. Vail uses a specially constructed operating table which he prefers to a bed. He always performs an operation, where the eyeball is to be opened, in the patient's bedroom, and for light uses a Sachs' illuminator. He thinks amphitheaters have no place in an operating room and very few, if any, outsiders should be allowed to witness an operation.

Hospital stretchers for ophthalmic patients. In all cases where it is desirable or necessary to have the patient carried to his bed and deposited there with the minimum amount of disturbance, one may employ a detachable stretcher, an example of which is immediately described. Such a convenience has been found to answer admirably the purpose for which it was designed.

Gordon Byers describes one made up of seven different pieces, two pieces of heavy white canvas, five and a half feet long by one foot wide; two side bars of oak, seven feet long, one and three-quarters by one and a half inches in size, provided with handles; two end iron rods, two feet long, with rings at the end of each and a thumb screw

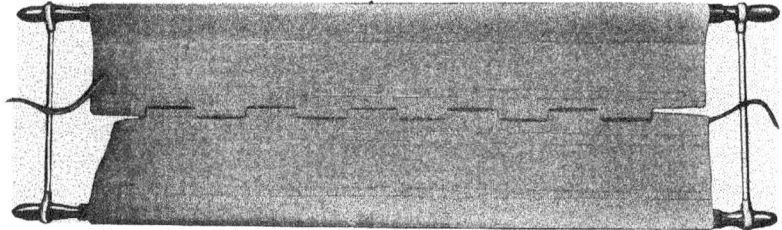

Detachable Stretcher for Conveying Patients to the Wards or to their Rooms from the Operating Theatre.

passing down through the iron rings; one strap eight feet long by three-quarters of an inch wide. The canvas is stitched over upon itself on the outer edges so as to make a loop through which the wooden side bars pass. The inner edges of the canvas are dovetailed so as to fit the one side into the other; and they are also stitched over upon themselves so as to form loops through which the long strap passes and binds the two pieces of canvas together as one piece. The iron rods with the rings at each end are the same length as the complete width of the stretcher, and keep it taut when placed in position by passing the rings over the ends of the side bars, where they are held in place by the thumb screws.

The stretcher is placed upon the table before the patient mounts upon it; and, following the operation, when the carrier containing the patient has been placed upon the bed, it is removed from beneath by disengaging the transverse bars, pulling out the lateral carriers, and extricating the central strap which unites the two halves.

OPHTHALMIC WARDS IN GENERAL HOSPITALS.

The great majority of ophthalmologists have not the opportunities that are offered by a hospital devoted entirely to their line of work and are consequently compelled to send their cases and do their operative, and especially their private operative, work in a general hospital.

In the general hospital the surroundings as well as equipment are not adapted for the care of ophthalmic patients unless some special provision has been made for their needs. In many general hospitals the eye department plays but an inconspicuous part. It is always advisable, when possible and when there are sufficient patients to warrant it, to have this class of cases in a section of the hospital by themselves. The wards need not be large; in fact it is preferable that each ward should contain very few beds. The operative cases should be kept entirely separate from the other patients, especially those of a contagious nature. The operating room should be used solely for eye surgery. It need not be large nor require the same amount of natural illumination as is desirable in a general operating room, but it should be equipped with the various features for obtaining the best of artificial illumination—a more important requisite than daylight. The same may be said of the light equipment in the wards where subdued light is to be desired, portable lamps of one kind or another being depended upon for illumination during examination and the application of dressings.

Some ophthalmic surgeons prefer to operate in the ward or private room, claiming that there is less danger of accidents while moving the patient from the operating room to the ward. Others go further and insist in performing the operation, especially where the eyeball is opened, without moving the patient from the bed. In such cases specially constructed operating tables are used which are easily movable from room to room and take up as little space as possible. For the same purpose beds are constructed that may be raised or lowered to suit the requirements of the operator. These have removable head and foot pieces, so that there is no obstruction about the field of operation.

One of the most important requisites of an eye service in a general hospital are house *surgeons or internes trained in ophthalmic work.* One or two of the House Staff should be assigned to duty in the eye department and should be held primarily responsible for the work of the department.

The ophthalmic nurse. The wards should be in charge of a permanent head nurse, with one or two assistant nurses. When it is not possible to have a permanent nurse one should be carefully selected from the other nurses and her period of service should not be less than three months, more if possible. She should devote her whole time to the service.

The duty of the ophthalmic nurse is to perform, personally, all the nursing necessary in her department. The nurse having charge of the contagious cases should, under no circumstances, come in contact with the operative cases for obvious reasons. She should always be on hand to make the rounds with the attending surgeon and the interne surgeon, and should carry with her a tray upon which is placed everything necessary for the daily dressing of the patients. She should not run here and there to get this bandage or that solution, but should remember that time is valuable and that everything must be close at hand. She should be able to vouch for the cleanliness, sterility and freshness of everything upon her tray and should give this matter her personal and earnest attention, remembering that while in general surgery a little suppuration in a wound need not necessarily prove disastrous, in ophthalmic surgery, particularly in cataract operations and iridectomies, perfect healing must be secured and the slightest infection will almost certainly bring ruin in its train. She should learn the knack of putting solutions and ointments into the conjunctival sac, of irrigating or cleansing the eye without injuring it, and of properly adjusting a bandage. She should understand how to use hot and cold applications; these and many other things too numerous to mention and so trifling as to appear insignificant and yet of great importance if the best results are to be obtained.

In the intervals between the visits of the attending surgeon the ophthalmic nurse should faithfully follow out his instructions, such as putting medicines in the eye, changing bandages, cleansing eyes, etc. She should so attend to her duties that she will inspire the attending surgeon with confidence that her duties are well and faithfully performed.

The ophthalmic nurse should also attend the surgeon when he performs operations. She should prepare the patient for operation and should have all dressings ready for application after the operation. Her duties are only second in importance to those of the surgeon.

A week or ten days before the nurse goes off duty the oncoming nurse should be assigned to the department, to make the rounds with both the attending surgeon and the retiring ophthalmic nurse, for by so doing she becomes familiar with the work and the establishment of new relations is accomplished with the least friction to all parties concerned.

One great advantage in the teaching of ophthalmic nurses in this way is the education of women in this line of work, so that after graduating surgeons can secure their services in private cases treated at home.

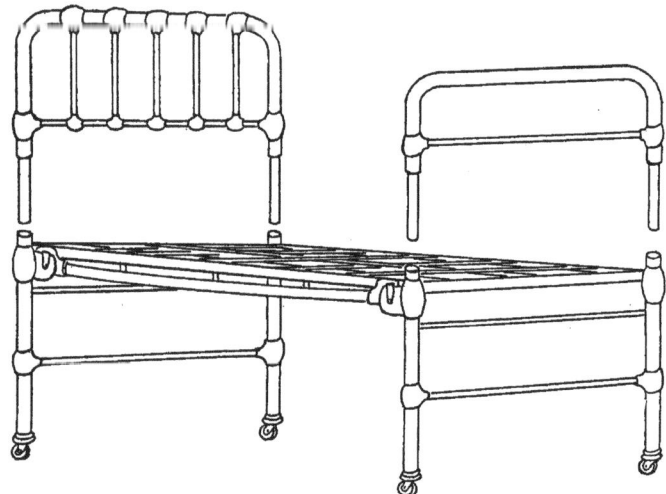

Aseptic Hospital Bed.

Operations in an amphitheater present advantages which to some extent offset the risks attendant upon removal of the patient after · operation from the operating room to his bed. A well-kept operating room needs, for example, very little extra preparation; it is aseptic; everything is handy and convenient for instruments, dressings and all appliances necessary for operative work. Moreover, when trained assistants do the work there is a minimum of danger from accidents during the removal of the patient from the operating room to the ward.

Sterilizers and sterilizing. A complete sterilizing outfit for an ophthalmic operating room should consist of: (1) An instrument sterilizer; (2) A dressing sterilizer; (3) A water sterilizer; (4) A sterilizer for pans, basins, irrigators, etc.

Instrument sterilizers. The boiling of such instruments as knives in water is recognized as the most satisfactory as well as the safest

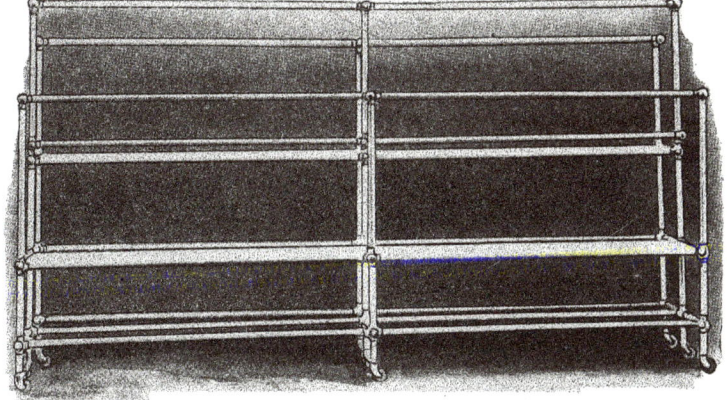

Observation Stand for Witnessing Ophthalmic Operations. Accommodation for
Eight Spectators.

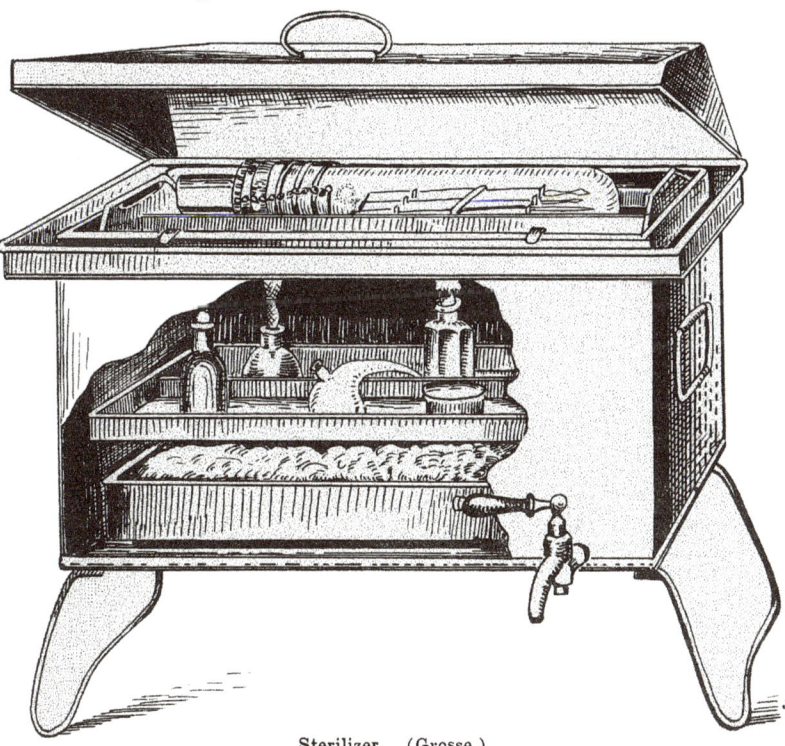

Sterilizer. (Grosse.)

and simplest method of sterilization.   Sodium carbonate or borax
(2 per cent.) added to the water will protect the instruments against
oxidization.   The instruments are placed in a perforated tray with
removable handle and set in the receptacle containing the water, which

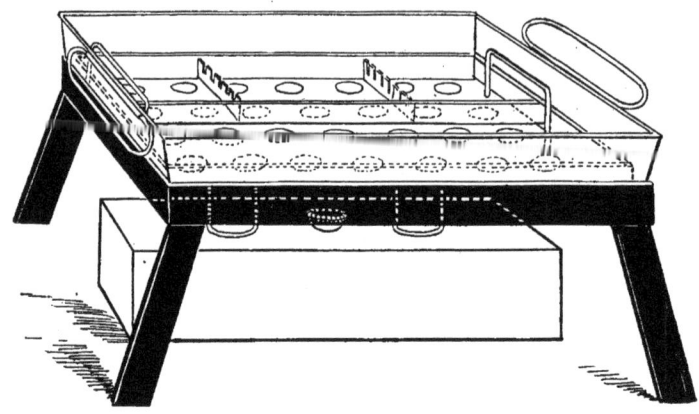

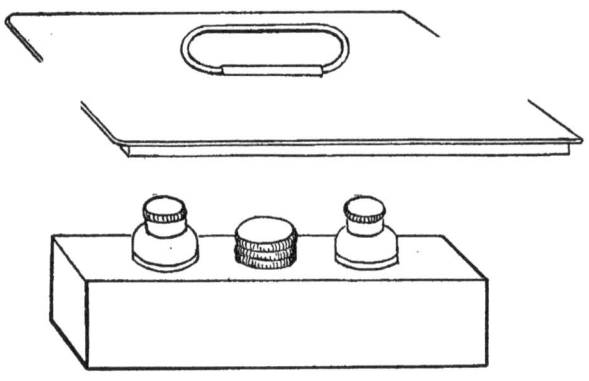

Portable Sterilizer for Eye Instruments.   (Veasey.)

is then brought to a boil, and the procedure continued for at least
twenty minutes.

Sterilizers for instruments are common to all hospitals.   They are
usually made of highly polished or nickel-plated brass or copper.
They can be equipped with steam heating coils connected with the

steam supply of the building, or they may be furnished with either electric, gas, petroleum or alcohol heating attachments. A detailed description of the large sterilizers employed in special and general hospitals is hardly in place here.

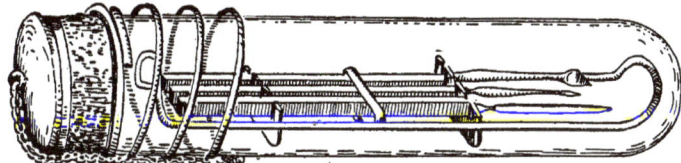

Ophthalmic Knife Sterilizer. (Grosse.)

Clarence A. Veasey (*Ophthalmic Record,* Vol. IX, page 80, 1900) describes a portable sterilizer for eye instruments. It is very compact and at the same time sufficiently large for all the instruments employed in the ordinary ophthalmic operations.

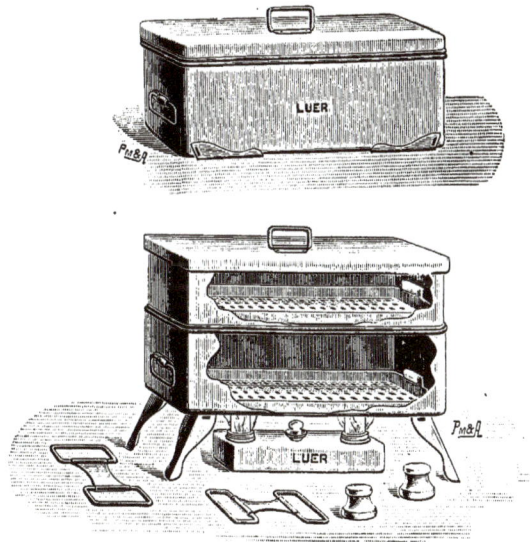

Luer's New Sterilizer for Ward Use.

The sterilizing pan is five inches wide, seven inches long and one and three-fourths inches deep, with a handle at each end and a closely-fitting cover to prevent the escape of steam. Inside of this is a perforated tray with handles for lifting, containing on one side a movable rack for the more delicate instruments. This tray rests upon small buttons in the bottom of the pan, allowing a free circulation of the water when boiling and preventing that injury which usually occurs to instruments when placed directly upon the bottom of a heated dish. The whole rests upon a skeleton stand, which, when not in use, is folded and fits tightly around the side of the pan. One of the best features of the sterilizer is the alcohol lamp. It is six inches long, one and one-fourth inches wide and one and one-eighth inches deep; has two large burners which bring water to the boiling point in five minutes and holds sufficient alcohol to keep it boiling for nearly two hours.

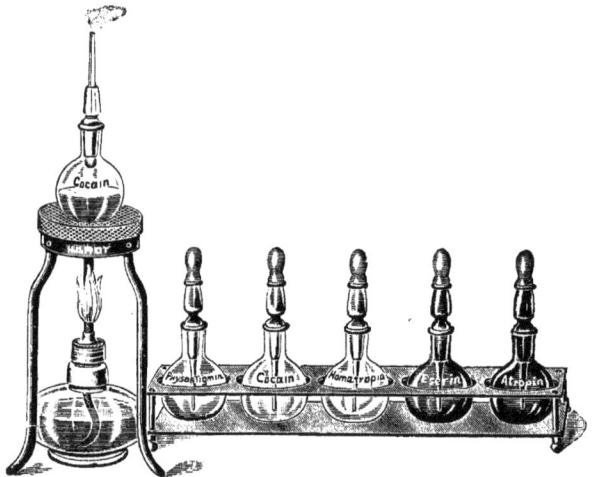

Stroheim Apparatus for Sterilizing Ophthalmic Solutions.

All cutting instruments should be boiled the minimum length of time in order to guard against injury to their edges. In order to avoid this knives may be sterilized by subjecting them to chemical sterilization. This may be accomplished by placing the knives in a tray containing 90 per cent. solution of carbolic acid with glycerine. They are allowed to remain for fifteen or twenty minutes, and after removal immersed in very hot water or 80 per cent. alcohol for the purpose of washing off the carbolic acid; then thoroughly dried with a sterilized towel. Exposing the knives to the fumes of formaldehyde is an effective method of sterilization. Formaldehyde gas is a powerful germicide, is readily diffused, has great powers of penetration, and quickly destroys all forms of micro-organisms.

H. O. Reik (*Phila. Med. Jour.*, Feb. 4th, 1899) describes a formalin sterilizer made of copper. It measures 7x12x12 inches, and has an air space of a little more than 1,000 cubic inches. The shelves are of heavy wide-meshed wire gauze, the upper one extending entirely across the chamber, while the lower two are only eight inches long, extending from the right side to an upright standard four inches from the left wall, thus leaving a space four inches wide by eight inches high, which is reserved for vaporizing the pastils. There is a small tray for carrying such instruments as cataract knives so as to prevent their cutting edges from coming into contact with anything. The sterilizer, when closed, must be air-tight, for if an interchange of gas and air is permitted the gas is diluted and fails to produce the expected results.

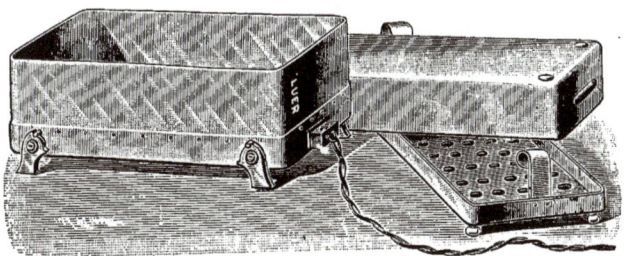

Wiart's Electric Sterilizer for Use in Ophthalmic Rooms and Wards.

Dressing sterilizer. The dressings, etc., are brought in direct contact with steam by placing them in chambers or cylinders and subjecting them to a pressure of superheated steam at 212° F. (100° C.) for twenty or thirty minutes. This produces thorough asepsis. Of the various methods of using steam for sterilization purposes that at high pressure is the most efficacious and it is generally used in all hospitals.

The autoclave is a form of high pressure sterilizer used principally by hospitals. It is used for the sterilization of both dressings and instruments. It consists of a boiler with inlet and outlet pipes surrounded with a jacket. The pipes are so adjusted that steam under any desired pressure may be admitted to the sterilizing chamber. Entrance to this chamber is effected by means of a cover or door, securely held in position by strong clamps, and provided with a registering gauge and steam valve.

Water to be absolutely sterile should be boiled at a temperature of not less than 250° F. for twenty minutes.

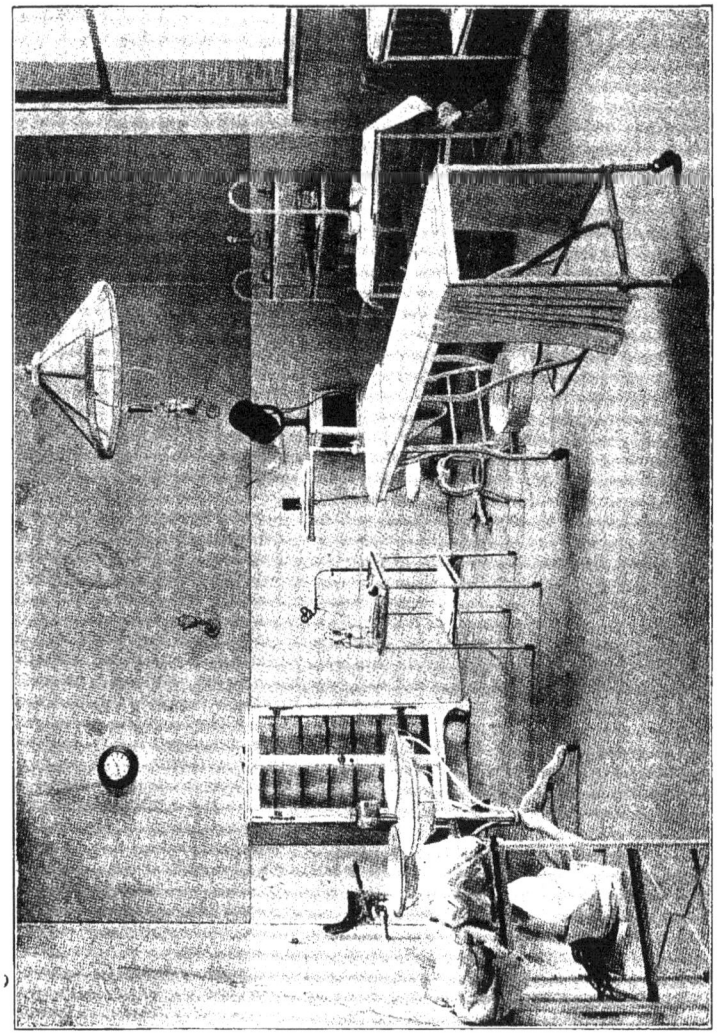

Eye Operating Room. Manhattan Eye, Ear and Throat Hospital.

. *Sterilization of pitchers, pans, irrigators and all utensils* used during an operation may be accomplished by placing them in a receptacle which has connection, by means of coils, with the steam boiler; or they may be submerged in water in a similar receptacle or boiler and the water heated to the boiling point from which the steam is generated. The source of heat may be gas, petroleum or electricity. The utensils may also be immersed in a trough containing such strong antiseptic solutions as corrosive sublimate, lysol, carbolic acid, etc.

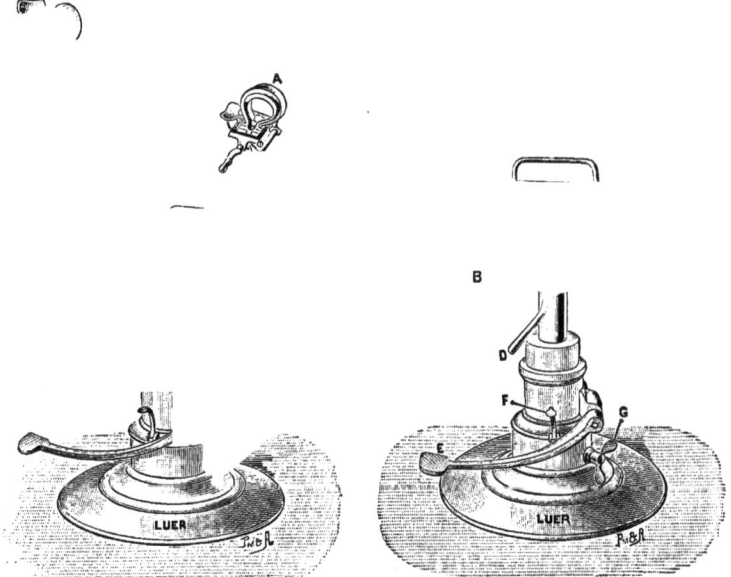

Luer's Chair-Table for Ophthalmic Hospital Operations.

The furniture of public ophthalmic operating rooms. In the Manhattan Eye, Ear and Throat Hospital the ophthalmic operating room is 16 by 18 feet, with a tile floor and tile base 5 feet high on the walls. The walls above the tiling and ceiling are painted light ivory and enameled; the windows are on the north side, on which are dark shades drawn during cataract operations, artificial light then being used exclusively.

There is no skylight. In connection with this room there is a "wash-up" room for surgeons with three sets of bowls, a small room with supply closets, etc., and a sterilizing room which is equipped like the corresponding room in a general hospital, i. e., with dressing-sterilizer, water-sterilizer and utensil-sterilizer. In the operating room are an ophthalmic operating table designed by the late Emil Gruening, an instrument cabinet, a cabinet for solution-bottles and other small articles, wall stand with four glass shelves for dressings, four glass top tables, stand with three basins for hand solution, one adjustable table for holding instruments, two white enameled stools, one two-step stool to enable patients to get on the operating table, one Haab magnet placed on a movable stand, small portable motor for cautery purposes, small gas sterilizer for instruments and a cluster of electric lights over the operating table provided with a steel-

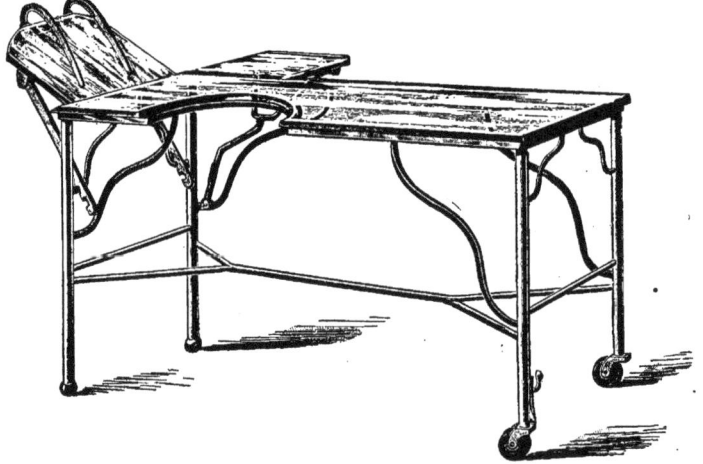

The Webster Fox Operating Table.

enameled hood over the lamps, from which, also, is a connection for a hand lamp.

All operations are performed on an operating table and the patients taken on a wheel-stretcher to their rooms. In operations in which the eyeball is opened there is placed on the table a canvas stretcher which is divided in the center and held in place by a long, flat, wooden pin, so that the patient can be readily moved to the wheel-stretcher. After being placed in bed the canvas is removed from under the patient by slipping out the wooden pin and allowing it to separate in the center.

The operating table should be of simple construction. The framework should be made of steel, mounted upon casters and capable of being moved to any part of the operating room without effort. The top should be of glass with or without an adjustable head-rest, some surgeons preferring the latter to assist in keeping the patient's head steady. The metal parts should be highly polished, or painted smooth with a thick coating of enamel paint, so that it can be scrubbed and sterilized without difficulty and without danger of rusting. Although any table that is used for general surgical work will answer the purpose, a number of tables have been specially constructed for ophthalmic surgery, their designers claiming certain advantages over the general surgical chair for this class of work.

A table designed by Charles H. May is made of steel and can easily be converted from an examining chair into an operating table. The center section or seat can be raised and lowered by means of a crank and endless screw, so that it always remains in a horizontal position. The head section or back is hinged at the junction with the seat and may be adjusted at any angle from the horizontal position upward. The foot section is hinged to the seat in a like manner and is capable of adjustment to any angle from the horizontal downwards. The table or chair is supplied with an adjustable head-rest that may be raised and lowered, moved forward or backward or inclined at various angles. It has two side pieces adjustable to any width, which can be turned back out of the way when not in use. A swinging glass tray for holding instruments, etc., is also provided and this may be attached to either side of the chair. Cushions add to the height.

L. Webster Fox uses a table for operating which consists of a brass frame mounted upon four legs, every one of which is provided with castors (locked if necessary) to facilitate movement from place to place.

Suitable braces are placed at each angle to render the frame-work firm and durable. The frame is made of rather thin, highly polished brass tubing, thus giving the entire table a neat appearance, a feature ignored in most tables. The height of the table is four and one-half feet, the width one and one-half feet and the length six feet. The top of the frame is covered by a single piece of thick plate glass, out of the left side of which, near the head of the table, a semi-circle is cut to enable the surgeon to stand more directly in front of the patient's face. A corresponding curve is made in the frame-work in this locality. A head-rest of metal and glass is provided which is raised or lowered to suit the convenience of the operator. The upper rim of the head-rest is longer on its under surface for receiving the extremities of the head clamps. These clamps are two long, thin, flat pieces of metal, one end of which is heavy, thick and grooved to fit snugly over the tongue of the head-rest. The clamps are made to slide along the rim of the head-rest until close to the patient's head, any movement of which will cause them to bend upon the rim and become more firmly fixed. A detachable leaflet for holding an instrument tray and dressings is also provided for one side of the table.—(T. A. W.)

Hospital trial frame. A name given to a simple lens holder whose pupillary distance and vertical and back and forward movement of the nose-piece is controlled by a rack-and-pinion movement.

Hot air therapy. Applications of dry hot air have long been acknowledged as most beneficial in a great many conditions, such as the

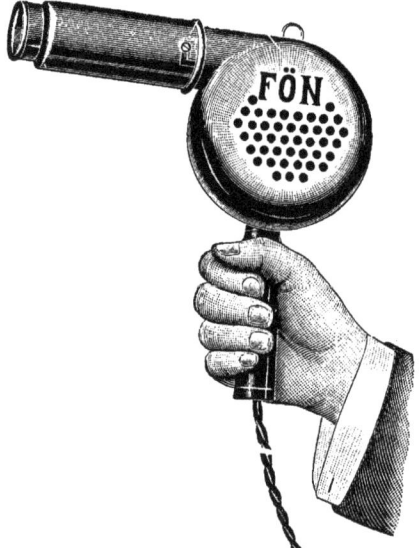

Foen Hot Air Apparatus.

treatment of acute eye diseases (especially iritis), headache, rheumatism, neuralgia, etc., due to the fact that a very decided local hyperemia is induced. With the Foen apparatus the desired amount of heat which can be borne by the patient may be applied under pressure. The equipment consists of a rotary fan, directly connected to a small motor, the blast of air being forced through a resistance wire, thus the air is heated in passing through the tubes. A switch is also provided for cutting out the heating unit where a cold blast is wanted. See, also, **Diathermy**; as well as **Heat.**

Hot eye. A name given by Jonathan Hutchinson to designate *episcleritis periodica fugax* (Fuchs). In this gouty or rheumatic affection patches of dusky, episcleral edema (with injection of the superficial vessels) show themselves, lasting a few days and then re-appearing at intervals of weeks or months. Swan Burnett called this intermittent or periodic form fugacious edema or *vasomotor dilatation of the vessels.*

Hotz, Ferdinand Carl. A famous ophthalmologist of Chicago, Ill., inventor of the well-known Hotz's operations for entropium, ectropium,

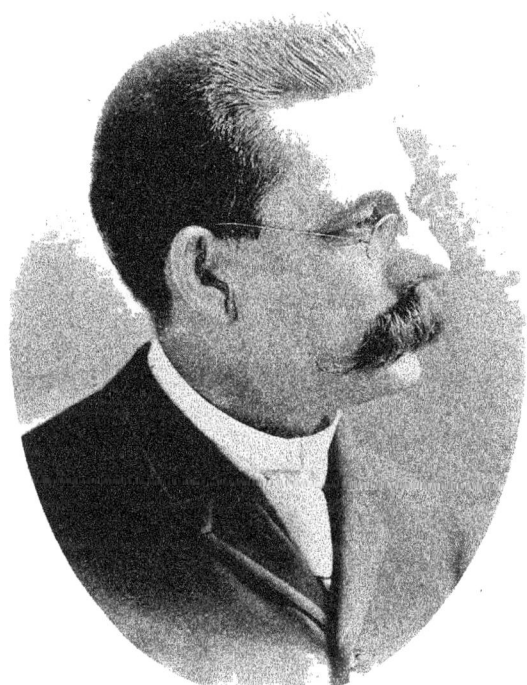

Ferdinand Carl Hotz.

trichiasis and trachoma. He was born at Wertheim, Baden, Germany, July 12, 1843. He received his early education in the Lyceum at Wertheim, his medical training at Heidelberg (1863-66) and Berlin (1866-67). His medical degree was conferred at Heidelberg in 1865. The teachers who chiefly influenced him at Heidelberg were Helmholtz, Simon, and Knapp; at Berlin, Graefe, Virchow, and Langenbeck. After a tour of study to Vienna, Paris, London, Edinburgh,

Glasgow, and Dublin, he came to America and settled in Chicago in 1869. He was ophthalmic surgeon at the Illinois Eye and Ear Infirmary from 1876 until his death. On the resignation by E. W. Holmes of the chair of ophthalmology and otology in Rush Medical College Hotz was appointed in his place, and this position he held for many years. For a time he also occupied the chair of ophthalmology at the Chicago Polyclinic.

Among his more important writings are: 1. Ein Fall von Strabismus Deorsum Vergens in Folge von Congenitaler paralyse der Rect. Sup. Geheilt durch Vorlagerung desselben. (*Archiv für Augen- und Ohrenheilkunde*, Bd. V, Abth. 2, p. 379, 1876.) 2. Two cases of Death Resulting from Aural Diseases. (*Transacts. of Ill. State Med. Soc.*, 1876.) 3. Notes on Intraocular Lesions Produced by Sunstroke. (*Am. Jour. Med. Sciences*, July, 1879.) 4. Two Cases of Chronic Blepharospasmus as Traumatic Reflex Neurosis. (*Ibid.*, Oct., 1879.) 5. Traumatic Aneurysm in the Eyelid, Following an Operation for Trichiasis. (*New York Med. Record*, June, 1879.) 6. Klinische Beobachtungen. (*Archiv für Augenheilkunde*, X.) 7. Eine Neue Operation für Entropium und Trichiasis. *(Ibid.)* 8. Die Ectropium Operation am Unteren Augenlid, Besonders bei Alten Leuten. (*Klin. Monatsblätter für Augenheilkunde*, 1880.) 9. Über das Wesen und die Operation der Sog. Ptosis Atonica. (*Archiv für Augenheilkunde*, Bd. I, 1880.) 10. Die Frühzeitige Perforation des Warzenfortsatzes bei Otitis Media Purulenta, Complicirt durch Acute Entzündung der Warzenzellen. (*Zeitschr. für Ohrenheilkunde*, IX.) 11. Schlimme Folgen einer Calomel-Einstaubung ins Auge. (*Archiv für Augenheilkunde*, 1882, IX.)

For a time Hotz was associate editor of the *Chicago Medical Journal and Examiner*.

In 1873 he married Emma, daughter of A. Rosenmerkel, Esq., of Chicago.

Dr. Hotz was a man of middle height, thick and stocky, with bushy hair and florid complexion; German to the core, versatile, contentious, sincere and hot-tempered. He was, withal, very unassuming and modest, and extremely helpful to all the younger men with whom he came in contact who were trying to succeed in ophthalmology. He was a hater of shams and quackery, and was thoroughly aroused and vehement whenever the subject came up. He was naturally inventive, and, even as he lectured to the students, would strike out one original idea after another. Dr. S. S. Bishop, of Chicago, declares, "I have never known a more constructive mind." And, similarly, Dr. Franklin Coleman: "In the plastic surgery of the eye, I know of no one who introduced so varied a number of operations as Dr. Hotz."

Hotz died March 20, 1908.—(T. H. S.)

Hotz's operation. See p. 4360, Vol. VI, of this *Encyclopedia.*

Hound's tongue. See **Cynoglossum officinale.**

Houppe nerveuse. (F.) A tuft-like termination of a fasciculus of nerves in a papilla.

Hour-circle. The graduated circle of an equatorial telescope which lies parallel to the earth's equator.

Hour-line. A line on which the shadow of the gnomon falls at a given hour.

House-leek. WALL PEPPER. *Sempervirum tectorium.* The juice of this plant was employed in ancient Greco-Roman times as a remedy for ocular ulcers and epiphora.—(T. H. S.)

Hovius, Jacob. This celebrated surgeon was born at Enkhuizen, Germany. The exact date of his birth (about 1675), as well as the place and date of his death, are unknown. He became doctor of philosophy, master of arts, and doctor of medicine, all at Utrecht. The date of conferring upon him of the last-named degree was June 13, 1702. On the reception of his medical doctorate, he presented a dissertation, entitled "De circulari humorum ocularium motu." This created a considerable stir in the ophthalmologic world—as well it might, for, therein, were first announced, or accurately described, two very important matters: (1) The influx and efflux of the ocular humors as well as a (very inaccurate) means of measuring these fluxions; (2) The "circulus venosus" which is formed by the venæ vorticosæ. This dissertation was published at Leyden in 1716, and again in 1740. In 1715 he published an *"Epistola Apologetica in Vir. Cl. DD. Fer-dericum Ruyschium."*

Hovius was one of the lesser opponents of the then new doctrine concerning the nature and seat of cataract. Throughout antiquity and the middle ages, and well on into the modern period, it was firmly believed that a cataract was a deposit of a corrupt and inspissated "humor" in a (wholly imaginary) space between the pupil and the lens. Quarré, about 1643, first theoretically taught the true doctrine, and Rolfinck, in 1656, confirmed his teaching by anatomical dissection. Then the matter simply sank into oblivion, until Brisseau and Maitre Jan, just after the beginning of the 18th century, re-discovered this most important truth and compelled the scientific world to accord it recognition. Before the recognition was accorded, however, a bitter controversy arose concerning the matter. The opposition to the new theory was led by Thomas Woolhouse, an English oculist resident in Paris. Among the followers of Woolhouse was Hovius.—(T. H. S.)

Hovius's canal. Canal of Fontana.

Howard, Henry. A well-known Canadian ophthalmologist, author of
the earliest text-book on the eye to be issued in the Dominion of
Canada. Born at Nenagh, County Tipperary, Ireland, Dec. 1, 1815,
he received his early education in his native town. He studied his
profession in Dublin, receiving the degrees of M. D. and M. R. C. S.,
the latter in 1838. After practising in Dublin for a very short time,
he emigrated, in 1841, to Canada. For a time he engaged in general
practice on Amherst Island, U. C., afterwards at Kingston. At length
he removed to Montreal, where he practised the eye, ear, nose and
throat exclusively, and where he was surgeon to the Montreal Eye and
Ear Institution. From 1845 until his death he contributed a number
of articles on the eye, ear, nose and throat to the *Dublin Medical
Journal.* He also wrote at some length and rather frequently for the
British American Journal of Montreal. About 1860 he wrote a
brochure entitled *"The Physiology of Insanity, Crime and Responsi-
bility."* In 1861 he was appointed medical superintendent of the
Lunatic Asylum, of St. John's, L. C., later situated at Longue Pointe,
Montreal, a position which he held until his death, Mar. 28, 1889.

The following is extracted from Dr. Howard's obituary notice in
the *Canada Medical Journal:* "Advancing years never took from
him the keen interest in scientific matters which he had pursued with
such zest as a younger man and nothing gave him such pleasure as
to take part in the discussions of our medical societies, or privately
with his younger medical friends. At such meetings the familiar
figure of the stately old doctor, with flowing patriarchal beard, will
long be missed. His kindly wit, free from all tinge of malice, his
animated discourse, his thorough honesty of purpose and his manly
straightforwardness made him respected and beloved by all who
knew him." The following passage is taken from a recent letter from
Dr. Frank J. Shephard, formerly Dean of the Medical College, McGill
University: "Dr. Howard, as the writer remembers him, was a tall,
thin old man with aquiline features and a long gray beard; his appearance was most dignified and he was blest with a fine Irish brogue and
a witty tongue; he was very fond of using long, fine-sounding words,
for instance, in speaking of some one of whose conduct he did.not
approve he said: 'There is some teratological defect in his psycho-
physical organization.' He was much beloved by his younger colleagues in the Montreal Medico-Chirurgical Society, and was always
ready to praise any original work they brought before the Society.
He was a personality and of a type of courteous physician now seldom seen."

One of Dr. Howard's sons graduated in medicine at McGill University in 1872, another was a member of the Provincial Cabinet of Manitoba.

The chief ophthalmologic writing of Dr. Howard was his justly famous text-book, entitled, *"The Anatomy, Physiology, and Pathology of the Eye;"* London: John Churchill; Montreal: Armour and Ramsey. 1850. In the preface to this work, the author says: "He [the author] has availed himself of the published opinions of the numerous distinguished writers who have 'explored the field of science in which he has labored; and he wishes in this place to state, not only his great obligations to them for the information which he has been enabled to derive from their writings, but also to express to those learned and respected friends who have contributed many valuable notes and suggestions, his sense of the service they have rendered to his inquiry; a service by which, in some instances, he has been enabled not only to enrich his work, but to confirm his own experience of the propriety of the treatment which he has successfully pursued; a treatment, which the author may be pardoned for stating, has not been suggested in any published treatise on the Pathology of the Eye which has come under his notice."

The peculiar treatment of the author's, thus indefinitely referred to in his preface, would seem to be that for cataract and glaucoma, which he thus describes, in the appropriate portions of the body of his book. Thus, at p. 354, speaking of cataract: "If the case be seen in the first stage of the inflammation, whether the cause be spontaneous or from an injury, the treatment must be antiphlogistic, but it should never be pushed too far. I generally begin with an emetic and purgative, followed up by cream of tartar drink, containing minute doses of tartarized antimony. I resort to local instead of general bleeding, keep the pupil under the influence of belladonna, and direct that the eyes have perfect rest, and be not exposed to strong light. If the disease run into the second stage, and the vascularity disappears, leaving the parts opaque (cataract in the incipient stage) the treatment must be altered at once, and recourse had to alteratives and tonics, such as calomel and quinine combined, or nitric acid, mixed in molasses so as to enable the patient's stomach to bear it in large doses. Benefit will also be derived from the internal use of the ioduretted iodide of potassium. The local remedies are, keeping the pupil dilated by means of atropine, or belladonna; fumigating the conjunctiva once every day with hydrocyanic acid, brushing the eye-lids and eye-brows with the solution of veratria, insulating the patient and drawing electric sparks from round the orbit and from the eye-lids, and keeping up a counter-irritation behind the ears by applying to these parts the tincture of iodine. It is just as necessary that the patient should avoid strong light, and every other exciting cause, as if it were acute inflammation that existed. By the above treatment, long persevered in, I have not only succeeded in curing hundreds of cases of incipient cataract, but have also in very many cases succeeded in giving to old people, who could not make their way alone, such sight as enabled them to read a moderate sized print.''

Thus, also, on p 362, speaking of glaucoma, which, to him, meant inflammation of the hyaloid membrane, he says: "The treatment which I pursue in glaucoma is the same as that which I adopt in inflammation of the lens and its capsule (incipient cataract).''

Just seven years later, von Graefe astounded the world by his application of iridectomy * for the cure of glaucoma, but, as to incipient cataract, who is there yet that can positively declare that the treatment of Howard (or something similar) will not suffice, at least in many instances, to establish an absolute cure? Have we not of recent years been far too much inclined to regard an incipient cataract as a matter to be merely watched and waited over?

The style of the book, as the reader can easily perceive in the passages quoted above, is simple, clear and mellifluous. The arrangement of the matter throughout the volume is no less excellent, and, in a word, this little book of Henry Howard's constituted a very auspicious beginning for Canadian ophthalmography.—(T. H. S.)

Howe, Samuel Gridley. The first American to devise (in 1830) an improved alphabet and to print literature for the sightless. See **Alphabet for the blind.**

Hubais. A distinguished Arabian ophthalmologist, nephew of Hunain and one of his most devoted students. He completed Hunain's *"Book on the Questions of Medical Science"* and wrote *"The Book on the Improvement of Purgatives,"* *"The Book of Simple Remedies,"* and the *"Work on the Pulse."* According to Halifa, he composed a book entitled *"The Volume of Explanations of Eye Diseases."* The ophthalmologic book is remarkable only for the fact that it seems to have contained a number of illustrations—e. g., of pterygium and pannus—and was, therefore, one of the very earliest of illustrated works upon the eye. This book, most unfortunately, is no longer extant.—(T. H. S.)

Hubbell, Alvin Allace. This well-known American ophthalmologist was born May 1, 1846, at Conewango, N. Y., the son of Schuyler

---

* The procedure itself had been devised by Beer in 1795 as a better means of forming an artificial pupil than the simple iridotomy of Cheselden.

Phillip and Hepzibah (Farnsworth) Hubbell. He studied medicine at Philadelphia, Penna., and at the University of Buffalo, receiving his degree from the latter institution in 1876. In 1896 he received the honorary degree of Ph. D. from Niagara University.

For a time he practised general medicine and surgery, and, in fact, performed in 1878 the operation of laparotomy for intestinal intussusception for the fourth time in the United States.

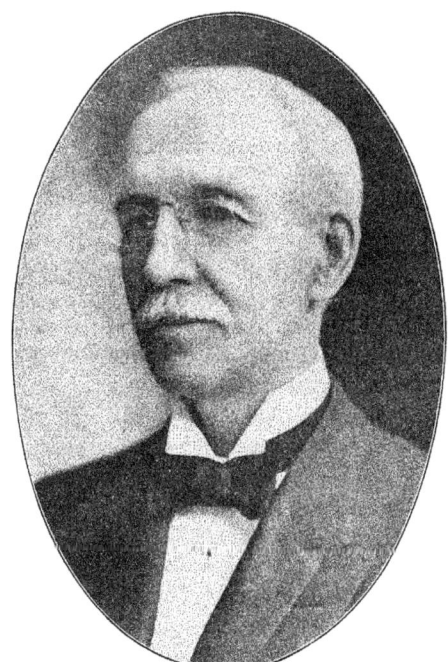

Alvin Allace Hubbell.

In 1883 he decided to limit his practice to ophthalmology and otology, and soon was known throughout the United States as an expert in these specialties.

He became ophthalmic surgeon to the Riverside Hospital, the Buffalo Hospital of the Sisters of Charity, the Erie County Hospital (of which he was one of the founders), and of the Charity Eye, Ear, Nose and Throat Hospital of Erie County, of which he was one of the founders and directors.

He was also one of the founders of the Medical Department of Niagara University, in which he became Professor of Ophthalmology and Otology and Secretary to the Faculty. In 1898 he accepted the chair of clinical ophthalmology in the University of Buffalo, a position which he held till 1911, when he was made Professor Emeritus.

He was a member of the Buffalo Academy of Medicine, the Buffalo Medical Union, the Buffalo Ophthalmological Society, the Erie County Medical Society, the Medical Association of Central New York (of which he was President in 1892), the New York State Medical Association (of which he was President in 1902), the Medical Society of the State of New York, the New York Academy of Medicine, the American Medical Association (of whose section on ophthalmology he was Chairman, 1908-09), the American Ophthalmological Society, the Pan-American Medical Congress, the Eighth International Ophthalmological Congress, held at Edinburgh in 1894, and of the Ninth, held at Utrecht in 1899. He was also a member of numerous historical and literary societies.

Dr. Hubbell invented a number of instruments and appliances, the most important of which, perhaps, is an improved electro-magnet for the extraction of attractable bodies from the interior of the eye.

In addition to numerous journal articles he wrote one of the sections in de Schweinitz's *American Text-Book of Diseases of the Eye* (Philadelphia, 1899); also *"The Development of Ophthalmology in America from 1800-1870"* (Chicago, 1908). He was associate editor of the *Buffalo Medical Journal* and of the *Ophthalmic Record*. At the time of his death he was engaged in writing a work on Daviel.

He married, June 26, 1872, at Leon, N. Y., Evangeline Fancher, daughter of Capt. William and Lydia (Mills) Fancher. Of the union was born one child, Bula, now Mrs. Everett Ward Olmsted, of Ithaca.

Hubbell died at the Lenox Hotel, Buffalo, Aug. 10, 1911, of general arterio-sclerosis.—(T. H. S.)

Huber, Francis. A celebrated and blind Swiss naturalist. He was born at Geneva, Switzerland, July 2, 1750, the son of a prominent soldier and natural historian, T. Huber, who was the author of a notable book, entitled, *"Observations sur le Vol des Oiseau"* (Geneva, 1784). The subject of this sketch would seem to have been myopic even in childhood, and when only fifteen years of age, he became totally blind.

Even before the onset of his blindness, he had shown a remarkable aptitude for natural history, and, when shut up in "the ever-during dark," his predilection rose to the point of an all-absorbing passion. His wife, Marie Aimée, was of great assistance to him in all his investigations. So, too, was his servant, François Burnens, who was trained by Huber to an almost marvellous power of observation. Huber even invented a glass bee-hive, through the walls of which his devoted helper could observe to a nicety the ways and works of his favorite bees.

Huber published: 1. Nouvelles Observations sur les Abeilles (1792; Eng. trans., 1806; 2d Fr. ed., 1814). 2. Mémoire sur l'Origine de la Cire (*Bibliotheque Brittanique*, tome xxv). 3. Lettre à M. Pictet sur Certains Dangers que Courent les Abeilles (*Op. cit.* XX, vii). 4. Nouvelles Observations rel. au Sphinx Atropos (*Op. cit.*, XXVII). In addition to these independent compositions, Huber assisted Jean Senebier in his "Mémoire sur l'Influence de l'Air, etc., dans la Germination" (Geneva, 1800).

Huber's name was given by De Candolle to a genus of Brazilian trees, *Huberialaurine*.

Huber was a wealthy man from the beginning to the end of his career. After a long and happy life (for he was always cheerful and contented) he died at Lausanne, Dec. 22, 1831.—(T. H. S.)

Hue. The quality of a color, distinct from its intensity.

Hueck, Alexander Friedrich. A celebrated Russian anatomist paleontologist, and archeologist, of some importance in ophthalmology. Born at Reval, Dec. 7, (19), 1802, he received the degree of Doctor in Medicine in 1826, his graduation thesis being "Diss. inaug. Physiol.-Med. de Mutationibus Oculi Interin Respectu Distantiæ Rerum." After a scientific journey to Berlin, Münich, Göttingen and Paris, he settled in Dorpat, where, in 1830, he became Prosector at the Anatomical Institute of the University. In 1833 he was made Full Professor of Anatomy. He died July 28, 1842, not quite forty years of age.

Hueck's ophthalmologic writings are as follows: 1. *Das Sehen, seinem Aeusseren Process nach Entwickelt.* (Dorpat and Göttingen, 1830.) 2. *Die Axendrehung des Auges.* (Dorpat, 1838.) 3. *Die Bewegung der Krystallinse.* (Leipsic, 1840; 4 plates.)—(T. H. S.)

Hueter, Karl Christoph. A German surgeon and obstetrician, who paid considerable attention to diseases of the eye. Born at Melsungen, Lower Hesse, Mar. 6, 1803, he received the degree of Doctor in Medicine at Marburg in 1824. After a year or more of study in various foreign universities, he settled in Marburg, as Privatdocent in Medicine, Surgery, and Obstetrics. He died of apoplexy, while in attendance on a patient, Aug. 18, 1857.

Hueter's ophthalmologic writings are as follows: 1. Ueber Ophthalmia Intermittens in Hinsicht auf ihr Vorkommen und den Zusammenhang mit dem Wechselfieber, etc. (v. Graefe and Walther's *Jour.*, vol. XII.) 2. Ein Fall von Ophthalmia Intermittens mit Achttägigen Typus. (*Ibid.*, vol. XIII.) 3. Die Katarrhalischen Augenentzündungen. (*Heidelberger Klin. Annalen*, Bd. V, VI.)—(T. H. S.)

Hügel. (G.) A prominence or tuberosity.

Huggins, Sir William (1824-1910). An English astronomer, born in London. He was attracted to the study of chemistry, magnetism, and allied branches of physical science. Having in 1855 built for his own private use an observatory at Upper Tulse Hill, near London, he began the study of the physical constitution of stars, planets, comets, and nebulæ. By researches on the sun's spectra and the spectra of certain comets, he ascertained that the luminous properties of the former are not the same as the luminous properties of the latter. Since 1875 he had been engaged photographing the ultra-violet parts of the spectra of the stars. He also determined the amount of heat that reaches the earth from some of the fixed stars. He was president of the Royal Astronomical Society (1876-78), president of the British Association (1891) and president of the Royal Society (1900).— *(Standard Encyclopedia.)*

Huile. (F.) Oil.

Huile de Herva. (F.) Castor-oil.

Huile de ricin. (F.) Castor oil.

Hulke, John Whitaker. A famous London ophthalmologist and President of the Royal College of Surgeons of England. He was born at Deal, England, in 1830, the son of a well-known general practitioner of that place. He studied at King's College, and was House Surgeon there under Sir William Ferguson.

He served in the war of the Crimea, and was surgeon at Smyrna and before Sebastopol. In 1857 he became a Fellow of the Royal College of Surgeons and Surgeon to Moorfields Hospital. Here he soon became a finished operator, ranking, in fact, almost as high as Critchett and Sir William Bowman. In 1862 he was appointed Surgeon to the Middlesex Hospital, and in 1890 was elected President of the Royal College of Surgeons.

Among his numerous writings, the following possess a maximum of ophthalmologic interest: 1. A Practical Treatise on the Use of the Ophthalmoscope; Being the Essay for which the Jacksonian Prize was Awarded in 1859 (London, 1861). 2. On the Morbid Changes in the Retina, as Seen in the Eye of a Living Person and After Removal from the Body (*Proceed. of the Royal Society,* 1865). 3. Anatomy of the Retina in Amphibia and Reptiles (*Proceed. of the Roy. Soc.,* 1865). 4. Anatomy of the Chameleon's Retina (*Philosoph. Transacts.,* 1866). 5. The Fovea Centralis of the Human Retina (*Ibid.,* 1867). Hulke was also a well known writer on geology, especially on paleontology. He died Feb. 19, 1895.—(T. H. S.)

Hulen's operation for cataract extraction. See **Cataract suction operation.**

Hülle. (G.) A cover; a covering.

Hüllenpilz. (G.) The generally poisonous mushroom, *Amanita*.

Hülsenwurm. (G.) Cysticercus cellulosæ.

Humeur hyaloïde. (F.) The vitreous humor.

Humid collyria. A name formerly applied to collyria consisting of liquid or almost liquid substances to distinguish them from solid varieties.

Hummer. (G.) Lobster.

Humor. (L.) Any fluid of the body. Of the old writers, a fluid supposed to be present in the body which by its excess gave the type to a certain disease. According to their ideas there were four humors, yellow and black bile, blood and phlegm. In popular language, a chronic skin disease attributed to disorder of the blood. See **Ophthalmology, History of.**

Humor, Black aqueous. See p. 1004, Vol. II, of this *Encyclopedia*.

Humor, Crystallinus. One of the synonyms for *crystalline lens*.

Humor hyalinus. HUMOR HYALOIDES. (L.) Synonyms of vitreous humor or body.

Humors of the eye. Aqueous humor, corpus vitreum, and crystalline lens.

Humor, Vitreous. See **Anatomy of the eye**; as well as **Histology of the eye.**

Humulus lupulus. (L.) The hop plant.

Hunain (full Arabic name, Abu Zaid Hunain b. Ishaq al Ibadi; the Latin name, Johannitius). A Christian physician (808-873 A. D.) who lived at Bagdad and practised as an oculist with conspicuous success. He wrote, among other treatises, *"The Work of the Ten Books of the Eye,"* which is highly important as being, so far as we know, the earliest ophthalmologic text-book produced in the Arabic period. According to the last "Book" of this work, the author had previously composed nine treatises on ocular subjects, and these he combined together, adding also certain new material, to form the present classic. Usaibia, in his work *"On the Classes of Physicians,"* says that the contents of the several books of Hunain's masterpiece are: "(1) Nature of the Eye. (2) Nature of the Brain. (3) The Optic Nerve and Vision. (4) Hygiene. (5) The Causes of Ocular Accidents. (7) The Virtues of Medicines. (8) Ocular Remedies. (9) Treatment of Eye Diseases. (10) Combinations of Ocular Remedies, Prescriptions." In certain manuscripts, there is given an eleventh book, devoted to Ocular Operations.

Hirschberg, to whom we owe so much that is valuable in the history of ophthalmology, has shown conclusively that this important work by Hunain still exists in two mediaeval Latin translations, as follows: *"Liber de Oculis translatus a Demetrio"* and *"Liber de Oculis Constantini Africani."*

Hunain also wrote for his sons, David and Isaac, "a work upon the eye in the form of questions and answers," nothing but fragments of which have come down to our day.

Hunain exerted a tremendous influence in Arabian ophthalmology for more than five hundred years. He is, in fact, always mentioned with a kind of reverence by the most important of the later Arabians, e. g., Ali b. Isa, Zarrin-Dast, Halifa, Al-Gafiqi, and Alcoati.— (T. H. S.)

Hunter, James. An Edinburgh ophthalmologist whose life-dates are unknown, but who flourished about the middle of the 19th century. He was for a time surgeon at the Edinburgh Eye Hospital. In addition to an article on presbyopia in a boy (*Edin. Jour.* No. 142, pp. 124-129) he wrote a book entitled, *"On the Influence of Artificial Light in Causing Impaired Vision"* (Edinburgh, 1840).—(T. H. S.)

Hunter, John. Though the achievements of this justly celebrated English surgeon relate almost exclusively to the general field of the healing art (and indeed to the borderlands thereof, as dentistry, botany, and comparative anatomy and pathology) still, his indirect relations to ophthalmology (through his investigations into the venereal diseases) require that a brief biography of the man should be inserted here. Born Feb. 13, 1728, at Long Calderwood, in the parish of East Kilbride, Lanarkshire, Scotland, of respectable and well to do parents, and the youngest of ten children, he at first displayed no extraordinary ability. Even when twenty years of age, he seems to have shown no very strong predilection for science, or even to have acquired an unusually good education. At about this age, however, he journeyed to London, there to join his brother, William, who had become a celebrated gynecologist. Stimulated by the example of his brother, he entered on the study of anatomy, and soon displayed a most extraordinary talent for this subject. He then proceeded to study surgery, first at the Chelsea Hospital, then at St. Bartholomew's. In 1756 he was surgeon at St. George's. For a time —from 1760-63—he was surgeon in the English navy. Returning to London, he became almost at once a famous man. However, he published nothing until 1771, when he was 43 years old. In fact the labor of writing seems always to have been for him extreme, and he never, even to the end of his life, attained to the clearness, force, and perfection of polish, which so plainly characterized the literary style of his far less painstaking brother. Nevertheless, he was a great observer and thinker, and he it was who, by directing attention to the underlying principles and facts of anatomy, physiology and pathology, established the surgery of England on a scientific basis. Hypothesis, with him, was in little estimation. He wrote to Edward Jenner, concerning a certain theory which the younger man had just proposed, "I think your solution is just; but why think? Why not try the experiment? Repeat all the experiments upon a hedghog as soon as you receive this, and they will give you the solution." It was also

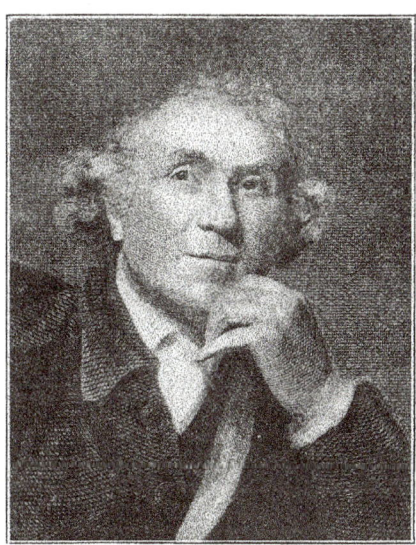

John Hunter.

largely due to Hunter's suggestions and stimulus that the validity of vaccination was established by Jenner on an eternal foundation of careful experiment and exact observation.

In fact Hunter's passion for observation amounted almost to mania. His own house at Earl's Court, Brompton, was almost literally "packed" with hedghogs, blackbirds, lizards, snakes, fishes, toads, partridges, pheasants, silk-worms, eagles, bees, and even leopards. Once he nearly lost his life by the escape of two leopards from their cages. These, however, he returned to their places alone and absolutely unassisted. Again, he was almost torn to pieces in a contest with a bull. Of course he did not know of the existence of the spirocheta pallida, but he calmly faced its ravages just the same—as will appear more plainly hereafter. For fifteen years he kept a flock of geese, and all this time he studied the embryology of the goose with most intense persistency. "It would almost appear," he said, "that this mode of propagation was intended for investigation." In the course of his toxicological experiments he poisoned, according to his own statement, "some thousands of animals." He succeeded in engrafting a human incisor tooth on the comb of a cock. He exchanged the spurs of a young cock and a young pullet. On the cock the small pullet spurs grew vigorously, while, on the pullet, the spurs of the cock either did not grow at all or grew very little. His experiments on the bones of animals with inserted shot, followed up by the feeding of madder, are among the most familiar facts of high-school physiology.

Hunter's most important writings are: 1. *Natural History of the Human Teeth, Explaining Their Structure, Use, Formation, Growth, and Diseases.* (London, 1771; 1778; Lat. trans., by Baddaert, Leipsic, 1775; Ger. trans., Leipsic, 1780.) 2. *On the Venereal Disease.* (London, 1786; Ger. trans., Leipsic, 1787; French trans., Paris, 1787.) 3. *Observations on Diseases of the Army in Jamaica and on the Best Means of Preserving the Health of Europeans.* (London, 1788; Ger. trans., Leipsic, 1792.) 4. *On the Nature of the Blood, Inflammation and Gun-Shot Wounds.* (London, 1794; Ger. trans., Leipsic, 1797-1800.) 5. *Observations on Certain Parts of the Animal Economy.* (London, 1787; Ger. trans., Braunschweig, 1803.)

In the work on the *Venereal Disease,* Hunter, though he contributed much to our knowledge of syphilis, soft chancre, and gonorrhea, yet did much harm because of the position which he took and most tenaciously defended, respecting the identity or non-identity of these three diseases. To him it seemed to be absolutely plain that all these three affections were one and one only. His belief, however, was by no means baseless, for, to determine the question, he had inoculated himself, on the prepuse and the glans, with gonorrheal virus, and, in consequence, had, at the usual intervals, developed not only gonorrhea, but also chancroid, and, finally, "Hunterian" chancre and syphilis. Until the beginning of the 18th century there had been no doubt at all concerning the essential unity of the venereal disease. Then there began to arise certain questioning voices. The matter remained in abeyance for a time, until, in fact, this work of Hunter's, when the question appeared to have been settled for all time. "No question," however, "is settled until it is settled right." So, from 1831 to 1837, by a vast series of inoculations, the immortal Ricord conclusively demonstrated that the three are by no means one, but that the one is by all means three.

In (5) *"Observations on Certain Parts of the Animal Economy,"* Hunter recorded his investigations into the ocular pigment and the functions of the ocular oblique muscles. He was the first to describe the muscular layer of the iris.

As a result probably of his self-induced syphilis, Hunter developed an aneurism of the aorta. Being a very irascible man, he was one day angered by a confrère, the aneurism ruptured, and Hunter passed almost immediately away. This occurred Oct. 16, 1793, when Hunter, though aged sixty-five, was still in the zenith of his powers and immense usefulness.—(T. H. S.)

Hura crepitans. (L.) The sand-box tree, indigenous to tropical America; known in Panama as *javilla,* and in New Granada as *ocupa* and *habille.* Its properties are similar to those of *Hura brasiliensis.* The seeds contain 50 per cent. of fixed oil, and this oil, when extracted, is used as a purgative. The seeds are employed in Mexico as a severe drastic cathartic, one seed sufficing to purge violently, and even to produce emesis frequently. Instances have been known of the juice of the plant causing destructive injury to the eyes. See, also, Lewin and Guillery (*Die Workung von Gift auf das Auge,* Vol. II, p. 702.)

Huschke, Valve of. See **Valves of the lachrymal canals.**

Husten. (G.) Cough.

Hutchinson facies. The facial expression of ophthalmoplegia.

Hutchinson patch. SALMON PATCH. Dull-red coloration of the cornea, with ciliary injection in interstitial keratitis.

Hutchinson pupils. Inequality of the pupils in meningeal hemorrhage.

Hutchinson, Sir Jonathan. A famous London syphilographer, dermatologist, and ophthalmologist. He was born at Selby, in Yorkshire, England, July 23, 1828. At first he studied in the York County Hospital and in the York School of Medicine and Surgery. In 1849 he entered Bartholomew's Hospital, London, and in 1854 was made full surgeon at that institution. From 1859-83 he was surgeon at the London Hospital, and, for many years, also surgeon at the Royal London Ophthalmic Hospital (Moorefields). In 1862 he became a Fellow of the Royal College of Surgeons, and in 1879 Professor of Surgery in the same institution. He was President of the Pathological Society in 1879-80 and of the British Ophthalmological Society in 1884-85. He founded in 1868 the Museum of the British Medical Association, and he was one of the organizers of the Medical Graduates' College, London. He received the order of knighthood in 1908.

Sir Jonathan Hutchinson was a man of great force and originality

—a fact which has linked his name inseparably with the very nomenclature itself of medicine. Thus we have "Hutchinson's Facies" (the facial expression of ophthalmoplegia); "Hutchinson's pupils" (inequality of the pupils in meningeal hemorrhage); "Hutchinson's mask" (the facial immobility of tabes); "Hutchinson's teeth" (the semilunation and notching of the free border of the permanent incisor teeth of the upper jaw in inherited syphilis); "Hutchinson's triad" (syphilitic teeth, labyrinthitis, and interstitial keratitis).

His most important writings are: "On the Form of Dyspepia which Usually Attends Phthisis" (1862); "Clinical Memoir on Certain Diseases of the Eye and Ear Consequent on Inherited Syphilis" (1862); "Surgical Diseases of Women" (in Holmes's "System of Surgery"); "On Constitutional Syphilis" (in Reynold's "System of Medicine"); "The Rectangular Catheter Staff for Lithotomy;" "Clinical Illustrations of Amaurosis;" "Lesions of the Eye in Connection with Injuries to the Fifth Nerve;" "Illustrations of Clinical Surgery;" "Clinical Lectures on Rare Diseases of the Skin."

Sir Jonathan died at his home in Haslemere, England, June 23, 1913. Regarding his career as a whole, Dr. James Moores Ball has said: "The death of Jonathan Hutchinson . . . removes from English medicine one of its most interesting and most versatile characters—a man who, forming part and parcel of the medical history of the 19th century, carried his influence, his studies and his intellectual vigor well into the present period. To few men is it given to follow the profession of medicine for more than sixty years, and to still fewer is it granted that even the latest of these years shall be fruitful."—(T. H. S.)

Hutchinson teeth. PEGGED TEETH. SYPHILITIC TEETH. The upper central permanent incisor teeth are "pegged," as well as notched on the cutting surface. This sign is noticed in about 65 per cent. of all cases of luetic interstitial keratitis. (See the figures.) In young subjects

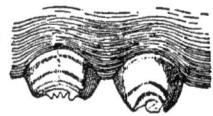 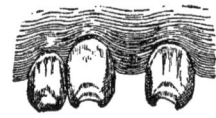

Hutchinson Teeth.

the incisors look as if a small peg had been driven into the center of each crown, but as time advances the pegged projection wears away and only the notch or cup remains. This appearance is due to lack of development not only of the tooth itself but of the enamel which normally covers it.

Hutchinson triad. Syphilitic teeth, labyrinthitis, and interstitial keratitis.

Hutchison, Edwin. A well-known American ophthalmologist, founder of St. Elizabeth's Hospital, at Utica, N. Y. Born at Utica in 1840, a son of Holmes Hutchison, he received his education in the arts and sciences at Yale and his medical training at the Long Island Hospital Medical College and at the College of Physicians and Surgeons in the City of New York. At the latter institution he received his degree in 1866. Having served throughout the war, and also having received his medical degree, he settled in New York both as general surgeon and as ophthalmologist, and, though his right forearm was anchylosed upon the humerus he soon had a wide reputation as an operator. In 1866 he married Miss Christina Rosswog. He died in 1887.—(T. H. S.)

Huygenian eye-piece. Designed by Huygens, consisting of a convexo-concave field-lens and a convexo-plane eye-lens, the focal length of the former being three times that of the latter; the distance between them being numerically equal to three times the focal length of the eye-lens. See also **Eye-piece.**—(C. F. P.)

Huygens, Christian. A celebrated Dutch astronomer, mathematician, mechanician and optician. He was born at The Hague, Holland, April 14, 1629, the second son of Constantine Huygens, Lord of Zelem and Zuylichem, and Secretary to the Prince of Orange. After his earliest instruction, which he chiefly received from his very learned father, he studied, first, at Leyden, mechanics and mathematics, and, later, at Breda, jurisprudence. Soon, however, he abandoned his legal studies, returning to mechanics, mathematics, and, by far the most important matter for our purposes, to optics.

In 1665 he invented a new and highly successful method of grinding lenses, and, by the aid of some of the lenses of his own production, he discovered a satellite of Saturn, and for the first time in history announced the existence of the Saturnian ring as well as its angle to the ecliptic, 20°. Prior to that announcement the changing phenomena of Saturn had given to that body the appellation of "the triple planet." Huygens also invented the pendulum-clock, a copy of which instrument he presented to the States General on the 16th of June, 1657. He also solved the problem of "the center of oscillation," invented cycloidal checks for clocks, as well as the "aerial telescope," which consisted simply of a series of lenses of very long focal distances, mounted on high poles.

In the field of optics his work was, if possible, more important and wide-sweeping still. He it was who established for all time the wave theory of light, which already had been propounded both by Grimaldi and by Hooke.

Huygens announced the results of his investigations as early as 1678 before the Paris Academy but it was not until 1690 that he published the little *"Traité de la Lumière."* Huygens also discovered the polarization of light, a phenomenon described in the same "Traité." Throughout the work, its distinguished author assumes the existence of a luminiferous ether, the fundamental principles of which he was first in history to propound. This theory was afterward further developed and firmly established by Euler, by. Fresnel, and, to much the same effect but independently, by **Young.** (See **Euler, Fresnel,** and **Young,** in this *Encyclopedia.*)

Huygens never married. He died in his native town, The Hague, June 8, 1695.—(T. H. S.)

Huygen's ocular. Same as Huygenian eye-piece.

Hyalin degeneration. HYALINE DEGENERATION. Owing to the confusion of this term with *amyloid degeneration* and especially with *colloid degeneration* the reader is referred both to page 332, Vol. I, and to page 2326, Vol. IV, of this *Encyclopedia,* where these subjects are fully discussed, depicted and differentiated.

Hyalitis. HYALITIS IN GENERAL. Inflammation of the vitreous humor, characterized mainly by failing vision and floating or fixed opacities in the vitreous, seen with the ophthalmoscope, and consisting of wandering lymphoid cells. It rarely occurs as a primary disease, but is usually secondary to some ciliary or choroidal disease, and should be studied with the cause that produced it. Straub (*Archiv f. Ophthalm.,* 86, I, 1913), however, believes that the vitreous is susceptible to inflammatory changes, and that it is perfectly justifiable to speak of "hyalitis." An irritant in the vitreous may produce chemotactic substances which attract leukocytes from the vessels of neighboring structures, and this process constitutes true inflammation; hence a distinction often can and should be made between inflammations arising primarily in the vitreous, and those arising primarily in the uvea. He thinks that, clinically, two forms of hyalitis are well known, namely, the conditions heretofore known as panophthalmitis and metastatic ophthalmitis. In both these conditions the organisms are introduced directly into the vitreous either by a perforating wound or by embolism of the retinal vessels. They grow here and attract lymphocytes or leucocytes according to the nature and intensity of the exciting cause. Besides these severe forms there are milder forms of hyalitis which either recover completely, or else lead to an early detachment of the retina through shrinking of the vitreous. These cases cannot be considered to be true cyclitis, because the bulk of the exudation and later new formation of vessels and fibrous tissue affect chiefly the vitreous, while the uvea as a whole is not affected.

Clinically it is possible to separate the cases of cyclitis from those of hyalitis. It is possible that the two conditions may occur together, but this appears to be very rare. Of course in all these cases the existence of collateral inflammation must be remembered. The vitreous will always suffer somewhat from a uveitis, on account of the diffusion into it of chemical irritants, but this will not be confused with a true inflammation.

As regards the diagnosis of hyalitis, the severe cases, such as panophthalmitis and metastatic ophthalmitis, present no difficulty, and the histological picture is characteristic. The hyaloid membrane is detached and the sub-hyaloid space is filled with fibrinous coagulum. In the centre of the vitreous there is a space filled with the same material. The leucocytic exudate is massed at certain definite spots, in front in the neighborhood of the ciliary body and iris, and behind in front of the papilla.

The milder cases of hyalitis are of an analogous nature. For instance cases of perforating wounds which show slight inflammatory signs, e. g., exudate in the anterior chamber and on the posterior surface of the lens and mild iritis. These eyes either recover or are enucleated for fear of sympathetic ophthalmitis. Histologically they show a mild hyalitis, the capillary layer of the uvea alone is infiltrated. The vitreous is detached and is infiltrated in the typical situations, near the ciliary body, the posterior lens surface, and the neighborhood of the papilla These cases of pure hyalitis never give rise to sympathetic ophthalmitis, and therefore a conservative line of treatment can be followed, but practically in any given case, it is difficult to exclude a focus of co-existent uveitis which might give rise to sympathetic trouble.

A second form of mild hyalitis consists of those cases in which the vitreous becomes infected through a wound to which the iris is adherent. These late infections can sometimes be cured by atropine and rigorous cauterization of the wound.

A third group of cases of mild hyalitis is furnished by the metastatic cases. There is generally a history of some mild general affection such as influenza. The eye becomes inflamed with raised tension, cloudy cornea, vessels on the iris and synechiæ. There is much fibrinous exudate in the anterior chamber. These cases yield readily to atropine. (A. Levy in the *Oph. Review*, p. 16, 1914.)

Hyalitis purulenta. SUPPURATIVE HYALITIS. An inflammation characterized by infiltration of the vitreous by large numbers of lymphoid cells, so that the vitreous is practically a large abscess. It may be circumscribed or diffuse, idiopathic or traumatic.

This is an exceedingly serious condition and is nearly always part of a general intraocular infection or inflammation. It is usually part of a panophthalmitis, generally the result of penetrating injuries of the eye, metastatic choroiditis and other lesions. The treatment is entirely symptomatic, the intraocular use of iodoform (q. v.) as well as the introduction into the interior of the eye of mercuric chloride, argyrol and chlorine water, may be mentioned—but without enthusiasm.

Hyalodecrysis. (Obs.) Escape of part of the vitreous humor of the eye.

Hyalodeitis. (L.) (Obs.) Hyalitis.

Hyalodeoglischrotes. (L.) (Obs.) Viscidity of the corpus vitreum.

Hyalodeomalacia. HYALODEOMALACOSIS. (L.) (Obs.) Softening of the corpus vitreum.

Hyalodeonyxis. (L.) (Obs.) Hyalonyxis, or puncture of vitreous body.

Hyalodeoproptosis. (L.) (Obs.) Prolapse of the corpus vitreum.

Hyalodes. (L.), adj. (Obs.) Hyaloid; as a noun, the corpus vitreum.

Hyaloid. Adj. Pertaining to the corpus vitreum; as a noun, the hyaloid membrane; also, as a noun, of Eimer, a clear zone surrounding the nucleolus of cells.

Hyaloid artery. In the embryo, a branch of the arteria centralis retinæ, traversing the vitreous humor to the posterior capsule of the lens. Its hyaloid sheath forms the canal of Cloquet. See p. 616, Vol. I, of this *Encyclopedia;* also **Congenital anomalies** and **Development of the human eye.**

Hyaloid artery, Persistent. See **Artery, Persistent hyaloid.**

Hyaloid body. Corpus vitreum.

Hyaloid canal. CANAL OF CLOQUET. An irregularly cylindrical canal running antero-posteriorly through the vitreous body, through which, in the fetus, the hyaloid artery passes to ramify on the posterior surface of the crystalline lens. See p. 292, Vol. IV, of this *Encyclopedia.*

Hyaloid capsule. Membrana limitans retinæ.

Hyaloid cataract. A false cataract supposed to be due to opacity of the anterior portion of the vitreous humor.

Hyaloïde. (F.) The vitreous humor or body.

Hyaloidea. (L.) Hyaloid membrane.

Hyaloideitis. (L.) Hyalitis.

Hyaloid fossa. The shallow, cupped depression on the anterior surface of the vitreous body on which the posterior surface of the lens rests. See **Anatomy of the eye.**

Hyaloidioproptosis. (L.) Prolapse or hernia of the corpus vitreum.

Hyaloiditis. (L.) A synonym of hyalitis.

Hyaloid membrane. The delicate, transparent envelope or limiting membrane of the vitreous humor, very thin behind, where it is intimately connected with the membrana limitans of the retina; thicker in the region of the ora serrata, where it goes to form the zonula of Zinn. It is a structureless membrane, which anteriorly lies in folds and here shows under the microscope a fine striation. Beneath it may be seen a more or less continuous layer of flattened epithelial cells. Cases of calcification (*Ophthalmic Record,* XIX, p. 459) of this structure have been reported, but they are very rare. See **Histology of the eye;** also, **Anatomy of the eye.**

Hyaloid vessels. The hyaloid artery and vein. See **Congenital anomalies;** as well as **Comparative ophthalmology.**

Hyaloma. (L.) (Obs.) A supposed conversion of the eye into a glass-like mass.

Hyalomeninx. (L.) (Obs.) A hyaloid membrane, especially that of the eye.

Hyalonyxis. (L.) (Obs.) Puncture of the corpus vitreum, as in keratonyxis.

Hydatid. A cyst with aqueous contents formed by the larva of a tenia, *Echinococcus polymorphus,* the larva of a small tapeworm, *Tenia echinococcus,* which, in its adult form (strobila) is known to infest only the dog and the wolf, while the larvæ (hydatids) are of frequent occurrence in man and other mammals. Three principal forms of hydatids are recognized, viz., exogenous, endogenous, and multilocular. The first is sparingly found in man, but is extremely common in the lower animals, whilst the second is most frequently developed in the human subject, the third kind being found only in man. (Cobbold.) The term hydatid is frequently, also, loosely applied to vesicular tumors and cysts of many kinds. Hydatids are most frequent in the liver, but are found in almost any tissue, even in bone.—(Gould.) See p. 4123, Vol. VI, of this *Encyclopedia.*

Hydatid buzzing. A symptom of echinococcus cyst of the orbit said to be elicited occasionally by tightly closing the eyelids.

Hydatis palpebræ. (L.) (Obs.) A rounded vesicle, as large as a pea, with pellucid contents, usually solitary, met with on the eyelids.

Hydatodeitis. (L.) (Obs.) Inflammation of the lining membrane of the anterior chamber of the eye.

Hydatodes. (L.) A term used by Hippocrates, meaning watery; of urine, limpid; of a person, dropsical. As a noun, the aqueous humor.

Hydatoid. Water-like. Resembling a hydatid. As a noun, the aqueous humor and its supposititious investment.

Hydatoïde. (F.) Resembling hydatids; Descemet's membrane; the vitreous body.

Hydatorrhea. (L.) Hydrorrhea.

Hyderiasis (L.) Hydropa.

Hydnocarpus wightianus. (L.) A botanical species found in India. An infusion of the seeds is used as a detergent douche after delivery, and an oil obtained from them is used like chaulmoogra oil—in ophthalmia.

Hydracetin. ACETYLPHENYLHYDRAZIN. PYRODIN. This poisonous, highly organized derivative is a colorless crystalline powder readily soluble in alcohol and hot water. It is antipyretic, analgesic and antiparasitic, and given in rheumatism and other febrile diseases in doses of from $\frac{1}{3}$ to 2 grains. It is used externally as an ointment in psoriasis and other skin diseases.

A few cases of amblyopia are reported, especially from its external application. Grünthal (*Centralbl. f. pkt. Augenheilk.*, p. 73, 1890) records one of these instances in which a 20 per cent. salve was rubbed over the whole body. This was followed, inside of 4 days, by cyanosis, albuminuria, hematuria and other general signs of intoxication and the appearance of a cloud before the eyes, which was explained by the discovery of a retinal hemorrhage (and a central scotoma) that persisted for four weeks.

Hydrargyri iodidum rubrum. See **Mercury, Red** iodide of.

Hydrargyri oxidum flavum. See **Mercury, Yellow** oxide of.

Hydrargyrophthalmia. (L.) A mercurial ophthalmia.

Hydrargyrum. (L.) See **Mercury.**

Hydrargyrum bijodatum, P. G. See **Mercury, Red** iodide of.

Hydrargyrum oxycyanatum, P. G. See **Mercury, Oxycyanide of.**

Hydrargyrum oxydatum, P. G. See **Mercury, Yellow oxide of.**

Hydrastinin. This is a yellow, crystalline powder derived from *hydrastis canadensis;* soluble in one part of water, and given internally in doses of from a quarter to one grain.

Although there is no recorded case of toxic amblyopia from this drug yet Meyer (*Arch. f. Exp. Pathol. u. Pharmak.*, Vol. 32, p. 115, 1893) noticed that after instilling a three per cent. solution of the sulphate into the eyes of pigeons, a marked miosis was produced in a very few minutes that lasted about half an hour.

Hydrastis. GOLDEN SEAL. YELLOW ROOT. INDIAN DYE. These and many more are the popular synonyms for *hydrastis canadensis,* a small shrub whose yellowish rhizome yields 2 to 3 per cent. of the alkaloid hydrastin, 4 per cent. of berberine (q. v.) and some canadine. The first is probably the active principle of the tincture, glycerite and fluid extract used in the eye. The best form, however, is hydrastin sulphate. Hydrastin occurs as white or colorless, odorless, tasteless prismatic crystals, although its salts generally have a bitter taste. It is sparingly soluble in water. It forms several salts, of which the chloride and sulphate are best known, the former, official in the U. S. P., being formed artificially. The sulphate is decidedly hygroscopic, has a bitterish taste, and like the chloride is very soluble in water. All the preparations of hydrastin are poisonous.

The *Extra Pharmacopeia* says that purulent ophthalmia neonatorum is occasionally treated by one per cent. hydrastin solution along with one-tenth of one per cent. morphin sulphate.

G. E. Dean uses the following collyrium in subacute conjunctivitis and in other diseases of the conjunctiva with profuse and purulent discharge: Fluid ext. hydrastis, U. S., m. iv; glycerini, m. xl; aquæ dest, ad, fl. ℥i.

J. W. Wright uses this drug with considerable satisfaction in the catarrhal forms of conjunctivitis. He prefers the agent known as the sulphate of berberine (q. v.), using as a solvent water and glycerine. He much prefers the yellowish crystal to the colorless form and gives the following formula, from which, in the Editor's judgment, the cocaine should be excluded: Hydrastin, gr. ss; acid. carbolic, gtt. i; morphiæ sulph.; cocain, mur. āā, gr. iv; glycerini, fl. ℥ii; aquæ dest., fl. ℥vi; mix and filter. A few drops in the eye three or four times a day.

Following the example set by genito-urinary surgeons in the successful treatment of urethral gonorrhea by this remedy, it has been prescribed for local use in gonococcus ophthalmia. The best known formula is F. X. Scott's mixture: Hydrastin sulphat.; acid boracic.; sod. boratis, āā, 0.3 gm. (gr. v); tinct. opii deodor., 2.0 c.c. (f℥ss); aquæ dest., 30.0 c.c. (f℥j); Filter. Sig: To be instilled every hour. This prescription is quite as effective without the opium; some have used it with considerable success in other forms of ocular blennorrhea.

Hydrastis, Glycerite of. See **Glycerite of hydrastis.**

Hydriatics. The systematic treatment of diseases with cold water.

Hydric chloride. See **Acid, Hydrochloric**; as well as **Hydrochloric acid.**

Hydroa. Large watery vesicles or bullæ. See p. 1328, Vol. II, of this *Encyclopedia;* also, **Conjunctiva, Pemphigus of the.** In hydroa there may be enormous bullæ upon the mucous membranes (mouth, lips, and tongue), as well as upon the conjunctiva. This affection usually recovers without corneal complications and without retractile

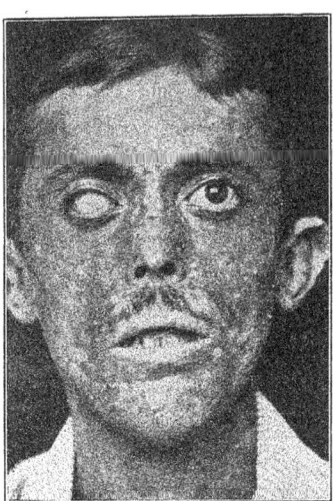

Kuhnt's Case of Pitting of the Sclera and Conjunctiva in Hydroa Vacciniforme.

cicatrices of the conjunctiva. One should then establish with care the diagnosis between bullous hydroa, harmless as regards the eye, and pemphigus, so grave and ending in symblepharon and blindness. See, also, p. 4515, Vol. VI, of this *Encyclopedia*.

Hydrocephalus, Ocular symptoms of. The ocular symptoms of this disease result from pressure on the optic chiasma by the distended third ventricle, namely: bitemporal hemianopsia, optic neuritis, and optic-nerve atrophy, the latter being secondary or primary according to the severity of the attack. Strabismus is not uncommon.

In one case occurring in a girl, æt. 16, who complained of headaches, impairment of vision and diplopia, Halben (*Practical Med. Series, Eye*, p. 212, 1910) found paresis of the left adducens, bilateral papillitis (with an elevation of 6 **D**.. i. e., 2 mm.), V. almost ½, pupils from 3.25 to 3.5 mm., nystagmus in extreme lateral fixation; tremor of head and hands. The patient had always had headaches, but more intensely during the last six months, in which period she had vomiting, lasting one to two days, three times. She was well-nourished, and there was no indication of lues, tuberculosis or spinal disease. The author made the diagnosis of chronic hydrocephalus of the fourth ventricle. As two punctures of the right lateral ventricle by Payr transiently reduced the papillitic swelling to 3.0 and relieved the headaches, the operation for permanent drainage of the ventricle was performed. After reflecting a skin-bone flap of the parietal bone, about 2 cm. from the longitudinal sinus, a trocar, 2 mm. wide, was introduced into the right lateral ventricle. At a depth of 5.6 cm. a stream of liquor spurted out. The trocar was replaced by a specially prepared and hardened calf's artery, which connected the venticle with the epidural and subdural spaces, the wound was sutured and the skull at this region fenestrated. Four weeks later all symptoms had disappeared, the discs were scarcely prominent, although they exhibited a dirty, slightly reddish-grey color, with somewhat indistinct borders. The lumen of the vessels was almost normal; vision was normal.

Hydrochinone. See **Hydroquinone.**

Hydrochloric acid. A description of hydric chloride will be found on page 69, Vol. 1, of this *Encyclopedia.* Organic lesions of the eye from its effects as an accidental cauterant are not so uncommon. Fehr (*Centralbl. f. prak. Augenheilkunde,* April, 1911), in connection with a case of injury, refers to the original experimental work of Guillery, who found that corneal injuries produced by the inorganic acids, such as hydrochloric, nitric, or sulphuric, were often complicated by opacities of the lens. These were not produced by acetic acid, or brine or alkalies. These opacities develop in a few hours after the application of the acid to the cornea, and affect chiefly the capsule and anterior cortex. If the quantity of applied acid be large, the equatorial portions are affected and also the posterior layers of the lens. Schmidt recorded a case in man in which such a development of cataract occurred, but the etiological connection was not absolutely certain.

Fehr's case is definite on this point. The patient, a man, æt. 47 years, had a large quantity of pure hydrochloric acid poured over his face as an act of revenge. After several hours the eyes were washed out, and twenty hours after the application of the caustic, he was brought to the eye clinic. The whole face was extensively corroded— the conjunctivæ were changed into dense greyish-white membranes with necrotic areas. The corneæ were less affected; there was diffuse cloudiness of substance, but the iris and pupil could be recognized. Both pupils were active, and both lenses were densely opaque. During the following days, large conjunctival sloughs became separated, but the corneæ cleared up in a remarkable manner. Eight days after the accident, the first signs of necrosis occurred. The eyes became soft, deep-yellow infiltrations formed at the corneal margin and spread rapidly over the whole surface, and soon the corneæ gave way and both eyeballs became shrunken, and owing to the extensive destruction of the lids, there resulted total symblepharon and ankyloblepharon. The final result was brought about not by the severe corneal injury, but by the destruction of the nutritive vessels of the eyeballs. The original injury to the corneæ was comparatively slight, but the lenses suffered much more, and it may be assumed that the extremely diffusible hydrochloric acid entered not only through the corneæ but also through the sclera and thus attacked the lenses from all sides, leading to the rapid development of complete cataract.—(*Ophthalmoscope,* October, 1914.)

Hydrocyanic acid, Amblyopia from. A description of this powerful agent is given on p. 70, Vol. I, of this *Encyclopedia.* Loss of vision from its use is, in spite of its extremely poisonous qualities, very rare. However, exposure to the vapor of dilute hydrocyanic acid has caused temporary amaurosis and hemiopia, due to disturbance either of the retinal circulation or of the cortical centres.

Hydrodiaskope. Another name (given by Lohnstein) for a modification of Batten's *hydrophthalmoscope* and Czermak's *orthoscope.*

Hydrofère. (F.) A method of giving a bath of water (simple or medicated) in the form of spray, the patient being seated in a box such as that used for fumigations.

Hydrogale. (F.) A mixture of water and milk.

Hydrogen dioxide. See **Hydrogen peroxide.**

Hydrogen peroxide. HYDROGEN DIOXIDE. H_2O_2. DIOXYGEN. PERHYDROL. The official liquid we familiarly call by this name is the Aqua hydrogenii dioxidi, U. S. P., and is a slightly aqueous solution of hydrogen dioxide, containing when freshly prepared about 3 per cent. by weight or 10 volumes of pure dioxide of hydrogen. It should be kept in a cool place and when uncorked the gas should escape with but slight pressure. Solution of the peroxide is a colorless, odorless liquid with a slightly acidulous taste. It decomposes readily into oxygen and water. It has powerful bleaching, disinfectant and oxidizing powers, foaming up and disengaging active oxygen or ozone during the process. In ocular therapy it is used as a disinfectant and cleansing agent in the treatment of wounds of the lids, especially after operations on the skin surface, as an application to corneal ulcer, in purulent conjunctivitis, dacryocystitis, etc. A proprietary solution of hydrogen peroxide, sold under the name dioxogen and said to contain 3 per cent. of H_2O_2, has been much advertised in the lay press, a fact that should be considered by physicians in ordering these preparations.

One obstacle that has until recently stood in the way of the general use of hydrogen peroxide has been the unstable nature of the product, as well as the fact that the ordinary commercial varieties are seldom, if ever, free from acid. Merck has overcome these drawbacks by the introduction of 30 per cent. "Perhydrol"—that is to say, an absolutely pure and acid-free hydrogen peroxide, not subject to spontaneous explosion, and capable of being kept almost indefinitely in the original bottles, which are lined with ceresite.

Solutions of hydrogen peroxide are incompatible with alkalies, albuminous compounds, carbolic acid, glycerine, hydrocyanic acid, iodides, permanganates and several other salts used in ophthalmic practice.

It may be used in its pure state or diluted with distilled water.

A. Jacqueau (*Semaine médicale*, No. 8, p. 94, 1907) has, in various corneal affections, used with advantage a solution containing 1.8 per cent. by weight = 6 per cent. by volume. He used this every day as a lotion or by instillation, and had satisfactory results, even in severe cases of keratitis. With this treatment, combined with cauterization and evacuation of pus from the anterior chamber, he obtained a complete cure, within a month, of traumatic corneal ulcers with hypopyon. In a case of corneal abscess the pain was relieved by the unaided use of perhydrol solution, and the pus soon disappeared. In perforating corneal ulcer the remedy also promptly assisted healing and cicatrization.

Hydrolat simple. Distilled water.

Hydrolé. (F.) An aqueous solution, decoction, or infusion of a medicinal substance.

Hydrology. That department or division of medical science which treats of the use of waters, especially mineral waters, for therapeutic purposes. See **Hydrotherapy.**

Hydrolysis theory. This is an attempt to explain the formation of cataract, and resembles the hydration hypothesis of L. Dor. See J. Burdon-Cooper (*Oph. Review*, p. 129, May, 1914) on this subject.

Hydromeningitis. A synonym of *keratitis punctata* or "serous" iritis.

Hydrometer. An instrument for measuring the density, etc., of fluids. Baumé's apparatus consists of a glass tube with a bulb blown in its end and loaded with mercury so as to float upright in a liquid. For determining the densities of liquids lighter than water the stem of the hydrometer is so graduated that 10° mark the level to which it sinks in distilled water, and 0° the level to which it sinks in a solution of 10 parts of salt in 90 of water; the graduation being continued upon the same scale up to the top of the instrument. For liquids heavier than water, the hydrometer is so made that the point marked 0° is at the top of the stem and indicates the level to which it sinks in distilled water; the lower part of the stem is then so graduated that 15° represents the level to which it sinks in a mixture of 15 parts of salt and 85 of water.—(Foster.)

In hydrometers of *constant volume* the stem is always immersed to the same extent, while the load which the hydrometer carries varies in each case and by the amount of its variation indicates the specific gravity.

Hydropathy. HYDROTHERAPY. HYDROTHERAPEUTICS. The use of water in the treatment of disease, or in the prevention of disease. Popularly, hydropathy has become attached to a special scheme of water treatment, while *hydrotherapy* refers to the less restricted and more scientific use of water as one of the many therapeutic weapons furnished by experience to the armamentarium of the practitioner of medicine. See, also, **Water**; as well as **Thermotherapy**; and **Cold, Application of.**

One of the most favorable adjuncts to ophthalmic treatment is the *sweat bath.* This should be given when the stomach is empty. The patient should be in bed and wrapped up to the chin in a woolen blanket and again covered with at least four woolen blankets. Under the latter six quart bottles containing boiling hot water should be placed. If used at all, pilocarpin or other adjuvant should now be given by the mouth or hypodermically. The patient is also given to drink at least a pint of very hot water, very hot and weak lemonade, or very hot tea, to be administered through a bent glass tube, while he is lying down. In a few minutes he should begin to break out in a profuse perspiration, which should continue for at least an hour, only stopping short of that time, if he shows any bad symptoms. At the end of one and a half or two hours he should be thoroughly dried and the skin rubbed with alcohol and then allowed to rest for another two hours, when he may go out if he wishes.

Hydrophilism. The theory or condition of edema of the eyeball.

In addition to the discussion of this matter under **Glaucoma** it may be stated here that Martin H. Fischer (Pflüger's *Archiv,* Vol. 127, 1909; also *Annals of Ophthalm.,* p. 360, 1913) regards that disease (especially the chronic form of it) as essentially an edema of the eyeball, and all the clinical signs of this pathologic entity are so explained. The eye, like any other tissue in the body, holds normally a certain amount of water. The amount thus held is determined by the hydrophilic colloids of the eye (the proteins chiefly) and the state in which these exist. Edema is a condition in which the amount of water thus held is increased. In glaucoma the hydration capacity of the tissues of the eye (including the vitreous and aqueous humors) is increased. Various conditions are able to increase the hydration capacity of a protein colloid and so to lead to an edema of the affected part. A most important factor in this regard is an increase in the amount of acid present in the part. Any circumstance which will lead to an abnormal production or accumulation of acid in the eye will lead to glaucoma. What are ordinarily classed as causes of glaucoma (arteriosclerosis, circulatory disturbances, kidney disease, hard mental or muscular work, worry, high protein diet, diabetes with acidosis, local circulatory disturbances in the eye, intoxications of a general or local type which affect the eye, injuries and operations affecting the eye, cold, starvation, etc.) all have this in common, that they lead to an abnormal production or accumulation of acid in the eye. In consequence of this abnormal acid content the hydration capacity of the ocular colloids is raised, and a glaucoma results, not because water is pushed into the ocular colloids, but because these suffer changes which make them suck in water from any available source. Obliteration of the filtration angle is not the cause of glaucoma, but a consequence resulting from the fact that in glaucoma the colloids behind the lens swell more than those in front, and so the lens and iris are crowded forward. As the swelling progresses the glaucomatous eye tends to make itself worse, for in swelling it compresses the blood vessels within the eye and so adds to its already precarious state the superimposed effect of a lack of oxygen due to defective blood supply; and so by the resulting further abnormal acid production and accumulation a vicious circle is established. Eserin and other drugs which by contracting the iris open up the vessels in the ciliary body and so give a better blood supply may, therefore, at any time be successful in removing a last straw which makes an eye just on the edge of a glaucomatous attack go over; on the other hand, atropin, cocain and similarly acting drugs have a reverse effect, favoring not only a compression of blood vessels, but adding a direct toxic effect which in the end leads to an abnormal production and accumulation of acid. In the treatment of glaucoma we must first get as clearly as possible before our minds all the conditions which in our patient are leading to an abnormal production or accumulation of acid in the eyeball. Rarely will only one etiologic factor be responsible. An abnormally high acid content may be induced in an eye quite as easily through an abnormal acid production which results from too hard muscular work, a leaking heart or a bad dietary regime; an arteriosclerosis that manifests itself especially in the circulatory apparatus of the eye, an inflammation of the ciliary body or a cataract extraction. When we have removed as many of these conditions as possible, we then meet the effects of those which we cannot remove. We need to give alkali to neutralize the acids present in abnormal amounts; we need to increase the salt content in the tissues of the eye, for all salts, including such neutral salts as sodium chlorid, decrease the amount of water that can be held by any protein swelling in the presence of an acid; and, finally, we need to give water to wash out the acids (and any other substance) which are capable of increasing the hydration capacity of the ocular colloids. In actual practice this is accomplished as follows: As the patient is usually in the midst of a glaucomatous attack at the time that we see him, we describe the handling of this picture first.

1. It is our purpose to dehydrate the swollen eye as rapidly as possible. To accomplish this we may use either local or systemic means or both. To obtain a dehydration of the eye by systemic means we stop the intake of water by mouth and inject slowly into the rectum by the drop method, having the patient retain a liter or, if necessary, two liters of the following alkaline, hypertonic sodium chlorid solution:

> Monohydrated sodium carbonate.......   4.1 grammes
> Sodium chlorid ....   14.0 grammes
> Distilled water ....   1000. cc.

When the injection is properly given the alkali and salt content of the patient's body is increased and the swollen eyeball shrinks. In from one to three hours the glaucomatous eye will then have returned to its normal tension. During the past year the writer named had found a proper utilization of this scheme of treatment so effective that he had relied upon it entirely and so has largely given up the use of subconjunctival injections of sodium citrate. Once the tension in a glaucomatous eye has been reduced the patient must be kept from getting renewed attacks by keeping metabolism constantly toward the alkaline side. This means that the patient must be taught how to inhibit his acid-producing factors while at the same time he is placed under the influence of a sustained administration of alkali, salts and water. Only in this way can an eye on the verge of a glaucomatous attack from such a condition as an arteriosclerosis of the blood vessels of the eye be kept from a frank attack, as the acid content in the eye is pushed beyond these tolerable limits by work, worry, dietary indiscretions, etc.

2. Local treatment in glaucoma, according to Fischer, resolves itself into an administration subconjunctivally of harmless salts to reduce the hydration capacity of swollen colloids. A freshly-prepared sterile sodium citrate solution (5.41 per cent. solution of the ordinary chem-

ically pure $Na_3C_6H_5O_7 + 11\ H_2O$) is used. Enough must be injected
to gently distend the subconjunctival tissue (ten to fifteen drops).
The short-lived pain following such an injection may be relieved by
alternate hot and cold compresses. Failure to get a prompt reduction
by such means indicates that the solution was of wrong composition,
or that enough was not injected, or that the systemic acid content was
so high that use of the salt subconjunctivally did not even temporarily
prove effective. He further maintains that what is known as glaucoma in the eye is identical with the series of changes which in the
kidney we call nephritis, and the principles of treatment governing
both conditions are the same.

Hydrophobia. The cases in which this disease affects the eye are
exceedingly few. According to Parsons (*Pathology of the Eye,* p.
1327) primary infection through the lid and conjunctiva is recorded.
The virus is found after experimental inoculation in the lachrymal
glands and vitreous. It is not under these conditions found in the
aqueous, though the animal can be infected by inoculation of the
anterior chamber.

Hydrophthalmia. BUPHTHALMUS OR BUPHTHALMOS. HYDROPS OCULI.
INFANTILE GLAUCOMA. CONGENITAL GLAUCOMA. HYDROPHTHALMOS.
A disease characterized primarily by a uniform spherical bulging of
the whole cornea. It generally takes the form of infantile or congenital glaucoma. See **Buphthalmia.** In addition to what is there
said about treatment of this serious disease Zentmayer (*Jour. Am.
Med. Assocn.,* p. 1103, Sept. 27, 1913) remarks that the proved value
of iridectomy, in glaucoma of the adult, has undoubtedly been the
reason for its selection by many operators in treating the congenital
type. Yet the anatomic conditions and the topography of the parts
are so different in the two types that what is a safe and satisfactory
procedure for the one becomes a dangerous and disastrous procedure
when performed for the other. This operation has the support, however, of a number of surgeons of large experience. Thus Hirschberg
reports a case in which sixteen years after the operation tension was
normal. There were macular changes, a flat excavation of the nerve-
head and a high myopia.

In Schoen's case (in which iridectomy controlled the process after
twenty years) a cystoid cicatrix had resulted, the cyst being almost as
large as the globe.

Schoenemann reports seven cases permanently arrested. He does
not consider the operation dangerous if performed early and after the
method of Schweigger.

Schmidt-Rimpler evidently does not share this view. He quotes von Graefe to the effect that "in the vast majority of cases the disease remains a *noli me tangere*" and adds that he has unfortunately too often seen the eye lost after iridectomy—"it did indeed become smaller, but from phthisis bulbi."

Fuchs emphasizes the dangers of iridectomy but adds that a series of favorable results have been obtained. Among the surgeons so reporting are Angelucci, Swanzy and Bergmeister. Haab states that if posterior sclerotomies are begun early enough infantile glaucoma can be cured. Stölting also advises this operation repeated so long as tension remains increased.

Schmidt-Rimpler sums up his study of the literature and the results of his own experience advising that, in advanced cases and in bilateral cases, only one eye be operated on and the result observed, in the meanwhile using miotics in the fellow eye. He is definitely of the opinion that these drugs at least delay the progress of the process.

An analysis of the experience of still others (American surgeons) shows that iridectomy gave fair results to 42 per cent., and poor results to 58 per cent. of the operators employing it. Sclerotomy gave fair results to 28 per cent. and poor results to 72 per cent. of the operators using it. Paracentesis of the anterior chamber with iridectomy gave unsatisfactory results to 100 per cent. of the operators using it. Sclerectomy gave satisfactory results to 40 per cent., encouraging to 20 per cent., and unsatisfactory to 40 per cent. of the operators employing it. Cyclodialysis gave unsatisfactory results to 100 per cent. of the operators using it. Miotic treatment was on the whole found to be unsatisfactory.

While the number of cases seen by the individual operator was small and the total for any particular operative procedure not large, a summary shows that the only method which gave satisfactory or encouraging results to the majority of surgeons employing it, was some form of sclerectomy.

Iridectomy and sclerotomy are the operations which have been longest employed, and it cannot be said that they have inspired confidence except when performed in the very earliest stage of the disease.

The dangers of iridectomy are patent. The sudden release of the intra-ocular tension in an eye in which the natural barrier between the vitreous and the wound has been weakened by disease, is always fraught with danger and often results disastrously. If the disease is to be arrested, the early age at which it is necessary to operate requires the use of a general anesthetic. Vomiting and the natural restlessness of the child after the use of a general anesthetic further increase the danger.

The objections to sclerotomy and to paracentesis of the cornea are that it must be often repeated and even then is often only preliminary to some other form of operation. Of the different ways of performing sclerectomy that of Fergus-Elliot is attended by the least hazard and is easiest of performance. It is inferior to the **Lagrange** operation in that the filtration area is not so extensive and the scar is not so well placed for permanent effect. The position in which the incision is made in the latter operation is, however, more dangerous. An operation which has been advised by several operators and performed by a few, and which seems to be well adapted to the conditions present in hydrophthalmos, is that of de Vincentiis. The deep anterior chamber in these eyes renders the operation less difficult of performance than in primary glaucoma for which it was devised. That the progress of the disease is sometimes naturally arrested must be taken into consideration in weighing the evidence presented favorable to any operative procedure. Limitation of the progress of the process is not however constant enough, nor does it as a rule occur early enough to justify tentative treatment. See, also, **Glaucoma.**

Hydrophthalmia anterior. Keratoglobus.

Hydrophthalmia cruenta. (L.) Hemophthalmia.

Hydrophthalmia postica. (L.) An enlargement of the eye due to an increase in the quantity of the vitreous.

Hydrophthalmia totalis. (L.) Hydrophthalmia which involves both the anterior and posterior portions of the eye.

Hydrophthalmion. HYDROPHTHALMIUM. (L.) Old terms for an edematous swelling of the conjunctiva.

Hydrophthalmoscope. ORTHOSCOPE. This is the name given by Batten (*Ophthalmoscope*, February, 1910) to a modification of the orthoscope. See p. 591, Vol. I, of this *Encyclopedia*. Batten has adapted it for clinical examination of the eye. The instrument consists of a metal cup resembling the ordinary eye bath, with two short metal tubes projecting from it, to which are attached pieces of India rubber tubing. To the upper tube is fitted a short piece of tubing closed with a clip; to the lower one a piece a yard long connected with a reservoir. The anterior surface is plane glass. For use the instrument is so applied as to hold up the upper lid. The reservoir is then raised and the clip opened, allowing the instrument to fill with water. The clip is at once closed, the reservoir is lowered when the instrument should be held in position by suction. It especially assists in the inspection of the iris and angle of the anterior chamber. The ophthalmoscopic examination may also be made through it. See p. 4752, Vol. VI of this *Encyclopedia*.

Hydrophthalmus. Hydrophthalmos. A synonym of buphthalmos. See **Hydrophthalmia.**

Hydropote. (F.) A water-drinker.

Hydrops chorioideæ internus. An old name for detachment of the retina.

Hydrops nerve optici. (L.) Dropsy of the optic sheath.

Hydrops oculi. (L.) Hydrophthalmia.

Hydrops sacci lachrymalis. Distension (large mucocele) of the lachrymal sac.

Hydrops subchoroidealis. An obsolete name for detached retina.

Hydroquinone. Quinol. Hydrochinone. Paradioxybenzene. $C_6H_6O_2$. This compound is made from quinone by reduction with sulphurous acid; it forms colorless crystals soluble in 17 parts of water, more soluble in alcohol and ether. It is decidedly antiseptic and is used in one to three per cent. solutions in all forms of conjunctivitis with much discharge. Solutions should be freshly made as old ones have an irritant, caustic action.

Hydrorrhea, Nasal. This peculiar disease, or rather symptom, is of interest to the ophthalmologist, owing to the ocular lesions that often accompany it. Although it generally falls, first of all, within the purview of the rhinologist and ophthalmic surgeon, it properly belongs to neither of these specialists. The tissue alterations that result in the serous discharge from the nose are almost invariably intracranial and should be the special property, not of the rhinologist but of the neurologist. It so happens, again, that this peculiar symptom is not infrequently associated with brain changes that affect the visual centers and give rise to eye symptoms.

The chief interest for the ophthalmologist in the discussion of nasal hydrorrhea lies in its etiology and in the fact of the occasional presence of marked eye complications. The literature of the subject is by no means extensive, and the histories of cases in which a continuous discharge of water from the nose was a symptom will compel one to conclude that it may, like atrophy of the optic nerve, be produced by different conditions.

Of the earlier cases one was evidently due to fracture of the base of the skull (Vieusse's case); it is an occasional accompaniment of general anasarca (Rees); of meningitis (Paget); of trifacial paralysis (Althaus); of hydrocephalus internus (Leber, who thought there had been bone absorption from pressure with escape of the cerebro-spinal fluid from the opening thus formed); while in some cases (Priestley Smith's and Nettleship's) the brain symptoms appear to have been very marked. On the other hand, in two cases reported by Bosworth, to whose valuable paper on the subject the Editor would refer the reader, this author believes the discharge to have been the direct result of a paresis of the sympathetic vasomotor nerves. Mules reports three cases in support of his theory that "the dropping is due to over-distended lymph-vessels of the pituitary membrane, which by their

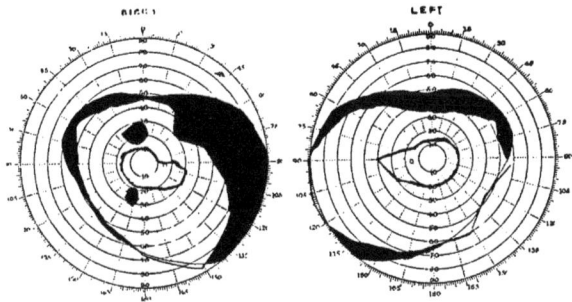

Nasal hydrorrhea.

Fields of vision; right eye; 5 mm. object; for red and white. Left, fields for white, red and green. (Casey Wood.)

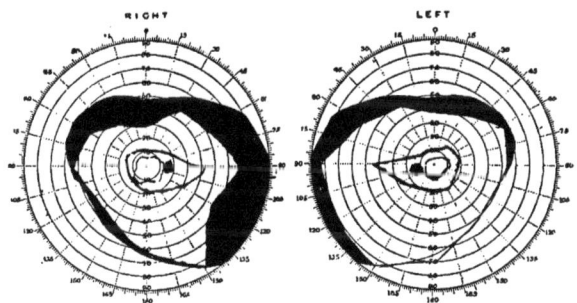

Nasal hydrorrhea.

Fields of vision; right eye; 5 mm. object; for white, red and green. Left, fields for white, red and green. (Casey Wood.)

bursting cause fistulous openings into the nasal meati." Mules concludes that the co-existence of optic-nerve atrophy with an abnormal watery secretion from the eye and nose is to some extent a coincidence. He explains the occurrence of the atrophy by suggesting that it may sometimes be due to the wasting character of the general disease, of which it and hydrorrhea happen to be symptoms. In some cases of hydrorrhea there is no atrophy, just as in other cases of atrophy there is no hydrorrhea.

A review of three cases by Casey Wood (*Jour. Am. Med. Assocn.*, September, 1912), as well as of others elsewhere reported, brings us to the following conclusions: The rather rare condition known as nasal hydrorrhea is not a definite disease, but is merely a symptom of one or more pathologic states.

In the majority of cases optic atrophy, more or less pronounced, accompanies or follows the discharge from the nose.

The visual involvement is, like the chief nasal symptom, generally a part of an intracranial disease that underlies the affections of both nose and eyes.

The discharge that flows so copiously from the nose is cerebro-spinal fluid, and it is just possible that when epiphora accompanies the hydrorrhea the lachrymal discharge may, in part at least, be of the same character.

The nasal hydrorrhea usually comes on without apparent reason, is generally intermittent as to amount and time, may disappear for a considerable interval or may cease entirely as quickly and mysteriously as it came.

If there be any organic disease of the nose it is, as a rule, merely a coincidence. Perhaps, however, some of the nasal lesions may be connected with the bony defects or minute fistulas through which the intracranial fluid finds its way into the upper nasal passages.

The underlying cerebral disease is frequently some form of hydrocephalus. The intracranial tension due to this disease finds relief by seepage of fluids through one or more basal openings (pressure-passages, congenital, natural or acquired) into the nasal meati or neighboring sinuses.

The course of the optic atrophy depends on the character of the brain lesion, and especially on the extent to which the visual centers are involved by the cerebral disease.

In every case of nasal hydrorrhea treatment of the brain alterations should first of all be considered; and, in this connection, lumbar puncture, or some decompression operation ought to be borne in mind.

Hydroscopy. HYDROPHTHALMOSCOPY. The examination of the interior of the eye when under water. See **Hydrophthalmoscope** and **Arlt's orthoscope.**

Hydrothalmos. See **Buphthalmos.**

Hydrotherapy in eye diseases. See **Hydropathy.**

Hydrous wool-fat. See **Lanolin.**

Hydrozone. This proprietary solution is intended to be a substitute for the U. S. aqua hydrogenii dioxidi. Although it is 3 times as strong as the official solution it loses very little of its hydrogen peroxide under ordinary conditions and may, therefore, be regarded as a fairly stable and useful preparation.

Hydryalos. (L.) Water-glass.

Hyetometer. A rain gauge.

Hyetometrograph. A self-recording rain gauge.

Hygidium. (L.) A collyrium suggested by Paulus Ægineta.

Hygiene, Marine. See p. 5038, Vol. VII, of this *Encyclopedia.*

Hygiene of the eye. This important subject has already been extensively discussed under such headings as **Illumination; Glaring; Dazzling; Eyestrain; Blindness, Prevention of; Eyes** of soldiers, etc., and particularly on p. 3186, Vol. V, of this *Encyclopedia.* The reader is referred to these captions.

Hygiene, School. See **Conservation of vision.**

Hygroblepharici. (L.) An old term for the excretory ducts of the lachrymal gland.

Hygroblepharismus. (L.) (Obs.) The watery eye; a more or less constant overflow of tears upon the cheeks, due to eversion, tumefaction or narrowing of the puncta lacrimalia, or to stoppage of the nasal duct.

Hygroblepharon. HYGROBLEPHARUM. (L.) A moist state of the eyelids. Hydroblepharon.

Hygrocataracta. (L.) An old term for a fluid cataract.

Hygrocollyre. (F.) A liquid collyrium.

Hygrodeik. A form of hygrometer.

Hygrograph. A self-recording hygrometer.

Hygroma of the orbit. A variety of exudation cyst, first described by Hyrtl, consisting in dropsy of the bursa of the tendon of the superior oblique muscle of the eye or of the bursa sometimes found between the levator palpebræ superioris and the rectus superior muscle. See **Bursa, Hygromatous degeneration of the orbital.**

Hygrometer. An instrument for determining the humidity of the atmosphere.

Hygrometric balance. A form of hygroscope.

Hygronhyalides. See **Galen.**

Hygrophanous. Transparent when moist and opaque when dry, as hydrophane.

Hygrophthalmia. (L.) An old term for irritation or inflammation of the eyeball or eyelids, accompanied by profuse lachrymation

Hygrophthalmic canals. Lachrymal canal.

Hygrophthalmique. (F.) Serving to moisten the conjunctiva.

Hyménoïde. (F.) Membranous.

Hymenophthalmia. (L.) An old term for membranous conjunctivitis.

Hymenopterygium. (L.) A name given by Petrequin to a "membranous or cellular pterygium."

Hyophthalmos. HYOPHTHALMUS. (L.) A person with small eyes, like a pig's.

Hyoscin. SCOPOLAMIN. This alkaloid is obtained not only from hyoscyamus but from many other plants of the *Solanaceæ*. Its best known salt is the hydrobromide which is official in the U. S. P. It occurs in rather large, colorless, transparent crystals that are odorless but have a bitter, acrid taste. It is soluble in 4 parts of water and 10 parts of alcohol.

When pure this drug is identical with scopolamin. Schmidt showed that chemically pure hyoscin produces physiological effects different from commercial hyoscin and that these differences are due to the presence in the latter of a left-turning hyoscin called atroscin. He it was who called the chemically pure product scopolamin. In the market we find two salts, scopolamin hydrobromide (Merck. $C_{17}H_2NO_4HBr +$ H_2O) in tablet-shaped, transparent, soluble crystals; and scopolamin hydrochloride (Rählmann, $C_{17}H_{23}NO_3HCl$ 3). Owing to the greater dilution of these salts in clinical use they do not so often produce irritative conjunctivitis and, it is claimed, much less increase of intraocular tension than atropia.

This drug is quite five times as powerful as atropia sulphate. The duration of the pupil dilation is about five days. It is believed (and the Editor has reason to concur in this belief) that it does not irritate mucous membranes as readily as atropia and is consequently indicated in persons exhibiting an idiosyncrasy against that drug. Owing to its brief and complete cycloplegia it is much preferred by some ophthalmologists as a routine agent for measuring refractive errors, in which case a solution of 1:500 generally suffices. At the same time it is a most powerful poison and its use should be carefully watched by the surgeon. The strength for home use in iritis, corneal ulcer, etc., is 1:1000.

In the literature of scopolamine and hyoscine and their salts it must be remembered that one is probably discussing identical therapeutic agents. Merck's *Index* mentions, in addition to the hydrobromide, the crystalline hydriodide, hydrochloride and the sulphate with the same actions and uses as hyoscine. The same authority also lists scopolamine hydriodide, hydrobromide, hydrochloride, methylbromide and sulphate, but states them to be identical in all respects with the corresponding hyoscine salts.

Adams uses a single drop in each eye of a one-half of one per cent. solution and considers the eye ready for refraction in one hour afterwards. The accommodation recovers in about three days. He regards the drug as thoroughly reliable and finds it seldom necessary to use a second drop.

The manufacturing chemist's point of view is well stated in *Therapeutic Notes,* May, 1915, as follows: The term "hyoscine" was first applied in 1871 to an alkaloid obtained from hyoscyamus. In 1880 the substance which we now know as hyoscine was extracted from the mother liquor from which hyoscyamine had been removed. At a later time a similar substance was extracted from the drug scopola, to which was given the name scopolamine. The identity of these two substances was a subject of bitter controversy among chemists for over thirty years, due to the fact that none of the substances extracted from solanaceous plants were in a chemically pure condition which would permit of determining their exact composition.

In the course of time, as the pure substances were separated and examined, it was found that they were isomeric—that is to say, they had the same chemical constitution; and it is generally admitted now that the proper chemical formula for both hyoscine and scopolamine is $C_{17}H_{21}NO_4$. For this reason it is very generally claimed that hyoscine and scopolamine are one and the same substance, whether they are extracted from hyoscyamus, scopola, belladonna, or any one of several other solanaceous plants.

Chemists further demonstrated another peculiar fact, and that is that both hyoscine and scopolamine can theoretically exist in three isomeric forms, and two of these have actually been produced and studied. In one form the alkaloid has the power of diverting a ray of polarized light to the left, or is levorotatory; in the second form it is dextrorotatory, having the power of diverting a ray of polarized light to the right; and finally there is an inactive or racemic form, which has no power of diverting a ray of polarized light. As intimated above, the levorotatory and the inert forms of these substances have been studied chemically and therapeutically, but the dextrorotatory form is as yet theoretical.

This discussion of optical rotation naturally leads to the next interesting point in the discussion, viz., that when hyoscine or scopolamine having a very low rotatory power upon polarized light is studied clinically, it is found to be less active and to have different physiologic effects than the same substances which have the power of diverting polarized light strongly to the left. Cushny and Peebles state that levo-scopolamine has double the action upon the terminations of the secretory nerves in the salivary glands and on the terminations of the cardiac inhibitory fibers of the vagus, as compared with the optically inactive scopolamine; that the levo-active and the inactive scopolamine produce the same effect in a like degree upon the central nervous system in man and mammals, and on the terminations of the motor nerves in the frog.

E. Hug, from experiments on cats and dogs, concluded that the action of levo-scopolamine on the vagus is three to four times as great as that of the optically inactive scopolamine; and that it acts twice as energetically on the oculomotorius.

Summing the matter up, therefore:

First, chemists have proved beyond any doubt that in an absolutely pure state hyoscine and scopolamine have exactly the same chemical constitution.

Second, in pure form their physiologic activity is undoubtedly very similar, and is claimed by many competent authorities to be identical.

Third, that form of the alkaloid or its salts which has a marked power of rotating a ray of light to the left is more active and perhaps differs in physiologic activity from the form which is optically inactive or which has less levo-rotatory power.

Fourth, there is reasonable evidence to warrant the conclusion that more or less of the scopolamine hydrobromide and hyoscine hydrobromide on the market is a mixture of the levo-active and the inactive forms of the drug, and hence care should be exercised to avoid the purchase and use of such admixtures.

Fifth, it is probably the custom among chemical manufacturers to supply the one substance either under the name of hyoscine or scopolamine, according to the wording of the requisition.

Reber (*Practical Medicine Series,* Eye, p. 18, 1909) has used a 1/10 per cent. solution of hyoscin hydrobromate, containing also 1/5 per cent. cocain in 2,000 refractive cases, and with much satisfaction. In about one case in fifty there is rather marked flushing of the face, quickening of the pulse and some slight vertigo, but not more than is sometimes seen with homatropin. Not once was pronounced "toxemia" noticed. Compression of the canaliculi immediately after instillation will prevent even the slightest constitutional reaction. The solution is instilled once or twice the evening before, and twice the morning of the examination. For office use cocain 2 per cent., warmed, is instilled, and the hyoscin dropped in, also warm, twice at intervals of a half hour. An hour later the testing may begin. Accommodation is sufficiently re-established for ordinary purposes at the end of 48 to 60 hours. It is not wise to attempt to hasten this by instilling eserin, as the benefit of the rest under a mydriatic is thus forfeited.

Hyoscyamin. This alkaloid occurs not only in *hyoscyamus niger* but in belladonna, stramonium and several other *Solanaceæ*. It is an isomer of atropin into which it is easily converted. Hyoscyamin crystallizes in colorless, odorless, slender, silky, anhydrous needles that have a disagreeable, acrid taste. It is slightly soluble in water, more so in alcohol, chloroform and ether. The official salts are the hydrobromide and the sulphate, both of which are to be preferred in ophthalmic practice to the basic alkaloid, owing to their ready solution in water, oil and other menstrua, and because they are more easily absorbed by the tissues. As they are decomposed by light and moisture they should all be kept in amber-colored or ''actinic,'' glass-stoppered bottles.

The action of these drugs is similar to that of atropin, although the mydriasis does not last as long in the case of hyoscyamin and the local irritation is likely to be greater. It is prescribed in from one-half to one per cent. solution. Merck's *Index* lists, besides the alkaloid and the U. S. P. salts, the hydriodide, the hydrochloride and the methylbromide, as well as pseudo-hyoscyamin, and several amorphous salts.

Alexander Randall prefers hyoscyamin (2 grains to the fluid ounce) as a cycloplegic. He has found it prompt and vigorous, holding the ciliary muscle firmly in its grasp for 72 hours, meantime giving complete, enforced rest. The cycloplegic effects practically disappear in 150 hours after the initial instillation.

Hyoscyamus niger. HENBANE. STINKING NIGHTSHADE. POISON TOBACCO. This plant belongs to the natural order *Solanaceæ*, having a five-toothed calyx, an irregular, funnel-shaped corollar and a capsule opening by a lid and enclosed in the hardened calyx. Henbane has become naturalized in America in waste places. The whole plant is covered with unctuous hairs, and has a nauseous smell, which gives warning of its strong narcotic poisonous quality.

This poisonous member of the *Solanaceæ* furnishes us with hyoscin (or scopolamin) and hyoscyamin, two of the most powerful and active of the cycloplegics. The extract is occasionally used as a collyrium: Ext. hyoscyami, 0.05 grm. (gr. 7-10); Aquæ dest., 10.0 (3iiss). It is one of the ingredients of the aqua nigra (q. v.) of von Graefe, who was also fond of using the extract of hyoscyamus as an ointment to the forehead and temples in painful diseases of the eyes.

Hypactique. (F.) Relaxing.
Hypagogue. (F.) Causing relaxation.
Hypaleiptris. HYPALEIPTRON. HYPALEIPTRUM. (L.) (Obs.) The implement or means by which an ointment is applied (to the eyes).

Hypalgesia. (L.) A term suggested by Eulenburg, for diminished sensitiveness to painful impressions.

Hypamaurosis. (L.) An old term for partial amaurosis.

Hypamblyopia. (L.) Slight amblyopia.

Hypasthenia. (L.) Weakness; slight loss of strength.

Hypemia. (L.) See **Hyphemia.**

Hypemia oculi. (L.) A synonym of hemophthalmia.

Hyperauxesis iridis. (L.) (Obs.) Extreme apparent increase in the size of the iris, causing it to seem also much darker, and resulting in contraction of the pupil.

Hyperbolic lens. A lens whose surface is generated by the rotation of a hyperbolic curve upon its axis, and designed to counteract the refraction of conical cornea. See, also, **Astigmatism.**—(C. F. P.)

Hyperboloid. A solid whose surface is generated through rotation of a hyperbola upon its axis. See, also, **Astigmatism.**

Hyperboloid lenses. Periscopic lenses having the curve of a hyperbola.

Hyperceratosis. (L.) (Obs.) A variant of hyperkeratosis or hypertrophy of the cornea, or conical cornea.

Hyperchroma. (L.) An old term for a red fleshy excrescence at the inner angle of the eye near the caruncle; also an (incorrect) term for the caruncle.

Hyperchromatism. Abnormally intense coloring.

Hyperchromatopsia. (L.) An old term for a defect of vision in which faulty ideas of color are attached to objects.

Hyperdacryosis. (L.) An abnormal increase in the secretion of tears.

Hyperemia, Collateral. In some cases of conjunctival or scleral congestion associated with circumcorneal or ciliary injection the former predominates, and to a large extent conceals the latter; in which case we have collateral hyperemia.

Hyperemia, Ocular. Congestion of the blood vessels, local or general, of the ocular apparatus is generally but a part of some other, more important, process. This symptom is considered under the various organs that it affects, or under the captions dealing with the diseases with which it is associated; thus, **Conjunctiva, Hyperemia of the.**

Hyperemia treatment. BIER'S CONGESTION METHOD. This therapeutic measure has not, especially in ocular diseases, proved to be unusually valuable, but many observers have recommended it in most chronic diseases of the lids and anterior eye segment. The Editor has employed for the purpose of obtaining ocular hyperemia both the Pynchon pump and the Victor suction apparatus and believes it has a place in ocular treatment.

Hoppe (*Münch. Med. Wochenschrift,* Oct. 2, 1906) uses an apparatus that consists of a small glass cup, rubber bulb and manometer. Applied to the closed lids of a normal eye, a 30 mm. mercury pressure produces hyperemia and serous infiltration of the skin and tarsal conjunctiva, the lids becoming of a violent hue. The congestion is the result of venous obstruction. The reaction is more marked when the lids are away from the eyeball. Lachrymation then becomes more intense, the secretion being of a sero-muco-sanguinous nature. The contents of the Meibomian tubules and goblet cells may also be expelled, although the bulbar and episcleral veins show no changes.

The marks of congestion disappear after removing the instrument. Conjunctival and cutaneous hemorrhages may occur, but only after exposing the lids to higher pressures. In such instances the lids may be discolored several days. Thirty to forty mm. pressures cause no pain. No disturbance of vision was noted.

Thirty cases of ocular disease were studied under the influence of the congestion apparatus. Six were chronic and three acute cases of purulent inflammation of the Meibomian glands, one chronic blepharo-conjunctival ulcer, one chronic hyperemia and thickening of the lid margin, two furuncles of the eyebrow, and one cold glandular abscess. The other cases included styes of various sizes and in various stages.

Treatment proved to be very satisfactory. Relief from pain was prompt, enabling the patient to attend to his occupation between treatments. Incipient inflammatory processes were checked, advanced conditions speedily regressed, often with the expulsion of a purulent core. Chalazia were less easily influenced by this treatment. Where pus had already formed, he did not hesitate to make small incisions before applying the instrument.

Thirty to forty millimeter pressures applied fifteen to thirty minutes at a time, two or three times daily, usually suffice. This method, he contends, should not be considered the only form of treatment but rather an additional remedy at our command; often used to best advantage in conjunction with other therapeutic measures. The apparatus should always be used by the physician himself. See, also, p. 950, Vol. II of this *Encyclopedia*.

Hyperesophoria. A tendency of the visual line of one eye upwards and inwards, but not sufficiently to cause strabismus. See **Heterophoria.**

Hyperesthesia, Ocular. Abnormal sensitiveness of an organ or of the nerve supply of an organ to irritants, or even to ordinary stimulants.

A good example is *hyperesthesia of the retina*—one of the developments of hysteria (q. v.).

Hyperexophoria. A tendency of either the right or left visual line in a direction upward and outward, but not to the extent of producing a hyperexotropia. See **Heterophoria.**

Hyperhidrosis. (G.) A spelling of hyperidrosis.

Hyperidrosis. EXCESSIVE SWEATING. This affection of the lid skin is noted in connection with the disease occurring on the face and body. It may be confined to the lids of one eye when there is unilateral facial hyperidrosis. In this case it indicates an irritation or lesion of the sympathetic nerve.

Hyperkeratosis. HYPERCERATOSIS. See **Conical cornea.** See, also, **Eye-lids, Hyperkeratosis of the.**

Hyperkinesis. Excessive motility of a muscle—an ocular muscle, for instance.

Hypermature cataract. Over-ripe cataract.

Hypermetrope. A person affected with hypermetropia.

Hypermetropia. HYPERMETROPY. HYPEROPIA. FARSIGHTEDNESS. HYPER-PRESBYOPIA. LONGSIGHTEDNESS. This refractive condition constitutes a form of ametropia in which the retina is situated in front of the focus

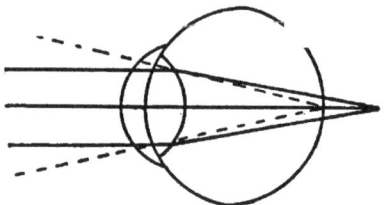

Diagram Showing Inability to Focus Parallel Rays of Light on the Retina of the Hypermetropic Eye.

of the dioptric system of the eye; and in such an eye, if it is in a state of rest, parallel rays form a circle of diffusion upon the retina. The rays, if they were to be continued, would come to a focus *behind* the retina. (See the figures.) The hypermetropic eye is sometimes called the "natural eye," or the "short eye." The word *hyperopia* (Helm-holtz), which is often used, is not as expressive of the condition as is *hypermetropia* (Donders).

The refraction power of the hypermetropic eye is so low, or its axis is so short, that, when the eye is in a state of rest, parallel rays are not united upon the retina, but behind it, and only convergent rays are brought to a focus upon that membrane. The *punctum remotum* of the hypermetropic eye is the point toward which rays should converge in order to be focused on the retina; but in the hypermetrope the *punctum remotum* is situated behind the eye, i. e., it is on the same side of the optical system as its image. Hence in this case the *punctum remotum* is negative (—R). Its distance behind the eye is equal to the focal length of the convex lens which corrects the hypermetropia. Since its retina is placed anterior to the focus of the dioptric media, the hypermetropic eye, in order to form an image, must have the object carried beyond infinity—an impossibility. Inasmuch as all objects reflect either divergent or parallel rays (there are no convergent rays in nature), such an eye is unable in a state of rest to see distinctly at any distance, unless it can add to its refractive power. This is accomplished by using its accommodation. It can then cause its lens to become more convex and thus refract the rays more strongly, thus making them convergent and thereby causing the principal focus to be thrown on the retina. (See the figure.)

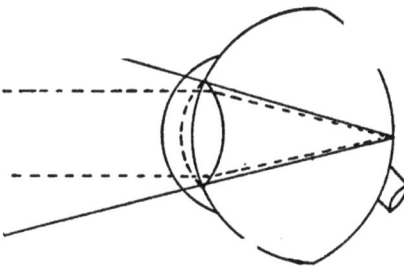

Accommodation is Necessary to Bring Parallel Rays on the Retina of the Hypermetropic Eye.

This additional convexity takes away a portion of the accommodation power merely to preserve a proper distant vision, leaving more or less of a minimum for purposes of accommodation. The result is that the near point will be farther removed from the eye; there will be a weakening of the dynamic or changeable power. Thus, in the figure the parallel, dotted rays have been sufficiently converged to be received upon the retina by the additional action of the lens, as shown by the dotted curve. A certain amount of lens action has been lost in this procedure. The remaining portion is useful only for accommodation. There being less dynamic play of lens-strength, the near point will be situated at a much greater distance than in either emmetropia or myopia.

A majority of hypermetropes have from 2 D. to 5 D. of error; cases of 6 **D.** to 8 D. are unusual. Rare instances of hypermetropia of 20 **D.** to 24 **D.** have been cited, without the presence of other anomalies, such as coloboma or microphthalmia.

The following table gives the amount of *shortening of the axial line in varying amounts of hypermetropia,* the axial line in emmetropia equaling 22.824 millimetres:

```
 0.50 D...............................0.16 mm.
 1.00 D...............................0.31 mm.
 1.50 D...............................0.47 mm.
 2.00 D...............................0.62 mm.
 2.50 D...............................0.77 mm.
 3.00 D...............................0.92 mm.
 3.50 D...............................1.06 mm.
 4.00 D...............................1.22 mm.
 4.50 D...............................1.40 mm.
 5.00 D...............................1.60 mm.
 6.00 D...............................1.90 mm.
 7.00 D...............................2.20 mm.
 8.00 D...............................2.60 mm.
 9.00 D...............................2.90 mm.
10.00 D...............................3.20 mm.
```

If the condition is due to a shortening of the eye, it is called *axial hypermetropia (Ha.).* If the length of the eye is normal and the lessened refraction power is due to a lack of convexity of the refractive surfaces, it is known as *curvature hypermetropia (Hc.).* If there is a reduction of the refraction-index of the aqueous humor and crystalline lens; or, if the refraction-index of the vitreous humor is increased, the state is one of *index hypermetropia (Hi.).*

The concealing power of the ciliary muscle and lens has given rise to the description of three clinical varieties, or types, of hypermetropia. When the defect is completely concealed by the accommodation in both far and near vision, it is known as *latent hypermetropia,* and has the symbol *Hl.* That portion which remains uncorrected and is exposed, giving rise to painful and indistinct vision of near objects, or misty outlines of distant ones, is designated *manifest hypermetropia,* expressed by the abbreviation *Hm.* In other words, it is that part of the defect that can be corrected by convex lenses without the use of a cycloplegic, whereas the latent part can be developed only by completely paralyzing the ciliary muscle. The entire amount of the error obtained by adding the manifest and latent parts is termed *total hypermetropia,* expressed by the abbreviation *Ht.*

Manifest hypermetropia is further divided into *facultative hypermetropia (Hf.),* which exists when objects can be seen accurately at infinity with and without convex lenses, and without any convergence being necessary; *relative hypermetropia (Hr.)*, in which there is only sufficient accommodation to neutralize the defect by an undue effort at convergence, and *absolute hypermetropia (Ha.)* when, even with the strongest convergence of the visual lenses, accommodation for near and far vision is impossible, objects being seen indistinctly at any distance.

The hypermetropic construction of the eyeball is congenital and often is hereditary. It is generally an imperfectly developed eye; the expansion of the retina is less, and there is a smaller optic nerve with a smaller number of fibres. The normal eyeball at birth is smaller in all the axes and there is an hypermetropia of about 3 dioptres, which is diminished by about one-third or one-half, not only by further development of the eye, but in many cases by pathologic change.

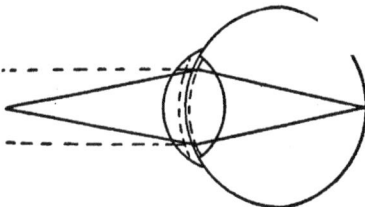

Additional Accommodation Power is Necessary to bring an Object at the Near Point upon the Retina of an Hypermetropic Eye.

The cornea in hypermetropia is more decentred than in emmetropia or in myopia; and the angles *gamma* and *alpha* are unusually large. The line of fixation passes to the inside of the visual axis through the center of the cornea, thus making the angle *gamma* positive. Donders has found that the macula in an hypermetropic eye is situated farther from the temporal border of the optic papilla than is the case in either emmetropia or myopia.

In addition to the ordinary congenital abnormality of having too short a visual axis, or too weak a dioptric apparatus, the shortening of the antero-posterior diameter of even an emmetropic or of a myopic globe, so as to produce a marked hypermetropia by pressure, has been attributed to augmentation of the retrobulbar contents of the orbit from vascular change, to excessive adipose tissue, to tumors, etc. Forward displacement of the retina in the macular region by the presence of an intra-ocular tumor, or by an exudate, may increase an already existing hypermetropia, or reduce a myopia or an emmetropia to an hypermetropia. Swelling of the nerve-head found in cases of optic neuritis will cause axial hypermetropia. Flattening of the cornea from traumatism and inflammation, and lid-pressure on the anterior part of the eyeball, are also causes. Reduction in the index of refraction of the cornea, aqueous humor, or crystalline lens will produce index hypermetropia. Aphakia, or absence of the lens, is one of the most frequent causes of acquired hypermetropia.

Hypermetropia is by far the most frequent of the errors of refraction, forming about 80 per cent. of cases of defect in school-children. Lawson, of London, found this error of refraction in 44 per cent. of all children over 7 years of age. At birth more than 90 per cent. of eyes are hypermetropic.

In many cases of hypermetropia the orbits are more shallow than in emmetropia or in myopia; the orbital margins are flattened and widely separated; the eyes are wide apart; the nasal bones are depressed, and the face resembles the Mongolian type. This relationship between the skull and the eye is emphasized in cases of facial asymmetry; here the eye belonging to the less-developed half of the head is often more hypermetropic than its fellow.

Many hypermetropes show congestion of the lids and conjunctivæ, with the formation of pustules along the margin of the lids—in the majority of instances associated with microbic invasion. Hordeola and Meibomian-gland cysts are of frequent occurrence. There is hypertrophy of the internal recti muscles. The sclerotic is thickened and dense. The circular fibres of the ciliary muscle are generally hypertrophied. In the higher degrees of hypermetropia the hypertrophy is so great that there is either a right angle or an obtuse angle formed at the junction of the anterior and the external surfaces. This is less in emmetropia. In high myopia the angle is often quite acute. The extra exertion put upon the ciliary muscle to overcome the optical defect causes an increased flow of blood to the eye. The optic disc at times exhibits a low-grade inflammation. The lymph-channels of the main retinal vessels are often thickened and opaque, while the veins may be somewhat engorged. The retina and the choroid are not infrequently congested, especially in the region of the macula lutea and of the optic disc.

The *symptoms* set up by the presence of hyperopia are (1) subjective and (2) objective.

Low and medium grades of hypermetropia are normal in the eyes of all the human race which are not excessively and constantly used for near work. It is only when the vision becomes indistinct or painful because of diminished power of accommodation, or in higher grades of hypermetropia, that the patient seeks relief.

In the lower grades of hypermetropia, especially in the middle-aged or in those using their eyes for observation of minute objects at close distances many hours daily, the patient complains of the eyes tiring easily. Such persons finally get sleepy, their lids become heavy, their eyes itch or burn, and the print begins to blur during continuous near work. They are compelled to stop, and a sense of relief is felt by pressing the eyes and forehead with the hands. Work is resumed, but the symptoms recur. This is repeated until the accommodation becomes exhausted (accommodative asthenopia) and the patient, as the result of continued eye-strain, is forced to discontinue work. The symptoms are always aggravated by artificial light. If work is persisted in, headache over the eyebrows and in the temples generally appears. In some cases the pain is referred to the back of the eye or to the back of the neck.

In the higher degrees of hypermetropia effort and strain on the part of the ciliary muscle are shown by pain in the eye or temple and forehead. In aggravated cases the pain shoots through the top of the head to the occipital region. Often the neuralgia is so intense that any change of tension in the ciliary muscle becomes painful, and reflex disturbances, usually consisting in sensations of dizziness and nausea, are developed. These symptoms are excited by work requiring rapid change of focus, as in bookkeepers, pianists who alternately glance at a sheet of music and the keyboard, or in those learning typewriting before the necessary manual movements have become sufficiently automatic not to require any fixity of gaze upon the variously placed characters. Less severe, but similar, symptoms occur in low grades of hypermetropia in persons who are convalescent from acute disease; or in those who have enfeebled or broken-down nervous systems; and in women with pelvic diseases, uterine displacement, etc., especially marked at the menopause, and during irregular menstruation, appearing after prolonged periods of abuse of the eyes, or during mental anxiety or undue fatigue. The symptoms are most severe soon after rising. The patient complains of pain in the back and top of the head, accompanied by great discomfort and dull pain deep in the orbits immediately back of the eyes. The ready fatigue of the eyes on very slight use and the neuralgia, discomfort, and blur caused by slight and moderate degrees of hypermetropia may also be very early symptoms of posterior spinal sclerosis.

In the hypermetropic eye the acuteness of vision is often diminished. In the slight degrees of error there is seldom any difference to be observed; but in the higher degrees of hypermetropia among the young, and in nearly every case in subjects who are beyond 45 or 50 years, visual acuity for both distant and near work is reduced.

In the very highest degrees of hypermetropia the retinal images become so small that the patients bring objects close to their eyes in order to make the images larger. At the same time they nip their eyelids so as to reduce the diffusion circles. This symptom may be mistaken for myopia, but can be distinguished by the want of uniformity in the distance at which the patient places his book. He holds the book far off, then again closer, and, even if the print is large and distinct, he is often unable to read fluently at any distance.

What properly characterizes the vision of the hypermetrope is not the diminished acuity of vision, but the recession of the near point, which is especially pronounced during monocular vision. The emmetropic person relaxes his power of accommodation as much as possible and then sees acutely at any distance; but the hypermetropic individual in order to see at a distance must bring his power of accommodation into action; consequently there is less power left to focus near objects, the lens reaches its maximum tension earliest, and for that reason the patient is forced to hold objects farther from the eye. This constant contraction of the ciliary muscle frequently produces a spasm of the accommodation, especially in neurasthenic individuals, giving rise to annoying blurring of distance vision. Both the near and the far point are brought nearer the eye, and vision is improved by concave lenses, which, of course, should never be ordered, as they would only increase the trouble. The condition simulates myopia, and might be mistaken for such by a careless observer, unless the eye is brought thoroughly under the influence of a cycloplegic.

The physiognomy which is often characteristic of hypermetropia, especially in the higher degrees, has been referred to. Not infrequently there is thickening of the conjunctiva, with stillicidium and epiphora, and a predisposition to herpetic disease of the cornea. Immediately around the cornea the sclera has a flat, slightly curved appearance. At the equator the eyeball is sharply curved and bulging. The cornea does not share in the imperfect development of the remaining structures, which prevents the hypermetropic eye from being classed as true microphthalmos. It has the appearance of being more convex, due solely to the shallow anterior chamber and small pupil.

In hypermetropia there is an apparent divergent strabismus when looking at a distance, due to the increased width of angle alpha,—the angle formed by the visual line,—which proceeds from an extraneous object directly through the nodal point to the macula lutea of the eye, and a line through the axis of the cornea, on the horizontal plane. The visual line in emmetropia passes to the nasal side of the axis of the cornea. The macula lutea in the hypermetropic eye is situated farther to the temporal side of the optic-nerve head than in emmetropia. Consequently the visual line cuts the cornea farther to the nasal side, increasing the angle alpha in high-grade cases to nearly double the width of that which is found in emmetropia; so that in hypermetropia in order to give a parallel direction to the visual line an extraordinary divergence of the visual axes is necessary, and, if in distance vision the necessary divergence of the corneal axes is insufficient, the convergence in looking at near objects will be relatively too great—a condition that facilitates the development of convergent strabismus.

In hypermetropia the patient must make an effort of accommodation to remedy the insufficiency of his static refraction. For every increment of nerve-force sent to the accommodation an equal amount is sent to the convergence, and, as an equal amount of nerve-force is sent to the accommodation and convergence of the two eyes, there must be an excess of convergence produced, which is still further exaggerated when the patient looks at a near object. This effort on the part of accommodation and convergence being in constant use in order for the hypermetrope to have clear vision, the habit of convergence is formed, which causes an increase in the development of the converging muscles with a corresponding weakening of the abductors, and the convergence becomes pathologic, but does not manifest itself at the same time in both eyes.

The nerve-force necessary to keep the eye directed upon the object is equally divided between the muscles of the two eyes, but in one it maintains the equilibrium between abductor and adductor muscles, while in the other, in which the sight is more feeble and the image is more easily suppressed, it goes entirely to the adductor, forming an angle double that which would be necessary if the convergence were symmetrical. Therefore we ordinarily see but one eye "squinting." Squint usually develops early in life, in poorly-nourished children, when they begin to fix their attention upon objects shown them or upon first entering school. It generally begins by being periodic, or alternating; later it becomes permanent and localized to one eye, generally the weaker, although it may alternate for years. It occurs principally in the medium degrees of hypermetropia. The higher degrees do not "squint," because good vision is out of the question under any circumstance.

Not all hypermetropes have strabismus, because of the innate tendency to binocular vision and the changeable relations between accommodation and convergence. Furthermore, it is now generally believed that the essential cause of squint .is a defect of the fusion faculty. Convergent strabismus from hypermetropia tends gradually to diminish as the patient grows older and often passes off spontaneously; so that it is rare after the age of forty. Of course, there are other causes of convergent strabismus which are discussed elsewhere in this *Encyclopedia*.

As has been mentioned, many hypermetropes show astigmatism, amblyopia, spasm of the accommodation, asthenopia, and strabismus. The small size of the cornea and shallow condition of the anterior chamber, with the relatively larger size of the crystalline lens, predispose the hypermetropic eye to attacks of glaucoma. The mental results of an uncorrected hypermetropia are shown in the languid, sleepy manner and in the dullness of intellect so often found in backward children. Remarkable improvement in facial expression and in educational progress often follows the use of proper glasses. Whether hypermetropia alone can cause epilepsy or chorea is a question which is still *sub judice*.

In examining an hypermetropic eye with the *ophthalmoscope* by the direct method, the fundus appears brilliantly illuminated; the ophthalmoscopic field is greatly enlarged, and a bright reflex, resembling watered silk, is often seen. An erect image of the fundus is visible at a distance of several inches, and the retinal vessels appear to move with the movement of the mirror. The low degree of magnifying power causes the optic disc to appear smaller than in emmetropia, and if the observer be emmetropic and his accommodation be relaxed, it will require a convex lens revolved before the sight-hole to render the image distinct. This is all that will be observed in low grades of hypermetropia.

In the moderate degrees, in addition to the appearance mentioned, there is increased redness of the optic disc, congestion, and tortuosity of the retinal veins, which is most marked near the disc. The thickening of the lymph-channels of the main retinal vessels produces a bright yellowish-white reflex, shifting with the motion of the mirror. Often the redness, slight swelling of the nerve-head, and blurring of its edges will simulate a beginning papillitis. This condition (hypermetropic disc, or pseudopapillitis) remains unchanged for an indefinite time and is probably of congenital origin. The epithelium of the choroid presents a smooth, hazy appearance. Frequently there is congestion of the choroid and retina, especially in the region of the optic disc and the macula lutea.

In the higher degrees of hypermetropia the media are clear and the disc, retina, and choroid appear nearly normal, because the patient cannot overcome his defect by increasing the accommodation to secure distinct vision. Therefore, with less physiologic action, less blood is sent to the eye, and the eye does not present the congested ophthalmoscopic picture of the lower grades, in which the patient can secure distinct vision by increasing the accommodation, thereby inviting an increase of blood to the eye.

The history of headaches coming on during or after use of the eyes; the usually slight impairment of distance vision, which may be improved by the addition of convex lenses; the removal of the near point farther from the eye than is proper for the age; the fact that the patient can read fine print through a convex lens at a greater distance than its principal focus; the characteristic mold of the face— the thickened and irritated conjunctiva, the small eyeball, sharply-curved at the equator; possibly a convergent strabismus; the narrow anterior chamber; the small pupil; the great width of the ophthalmoscopic field and small image in the direct method; the fundus-image test, and the fundus-reflex test all determine the presence of hypermetropia.

In all persons below middle age, provided the intra-ocular tension is normal, a cycloplegic should be used. This permits the surgeon to measure the amount of total hypermetropia. Prior to using a mydriatic the manifest hypermetropia should be measured. The strongest convex glass with which the patient gets vision of 6/6, or better, or with which he gets the greatest acuteness of vision, is the measurement of the manifest hypermetropia. With the eye under a cycloplegic, preferably atropin, the total hypermetropia may be measured by the use of trial lenses, by retinoscopy, or at times by ophthalmoscopy. With the accommodation completely paralyzed, the strongest convex lens with which the greatest acuteness of vision is obtained will indicate the amount of total hypermetropia. The findings by different tests should be compared; if discrepancies exist, the cause should be sought. Of the tests mentioned, retinoscopy and the use of trial lenses are universally employed. In every case of hypermetropia search should be made also for astigmatism.

Hypermetropia cannot be cured. It admits only of palliative treatment—the wearing of convex lenses. Since hypermetropia is the normal state of most eyes, the condition calls for treatment only when it produces discomfort or causes definite symptoms. Theoretically we should make such eyes artificially emmetropic by means of convex lenses; but practically this is impossible, since most hypermetropes will reject glasses so long as they can see distinctly without asthenopia.

Having measured the total hypermetropia under cycloplegia, the questions are: What shall we order? Shall we give the full correction? If not, what proportion of the error shall be left uncorrected? The full correction placed before the eye while under a cycloplegic will give normal acuity for far vision, but the use of the same lens after the effect of the drug has passed will often cause dimness of distance vision and may produce asthenopia. In this dilemma one of two courses may be pursued: (1) The full correction may be worn for a short time, and, after the accommodative power has returned, a post-cycloplegic test can be made, the strength of the sphere being reduced according to the findings. (2) Less than the full correction may be ordered. The amount of reduction will depend on several conditions:

1. If the patient is young and in good health, his accommodation will care for a not inconsiderable part of the hypermetropia. In such subjects, with from 2 D. to 4 **D.** of error, we subtract from 0.50 D. to 1 **D.** If astigmatism is present, its full correction is added to the spheric lens.

2. The amount of manifest hypermetropia will have an influence on the under-correction. The less the manifest error in proportion to the total hypermetropia, the more need will there be to under-correct. For example, in a case showing 1 D. of manifest hypermetropia and 3 **D.** of latent error (total 4 D.), usually we would order a + 3 **D.** lens for constant use. For a patient with 1 D. of manifest and 1 D. of latent hypermetropia (total 2 D.), most surgeons would order a + 1.50 sphere for constant use.

3. The patient's vocation will have a bearing. If he leads a sedentary life and does a large amount of work at near points, more of the error should be corrected than if the same individual were engaged in farming or in other out-door vocation.

4. The patient's symptoms must be considered. The greater the intensity of asthenopia, the greater will be the need of a full, or of nearly a full, correction.

5. The state of the muscle-balance must be noted. If there is insufficiency of convergence (exophoria) present, full correction is contra-indicated, whereas if there be esophoria, full correction will be worn with greater comfort.—(J. M. B.) See, also, **Refraction and accommodation.**

Hypermetropia acquisita. Acquired hypermetropia.
Hypermetropia, Transitory. See p. 3929, Vol. V, of this *Encyclopedia.*
Hypermyopia. (F.) Excessive myopia.

Hypernephroma. A tumor derived from suprarenal tissue and found in the kidney region. It may occur—an exceedingly rare accident—as a metastasis within or about the eyeball. The primary neoplasm is generally small, benign and unproductive of symptoms, while the

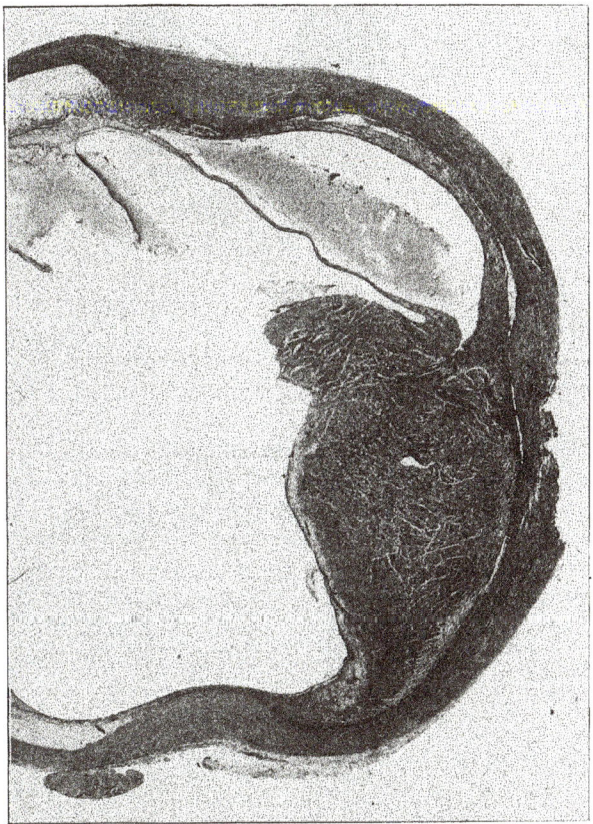

Probable Metastatic Hypernephroma of the Choroid with Microscopical Findings. (C. P. Small.)

metastatic deposit may develop into large and malignant masses. C. P. Small (*Ophthalmic Record,* Feb., 1908) gives an account of a (probable) metastatic *hypernephroma of the choroid.* The accompanying figures illustrate the findings. Histologically, the tumor cells are epitheloid in appearance; small, sharply-outlined nuclei; a few granules and nucleoli in some cells; protoplasm clear. In some cells,

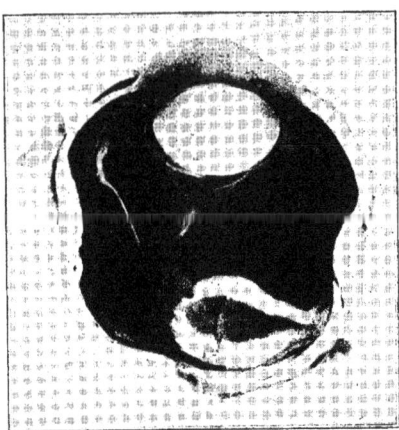

Probable Metastatic Hypernephroma of the Choroid with Microscopical Findings. (C. P. Small.)

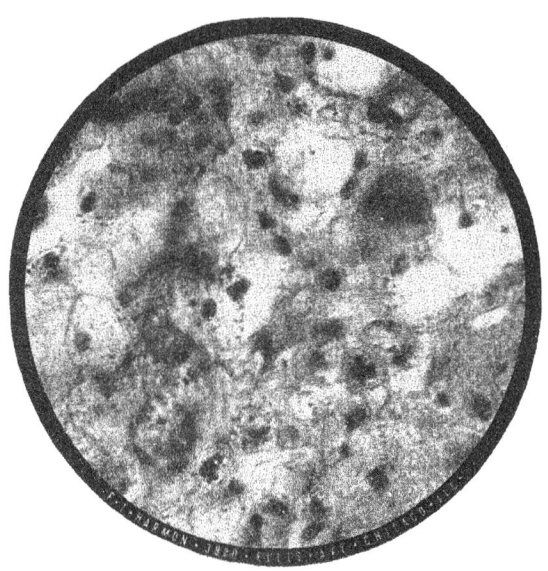

Probable Metastatic Hypernephroma of the Choroid with Microscopical Findings. Microphotograph. (C. P. Small.)

especially near the choroid, are some melanotic pigment granules. Capillary blood vessels are throughout the tumor among the cells, between which the cells are arranged in strands or cords. The capillaries show only an endothelial wall. Towards the vitreal surface the membrane is composed of long, spindle-like cells, with long, rod-shaped nuclei—possibly the endothelial cells of the capillaries—outside of these are round pigment cells, resembling degenerated retinal cells. A sharp line of demarcation exists between the tumor cells and the necrotic mass, but nuclei are numerous along this line of demarcation. The vitreous surface is sharply-outlined, the other surfaces have a gradual transition into the pigmented choroid and sclera.

The yellow pigment in the medulla of the tumor produces negative results under tests for bile, blood pigment, iron test, glycogen, cholestrin, or corpora amylacea. The light, canary-yellow color excludes melanin.

Hyperopia. A term proposed by Helmholtz for hypermetropia.

Hyperopsia. (L.) Exposure of the eyes to too great light.

Hyperoptic. Hypermetropic.

Hyperostosis, Ocular. This hypertrophic condition is of course confined, in an ocular sense, to the bones of the orbit, although eye symptoms sometimes arise from the same alteration in the sphenoid. It is a very rare disease having been noted by Bull but four times in about twenty thousand cases. It is characterized by an increase in the diameter of the bone, and is primarily a disease of the bone itself. Such a condition could, of course, cause marked and curious deformity. Syphilis is rarely a cause of the disease. See, also, **Orbit, Tumors of the.**

Hyperphaes. (L.) Abnormally clear or light. Of some modern authors, produced by excessive light.

Hyperphoria. A tendency of one of the visual axes upwards. See **Heterophoria**; as well as **Examination of the eye; Muscles, Ocular,** and p. 3954, Vol. V, of this *Encyclopedia.*

Hyperplasia. Increased growth of the volume or number (or both) of the normal elements, with often additional deposits or formations, in an organ or part. For example hyperplastic conjunctivitis, or retinitis.

Hyperpresbyopia. (L.) Extreme presbyopia; also an obsolete term for hypermetropia. Gottheff Kaestner, of Leipsic, is said to have described hyperopia under the name hyperpresbyopia in 1755.

Hyperpresbytia. (L.) Hyperpresbyopia.

Hypersarcosis oculi. (L.) Lachrymal caruncle.

Hypertension. This term is most frequently applied in ophthalmology to increased intraocular tension, but it is more generally used to designate an abnormally high arterial pressure. See p. 610, Vol. I, as well as p. 5425, Vol. VII, of this *Encyclopedia.*

L. C. Peter (*Ophthalmology,* April, 1911) believes that: 1. Arterial hypertension is the chief cause of the eye-ground phenomena observed in chronic interstitial nephritis and arteriosclerosis. 2. Similar vascular changes in the retina may be observed at times associated with higher blood pressure, before these diseases are diagnosed by other clinical symptoms. 3. It frequently acts as a cause for subconjunctival hemorrhage and is so closely associated with glaucoma that it should be regarded as an active factor in the development of the disease. 4. It probably will help to explain the phenomena of intraocular hemorrhage after cataract extraction. 5. In order to prevent the more serious eye conditions and to treat rationally, routine blood-pressure studies should be made in all cases of intra-ocular diseases not traumatic in origin.

Hypertonus. HYPERTONY. (L.) That condition of the eye in which the intra-ocular tension is increased. See **Hypertension.**

Hypertrophic conjunctivitis. Chronic catarrhal conjunctivitis with hypertrophy of the conjunctival papillæ.

Hypertrophy. (HYPERPLASIA.) The morbid enlargement or overgrowth of a part. This condition, as it affects the various ocular tissues and organs, is described under such appropriate captions as **Tarsus, Hypertrophy of the.** In *numerical* hypertrophy there is an increase in the *number* of the elements, a condition sometimes called simple hypertrophy. In quantitative hypertrophy, or hyperplasia, there is an increase in the *amount* of tissue structure.

Hypertropia. A form of strabismus in which one eye turns up. See **Muscles, Ocular.**

Hypesthesia. Diminished sensitiveness; partial loss of capacity for sensation.

Hyphema. The blood deposit or sanious exudate seen in a hemorrhage

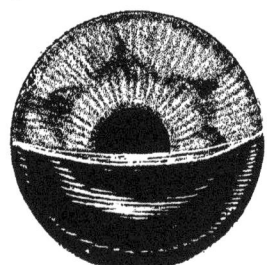

Hyphema.

into the anterior chamber (hyphemia). Blood in the anterior chamber is not infrequently seen after ocular traumatisms, operative and other. It is also occasionally found in severe iridocyclitis, in intraocular neoplasms, splenic leucocythemia, in hemophilia, and in hemorrhagic glaucoma. As hyphema is but a symptom, its treatment is naturally bound up with the conduct of the cause of the hemorrhage.

Hyphemia. OLIGEMIA. HEMOPHTHALMIA. The condition of hemorrhage into the anterior chamber. The blood or sanious deposit itself is a *hyphema;* although these terms are often confounded. This name has also been applied to ecchymosis of the conjunctiva, as well as to hemorrhages into *any* chamber of the eye. See **Hemorrhages, Ocular;** also **Injuries of the eye.**

A unique case of *alternating hyphemia* (the result of concussion of the eyeball) is reported by A. J. Ballantyne (*Ophthalmoscope*, June, 1914) in which the blood deposit disappeared on fixation of a near object and reappeared on relaxing the accommodation.

The feature of the case which at once arrested attention was that if the patient directed his gaze to a finger held seven inches from his face there was at once a considerable fall in the level of the hyphema, and then a more gradual fall until, in the course of about five to ten seconds of maintained fixation, all trace of blood had gone from the anterior chamber, leaving merely a little greenish staining of the lower part of the iris. When he was instructed to look again into the distance, the blood rapidly re-appeared, apparently from the lower angle, and after one or two repetitions of the experiment was actually greater in amount than at the first examination. The phenomenon occurred even with the fixation object directly in front of the affected eye, so that accommodation was not accompanied by any lateral movement of the eye. Digital pressure on the globe, either on the cornea or on the sclera, produced no change in the amount of the hyphema. The disappearance and re-appearance of the blood with near and far fixation was demonstrated many times in the course of this first examination, and there could be no doubt that the phenomenon depended on the contraction and relaxation of the ciliary muscle. Beyond all doubt the blood left and returned to the anterior chamber through an opening of limited extent.

The injury seems to narrow itself down to a choice between the two lesions, namely, detachment and splitting of the ciliary body.

Hyphemia oculi. (L.) Hemophthalmia.

Hyphomycetes. A group of fungi, including the molds, some of which are pathogenic, found, under various names, in the tissues of the eye.

The streptothrix, that grows in the lachrymal passages, and the trichomycetes, found in the same region, furnish examples of these plants.

Hypnesthésie. (F.) The feeling of or the desire for sleep.

Hypnosis. See **Hypnotism.**

Hypnotic suggestion. See **Hypnotism.**

Hypnotism. HYPNOSIS. PSYCHO-THERAPEUTICS. SUGGESTION. ANIMAL MAGNETISM. Long tabooed as superstition by the medical profession, this form of therapy is now used as a legitimate agent in treating disease. It is still necessary to write very guardedly upon the subject, as its action when used for the cure of disease is imperfectly understood; but that it is useful as a method of treatment is demonstrated by many cures which have been thoroughly investigated by the highest scientific men. The chief reason why hypnotism cannot be universally employed as a therapeutic agent is the fact that only a certain proportion of persons can be hynotized. The proportion, however, of persons insusceptible to its power is much less than was at one time thought; and, when used therapeutically, somnambulism, the deepest stage of hypnotism, is not necessary.

There are four main methods of inducing hypnotism, all originating in France. These are as follows: *Charcot's method,* which consists in making gentle pressure over the eyeballs, and, finally, rubbing the top of the head. *Luys' transference method,* wherein the hypnotism is induced by having the patient sit with his back to the light and look steadily at a rapidly-revolving mirror placed two or three feet from him, on which the light is directly shining. The constant flash of the light soon wearies the eyes and produces sleep. The *Nancy method,* in which hypnotism is induced by means of suggestion entirely, the patient submitting to the will of the operator. And *Voisin's method,* Braidism, where the patient lies upon the broad of his back and gazes steadily at a bright, silvered ball, suspended from the ceiling and at a distance of about nine inches from his eyes. The method of *fascination* is also used, the operator gazing fixedly in the subject's eyes at a distance of about a foot.

Hypnosis may be used as a remedy to induce simple sleep, and sleep when produced without the action of drugs is often of great importance, and of itself aids in treatment. Again, in many cases when the person is asleep, suggestions may be made to him which will abolish pain, and which in some diseases will bring about either the relief of symptoms or the cure of the disease. The patient being placed in a hypnotic sleep, his attention is directed to various parts of the body, and very often the effect is increased through local stimulation by means of passes or rubbing. During the hypnotic sleep the patient is uninfluenced by his surroundings, and therefore he is all the more open to suggestions, and no disturbing influences diminish his powers of concentration. By means such as these neuralgic or rheumatic pains may frequently be removed; headaches may often be cured, and so may some forms of dyspepsia, as well as the various manifestations of hysteria and hypochondriasis, and even functional paralysis. It is found, too, that hypnotism is useful in dipsomania and in treating persons addicted to opium-eating and other depraved tastes. At present it cannot be said that hypnotism is of use in any disease having an organic origin, although in such diseases various symptoms, especially those of pain, may be removed successfully. It is quite possible for operations to be performed upon persons under hypnotic influence without the slightest pain being felt by the patient; but as various other anesthetics are more easily employed, it is only in but few cases where these are contra-indicated that hypnotism will be used in this connection.

It is a mistake to suppose that hypnotism can only be used successfully in treating nervous or hysterical persons. Such people are often difficult to hypnotize, and there is always a danger of either increasing their troubles or in some cases of inducing insanity. Ordinary individuals, especially those who have learned to obey, are the subjects whom a hypnotist would prefer to treat. Children at school, soldiers and sailors, and officials of all ranks, are the classes from which the most successes have been obtained hitherto in treating disease. In many cases of insanity hypnotism may be used with advantage as a therapeutic agent.

Although hypnotism has power for good when properly used by medical men, it is an exceedingly dangerous weapon in the hands of the unskillful or unscrupulous. Crimes have been committed by persons who have been hypnotized. Just as a person when hypnotized is rendered extremely impressionable, and therefore capable of receiving beneficial suggestions, so he is nearly as liable to receive suggestions for evil; and it is quite possible for him during the hypnotic sleep to be impressed with the belief that he is to commit some act after he has awakened from the sleep—an act he is safe to do, acting at the time as an automaton. In this connection is may be said that suggestion has, indeed, been used, consciously or unconsciously, by certain people in all ages, and the magicians of the East are probably aware of what may be done by it, and can make the more impressionable peoples of those countries perceive what is merely suggested.

The *glamour* of the past is the *suggestion* of the present, and illusions and delusions of all kinds, including apparitions, formed part of the mysteries of the past.

It is absolutely impossible for a person to be hypnotized unless he has the idea of what is going to happen. It is a psychical and not a physical influence which brings about the condition. It should be added that in more recent years hypnotism has not realized the expectations of its protagonists.—(Abstracts from Foster's *Dictionary* and the *Standard Encyclopedia*.)

Hypoblepharon. An artificial eye; also a swelling under the eyelid.

Hypochromia. Deficiency in color or of pigmentation.

Hypochyma. (L.) A term applied by Galen to cataract. It was also used to designate glaucoma.

Hypochysis hematodes. (L.) Hemophthalmia.

Hypocœlis. (L.) An old term for the lower eyelid.

Hypocœlon. HYPOCŒLUM. (L.) An old term for the hollow under the lower eyelid.

Hypoconchia. A form of orbit which Stilling believed to predispose to myopia.

Hypocranium. The parts situated between the cranium and the dura mater.

Hypoderma bovis. See **Beef worm.**

Hypoderma hominis. See **Beef worm.**

Hypodermatoclysis. HYPODERMOCLYSIS. A method of supplying fluid to the body to replace that lost through excessive hemorrhage; or through diarrhea, as in cholera. It consists of subdermal injections of normal saline solution.

Hypodermic injections. HYPODERMATIC MEDICATION. Although the hypodermatic use of drugs in eye diseases does not differ in its technique from the same method employed as a part of general treatment, yet the ophthalmic surgeon should be impressed with the remarkable efficacy of this kind of medication. Especially in the use of powerful drugs like strychnia, cocaine, brucine, the mercuric cyanides and iodides, atropia, pilocarpine, thiosinamine, morphia, enesol, etc., the ophthalmologist should exercise the greatest care in performing this apparently simple operation. They generally exert their influence on the eye through the general organism and as such are probably no more effective when given in the temple than in the gluteal region.

It may be necessary to use hypodermics for several weeks or months at a time, and we should remember that everything connected with them should be conducted with special reference to accurate dosage and asepticism.

Whether the injections be given for their local effect, e. g., for anesthetic purposes (in the removal of chalazion, the expression of granulations or as deep, massive intramuscular medication) the results will to a large extent depend upon an accurate dosage and care in making the injections. When possible, superficial veins and nerves should be avoided, the needle should be very sharp and as small as possible, and successive injections should not be given within the same area or, for that matter, upon the same limb when the extremities are used. When a solution of cocain is injected deeply into the muscular tissue it largely passes into the general circulation and is lost so far as local action is concerned.

This is the reason for the combined use of a vaso-constrictor and a local anesthetic. The injection, especially after the Schleich method, of the solution of a suprarenal alkaloid brings about a local vaso-constriction that in turn prevents the too rapid absorption of the cocain solution into the general circulation, and also prevents, for the time being, the hemorrhage that is so objectionable in ophthalmic operations.

Lanceraux (*Medizinische Klinik*, 1907, p. 370) has reported a case of aneurism of the ophthalmic artery cured by deep orbital injections of gelatine. The patient had exophthalmus, diplopia, headache and a rumbling noise in the head; the latter symptom left off entirely two hours after the first injection of gelatine, reappearing seven hours later and then disappeared again after a renewal of the injection. The tinnitus returned with diminished intensity after the effect of each gelatine injection had passed off. After thirty-nine injections it altogether disappeared, the aneurism having completely filled with blood clot.

In retinal hemorrhage Wuillomenet (*Ophthalmology*, October, 1907), in addition to other remedies, prescribes subconjunctival injections of a sterile, 2 per cent. solution of gelatine with successful results.

Sydney Stephenson (*Ophthalmology*, October, 1908) gives the following review of the employment of injections of alcohol for the cure of angioma of the conjunctiva and blepharospasm.

H. Gifford (*Ophthalmic Record*, December, 1906) cured an angioma, one-fourth inch thick, extending from the caruncle to the fornices and cornea, but not invading the palpebral conjunctiva or the skin, by injecting on several occasions two or three drops of absolute alcohol into the substance of the tumor.

In the course of 1905 Valude claims the instantaneous cure of two cases of tic non-douloureux by injection over the stylo-mastoid foramen of 1.5 cc. of 80 per cent. alcohol with a little added cocain. One injection only was employed in each instance. The injection, as usual, was followed by temporary facial paralysis. In one of Valude's patients the spasm had lasted for three, and the other for ten, years. Abadie and Dutemps (*Archives d'Ophtalm.*, February, 1906) reported a successful case in a woman of 56 years, in whom unilateral facial spasm had persisted for sixteen years, and for five years had been so severe that she had been compelled to give up her occupation, that of a dressmaker. De Speville reported the cure of hemifacial spasm in a woman, aged 62, after the injection of 1 cc. of 80 per cent. alcohol with 1 cc. of stovain. Noceti treated with success three cases of clonic hemi-spasm by the injection of from 1 cc. to 1.5 cc. of 80 per cent. alcohol, containing from 1 cc. to 1.5 cc. of cocain hydrochloride. The injections numbered two and three. Valude has reported three cases of blepharospasm cured by alcohol injections and has taken the opportunity to discuss the question of the treatment of the condition by alcohol. Valude has now replaced the cocain, used formerly, by stovain. One cc. or 1.5 cc. is the proper amount of the liquid to inject, and the point of the needle should be moved gently to and fro while the fluid is being injected in the neighborhood of the exit of the facial nerve from the stylo-mastoid foramen.

Hypodermic syringes. In ophthalmic surgery it is important that syringes for special use should be employed and not one syringe for all purposes. The *Extra Pharmacopeia* divides hypodermic syringes into the following classes:

1. Metal or vulcanite mounted (capacity 15 or 20 minims), with glass barrels. 2. All glass. 3. All metal, graduated in 20 minims. 4. Antitoxin, capable of thorough sterilization, capacity 3, 5 and 10 cubic centimeters, in plated metal cases. The tightness of the piston is adjustable. 5. Syringes with bent, blunt needle having wide lumen, suitable for injection of sterilized paraffin in plastic operations. 6. Eucain syringes for use with beta-eucain solution for infiltration.

Hypodermic cups, of glass, are intended for holding the solution for injection while drawn up into a hypodermic syringe, or for dissolving a tablet with the aid of a glass rod as a pestle.

Hypoesophoria. An abnormal tendency of one visual line downward and inward. See **Muscles, Ocular.**

Hypoestes triflora. (L.) A species of plant growing in the mountains of Arabia; used in coughs and in eye diseases.

Hypoesthesia. Defective or subnormal sensibility.

Hypoexophoria. An abnormal tendency of one visual line downward and outward.

Hypogala. (L.) An old term for a supposed effusion of a milky fluid into the anterior chamber of the eye; a hypopyon.

Hypoglobulie. (F.) Deficiency of red blood corpuscles.

Hypokinesis. HYPOKINESIA. Defective motor response to a stimulus, as in the case of the ocular muscles, for example.

Hypolympha. (L.) (Obs.) An effusion of plastic lymph into the anterior chamber of the eye.

Hypometropia. (L.) An old name for myopia.

Hypomuqueux. (F.) Situated immediately beneath the mucous membrane.

Hypomyosthénie. (F.) Muscular weakness.

Hyponervia. HYPONEURIA. (L.) Nervous atony. A partial paralysis.

Hypophasis. A condition in which the patient's eyes are half shut, only the whites being visible.

Hypophoria. A condition of extrinsic oculomuscular imbalance in which one visual line has a downward tendency. See **Muscles, Ocular.**

Hypophthalmia. (L.) An old term for hypopyon.

Hypophthalmion. A term employed by Hippocrates and others of the old writers to indicate the parts under the eye where edema generally begins in certain chronic diseases and cachexiæ.

Hypophyseal. Referring to the hypophysis or pituitary body.

Hypophysis, Ophthalmic relations of the. See **Pituitary body, Ophthalmic relations of the,** under which caption this important subject will be considered. Here it may (briefly) be said that our present knowledge of the anatomy and functions of the pituitary gland is well stated by Sutherland Simpson (*Ophthalmology,* July, 1913; abstract in *Ophthalmoscope,* p. 479, Aug., 1914). The *hypophysis cerebri* (pituitary gland or body) is a small, reddish, elipsoidal, double-lobed, organ situated in a depression—the *sella turcica*—of the sphenoid bone. It is attached to the brain by a pedicle.

In man, monkeys, and some other mammals, the body and neck of the gland are solid, and the posterior portion or *pars nervosa* is only partially surrounded by the epithelial portion. The latter is divided into the pars anterior, which forms the anterior lobe, and the pars intermedia, which forms part of the posterior lobe. The pars anterior consists of epithelial cells arranged in columns, between which are the blood channels. The pars intermedia is composed of finely granular epithelial cells arranged in layers closely applied to the pars nervosa. The latter consists of neuroglia and ependymal cells. Colloid material produced by the cells of the pars intermedia passes through the pars nervosa into the third ventricle, where it mingles with the cerebro-spinal fluid. The pituitary may therefore be said to have an external secretion from the pars intermedia into the third ventricle, and an internal secretion from the pars anterior into the blood.

Extracts of the *posterior lobe* stimulate plain muscle in the walls of blood vessels, in the uterus, intestine, and elsewhere, produce dilatation of renal blood vessels and stimulation of the renal cells, and excite the secretion of the mammary gland. How many hormones take part in these effects is not known.

Extracts of the *anterior lobe* are physiologically inactive. Experimental extirpation of the anterior lobe usually causes death. Partial removal leads to nutritional changes in the skin and its appendages, disturbances in carbohydrate metabolism, body temperature, growth and renal function, mental dullness or irritability, sexual inactivity or atrophy of the reproductive glands, and microscopic changes in the other ductless glands. More light has been thrown on the functions of the anterior lobe by cases of diseases, e. g., acromegaly, of which changes in the anterior lobe are supposed to be the cause. Generally, this disease is supposed to be due to functional overactivity of the anterior lobe, the assumption being that this part normally produces a secretion which promotes the growth of the skeleton and soft tissues. The group of symptoms known as "dystrophia adiposo-genitalis" is associated with tumor of the hypophysis and on the same ground would be considered the result of hypopituitarism, a view supported by the results of Cushing's partial removal experiments.

It is known that functional and anatomical changes in the pituitary lead to changes in the thyroid, suprarenal, and reproductive glands, but the significance of these relationships is not yet understood.

As regards the *symptoms, pathology and treatment of hypophysis tumor,* Geo. Coats gives a review of Fleischer's (*Klin. Monatsbl. f. Augenheilk.,* 52, I, p. 626, 1914) work based on an analysis of 15 cases. In three of these the diagnosis was confirmed by operation, in one by autopsy. In eight the clinical features of the cases were so characteristic as to leave little room for uncertainty. Acromegaly was present in 11, dystrophia adiposo-genitalis in 2, simple optic atrophy in 14, post-neuritic in 1; the sella turcica was enlarged in 9 out of 13 cases submitted to radiography. An enlargement of the sella, however, is not absolutely diagnostic of neoplasm of the hypophysis itself, having been observed in other basal tumors, and even in hydrocephalic expansion of the third ventricle. The series is valuable on account of the prolonged period—up to 15 years—during which some of the cases were under observation. Fleischer is of opinion that although remissions may occur, simple tumors of the hypophysis lead almost inevitably in the end to blindness; rapid deterioration of sight may, of course, result from involvement of the macular fibres. In one case, after rapid deterioration, a small area in the nasal field of vision was preserved for ten years.

Bitemporal hemianopsia was present in every case, either complete, or, more commonly, in the form of irregular defects; typical complete bitemporal hemianopsia is only a passing stage in the evolution of the disease. In some cases the temporal defect began as a progressive contraction from the periphery; in others, however, it first appeared as a temporal paracentral scotoma, which expanded towards the outer limits of the field, a condition to be explained by a lesion of the crossing macular fibres, due either to their greater vulnerability or to their position on the dorsal surface of the posterior part of the chiasma. Yet at first sight this would seem to be a protected rather than an exposed situation; the explanation that the tumor in these cases may arise from the pituitary stalk, or from the infundibulum rather than from the hypophysis itself is plausible, but lacks post-mortem confirmation. It should be remembered, however, that the growth of true hypophysis tumors is frequently irregular, and that some of their effects are probably produced by stretching rather than by direct compression. The author emphasizes the great importance, especially in equivocal cases, of a painstaking investigation of the color fields; considerable constriction for color may be found while the limits for white are still normal, and characteristic bitemporal color defects may antedate contraction of the field for white. Irregular defects in the fields in the presence of unexplained neuritis or optic atrophy should always suggest the possibility of a pituitary growth.

In the three cases which were operated upon Fleischer was much pleased with the result. In the first the patient was free from all the distressing symptoms of the disease for three years, the visual acuity underwent no deterioration, and the field of vision improved. In the second case there was enlargement of a field which was almost lost. The third patient, in whom vision had not sunk much, remained in good health, and capable of a full day's work. Fleischer agrees with the view of most modern authorities that transcranial should be given up in favor of endonasal methods, with or without temporary resection of the cartilaginous nose. Cystic simple tumors give the best results. In his recent Bowman lecture Uhthoff spoke somewhat less enthusiastically of operation. Even the most recently published results show a mortality of 11.5 to 13 per cent., while surgeons of great experience have recorded 25 per cent. to 37 per cent. of deaths. In view of the prolonged and often intermittent course of the disease, therefore, it is evident that surgical interference should not be adopted without some hesitation. Most authorities seem to agree in thinking that the chief indication for operation should be deterioration of vision.

Hypopion. A term applied by Hippocrates to the part of the face below the eye. Of Galen, a subocular bloody effusion or suggillation; an ecchymosis of the lower lid. An erroneous spelling of hypopyon.

Hypopyon. Hypopyum. The formation of a purulent or pus-like fluid in the anterior chamber, generally as the result of some forms of iritis, iridocyclitis, corneal ulcer, etc. See, for example (and especially), p. 3449, Vol. V, of this *Encyclopedia*.

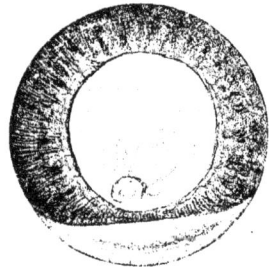

Hypopyon Keratitis, Ulcer, Striate Keratitis. (Würdemann.)

The origin of hypopyon has been the subject of much controversy. Ewing states that it has been attributed to the direct passage of leucocytes through Descemet's membrane; to the traveling of leucocytes around Descemet's membrane and their passage into the anterior chamber *via* the ligamentum pectinatum; to leucocytes originating in the endothelium; to direct rupture of Descemet's membrane; to leucocytes from the canal of Schlemm and small, deep, circumcorneal vessels; and to exudation from the iris.

Uhthoff and Axenfeld, after a series of careful investigations, doubt the origin of hypopyon from the cornea, and attribute it to the iris and ciliary body. Their conclusions have been generally accepted by modern ophthalmologists. Elschnig has attributed the breaks in Descemet's membrane to erosions produced by chemotactic changes in aggregations of leucocytes on the posterior surface of the cornea, the leucocytes being derived from the iris, ciliary body, and ligamentum pectinatum. Two points in favor of this view are the absence of bacteria in hypopyon and its frequent occurrence with intact membrane of Descemet. Onyx, a term much used by the older writers to describe the shape of an hypopyon, is now applied to a collection of leucocytes in the corneal stroma or beneath Descemet's membrane.—(J. M. B.)

The *treatment* of hypopyon is, of course, bound up with the conduct of the disease of which it is a sign and of which it forms a part.

Hypopyon intermittens. (L.) A periodic hypopyon assumed to be due to malaria.

Hyposcope. PERISCOPE. The optician has made modern warfare possible. He has given the submarine eyes so that it can see above water, while the torpedo laden craft is safely under water. He has brought the enemy close up with the field glass and telescope so that he cannot find safety beyond the vision of the naked eye and can destroy his opponent with long range fire. He has made it possible to see around corners. In the lines of trenches in France and Belgium he has made it possible for the opposing sides to watch the enemy and not be seen. He has made it possible for a soldier to aim his rifle without exposing any part of his body, not even the top of his head or eye. Instead of raising his head above the breastworks the present day soldier puts his periscope or hyposcope, as the land instrument is called to distinguish it from that used on the submarine, and which can be turned to every angle of the horizon, above the top of the trench, and gets a clear view of what is going on in front of his position.

Field glasses and telescopes are also equipped in the same manner and instead of looking directly at the image, the military observer of today looks at it through a series of prismatic mirrors and lenses, or, in the simpler instrument, plain mirrors. A haystack, a tree, a little tuft of shrubbery will conceal the observer and only the small opening of the periscope or hyposcope will be in the line of vision of the enemy.

The fundamental principle of all these devices was discovered in the sixteenth century by Giovanni Battista della Porto, a Neapolitan. He had noticed that when his window shades were drawn almost to the bottom to exclude the bright sunlight, objects passing in the street below were clearly depicted with all their colors upon the ceiling of his room, but in an inverted position. That gave him an idea for a little toy, known as the ''camera obscura,'' in which he developed the natural principle that light travels in a straight line and bears with it the color of the object from which it is reflected. He overcame the inversion of the image by a system of mirrors and lenses, which today in all essentials is the periscope and hyposcope of modern land and naval warfare.

The object to be gained in all these devices is to see what is going on and still keep out of sight. A description of the elementary periscope of the submarine will illustrate readily enough how a simple apparatus may be operated from below the ridge of the trenches. When the submarine is submerged a tube is left protruding above the surface of the water. At the top of the tube is a cylinder which, by manipulating a button below, may be turned in any direction, sweeping the surface of the water.

This cylinder contains on its face a convex lens; within, a mirror, and at its base a concave lens. Thus the rays of light bearing the images of the objects from which they are reflected enter the cylinder through the convex lens and are reflected downward by means of the mirror through the concave lens upon a white surface in a darkened chamber beneath, where sits the observer. As this surface is marked with perspective lines it becomes perfectly plain that, the size of the object being known—a battleship, for instance—its distance from the submarine may be easily calculated. Hence the periscope of the submarine also performs the office of range finder.

The simplest form of periscope or hyoscope used in the trenches is an oblong box held at the bottom by the hand. There are no lenses. The light enters at the side near the top and the images carried with its rays are reflected by a mirror downward upon a white surface at the bottom of the box, where they are observed by the holder looking through carefully shaded eye holes.

These hyoscopes can be used in connection with field glasses, giving the observer a greater range of vision and a concentration of images.

There is also a hyoscope that fits the soldier's rifle stock with which he is able to aim at an enemy while his eye and head are concealed below the trench or breastwork. This device is the invention of William Youlton, an Englishman. Some excellent rifle scores have been made by marksmen using hyoscopes. (*Chicago Tribune*, March 8, 1915.)

Hypospathismos. Hypospathismus. An ancient operation which consisted in making three incisions through the skin of the forehead and passing a spatula under the skin; used in cases of chronic eye-diseases and chronic headaches.

Hyposphagma. (Obs.) Subconjunctival hemorrhage.

Hyposthenia. A state of diminished strength.

Hypostoma. The face of insects, or that part which extends between the eyes and the base of the antennæ.

Hypothermal. Tepid; denoting a temperature placed arbitrarily between 59° and 68° F., or 15° and 25° C. Also, pertaining to the reduction of the temperature of the body.

Hypotonina. A liquid composed of sodium iodide, nitrite and nitrate of sodium, sodium bicarbonate, citral and lobelin. Its hypodermic use has been recommended (under its Italian form, *ipotonina*) by Ricca (see *Oph. Year-Book,* p. 172, 1913) for reducing abnormally increased intraocular tension.

Hypotonus. HYPOTONIA. HYPOTONY. That condition of the eye in which the intra-ocular tension is below normal, sometimes without being of necessity accompanied by organic disease of the eye-ball. On the other hand, as Ball (*Modern Ophthalmology,* p. 583) says, it generally indicates a reduction in volume of the ocular contents and follows perforating wounds or ulcers, and occurs in cases of atrophy of the globe after iridocyclitis. It is found after injury to the cerv. ical portion of the great sympathetic nerve or after removal of its ganglia. Slight reduction of tension follows the use of a bandage which has been tightly applied to the eye. It is a common symptom in detachment of the retina and in keratitis. The local use of cocain causes slight hypotony. Dionin is said to produce a similar effect.

Hypotony. HYPOTONIA. See **Hypotonus.**

Hypotropia. This is a synonym of *strabismus deorsumvergens,* or vertical squint. It may be either left- or right-sided.

Hypsicranius. Lissauer's term. for a skull having the ratio between length and height of 82.5° to 90.4°.

Hypsometer. A thermometric appliance used in measuring altitudes.

Hypsopisthius. Lissauer's term for a skull in which the angle included between the radius fixus and the line joining the hormion and lambda is between 33° and 41°.

Hyssop. *Hyssopus officinalis.* In the times of Archigenes and Dioscorides, hyssop was used as a poultice in various diseases of the eyes. The plant was first bruised, then enclosed in a canvas cloth, and steeped in hot water.—(T. H. S.)

Hysteria, Ocular manifestations of. Although the ocular relations of this neurosis have been to some extent treated on page 299, Vol. I; p. 1131, Vol. II; p. 3334, Vol. V; p. 3305, Vol. V, of this *Encyclopedia,* the subject may be somewhat further discussed here.

Hysteria, although very generally classified in our modern textbooks with the neurologic clinical entities, is, properly speaking, a mental disorder, a psycho-pathological condition. No one who has seen much hysteria will fail to appreciate how striking and interesting among the clinical features of this protean malady may be the disturbances of vision.

For example, *hysteric alopecia* is sometimes seen in hysterical children and neurotic females who systematically pull out their cilia.

Hemianopsia has been frequently noted. It is usually transitory. It may assume the homonymous, the bitemporal, and even the binasal form. Janet believes there is a stage between hysterical amaurosis and recovery which may appear as an hemianopsia.

Hysterical spasm of accommodation, or cyclospasm, is one of the most frequent manifestations of hysteria. It produces an apparent paresis of accommodation for near vision and an apparent myopia for distance. In other words, the punctum proximum recedes and the punctum remotum advances. A convex glass would be required to regain the near point, and a concave glass to regain distant vision (Parinaud). Such spasm may be unilateral or bilateral. A similar condition can be produced by eserin.

Hysterical paralysis of accommodation is not as common as the preceding. It is usually observed in young people. They are unable to read fine print at the usual distance. In hysterical convergence weakness, or paralysis, the near-point recedes and the far-point advances. If the patient is able to converge to the usual near-point he does so only momentarily. Convergence spasm and convergent strabismus are rather frequent in hysteria. They are usually associated with spasm of accommodation. When diplopia occurs there is not the usual separation of the images when the test-object is moved from side to side.

Hysterical pseudoptosis, or pseudoparalytic ptosis (Parinaud), is due to a partial spasm of the orbiculares, and not to a paresis of the levator. If the patient's attention is diverted, he may raise the lid. If the lid is raised for him, there is some resistance, and when released the lid does not fall as readily as in paralytic ptosis. Charcot and Landolt observed that in pseudoptosis the brow is depressed by the contraction of the orbiculares instead of being elevated by a contraction of the occipito-frontalis, as it is in true ptosis. A number of cases of true ptosis of hysterical origin have been reported, but they are much rarer than pseudoparalytic ptosis.

Many cases of *palsy of the external ocular muscles* have been reported. Voluntary ocular movements cannot be made, although movements may occur unconsciously.

Monocular diplopia and polyopia not infrequently complicate hysteric amblyopia. They are, however, rarely complained of by the patient, and are elicited only after a careful test. The phenomena are really due to different images being thrown on the retina when the eye is unable to focus, while there is a spasm of the accommodation. Each sector of the lens possesses a focal point of its own capable of throwing a distinct and separate image of the same object on the retina. Paralysis of associated ocular movements has been reported. Nystagmus has been noted. In most cases of hysteric amaurosis the pupil reacts normally to light. This may serve to differentiate hysteria from other forms of blindness. There may be spasmodic or paralytic mydriasis or miosis. The paradoxic pupil reaction, in which the pupil dilates under the influence of light, has been observed by Westphal and by Lépine. Hippus has also been observed.— (J. M. B.)

Four cases of hysteric *defect of the visual fields* have been described by Rönne to illustrate the fact that the defects in hysteria do not invariably follow the typical arrangement of a concentric contraction. In one case the field taken with a large test object was three or four times smaller than that taken with an object of half the size. In the second case there was a large paracentral color scotoma. In the third there was a quadrant defect. The fourth patient showed a large absolute scotoma in the lower temporal quadrant and a small relative scotoma beginning at the blind spot. Rönne considers that in this class of cases the examiner finds reflected in the visual field of his patient his own thoughts and method of examination; a condition which is all the more deceptive in that the physician, having already formed a diagnosis in his own mind, is concerned merely with controlling his result. Thus concentric narrowing of the field has its origin in the customary meridional movements of the test object, and it is not improbable that a horizontal cleft-shaped field might be produced by moving the test object up or down towards the horizontal meridian.

The *simulation of blindness* is not infrequently an hysterical obsession; the tricks and antics of the hysterope to deceive his or her friends are quite well-known to the oculist. For example, a patient, aged 16, was an inmate of the Chicago Refuge for Girls. She complained, reported Heath (*Ophthalmic Record,* April, 1907) of having gotten some pieces of glass into her left eye on the day before through the breaking of one of her lenses. Five pieces of glass were removed by one of the attendants. Considerable attention was given the girl and she was taken downtown to see the oculist, and in order to continue in that rôle she repeatedly put small pieces of glass in the conjunctival sac, which were removed by the attendants as well as the oculist. Examination of her visual fields showed them to be contracted for white with reversal for colors.

General examination revealed her to be a subject of characteristic hysterical attacks. She had areas over the body and extremities of hypalgesia and hyperalgesia, as shown by the accompanying cuts.

The date the patient was sent to the writer (Dec. 17th) may, he thinks, have been a factor in the case, because she probably enjoyed the trips to his office, as the downtown streets were crowded at that season and the shop windows were attractively filled with Christmas displays.

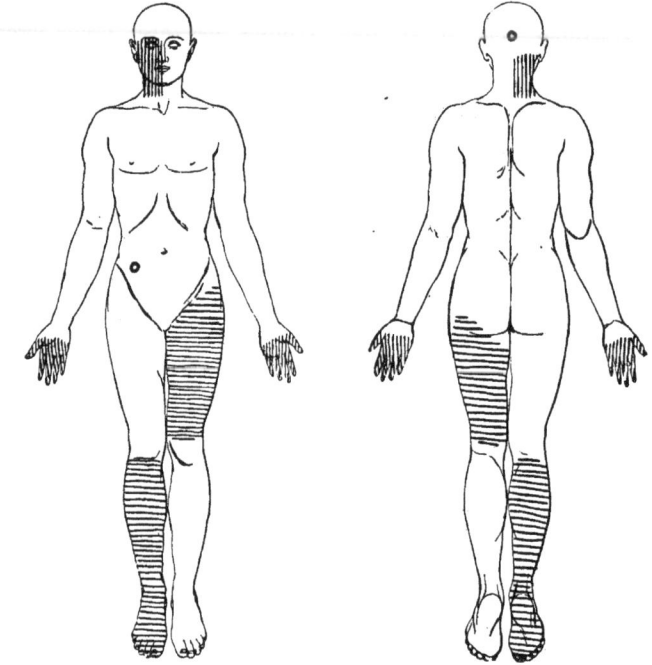

Heath's case of Hysterical Trauma.

The patient's vision is 3/50 in each eye and she wears — 8 D. lenses, with which she gets the very fair vision of 6/10.

The perimeter charts show that the red field overlapped the blue on one occasion and the red and green fields were interchanged on another day, demonstrating an inversion of the color fields, and a marked variability in the fields of vision.

For a more detailed examination of the patient's nervous condition Heath referred her to Dr. Julius Grinker, whose findings were substantially as follows: The patient is of medium-size, well-nourished and presents no signs of organic disease. She has been a nervous girl all her life. The examination was naturally directed toward hysteria, and she was found to present a typical case of that affection. The patient has had characteristic hysterical attacks, beginning usually with a fluttering in the region of the heart, and peculiar sensations about the throat, which would conclude with throbbing pains in the head. In addition, there were occasional convulsive attacks, consisting of a state of tonic rigidity, not accompanied by loss of consciousness. Nervous tremblings, so-called "nervous chills," brought

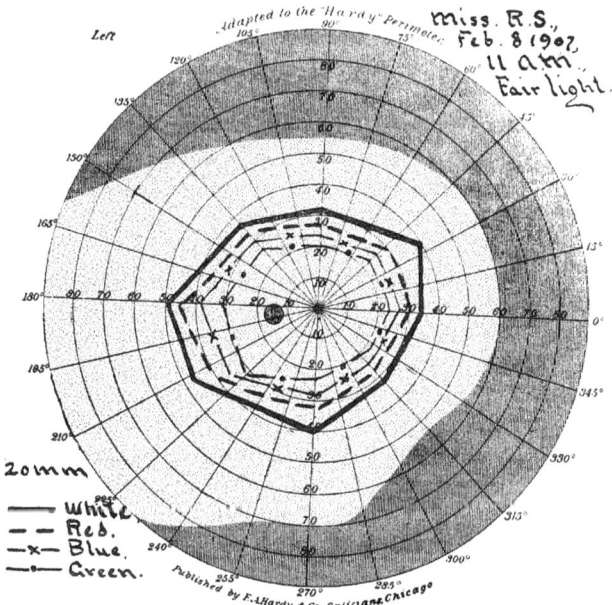

Heath's case of Hysterical Trauma.

on by emotional causes, have been quite frequent with the patient. A search for hysterical stigmata revealed a distinct degree of hypalgesia, affecting the whole right half of the neck and face below the eyebrows, beginning exactly in the median line anteriorly. In addition, the right lower extremity below the knee was hypersensitive to pin pricks, while the left lower extremity showed a marked degree of hypalgesia above the knee, both anteriorly and posteriorly. A relative degree of analgesia was noted in both hands, stopping two fingers' breadth below the wrist, and involving both palms and dorsum. A hyperesthetic zone was easily located in the right iliac region, the so-called "ovarie" of French authorities. Another point of tenderness was found over the occipital lobe, about the size of a half dollar. The reflexes were all moderately exaggerated, except the faucial, which was abolished. The corneal reflex was normal, but the conjunctival was somewhat retarded.

From the absence of symptoms denoting organic disease and the presence of the stigmata characteristic of hysteria, the diagnosis is placed beyond a doubt.

Russell (*Brit. Med. Journal*, March 14, 1908) reports a case of *hysterical somnambulism* in a woman aged 29. During the attacks she showed a condition of hyperesthesia in which she could read, write, and crochet in a light so dim that normal persons could not see to do anything; and on awakening she was unable to do the same things by such a light. Charles has made a study of the relation of monocular diplopia to hysteria, based upon recorded cases. He concludes that monocular diplopia may be due to physical causes (irregular refraction), may result from simultaneous activity of a pseudo-fovea and anatomical fovea, or may be associated with a cerebral lesion. But there is also a form only accounted for by the hypothesis of cortical disassociation, the basis upon which hysteria is explained by modern neurologists. In discussing Hansell's case, where blindness, bloody diarrhea, rectal fistula and appendicitis were all ascribed to a scratch of the cornea, Sweet, Posey, de Schweinitz and Pyle called attention to the fact, that even where the visual test proved vision in the eye supposed to be blind, this did not prove that the patient was malingering. A true disassociation, or exclusion of sensations from consciousness, may result from hysteria or traumatic neurosis.

As an exception to the rule that *hysterical amblyopia is usually bilateral* E. Valude (*Annales d'Ocul.* 145, p. 87, 1912) gives an account of a girl of 16 years who complained of having completely lost the sight of the left eye for a period of eighteen months. Since the age of 12 years the patient had been subject to attacks of loss of consciousness lasting ten minutes. The left eye was slightly deviated outwards, but appeared otherwise normal, including especially the pupil reactions. There was no light perception, nor did tests with a strong convex sphere over the right eye, or with the diploscope, furnish any evidence of simulation, or of binocular vision. Use of the giant magnet while the left eye was kept shut; and simulated operations on the left eye, were followed by improvement to a visual acuity of 1/10. But no binocular vision could be demonstrated with the diploscope, and the vision of 1/10 in the left eye was only obtained when the right eye was covered by a black disc, the use before the right eye of a strong convex sphere being attended with return of complete amaurosis of the left eye. The writer is satisfied that the patient's statement of amaurosis was honestly made, although the blindness wâs of hysteric origin.

Hysterical amblyopia or amaurosis following injuries—generally slight injuries or concussions—forms one of the most curious manifestations of the neurosis. Oddone (*La Practica Oculistica,* September, 1913) gives the history of two cases of this condition; in both the amaurosis was complete. In the first, the patient, an officer, a strong robust man, was attacked by acute pneumonia

After a slow resolution, the pneumonia was followed by empyema, and it was found advisable to make an incision to drain this. The operation was not apparently the cause of much mental distress, and no untoward symptoms were noted until the second dressing, on the following day; at this dressing he expressed his dislike to an orderly in violent language; this was noted by the medical attendant, but it was not thought to have any bearing of importance. At the fourth dressing, without warning, the patient, saying he felt ill, threw himself violently back in the bed and went into violent tonic spasm of the whole body. This lasted about ten minutes, at the end of which time he suddenly announced that he had gone blind. The eyes were immovable and the pupils were dilated and inactive to light. Examination of the eyes showed nothing abnormal either in the dioptric media or in the fundi.

Thirty-six hours after, during another dressing, the vision was suddenly restored and with the restoration, all the other hysterical symptoms, which had appeared (the nodus hystericus, varying zones of anesthesia, etc.) disappeared also.

Before the patient was discharged the visual fields were carefully examined; the field for white was slightly contracted and the perception for violet was a little altered.

The second case was that of a young and healthy man, who after a long distance bicycle contest noticed a lump in the groin. This became an abscess and was opened and drained. At the time of operation the patient was seized by tonic spasm, and this was followed by muscular relaxation during which the subject was half-conscious, fulfilling certain suggestions, which were made with a loud voice to him.

There followed a stage of excitement, and on return to complete consciousness, the subject announced that he was completely blind.

The fundi were normal and the pupil reflexes (which were lost in the preceding case) were in this preserved.

On the fourth day, at the stimulus of a little pain in the dressings of the wound, the vision was suddenly restored. The visual field again showed slight contraction for white, the color sensations were more disturbed; the man was color-blind for violet, and dark-red was confused with black.

These cases are very rare; and especially those in which the pupil reflex is altered. Diagnosis depends on the negative ophthalmoscopic findings, on the sudden onset, which distinguishes them from retro-ocular neuritis, and the absence of any cause apart from mental shock.

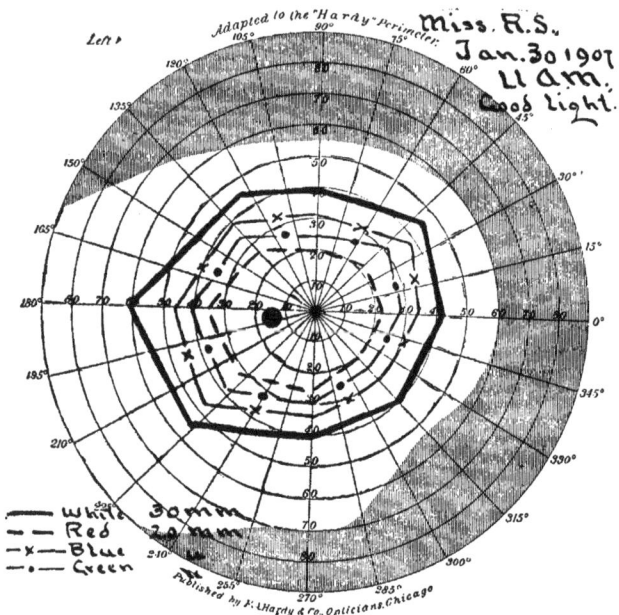

Heath's case of Hysterical Trauma.

The mechanism of the disturbance seems to be an inhibition of the stimuli which have been received by the cells of the retina, but are not passed on the cortical centres.

As hysteria reflects a morbid state of mind, which may give rise to a very great number and variety of physical symptoms, all of them, however, functional in character, it will readily be seen that the plan of *treatment must be mainly psychic.* Success will depend upon the mental acumen and personality of the physician, together with such novel measures as he may initiate with promptness, decision and power.

The early recognition of the symptoms as hysterical is a most valuable prerequisite to the successful treatment in any case. Wavering, dilly-dallying, trying first one remedy and then another in a vain endeavor to relieve a distressing symptom constitute a tacit admission in this class of cases of the physician's inadequacy or unfitness, and it is not calculated to inspire patients with the degree of confidence necessary to the accomplishment of a cure. With no intent to deprecate the talent and skill of the general practitioner, let it be said that he is not the best nor, as a rule, the last adviser in hysterical cases. Hysteria is not a grateful disease for the general practitioner to treat. A strange physician, a specialist for the eye, if that sense organ is involved, or a neurologist familiar with hysterical ocular manifestations is in a better position to institute appropriate and effective treatment.

The physician undertaking to cure a case of hysteria must feel assured of the fullest co-operation and obedience on the part of the patient. The meddlesome interference of anxious relatives and interested friends must not be tolerated. If it is impossible to restrain these pernicious influences, a new environment far removed from familiar scenes and faces is indicated and indeed almost indispensable to the welfare of the patient. In new and strange surroundings patients yield more gracefully to authoritative control and are more amenable to the reassurances of a cure.

Isolation, reducing as it does to a minimum extraneous psychical annoyances and facilitating in the highest degree bodily rest, is to be commended in extreme cases. When malnutrition is a feature, a modified or complete rest cure is beneficial.

The premises favorable, every effort should be made to destroy the obsession or fixed idea that is so deeply implanted in the mind and **capable of distorting, even paralyzing,** bodily **functions.**

Hypnotism as a general therapeutic agent in cases of hysteria has met with growing disfavor, and is by many regarded as a dangerous procedure.

Of especial significance to the oculist is the treatment of hysterical amblyopia, asthenopia, and the rarer condition of amaurosis, the anomalies of eyelid and eye muscle movement, hysterical ptosis and blepharospasm. Any of these conditions may have their origin in a trivial local irritation, a fright, insignificant injury, grief, menstrual disorder, or excessive emotionalism. To dislodge the deep initial sensory impression, awaken confidence and arouse the patient to an attitude of expectation and hope will go a very long way toward the restoration of normal vision, and it matters little whether the cure is effected by leeches, magnets, the static breeze, faradization, or any of the forms of waking suggestion. A single act or word not infrequently dispels a most distressing symptom-complex. There is little need to more than mention hydrotherapy, medicinal agents, massage, etc. All these may be valuable adjuvants with which to impress and encourage the patient.

Hysterope. A name suggested by Casey Wood to designate one who presents the ocular signs or symptoms of hysteria.

Hysteropia. A name suggested by the Editor of this *Encyclopedia* for the ocular manifestations of hysteria.

I. The symbol for iodine. In some old English and modern German words it is employed indifferently for *J*, and *vice versâ*.

Iaborandi. Another spelling of jaborandi.

Ianthinopia. Violet vision. See **Colored vision.** See, also, p. 2198 and p. 2202, Vol. III, of this *Encyclopedia*.

Iater. (L.) A physician.

Iatrion. In ancient times, the operating room or surgical laboratory of a medical man.

Ibn Abi as-Sajjar. An Arabian ophthalmologist of the Middle Ages, whose name is mentioned in Halifa's *"Book of Sufficiency in Ophthalmology."* Nothing else is known about him.—(T. H. S.)

Ibn Mendeweih al-Isbahani. An Arabian physician of the 11th century, who, in addition to a number of works on general medicine, composed a special (but unimportant) book entitled, *"On the Ocular Membranes and the Dilatation of the Pupil."*—(T. H. S.)

Ibn Serafiun. See **Serapion the Elder.**

Ibn Sina. See **Avicenna.**

Ibn Wasif. A famous Sabæan physician who flourished at Bagdad in the middle of the 10th century. He was far and away the most noted oriental ophthalmic operator, and was besieged by patients not only from India and Egypt but from far Andalusia and Gaul. He was also a famous teacher, but he left no writings.

It is related that on a certain day seven cataract-patients came in a body to Ibn Wasif's door. Of these, one offered him for an operation 80 drachma, pretending that this amount constituted his entire fortune. But just at the critical moment, the patient's girdle broke, strewing the whole floor with glittering gold-pieces. In anger, Ibn Wasif arose and drove the liar from his house. All of which shows that patients have always been as tricky and oculists as easily imposed upon and, withal, as uncalculatingly irritable as is the case today.—(T. H. S.)

Ibn Zuhr, Abu Bekr Muhammed b. Abd al-Malik. This fairly famous physician in general and excellent ophthalmologist in particular was born at Seville, A. D. 1113, and died in Morocco, 1199. Son of the famous Avenzoar, he was body-physician to the king and a well-known poet. He is said to have written a volume on the diseases of the eye, which enjoyed an excellent reputation during its author's lifetime, but which, to all appearances, has been irrecoverably lost.—(T. H. S.)

Ibn Zuhr, Abu Muhammed Abdallah b. Abu Bekr Muh. This well-known grandson of the much more famous Avenzoar would seem to have been an excellent practical oculist and writer on diseases of the eye. Nothing from his pen, however, is extant.—(T. H. S.)

Ice. Water in the solid form. It is specifically lighter than water which is just about to freeze, and therefore floats in it. Water, in becoming solid, expands about 1/11th in volume, and thus acquires

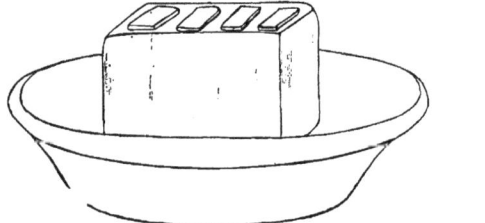

Eye Pads on Ice for Application of Extreme Cold. Small Ice-bag for the Eye.

a density equal to 0.91674 (water at 0° C.=1.00). The formation of ice takes place generally at the surface of water. This is owing to the peculiarity that, when water has (at the ordinary atmospheric pressure) cooled down to within 3.9° C. of freezing, it ceases to contract with increase of cold, and begins to expand until it freezes; this causes the coldest portions of the water to float always on the surface. In some circumstances ice forms at the bottom of rivers, and is called *ground-ice* or *anchor-ice*.

Water in ordinary cases freezes at the degree of temperature marked 0° on the Centigrade and Réaumur's thermometers and 32° on Fahrenheit's; but if it is kept perfectly still it may be cooled to nearly —5.5° C. below freezing (=22° F.) and still remain liquid. Sea-water and salt water in general freeze at a lower temperature than pure water. To melt a pound of ice it is necessary to communicate to it as much heat as will raise 80.025 pounds of water 1° C. This measures the "latent heat," of ice.

The accompanying figures depict the usual methods of applying extreme cold, in the form of ice, to the eye.

Ice-blink. A luminous appearance on the horizon due to the reflection of light from a surface of ice.

Iceland spar. CALCITE. A transparent crystalline form of calcium carbonate, and at one time found in great quantities in Iceland. It crystallizes in many forms, each of which may be reduced, through cleavage, to a rhombohedron, bounded by six similar parallelograms with angles equal to 101° 55′ and 78° 5′. Two opposite solid angles are encompassed by three obtuse angles, whereas each of the remaining solid angles is encompassed by one obtuse angle and two acute angles. The diagonal line, through the crystal, which connects the corners containing the three obtuse angles, or any line drawn parallel to it, is termed the axis of the crystal, in which no double refraction occurs. See **Axis**; also **Double refraction.**—(C. F. P.)

Ichthargan. Silver ichthyolate. Soluble silver sulphichthyolate.

Ichthyol. AMMONIUM ICHTHYOLSULPHONATE. DESICHTOL. AMMONIUM ICHTHYOL. AMMONIUM ICHTHYOLATE. The source of this valuable remedy is a crude fish-oil obtained from fossil rocks in the Tyrol. It is a transparent, yellow-brown liquid with a peculiar, fishy odor. What we know as ichthyol is a syrupy, reddish-brown, transparent liquid of a bituminous odor and taste, soluble in water and glycerin and made by the action of ammonia on an ichthyol derivative. In the same way we have a sodium-zinc-and calcium ichthyol. Deodorized ichthyol is known by the trade name of desichtol.

Were it not for its disagreeable odor and dark color this compound would be more generally employed in blepharitis and allied diseases. It has been successfully employed as a one per cent. mixture with lanolin, cold cream and petrolatum. Von Schlen advises the following formula in blepharitis eczematosa: Ichthyol, 0.03 gm. (gr. ½); amyli, zinci ox. āā, 10.0 gm. (ℨiiss); vaselini, 25.0 (ℨvi, gr. xxv). Another formula by Michel is: Ichthyol, zinc. ox., gelatini, āā, 5.0 gm. (ℨj 1-3); glycerini; aquæ dest. āā, 25.0 c.c. (fℨvi. mxxv). To be warmed before applying.

C. T. Caldwell advises the following ointment in angular conjunctivitis and corneal ulcer due to the diplobacillus: Ammonii ichthyol., 0.15; zinc. oxid., 5.00; vaselin, alb., 15.00. To be thoroughly mixed and applied both to the inside and outside of the lids.

Ichthyosaurus. This extinct "fish-reptile" constitutes a remarkable genus that inhabited the prehistoric seas during the deposition of the Mesozoic strata. Like the modern Cetacea, their structure was modified to suit their aquatic life. The body was shaped like that of a fish, the limbs were developed into paddles, and the tail, long and lizard-like, was furnished, it is believed, with a fleshy fin, as in the dolphin, except that its position was vertical. The head was large, and protruded into a long and pointed snout, resembling that of the crocodile, except that the orbit was much larger, and had the nostril placed close to it, as in the whale, and not near the end of the snout. The jaws were furnished with a large series of powerful conical teeth, lodged close together in a continuous groove, in which the divisions for sockets, which exist in the crocodile, were indicated by the vertical ridges on the maxillary bone. The teeth were hollow at the root, sheathing the young teeth, which gradually absorbed the base of the older ones, and, as they grew, pressed them forward, until they finally displaced them. The long and slender jaws were strengthened to resist any sudden shock by being formed of many thin bony plates, which produced light and elastic as well as strong jaws. *The most remarkable feature in the head was the eye, which was not only very large—in some specimens measuring 13 in. in diameter—but was specially fitted to accommodate itself for vision in air or water, as well as for speedily altering the focal distance while pursuing its prey.* The structure, which thus fitted the eye so remarkably to the wants of the animal, consisted of a circle of thirteen or more overlapping sclerotic bony plates surrounding the pupil, as in birds. This circle acted as a sort of self-adjusting telescope, and, assisted by the extraordinary amount of light admitted by the large pupil, enabled the ichthyosaurus to discover its prey at great or little distances in the obscurity of the night, and in the depths of the sea. The neck was so short that the body was probably not in the least constricted behind the head. The backbone was fish-like; each joint had both its surfaces hollow, making the whole column very flexible. The small size of the paddles compared with the body, and the stiffness of the short neck, seem to suggest that the tail must have been an important organ of motion.

The remains of the ichthyosauri are peculiar to the Mesozoic strata, occurring in the various members of the series from the Lower Lias to the Chalk, but having their greatest development in the Lias and Oolite.—*(Standard Encyclopedia.)*

Ichthyosis, Ocular. See **Conjunctivitis entomotoxica,** on p. 3101, Vol. IV of this *Encyclopedia.*

Ichthyosis palpebrarum. Ichthyosis affecting the eyelids.

Iconantidiptychon. (Obs.) A lens giving a double image of an object, but with one of the images inverted.

Iconic. Iconical. Of the nature of, or pertaining to, an image or a portrait.

Iconograph. A pictorial representation.

Iconographie. (F.) Photography.

Iconograms. A word coined by Faxton E. Gardner, of New York, and used as the title of a book which is a collection of colored plates illustrating surgical conditions.

Iconometer. Literally, an image-measurer, but as generally understood, an optical instrument for finding any one of the following data when the other three are known: (1) the size of an object; (2) that of its image cast by a photographic lens; (3) the character of the lens, and (4) the distance of the object from the image.

Iconoscope. An instrument devised by Javal for testing binocular perception of depth. It resembles an inverted telestereoscope (q. v.).

Ictère. (F.) Icterus; jaundice.

Icterus neonatorum. When this infantile disease is complicated with purulent ophthalmia the pus—but never the tears—is stained yellow.

Identical points of the retina. See p. 3539, Vol. V of this *Encyclopedia*.

Identical visual directions. The law of identical visual directions, elaborated by E. Hering in 1861, and that of J. Mueller of identical retinal points, Milutin (*Doctorate Thesis*, Berne, 1914) regards as the most important discoveries in the physiology of the senses. As these laws are not generally accepted, Milutin wished to extend the previous experiments for a larger number of corresponding retinal points, which she did under the guidance of Asher, of Berne. She describes a method for demonstrating the law of the identical visual directions and for keeping a graphic record of them. The validity of this law was demonstrated in the primary position for a larger number of eccentrical retinal points, and also in secondary positions (raising the eyes, lateral movements of the head, etc.) for central and eccentric retinal points. The difference of direction which results between exact and approximately identical visual objects is distinctly noted. This was demonstrated by using the true horopter as the position of the fixed points. Care was taken that objects intentionally put next each other did not produce mistakes. The results found support the theory that the observation of the visual directions is the result of stable conditions in the retina.

Identity, Ocular signs of. See **Legal relations of ophthalmology,** in middle third of section.

Idiacoroiris. (L.) A term, suggested by G. P. Poggi, for the formation of an artificial pupil.

Idiocy. AMENTIA. This cerebral defect is defined by Ireland as ''mental deficiency or extreme stupidity depending upon mal-nutrition or

disease of the brain occurring either before birth or before the evolution of the mental faculties in childhood; while imbecility is generally
used to denote a less decided degree of such mental incapacity.'' The
difference between both conditions and *dementia* is that the dement
was once sane and responsible, the idiot and the imbecile never
developed mental capacity at all; they remained arrested children.
There are great varieties of idiocy and imbecility. Some of the lowest
have no speech, no power of distinguishing between one person and
another, no affection or hatred, no feelings of pleasure or pain, no
power to take care of themselves, and can never be taught any of these
things. In body such idiots are dwarfish, misshapen, ugly, with the
features and expression of face often of the lowest of the lower animals, with no power of walking. This being the condition of the lowest varieties, they rise gradually in the scale till many imbeciles are
beautiful in features, and reach normal bodily development, but are
slightly wanting in some essential mental faculty, in intelligence,
affection, control, or self-guidance. The mental deficiency is in by
far the majority of idiots and imbeciles accompanied by corresponding bodily weaknesses of some sort.—(Abstracted from the *Standard
Encyclopedia.*) See **Amaurotic family idiocy**; also **Familial diseases**;
as well as **Heredity in ophthalmology**; and **Imbecility.**

A. W. Ormond (*Ophthalmic Review*, p. 379, Dec., 1911) reports of
43 Mongolian idiots that they had a certain liability to particular
ophthalmic diseases. Over 50 per cent. had a defect in their lenses,
and almost all had some ocular defect. Sometimes Mongolians could
be recognized as early as the second year. When seen later they were
short of stature, due mainly to the shortness of the limbs. The head
was round and the occipital protuberance of the skull ill-developed.
The hands were small and the thumbs squat, the little finger being
incurved. The foot was flat, and the subjects often sat tailor-fashion.
They had a difficulty in pronouncing certain consonants. They were
imitative, fond of music and affectionate. Most of them died from
tuberculosis, and they did not often attain adult life. There was
almost constantly some ocular trouble present—blepharitis, ectropion,
squint, nystagmus, or lens opacity. Blepharitis and conjunctivitis
might be primarily due to dirty habits, and might be kept up by
uncorrected errors of refraction. A more certain cause of the inflammatory condition of the lids was a dry, glazed condition of the skin
of the lower lids, which, by its contraction, caused a slight degree of
ectropion. In more than 50 per cent. of his cases, some form of lens
opacity was present, and with such a high proportion, it might be
regarded as an aid to diagnosis. The cataracts were of the incomplete

form, and most of them of the "dot" variety, in the position common for lamellar cataract. These dots, when slight were often translucent, and so could not be seen by transmitted light. The opacities did not reach to the periphery of the lens in any direction, and consisted of numerous small discrete dots. The posterior pole of the cataract was often marked by a star-shaped opacity. Though the teeth of these people were defective, they did not show the honey-combed condition so frequent in cases of lamellar cataract. Ormond could not record accurately the visual acuity, as the children were not sufficiently controllable to be trusted with glasses. The youngest of the patients showing cataract was aged 6½ years, and the oldest 43. Mongolian imbeciles were, in many cases, the children of old parents, or the last child in a large family. Of his 42 cases, 32 were males, and 10 females. The average was 14¾ years. Twenty-three had the interpalpebral fissure directed upwards and outwards, 5 had nystagmus, 9 had squint, 18 had either blepharitis or ectropion, or both, 11 had epicanthus, and 25 had some lens opacity.

Idiocy, Amaurotic family. TAY-SACHS DISEASE. See **Amaurotic family idiocy**; also **Familial affections**; and **Idiocy.**

Idiopathic. Originating from within; designating a disease not due to external or evident causes.

Idiophanous. A term applied to certain types of crystals which exhibit axial interference figures without necessitating the use of a polarization apparatus.

Idiopt. A term proposed by Professor Whewell to designate a person having a peculiarity of vision now universally known as color-blindness.

Idiosyncrasy. See **Disposition.**

Idiot. See **Idiocy.**

Idrocefalo. (It.) Hydrocephalus.

Idrope del sacco lagrimale. (It.) Hydrops of the lachrymal sac.

Idrottalmo. (It.) Hydrophthalmus.

Ignescent. Emitting sparks; scintillating.

Ignipuncture. A method of treatment which consists in making punctures with a cautery.

Ilamides. (F.) The meninges.

Ilingos. ILINGUS. (L.) An old name for vertigo.

Illacrymatio. (L.) Excessive involuntary weeping; epiphora.

Illaqueation. An ancient operation, probably devised by Celsus, for restoring the position and direction of a single cilium in distichiasis by passing a fine needle and thread through the border of the lid and around the misplaced follicle, and drawing it into its normal position through the puncture made by the needle.

Illis. (L.) A term, attributed to Galen, for one who squints.

Illiterate charts. See **Examination of the eye.**

Illiterate test chart. KINDERGARTEN TEST-CARD. OBJECT TEST CHART. See p. 2022, Vol. III, and p. 4653, Vol. VI, of this *Encyclopedia.*

Illosis. (L.) (Obs.) Strabismus.

Illuminated bodies. Bodies which reflect, but not emit, light.

Illuminating apparatus, Office. See p. 4603, Vol. VI, of this *Encyclopedia.*

Illuminating gas, Ocular symptoms of poisoning by. These are: diminution of visual acuity, with contraction of the visual field; dilatation of the retinal veins and contraction of the arteries. Persistent bilateral hemianopsia after recovery, has been recorded. There is sometimes paralysis of the various ocular muscles, extrinsic and intrinsic, accompanied or unaccompanied by exophthalmia. When the recti are paralyzed, there is always exophthalmia. See **Legal relations of ophthalmology,** in middle third of the section. See, also, **Toxic amblyopia.**

Illumination. INTERIOR AND EXTERIOR LIGHTING, OCULAR RELATIONS OF. As civilization advances there is an increasing amount of close visual work in offices, factories and homes, and a tendency to arrange buildings so that the natural light is restricted and artificial light must be used to an increasingly greater extent. It is by virtue of the illumination or light upon various objects that vision is made possible. A study of the conditions of illumination both by daylight and by artificial light which are best for the comfort and health of the eyes, is of tremendous importance to the human race. The intelligent study of methods of illumination and their bearing on the conservation of vision has only recently begun to be given the serious attention which it deserves.

Illumination is that which renders objects "bright" or visible. We see ordinary non-luminous objects because of the various intensities and colors of light which are reflected into the eye from the different parts of such objects and their surroundings. In other words we see them by reason of variations or differences in the brightness and color of their surfaces and their background. It is only by virtue of such differences that images are thrown upon the retina of the eye. The study of good and faulty illumination conditions therefore is a study fundamentally of brightness produced within the range of vision by illumination of different kinds.

That the brightness of objects resulting from the illumination must be sufficient to enable objects to be seen clearly enough for the purposes in hand is evidently one of the first requirements. In common language there must be light enough to see 'by. Insufficient brightness of the visualized object may be merely annoying; or if eye work is attempted under such conditions for too long a time it may produce well-defined eye-fatigue and strain.

A second essential to good illumination is reasonable steadiness; that is, avoidance of flicker.

Both these foregoing requirements are easier to meet than the third, which affords a fertile field for study in the elimination of faulty illumination conditions, namely, the avoidance of glare in its various forms. The study of glare involves the study of the relative distribution of brightness within the field of vision. That is, when glare is . present certain portions of the field of vision are excessively bright as compared to other portions. (See **Glaring.**) So much depends upon the existence or non-existence of glare within the field of vision and the question of sufficient quantity of illumination on the visualized object is so interrelated with it that glare, or distribution of brightness within the range of vision, will be taken up first.

Glare or distribution of brightness. Glare has been defined by the 1915 Committee on Glare of the Illuminating Engineering Society as follows: (1) Brightness within the field of view of such excessive character as to cause discomfort, annoyance, or interference with vision. (2) Excessive brightness of or flux of light from the whole or any portion of the field of view, resulting in reduced vision, fatigue, or discomfort of the eye. (3) Light shining into the eye in such a way and of sufficient quantity as to cause discomfort, annoyance, or interference with vision.

These definitions recognize that glare includes three different effects on the eye, viz., mere annoyance; measurable or observable fatigue or strain; and finally the "blinding effect" or positive interference with visual acuity which takes place with some conditions of glare. These three effects are discussed later under the head of "Effects of glare on the eye."

Various kinds and degrees of glare have been defined and enumerated by the committee referred to.

Brightness glare is a term which may be used as applying to glare caused by an area of brightness within the visual field which is above the maximum limit of full brightness accommodation of the eye. The most notable example of this is the glare from the sun. In this case the brightness is of a high order of magnitude and comes from a very small portion of the field of view. Another example is the glare from a very powerful electric lamp close at hand. Brightness glare from such powerful restricted area light-sources is so obviously annoying and dangerous that it is instinctively avoided and hence little need be said of it in connection with the practical effects of illumination upon the eye. The less pronounced glare effects which are slow-acting and therefore more insidious require more careful study on the part of the oculist and the illuminating engineer.

Sunlight reflected from a large snow field or light desert sand is another example of brightness glare. In this case while the bright-ness of any one patch of snow is not intolerable the total flux of light from the large field (entering the eye from below which is an unac-customed angle) is sufficient to produce all the effects of glare. This also is an abnormal and instinctively avoided condition of illumination.

Contrast glare is a term which may be used to apply to excessive contrast of brightness within the field of view. Contrast glare is at the bottom of the majority of the defects or faults in artificial light-ing and also defects in natural or day-lighting of interiors where the lighting is unsatisfactory for reasons other than insufficient quantity. In a case of pure contrast glare the brighter surface which causes the trouble is one which could be comfortably viewed amid lighter or brighter surroundings. However, when viewed on a much darker background it causes one or all of the bad effects upon the eye enu-merated. One good example of contrast glare is a small patch of sky seen through a window from the rear of a dark room. This sky brightness which would be perfectly comfortable out of doors in the open for a normal healthy eye, causes discomfort when contrasted with the dark field or surroundings of the darkened room. Another example of contrast glare is the globe of a lighted electric or gas lamp which may be scarcely brighter than a hazy sky and hence unnoticeable in the day-time out of doors when the eye is adapted to the general level of brightness prevailing outdoors. The same globe indoors at night amid a lower general level of brightness, and in particular against a background much less bright, may be very annoying and possibly fatiguing if faced continuously.

Temporary glare is a term which may be used for glare caused by sudden introduction of brightness within the field of vision before the eye has had an opportunity to accommodate for the change of brightness conditions. When there is flicker there is a rapid repeti-tion of this.

Veiling glare is glare caused by reflection or diffusion of light form-ing a light veil obscuring the object viewed. Examples are glare from glossy paper, landscape viewed through a haze, objects seen through dirty windows upon which the light is shining or the oiled paper of a window envelope when viewed at certain angles. The interference with vision is caused by specular or diffuse reflection from the veil.

Contrast glare effect in a preceding paragraph has been charged with many of the troubles connected with faulty illumination and it has already been defined in a general way. In order to define it specifically, however, we must determine the limits of tolerance, or in other words the maximum contrast, which the eye will tolerate without annoyance, discomfort, eye-fatigue or interference with vision. In the practical lighting of interiors to avoid contrast glare effects it is essential to determine what contrast ratios of brightness of adjacent surfaces the eye can tolerate continuously without suffering any of the fatiguing or annoying effects of glare. While the experimental data are not perhaps as complete as might be wished, enough has been collected to set a tentative limit of good practice. In sunlight, out-of-doors brightness ratios of adjacent surfaces (excluding, of course, the sun which is avoided by the eye) are not usually over 1 to 20, and generally much less. The largest contrast ratios are on bright days when the contrast is between surfaces in full sunlight and those in deep shadow. We know that the eye is adapted to ordinary outdoor conditions without suffering the effects of glare. For indoor conditions the data so far obtainable on the effects of glare consist of measurements of brightness taken both in rooms where conditions are known to have been such as to produce glare effects because of the complaints of the occupants, and also measurements in other rooms where no such complaints have been made. We also have brightness measurements in rooms used in a limited number of tests made for eye-fatigue by the Ferree method (which is described more fully later) under conditions which produced varied amounts of eye-fatigue. A study of this data shows that usually where the bad effects of glare have not been observed, the contrast ratios between the brightest surfaces within the range of vision and the surfaces surrounding the brightest surfaces in the field of view are not over 1 to 100. Of course the contrast ratio taken in this case is that presented to the eye.

For a tentative working limit for the present, after considering the facts with both natural and artificial lighting, it looks probable, as stated by the Glare Committee report, already quoted, that the comfortable limiting ratio between the brightest surface and its surroundings lies somewhere between 1 to 100 and 1 to 200, and preferably until we have more evidence the contrast in brightness of adjacent surfaces should if practicable be kept below the 1 to 100 ratio, where long-continued work is done.

The accompanying table gives the brightness of various sources of light and also the brightness of some common reflecting surfaces illuminated with common quantities of illumination.

APPROXIMATE BRIGHTNESS OR INTRINSIC BRILLIANCY OF VARIOUS PRIMARY AND SECONDARY LIGHT SOURCES:

Light Source	Millilamberts *
Sun at zenith (rough equivalent values, taking account of absorption)	292,020,000
Sun at 30° elevation (rough equivalent values, taking account of absorption)	243,500,000
Crater, carbon arc	40,800,000
Flaming arc, clear globe	2,435,000
Calcium light, clear globe	2,435,000
Magnetite arc, clear globe	1,945,000
Nernst glower, unshaded	1,460,000
Gas filled tungsten electric lamp filament	1,400,000
Sun at horizon, rough equivalent value, taking account of absorption	973,400
Incandescent electric tungsten, 1.25 watts per candle	516,000
Quartz tube, mercury vapor arc .... 486,700 to	292,000
Incandescent, electric, graphitized carbon filament, 2.5 watts per candle	365,000
Incandescent electric tantulum filament, 2 watts per candle	282,400
Incandescent electric carbon filament, 3.1 watts per candle	236,000
Incandescent electric carbon, 3.5 watts per candle....	194,500
Incandescent electric carbon, 4 watts per candle	158,100
Enclosed electric arc, opalescent inner globe—36,500 to	73,000
Melting platinum	62,750
Welsbach (mesh)	27,250
Acetylene flame (1 foot burner)	25,800
Acetylene flame (¼ foot burner)	16,050
Welsbach mantle	15,080
Cooper Hewitt glass tube mercury vapor lamp	6,800
Kerosene flame .... 1,946 to	4,380
25-watt frosted tungsten lamp, side	2,920
Candle flame .... 1,460 to	1,945
White paper in full sunlight	10,000

---

* 1 candle-power per sq. in. equals 486.7 millilamberts.

Light Source	Millilamberts
Sky, with light clouds............................	2,075
Sky, clouds predominating, generally cumulus........	1,887
Sky, blue predominating, clouds cirrus..............	1,484
Gas flame (fish tail)............................	1,314
Sky, cloudless, either clear blue or hazy..............	1,046
25-watt frosted tungsten lamp, tip..................	812
Sky, cloudy, storm near or present............676. to	73.
Moore tube ....486 to	243
10-inch opal ball, over 100-watt tungsten lamp........	306
Walls, typical rooms, ordinary range, diffused daylight through window ....48.6 to	0.973
Ceilings over indirect lighting fixtures (usual range, brightest part as viewed by occupants of room)..... ....73. to	4.18
Glass bowls used for semi-direct lighting......1000. to	35.
White paper illuminated to 5 foot candles (diffuse reflection)	4.04
Walls of typical small rooms with ample artificial light ....3.00 to	.0073

BRIGHTNESS VALUES IN AN OFFICE EQUIPPED WITH EIGHT SEMI-DIRECT UNITS OF PROPER DENSITY AND LIGHT-COLORED WALLS (DURGIN AND JACKSON) :

	Millilamberts	
	Mean	Maximum
Bottom of glass bowl...........................150		190
Side of glass bowl 60		90
Ceiling above bowl............................. 55		60
Ceiling at center of four unit square.............	1.2	1.4
Ceiling at middle of side of four unit square........	2.8	3.0
Side wall 6 ft. from floor........................	2.6	2.6
Side wall 4 ft. from floor........................	1.8	2.2

It is not claimed that it is feasible or desirable to keep all contrasts with artificial illumination below the 1 to 100 limit, as that would practically prohibit all present feasible methods of street lighting and make unnecessarily expensive some artificial lighting of interiors. Where the brightest surfaces are not to be faced continuously for considerable periods of time the only bad effects of the glare are discomfort and annoyance of a very temporary nature and in many cases not even annoyance would be felt. The bad effects would come from

long-continued subjection of the eye to contrast conditions in excess
of the figures named.

The practical effects of limiting contrast ratios to 1 to 100 or less
in interior artificial lighting at the present time would be to limit the
brightness of bowls and globes in locations where they must be faced
continuously to an approximate value of 250 millilamberts (about
¼ the brightness of a blue sky) for rooms with light-colored ceilings,
and walls with an illumination on desks and tables of about 4 foot-
candles. Practically all of the lamps and their globes used for direct
lighting, and a majority of those used for semi-direct lighting are, at
present writing (1916), in excess of this value (see Brightness Table)
so that great care should be taken in this respect.

In order to secure the most comfortable lighting conditions with
artificial light it is usually necessary to obtain most of the useful
illumination by reflection from a ceiling, permitting only a small percentage of the light to come directly through the glassware of the
fixture. In some interiors this is, of course, impracticable.

With daylight the brightness of the sky is to be dealt with. Too
great a contrast between the sky brightness as seen through the window and the brightness of the window casing and surroundings in the
room will cause contrast glare and its consequent bad effects. The
contrast will be most pronounced when the window surroundings
receive but little light by reflection from the interior of the room.
This is the case when the room is very deep in proportion to the window area. It is still further accentuated when ceiling, walls and floor
are dark in color. This is one good reason for certain school building
regulations which have been proposed and enacted from time to time
requiring a minimum amount of window area to floor area, although
this is not the main reason for such regulations.

Veiling glare effects caused by specular reflection from glossy paper
are common and well-known sources of eye-strain. Although it is due
primarily to the smoothness of the surface of the paper rather than
to the illumination, nevertheless the character of the illumination
(that is, the direction from which the light comes and the size of the
source of light) has much to do with the magnitude of the veiling
glare effect experienced. The more concentrated the light source the
more pronounced the glare. The annoyance of veiling glare from
glossy papers is caused by two things. The blurred image of the
source of light as seen reflected from the paper is brighter than the
surrounding paper. From the latter the eye receives diffuse reflection only as distinguished from the specular and diffuse reflection
received from the glare spot. The glare spot may be brighter than
the surrounding paper by 1.5 times or more. While such a ratio of

brightness would hardly be noticeable in many locations in the field of view, it is very annoying when it occurs on a printed word upon which the vision is centered. In such cases it may be sufficient to wholly or partially obliterate the print and the effort to see in spite 'of this is, of course, conducive to strain. Combined with this is another effect, namely, that the specular reflection from the printer's ink or from a pencil mark may be so great as to make it appear equally bright with the surrounding light-colored paper, so that really there is no way for the eye to distinguish the mark. This can be simply demonstrated by taking a paper on which there are glossy indelible pencil marks and holding it at various angles with reference to a light. When the angle of incidence of the light on the paper equals the angle of reflection into the eye, the pencil marks may be brighter than the page. At certain positions they will be equally bright, in which case they disappear altogether until the paper is turned to another angle. In office lighting glare from paper and desk tops is to be especially guarded against. The general method of treatment is taken up under practical conclusions.

When the eye is shaded from excessively bright surfaces but the paper is not, as in the case of localized lighting with a shaded desk-lamp, there is still likely to be considerable trouble as it is almost impossible to so locate an individual desk-lamp as to avoid this glare.

Effects of glare on the eye. Although the physical conditions known to cause glare effects upon the eye have been briefly defined in preceding paragraphs we have yet to take up the observed effects of glare upon the eye. These are (a) Interference with vision, (b) Measurable or observable eye-fatigue or strain, (c) Annoyance.

Interference with vision. The first and most pronounced of these effects is known among some illuminating engineers as the "blinding effect" and is included in the foregoing definitions of glare as an "interference with vision." Of all the effects of glare this is the most pronounced and best-known and probably the easiest to determine quantitatively. It should be a matter of common knowledge, but it is often overlooked, that when a bright source of light is introduced but a few degrees removed from the center line of vision there is a marked reduction in the ability to see clearly the objects upon which vision is centered. In some places the glare completely obliterates the surroundings as far as the observer's eye is concerned.

The amount of interference with vision or blinding effect so caused will depend on the nearness in angular position of the bright light to the center line of vision; that is, upon the angle between the line of vision and a line from the eye to the light. It will also depend upon the relative brightness of the light and the surface viewed, although a light source is usually so much lighter than its background that this factor need not be reckoned with.

The blinding effect or interference with vision caused by the intrusion of the glare of a lamp within the range of vision has been investigated in a pioneer way for certain specific conditions by A. J. Sweet. His paper entitled "An Analysis of Illumination Requirements in Street Lighting" in the *Franklin Institute Journal*, May, 1910, gives the result of laboratory investigations of this phenomenon. In these tests the observer or subject looked at a test object consisting of a black square on an illuminated background. The test was conducted in a dark room. The brightness of the background which the observer required to certainly distinguish the test object, with and without glare present, was taken as a measure of the interference with vision or blinding effect. The interfering source of glare was about 50 square inches in area. The candle power was changed for different tests from 12.5 to 400. The glaring light source was placed directly above the line of vision of the observer at a distance of 10 feet. It was found under these conditions that when the source of glare was brought within about 25° of the center line of vision the interference began to be apparent or measurable in the shape of increased illumination required by the test object to make it just visible. This effect rapidly increased the nearer the interfering light source was brought to the line of the test object.

With an interfering light source of 400 candle power he found that the amount of illumination required on the test object to make it just visible with the light 2° above the line of vision, as compared with the illumination required to make it just visible with the surroundings dark, was in the ratio of 100 to 20. In the case of a 12.5 candle power source this ratio was 100 to 55. Somewhat similar results are reported by Preston S. Millar in the *Illuminating Engineering Society Transactions* for 1910, page 668. Stating Mr. Sweet's results another way the introduction of a 400 candle power light source of this size within two degrees of the line of vision at the distance of 10 feet would be equivalent to reducing the effective illumination on the visualized object to 20 per cent. of the value which would make the object equally clear were the interfering source of glare removed. This of course assumes that the interfering source of glare is so placed that it does not give any added light on the visualized object as the light source is moved nearer the center of vision. This latter condition is one which frequently does not exist in practice. These laboratory tests are of value as indicating how much increased illumination is necessary to compensate for the introduction of a light source nearer the

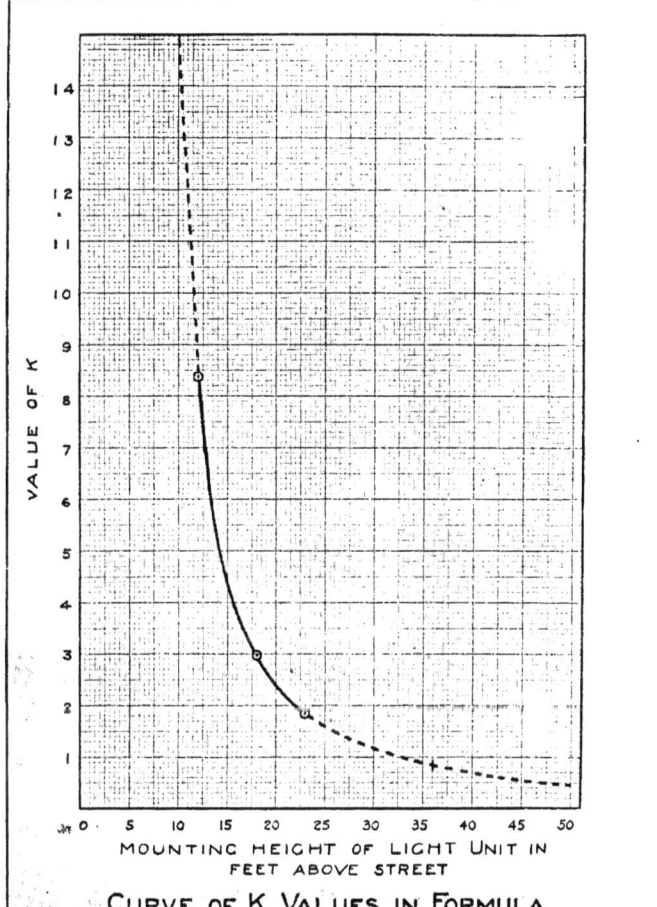

CURVE OF K VALUES IN FORMULA

BLINDING EFFECT = K √CANDLE POWER

BLINDING EFFECT being measured in Per Cent Increased Illumination
for Equal Clearness of Vision as compared with conditions where Blinding
Effect is absent and
CANDLE POWER being taken as the average Candle Power emitted by the
Light Unit between the angles of 75° from the Nadir and 85° from the Nadir
inclusive.

C 983

line of vision. It must be remembered that these tests do not in any way indicate the fatigue or eye-strain which may be caused by the efforts of the eye to adapt itself to see under these adverse conditions. They simply relate to actual interference with vision before fatigue has had time to influence the results.

Mr. Sweet has also investigated the same subjects with certain street-lighting installations made for experimental purposes at the University of Wisconsin and reported in an article entitled "Glare as a Factor in Street Lighting" in the *Electrical Review*, March 6, 1915. From this investigation he drew as one conclusion, that for the street-lighting conditions investigated, which were common, typical conditions, the blinding effect is proportional to the square root of the candle power of the light unit emitted in the direction of the eye, multiplied by a constant. This constant for which he gave the curve shown herewith is dependent upon the height of the lamps above the street and possibly on their spacing also. The blinding effect according to his curve increases very rapidly when the lamps are below 16 feet in height. He also concluded that although ocular discomfort or annoyance caused by the glare from a lamp may be reduced by surrounding the lamp with a diffusing globe, such diffusing globe does little or nothing in reducing the measurable blinding effect, so that the blinding effect and discomfort caused by the glare from a lamp are really separate phenomena. A practical conclusion from this work was that insofar as other considerations permit lamp heights of less than 20 feet should be avoided and in no ordinary case should lamp heights less than approximately 15 feet be employed.

Annoyance or temporary discomfort caused by glare in the eyes, although a matter of common observation, especially on the part of individuals having already slight irritation of the eyes from any cause, is not a thing which can be measured at present writing. The discomfort experienced under a given set of conditions will vary considerably with individuals, some of them being indifferent to conditions which would prove very trying to others.

The physiological effects of glare in producing discomfort, fatigue or strain are not understood at the present time. However, methods have been devised for quantitatively measuring the effects of fatigue or tiring of the eyes when working for some time under different illumination conditions. Before the invention of such methods there was necessarily much guesswork as to the effect of illumination on the eye.

The Ferree test for eye-fatigue (or loss of eye efficiency after a period of work) was devised by C. E. Ferree, professor of Psychology at Bryn Mawr College; this work being taken up at the solicitation of a committee of the American Medical Association desiring a method of testing the tiring effect upon the eye of various conditions of illumination. This test was devised in 1911 and publicly reported upon by Dr. Ferree at the conventions of the Illuminating Engineering Society in 1912, 1913, 1914, and 1915. (See *Transactions Illuminating Engineering Society* for 1913, 1914, and 1915.) Previous to the invention of this test, most tests for visual acuity and the like depended upon momentary judgment of the subject. Dr. Ferree points out that after a period of tiresome work with the eyes the eye may be forced to make a momentary judgment as accurate as that made by the fresh eye, just as a runner may be able to spurt at the end of a race. Dr. Ferree's test is therefore devised so as to require the continuous and strenuous effort of the eyes over a period of time.

The subject is given the following test immediately before or after a period of work of several hours under the conditions of illumination to be tested. The subject is required to gaze steadily at a certain small test object placed at a given distance from the eye for a period of time (usually 3 minutes) and to record during that time, on a chronograph or stop watch, the intervals when the test object appears blurred. This is done easily by simply having the subject press a button when a period of blurr occurs and release the button when the object again appears distinct. A number of short periods when the object appears blurred will occur during the period of the test if the test object selected is of the proper size and is at the proper distance from the eye. The test object preferred by Dr. Ferree is a white card with the letters li printed upon it. Before beginning such a series of tests on a given subject it is important to determine the proper distance from the test card to the eye for that given subject. Dr. Ferree aims to select a distance at which the ratio of time seen clear to time seen blurred is as 3.5 to 1, when the subject is fresh before a period of tiring work. After this test distance has been determined for a given subject that distance is used for the subject on all subsequent tests. The sensitivity of such a test is considerably influenced by the selection of a correct distance for a certain subject at the beginning, as too great a distance will cause the object to appear blurred all the three minute test period after the eye is tired, while on the other hand if the distance is a little too short the test imposes so little effort on the eye of the subject that small differences in fatigue are not detected. In most of Dr. Ferree's work the subject under test worked three hours under the arrangement of illumination selected for test. Tests were repeated many times and various precautions common to careful scientific research were taken which it is impracticable to give here.

The time which the subject sees the test object blurred during the test made after three hours of work is compared to the time the test object was seen blurred in the test made just before the period of work. The increase in the time the object is seen blurred in the test made at the close of work over the test made at the beginning of work, or the increase in the ratio of time seen blurred to time seen clear, is taken as a measure of the eye fatigue, and by comparing the results obtained with different systems of illumination a quantitative measure of the fatiguing effect of the conditions of illumination upon the worker is obtained.

In comparing systems of illumination it is obviously necessary that the kind and duration of work be the same if comparisons are to be made. In the first work done by Dr. Ferree, four given lighting conditions were tested, the illumination on the reading page of the subject being adjusted to the same values in each case. The tests were made in room 30.5 feet long, 22.3 feet wide and 9.5 feet high with white ceiling and walls. A row of three windows was along the side of the room. The amount of daylight for the test of daylight illumination was regulated by screens. The 4 systems of illumination tested were distinctly different and were as follows: (1) Daylight coming from one side through the windows. (2) A very bad system of direct artificial lighting using exposed clear bulb tungsten lamps under flat reflectors with two rows of fixtures 6 feet apart; 8 fixtures in all. (3) An indirect system of artificial light in which the light was received from the illuminated ceiling over each fixture. (4) A semi-direct system of artificial lighting in which white Alba glass reflectors were pointed upward so that part of the light came by reflection from the ceiling and part came directly through the reflector. The subject was seated so as to face lengthwise of the room with the windows at one side. The sources of light on or above the fixtures were within the range of vision continuously. The work performed between tests was mainly reading on a given print and paper. The conditions in general were fairly representative of conditions in many offices and reading rooms.

Ferree found for the conditions of illumination enumerated before, that the least eye-fatigue is shown by the tests after working under daylight and a slightly greater eye-fatigue under the indirect artificial light. For the direct and semi-direct lighting systems enumerated there was a very marked eye-fatigue.

Later Ferree carried his investigations further to determine the difference between lighting equipment and conditions in which there was less marked brightness contrast presented to view. As a large number of equipments are sold under the name of semi-indirect lighting in which the brightness of the bowls varies over a wide range, an attempt was made to determine at what point the brightness of the bowls or glassware used in semi-indirect lighting becomes inoffensive. While it is impossible to review his tests along this line here, it may be said in general that only a few of the most dense glass bowls tested resulted in negligible eye-fatigue. In general the contrast ratio of 1 to 100 of the illuminated glassware with its background already given in this article as a safe practical limit was confirmed.

Another interesting point brought out by some of Dr. Ferree's tests is that the contrast introduced in the range of vision by a dark-colored eye-shade introduces measurably more fatigue than a light-colored eye-shade, and that the use of any eye-shade at all is more fatiguing than its non-use, provided the system of illumination is such that there is no glare in the eyes from the sources of light. The practical conclusion is that eye-shades should only be used where there are exposed bright sources of light and then they should be light in color and preferably somewhat translucent so as to avoid the sharp contrast of light and dark areas within the field of vision.

The Ferree test has also been somewhat extensively experimented with by the writer (see "Some Experiments With the Ferree Test for Eye Fatigue," by J. R. Cravath, *Illuminating Engineering Society Transactions*, 1914, page 1033) with results which confirm the usefulness of the test as an indication of relative eye-fatigue with different conditions of illumination. In these experiments the additional fact was brought out that the test is also influenced by various other physical conditions which are well-known to affect the eye, such as headache, general bodily or mental fatigue, and irritation of the eyes by dust. Many tests were made in regular commercial office work just before and after the morning and afternoon working period. Recuperation of the eye after the noon hour was always indicated. After unusually long and strenuous typewriting work a test was made and after 15 minutes of rest and light gymnastic work another test showed a very marked recuperation of the eye. This sensitivity to other than illumination conditions does not detract from the value of the test for indicating fatigue caused by different illuminating conditions if used with proper precautions, but rather indicates its sensitiveness to the condition which affects the eye, of whatever kind.

Another test for eye-fatigue has been devised by Prof. F. K. Richt-myer and **H**. L. **H**owes, of Cornell University, and described in a paper entitled "A Method of Studying the Behavior of the Eye under Different Conditions of Illumination," presented at the Illuminating Engineering Society Convention at Washington, D. C., 1915. This test is applied like the **F**erree test before and after a period of work under given conditions. The test itself consists in reading backward a number of words of selected length and the fatigue is compared on the basis of the relative time required to read the given number of words. With proper precautions the method looks promising but at present writing very little experimentation with it has been recorded.

Annoyance. As to the amount of glare which will cause annoyance there is considerable difference between individuals. If the eyes are slightly irritated from any cause whatever or if the general physical condition is subnormal conditions of illumination are likely to cause annoyance and ultimately fatigue that would not be noticed by a normal, perfectly healthy eye. General mental and bodily fatigue also has an important influence. It looks reasonable and appears to be true that eye muscles and retina, like hand muscles and skin, may become hardened to conditions of work that for the novice at a given task would cause great fatigue and irritation. Interesting examples of this can be found in incandescent lamp factories in certain departments where the employees are exposed almost continuously in some processes to the unshaded light of tungsten lamps of various candle power. These employees prefer not to be hampered with shades or dark glasses as their eyes become accustomed to working with bare unshaded lamps. New employees are usually troubled with inflamed eyes and swollen lids for a time, but if their eyes are strong enough to survive the first ordeal this trouble is said to disappear after a few days.   .

However, on account of the large number of eyes which are required to do close work which are somewhat inflamed or subnormal because of overwork or other causes, such as the constant irritation of dirt in our large cities and slight refractive errors, the wise course to pursue is to remove as far as possible all defective conditions of illumination which have been shown to produce a measurable fatigue or conscious annoyance. It must be remembered, however, that frequently the subject ascribes the annoyance to something other than the real cause. Sometimes the complaint is of insufficient light when really the trouble is the presence of too much glare. At other times the general system of lighting is blamed when really it is nothing but a case of insufficient illumination on the work. The latter is especially likely to be the case where an indirect system is used and insufficient candle power of lamps is provided.

Brightness table. A table of brightness values accompanies this article in order that the reader may judge how far many modern artificial light sources when unshaded and undiffused, exceed the conservative safety limit of brightness for use in places where they are exposed continuously to the eye. By comparing brightness of walls and ceilings with brightness of various sources of light an approximation of the probable contrast presented to the eye can be reached by study of the table, although of course exact data can only be obtained by measurements on any given installation. It is seen that most modern illuminants undiffused are much brighter than the sky to which the eye is accustomed. By insertion of diffusing glass, such as opal or ground glass shades, the brightness of the artificial sources can be reduced to that of the sky. However, these artificial sources are usually seen amid much darker surroundings than is the sky. Consequently their brightness as ordinarily used needs to be reduced still more, as previously explained under *Contrast glare.*

Quantity of illumination. The quantity or intensity of illumination necessary to produce a brightness of surfaces such that the eye can perform its functions covers an enormous range. Although strictly speaking it is brightness with which the eye is concerned the subject is usually discussed on the basis of the illumination which is incident upon objects rather than the brightness which is reflected from them as a result of the incident illumination.

Intensity of illumination upon a given surface is commonly measured and expressed in the United States and England in terms of foot-candles. In purely scientific work the meter-candle, or lux, is used. A foot-candle is the illumination incident on a surface at right angles to a ray of light emitted from one standard candle one foot distant from the surface. The illumination varies inversely as the square of the distance from the light source to the surface.

To show the great range of illumination within which the eye works the following results are quoted from tests made through 24 hour periods on the roof of a building in New York City and reported by L. J. Lewinson in a paper before the Illuminating Engineering Society convention in 1908. (See *Transactions Illuminating Engineering Society,* page 482, 1908.) These observations were made in September. Daylight illumination measured on a horizontal plane varied in intensity from 2000 to 8000 foot-candles (in sunlight) between 8 a. m. and 4 p. m. Moonlight illumination was from .01 to .02 foot-candles. Illumination from stars and sky at night with no moon was about .001 foot-candles.

Daylight illumination near a window not in direct sunlight may be 300 foot-candles or more. A short distance back from the window it may fall to 50, and further back in the room as low as 4 or 5 before it appears dim for reading. There is also a great variation from moment to moment in the illumination on any cloudy or partly cloudy day. This depends upon whether light clouds, dark clouds, or blue sky are occupying the visible window space. Artificial illumination values are very low in the case of much of our street lighting and in the lighting of interiors simply for the purpose for seeing about. The

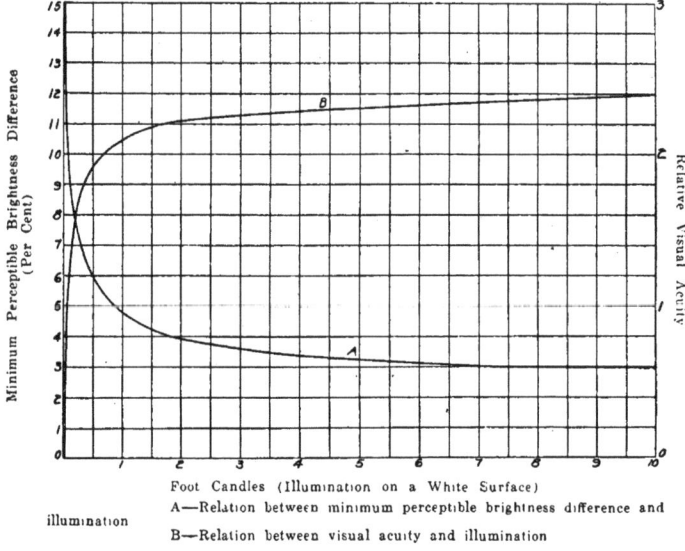

Foot Candles (Illumination on a White Surface)
A—Relation between minimum perceptible brightness difference and illumination
B—Relation between visual acuity and illumination

illumination values common for artificial lighting for close work range from .5 to 20 foot-candles.

Fechner's law relating to sensation when applied to vision tells us that within very wide limits of illumination the brightness differences of adjacent surfaces are equally distinct provided the ratio or percentage of difference in brightness of the two surfaces remain constant. Applying this law to such visual work as reading black letters on a white page it means that we can see the contrast between the black and white equally well over a wide range of illumination on the page because the contrast of brightness is always the same ratio as the relative reflecting powers of the black ink and white paper and this ratio remains the same. The actual ratio of brightness on this page is probably about 75 for the white paper to 3 for the black ink.

That is, the paper diffusely reflects about 75 per cent. of the incident light and the black ink about 3 per cent. Now this ratio will hold constant whether there is 1 foot-candle or 1000 foot-candles.

The accompanying curve, by M. Luckiesh, shows the variation of visual acuity with illumination over a limited range, based on the published tests of König.

In artificial illumination where economy is some object it is important to know the limits below which the illumination on the page cannot be carried without reducing the ability of the eye to quickly and easily distinguish this difference in relative brightness. It is evident from what has been said before that various adverse glare conditions of illumination within the range of vision and the tiring effect of such glare may have a decided influence on the minimum amount of illumination required for comfortable work.

A considerable number of tests have been made to determine what illumination is required by the average person for ordinary comfortable reading where adverse glare conditions are not present to any great extent. The method used in most of these tests has been to start with the room almost in darkness and gradually increase the intensity of illumination as requested by the subject (who is reading a given newspaper or magazine held in a comfortable position) until the subject decides that the illumination is ample for continuous reading. In most of the tests which have been made this process has been repeated 10 times in each sitting and the average of the 10 readings taken. The 10 trials usually do not vary much from the average, the majority falling within 25 per cent. of the average.

The first tests of this kind were reported by Preston S. Millar in the *Illuminating Engineering Society Transactions* for 1907, page 590. The room used had light walls and was lighted with lamps equipped with prismatic reflectors on a chandelier. The 10 subjects tested by Mr. Millar averaged 2.7 foot-candles with a maximum of 3.7 for the highest subject, and 1.85 for the lowest subject.

The writer, J. R. Cravath, tested 12 subjects as reported in the *Illuminating Engineering Society Transactions* in 1911, page 793. Under 5 different conditions of illumination the average was 1.73 foot-candles. The maximum required by any one subject during any one test was 11.96, and the minimum .39. In these tests the direction and diffusion of the light on the paper was found to have an important influence on the amount of light asked for by a subject, as will be explained later.

Extensive tests of this kind were carried on in a U. S. postal car in 1912 under the supervision of A. J. Sweet and others to determine the standard specifications for the lighting of railroad postal cars. The subjects tested consisted of men in railway postal service and railway electrical engineers. Some 23 different arrangements of lamps and reflectors were tested. The arrangements were chosen which it was proposed to use in postal service and the tests were conducted in a postal car. Those for which the results are here given were not made with the car moving. Eleven subjects underwent 23 of the tests and a number of other subjects took part in the tests. The average of 204 such tests, each consisting of 10 trials, showed 2.9 foot-candles as ample and 1.98 foot-candles as a minimum selected by the subjects as satisfactory illumination for newspaper reading. The maximum required by any of these subjects on any test was 6.66 and the minimum considered ample was 1.04 foot-candles. As a result of these tests the United States government now specifies a minimum illumination of 2.8 foot-candles at points where reading of letter addresses is to be done by postal clerks.

One striking thing about all tests of this kind is that there is so so much difference between the averages of different subjects, although each subjcet is consistent as regards any one test and shows small mean variation from his average. This may be due partially to the difference in the reading illumination to which different subjects are accustomed. In general the younger subjects require the least light. Those of low vitality or in poor health are apt to require higher illumination than the average. If refractive errors in the eye are not properly corrected with spectacles the subject is apt to require high illumination. There is also good reason to believe that on days when the subject is below normal, either in general physical condition, or as regards his eyes, his judgment as to sufficient illumination is modified thereby.

The tests by the writer were mainly of value as bringing out the very decided influences that the direction and diffusion of light have upon comfortable reading conditions. In these tests the average amount of light required by the subject was lowest for the conditions in which the direction and diffusion of light were such as to cause the least glare from the paper. Where light came upon the reading page from the ceiling above four indirect lighting fixtures located sufficiently in front of the reader so that the glare of the paper was the least, the subjects required the lowest intensity of illumination called for in the series of tests. The test indicating the least satisfactory lighting condition as shown by the highest required illumination was the one in which a shaded desk-lamp was placed close down over the work and the surroundings were dark. In this latter case there was the greatest amount of glare from the paper. These results were obtained in spite of the care used to select a paper for the subjects to read which was almost free from noticeable glare effects. For one who is expert in looking for glare effects from paper it is easy to detect differences between comfortable and uncomfortable conditions that would be unnoticed by the ordinary person.

It is agreed by those who have conducted the reading tests mentioned here that it should not be assumed from such results that the illumination is equally satisfactory to the subject in all cases when it has reached the values which he selects. This is due to the fact that in the process of·being tested the subject naturally calls for more and more illumination until he finds that additional illumination fails to improve the comfort with which he can read. Now if the illumination on the page is of a character which makes thoroughly comfortable reading impossible, as for example when there is an annoying glare from the paper caused by the improper direction from which the light is received on the paper, the conditions will be unsatisfactory and the subject will keep calling for more light with the idea that it will enable him to see better, until he has called for more light than he requires and has become thoroughly satisfied that the increase is not improving conditions. When, on the other hand, the illumination is satisfactory in direction and diffusion the subject will decide that he has enough illumination as soon as it is sufficient to enable him to see clearly, and he does not feel the need of calling for more in the effort to get satisfaction. If the subject could select by direct comparison which of the two conditions were more satisfactory he would probably in most cases select the conditions under which he called for the least value of illumination. To state the matter in another way no amount of increase in the illumination on a reading page can render its illumination comfortable and satisfactory if the illumination is such that glare is received from the page.

While there is little difference in the ability of the eye to work and distinguish detail, over a large range of daylight and artificial light for practical purposes, say from 3 foot-candles, upward, for most kinds of work, there is nevertheless considerable difference in retinal sensibility between the highest and lowest illumination or brightness with which the eye deals. The following table calculated by P. G. Nutting from his own measurements and those of A. König (see "Retinal Sensibilities Related to Illuminating Engineering" by P. G. Nutting, Illuminating Engineering Society Convention, 1915; and König and Brodhun in *Gesammelte Abhandlungen zur Physiolo-*

gischen Optik, pp. 116-143, July 26, 1888) shows this for four typical conditions:

	Average brightness level; milli-lamberts	Perceptible percentage Difference in brightness	Relative * retinal sensibility to a given number of units difference in brightness
(1) Exterior daylight	1000	.0176	1
(2) Interiors in daylight	10	.030	59
(3) Interiors at night	0.1	.123	1430
(4) Exterior at night	0.001	.79	22300

Color of artificial light. While there has been much discussion of the color of artificial illuminants very little is known at present writing as to their effects upon the eye. This is independent of the fact that many consider yellow illuminants, such as the candle, kerosene lamp, open gas flame and electric incandescent lamps more pleasing from a psychological and artistic standpoint than illuminants in which more green than yellow is present, such as the gas mantle burner and mercury vapor lamps.

There is some good evidence that nearly monochromatic light is better for seeing fine details than light containing many colors of the spectrum. Experiments of Louis Bell, reported in the *Electrical World* of April 14, 1910, and those of M. Luckiesh, reported in the *Illuminating Engineering Society Transactions* for 1912, pp. 135 to 152, indicate that monochromatic light produces a better defined image on the retina than light of an extended spectral character. This is due to the chromatic abberation of the eye. Consequently such illuminants as the mercury vapor lamp (which emits most of its light in a certain narrow region of the spectrum) are superior for use in distinguishing fine details.

Ultra-violet light or radiation. No trouble need be feared from the effects of ultra-violet light upon the eyes with any of the common illuminants in use at the present time. An impression seems to have got abroad that there is considerable danger from this source with certain illuminants, but the amount of ultra-violet light obtainable from commercial illuminants is so small compared with that to which the eye is subjected constantly in daylight that it can be left out of account. It is true, however, that the radiation from a mercury

---

* Indicates for example that a sign-board in broad daylight requires 22,300 times the illumination to make it as legible as at night. In this column "contrast" means the difference between the brightness of two surfaces as expressed in absolute units, such as millilamberts, rather than the ratio of brightness of the two surfaces to each other.

vapor quartz lamp not protected by a glass globe kills living cells and tissues. This fact is made use of in certain sterilizing operations, but it has very little practical bearing on commercial illumination and its effect upon the eye. An interesting paper, ''Ultra-Violet Radiation and the Eye,'' was presented by W. E. Burge at the Illuminating Engineering Society convention, 1915.

Brightness of surroundings. In the past there has been considerable difference of opinion as to whether visual acuity is best with the surroundings brighter or less bright than the object on which the vision is centered. Dr. Percy W. Cobb, in the *Psychological Review,* Vol. 20, p. 425, and in the *Transactions of the Illuminating Engineering Society,* 1915 convention paper, ''Vision and the Brightness of Surroundings,'' sums up the results of several years' work on this question. His results indicated that visual acuity is best when the surroundings are of about the same brightness as the test object. Considering the conditions under which the eye has been evolved this seems quite natural, as the eye in its daily work is constantly called upon to scrutinize objects which are of about the same relative level of brightness as their surroundings. It is only when artificial conditions are introduced by means of artificial lighting that this is changed.

Analysis of illuminating conditions. Natural illumination or daylight covers a great variety of illumination conditions and the same is true of artificial light.

Outdoors with a clear sky, while the sun is up, we have a combination of light coming directly from a small, intensely bright surface, the sun, and a considerable amount of light coming indirectly by reflection and diffusion from a very large blue surface, the sky. When the sky is overcast with clouds all of the light comes from the large surface of the sky by the reflection and diffusion of the sunlight by the clouds.

The natural illumination of interiors is usually through windows, in which case the source of light is the patch of sky exposed by the window, except of course when the sun is also shining through the window. Some illumination may also be received by reflection from nearby buildings and from the ground. As to whether the sky, which is the principal source of illumination, is visible to the eyes of the occupants will depend upon the positions of the occupants and whether the window-shades are pulled down far enough to hide the sky. It is evident that the essential conditions of natural illumination through windows are: First, a large area of light-giving surface; and second, light coming from an oblique angle. The main source of light, the sky, may or may not be shaded from the eye. It is not at all essential that it be shaded from the eye, provided the brightness of the interior of the room within the range of vision is of sufficient value so that a great enough contrast is not introduced to cause contrast glare.

Natural illumination of a room from a skylight is practically illumination from a large, low intensity light source with the general direction of the light from above. The source of light is not shaded from the eye unless the head is inclined so that the eye-brows shade the eye or the subjcet is seated near a wall.

Certain terms and classifications have come to be applied to methods of artificial lighting, which while not scientifically exact, convey fairly definite meanings to those in illumination work.

Direct illumination from an artificial light source, such as electricity, gas or oil, is commonly understood to apply to a method of illumination in which a considerable portion of the light obtained for useful purposes comes direct from the lamp and its equipment. This lamp equipment may consist of a globe which surrounds the lamp for the purpose of ornament or for softening or diffusing of the light, or it may consist of a reflector, either translucent or opaque, placed over the lamp for the purpose of reflecting the light in directions where it is needed. The lamp, together with its equipment, however, comprises a light source of relatively small area, usually much brighter than anything else within the range of vision. At the same time considerable light may be received by reflection from ceiling, walls and floors; the amount so received depending on the amount of light striking these surfaces and their reflecting power.

Localized direct lighting is a term applied to the plan of placing a shaded lamp over or near the work to be done. In such a case there is a strong light from one direction which may be either from above or from one side, and the brightest surfaces within the range of vision are below the eye rather than above, as in some of the other cases.

Indirect illumination is a term commonly used for a system of artificial lighting (sometimes called inverted lighting) in which reflectors are placed under the lamps, so that the lamps are not visible, and the light is directed toward a light-colored ceiling from which it is reflected and diffused for useful purposes down into the room. Essentially as far as the effect on the eye is concerned this is lighting by large area, low intensity light sources from above. It is similar in general effect to daylight received through a skylight.

The reader should here see the illustrations under **Conservation of**

vision, pp. 3218 to 3229, Vol. V, of this *Encyclopedia,* as well as the figure on p. 3189 of the same volume. A number of appropriate cuts are also to be found under the heading **Hospitals, O**phthalmic.

The terms semi-direct and semi-indirect illumination have been used to describe a number of different methods. At the present writing they are most commonly used to describe a system in which translucent glass bowls are placed under the lamps; some of the light going through the bowls and some being reflected by the bowls to a

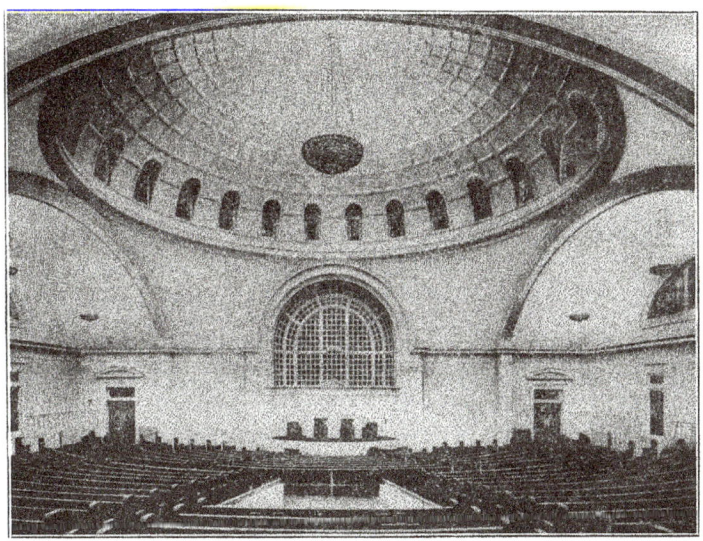

Indirect Lighting.

light-colored ceiling. The bowl usually constitutes a light source of moderately high surface brightness of small area, while the ceiling above it constitutes a large area light source of low surface brightness. The bowl brightness, however, may be easily regulated by the application of proper engineering principles. See illustration and table.

Another artificial lighting arrangement to which various names have been applied is that of placing lamps above a diffusing skylight. The resultant effect is different from daylight coming through a skylight and is also different from indirect light from light-colored ceilings because the artificial light coming through the skylight is seldom as well diffused as the daylight or indirect light. The effect is that of light coming from above, principally from areas of rather small size and high surface brightness.

Any one of the foregoing systems of artificial lighting may be carried out with any one of several common illuminants such as electricity, gas or oil, with about the same results as far as effects on the eye are concerned, provided means are employed whereby the brightness of the principal sources of light are reduced to the same intensity and the total quantity of light is the same. However, in practice there are differences in the way different illuminants are commonly used which may make great differences in the effect on the eye.

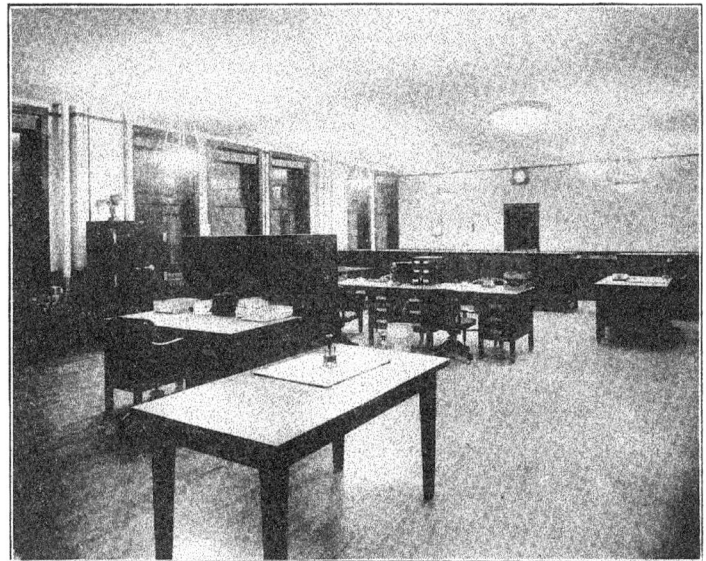

Semi-direct Lighting.

Practical conclusions. A study of the facts which have been presented here, together with the brightness values given in the subjoined table, lead to the following practical conclusions as to precautions which should be taken to avoid the annoying, fatiguing or blinding effects of improper illumination conditions upon vision. The extent to which the precautions recommended in the following paragraphs should be followed depends very much upon whether the eyes of one or more persons are likely to be subjected to the defective conditions for considerable periods of time.

As a first precaution no artificial light should be placed so that its undiffused light will shine directly in the eyes of the user for any considerable length of time. The more fixed the position of the user the more important this is. As a first step, the least that can be done is to use diffusing glass globes, reflectors or shades between the eye and the light. This improves conditions somewhat, as the Brightness Table will show, but, in order to reduce the contrast of brightness within the range of vision below the desirable limit of 1 to 100 so as to afford the best conditions for the eyes the most practicable method in most cases is to adopt indirect lighting or semi-direct lighting in which the brightness of the bowls is reduced below 250 millilamberts. This latter involves the use of bowls of very dense glass, which preferably should be highly polished on their interior surfaces so as to efficiently reflect a considerable percentage of the light to the ceiling for indirect lighting.

Localized lighting with opaque reflectors which put most of the light in spots under the reflectors and leave the rest of the room dark should only be used in connection with some good general system of lighting, for it is well established that it is not comfortable for the eye to work for a long time on a brightly illuminated surface amid very dark surroundings. Another objection to purely localized lighting is the glare from paper or machine-work which is emphasized by the absence of a considerable amount of general lighting. At best it is difficult to locate a desk-lamp where it will not cause glare from the paper to the user's eye from some part of the desk, even though it may not be the exact part where reading is being done. The majority of desk-lamps are placed so that they cause considerable eye-strain, for the usual position is directly in front of the user so that the angle from some part of the paper to the lamp and to the eye is equal. The best position is at the left of the user, if he is right-handed.

One of the most important problems in illumination where close visual work is performed is to get the light from the proper direction to avoid the glare of reflection from papers and polished surfaces. One of the superiorities of natural light from windows over artificial light is due to the fact that it is light from a large source that strikes papers and desk tops at an angle which is usually such that the glare from papers is reduced to a minimum.

For natural lighting through windows the windows should be as large a percentage of the total wall area as possible. The smaller the windows in relation to the wall area the greater the contrasts of brightness which are introduced within the range of vision for anyone who is obliged to sit facing or nearly facing a window. Window shades and curtains used to reduce the amount of light entering a room, if made of dark opaque materials, are likely to be misused by being carelessly left so that they obstruct an unnecessarily large part of the total window space at times when they are not needed to keep out direct sunlight. The result is that bad contrast glare effects are introduced in the room, and in addition the appearance of the room is likely to be gloomy. Translucent shades are better for such purposes. Ground glass and the like should be avoided in window sashes which are below the level of the eye, as they introduce a brightness equal to or greater than that of the sky on a part of the retina which is unaccustomed to such brightness in such a location, and the contrast with the adjoining wall and floor brightness is likely to be too great.

Another phase of this same matter is the effect of light from an unusual direction upon patients lying in bed in sick rooms and hospitals. If the foot of the bed is toward a window or toward an artificial light, no matter how well diffused, the greatest amount of light is sure to fall on the part of the retina least accustomed to it and cause discomfort or worse, aggravated further by the subnormal condition of the patient which usually exists at such times.

It is very often desirable both for economical and hygienic reasons to equip the lamps in a direct lighting system of interior lighting with rather deep reflectors. Such reflectors accomplish the double purpose of economizing light by reflecting more of the light of the lamp down where it is useful and shading the naked source of light from the eye.

Eyebrows play an important part as shades for the eye from artificial light indoors as well as from the sun outdoors. With the head in an upright normal position the eyebrow of the average person will shade the eye from light coming from above at an angle of less than about 25 degrees from the vertical. Slight inclination of the head or abnormally large eyebrows will increase this figure. Reflectors or shading devices used with lamps placed above the head of the users should be constructed with this fact in view if complete shading of the eye from the direct light of the lamp is desired. That is, the shade should intercept the light emanating from the lamp at all angles more than 25 degrees from the vertical.

The annoyance caused by shadows, if any, is likely to be dependent upon the sharpness of the shadows. With light coming from large sources, such as the sky or illuminated ceiling, the shadows are rendered unnoticeable, although it should be remembered that they still exist to some extent and that the illumination in the shadow is not equal to that which is obtained elsewhere.

Dark-colored finishes, walls and ceilings of rooms should be avoided if the best eye comfort is desired, as the illumination, both natural and artificial, of such dark-colored rooms is more apt to introduce glaring contrast than in light-colored rooms.

—(J. R. C.)

Illumination, Oblique. See **Examination of the eye.**

Illumination of the eye. See **Examination of the eye.**

Illuminator. A lens or mirror, or any other optical apparatus, for concentrating light on an object or area. A number of these, for ocular illumination, are described and pictured under the heading **Examination of the eye;** as well as under **Hospitals, Ophthalmic.** To this matter may be added references to a few other illuminators.

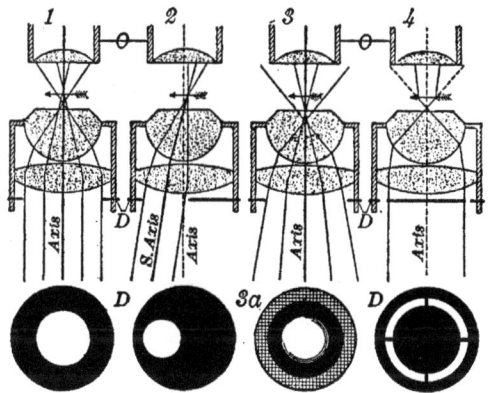

Abbé's Illuminator.

1, section of the illuminator with central parallel rays; 2, illuminator receiving oblique parallel rays; 3, section showing that a central converging beam is brought to a focus within or at the surface of the front lens and that the object is lighted with widely diverging rays; 4, section showing the production of dark-ground illumination by the use of a diaphragm shutting off all but the marginal rays, the angle of which is so great that, as shown by the dotted lines, they cannot enter the objective unless changed in direction by a suitable object. The appearance is that of a self-luminous object in a dark field; 3a, the upper front or end view of the illuminator; D, D, D, D, diaphragms seen in section in the illuminator, face views below; O, O, front of the microscopic objective. As shown in the figures, the illuminator is centered when the axis coincides with the axis of the microscope.

A form of illuminator of interest to the microscopist and ophthalmologist is Abbé's wide-aperture lens combination. It is not achromatic; the form of 1.20 numerical aperture consists of two, while the form of 1.40 numerical aperture consists of three, lenses. As shown by the arrows in the figures, the object should be placed in or very near the focus and, except for low powers, parallel or approximately parallel, rays should be reflected on it from a plane mirror. For

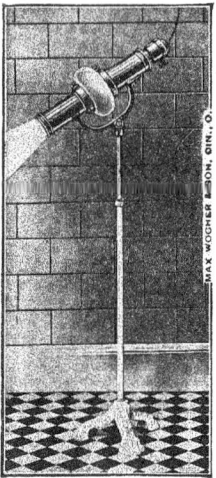

Coakley Electric Light Illuminator.

refraction images, as in studying histology, a diaphragm with small opening is used, but for color images, as in studying stained microbes,

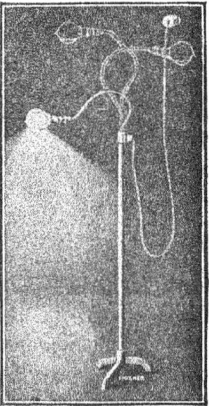

The Goose-Neck Electric Illuminator.

either a large-holed diaphragm or none at all is used. In employing the best high-angled objectives a drop of water or homogeneous immersion fluid is placed between the illuminator and the slide.

Of *ocular illuminators* the Coakley electric light apparatus (see the figure to the left in the cut) is a useful one. It consists of an adjustable stand with a 50 c. p. spiral filament lamp mounted on it.

The so-called *goose-neck electric illuminator* (see cut) is supplied with a spiral filament bull's-eye lamp (giving a concentrated light) and a swivel socket, which allows the lamp to be revolved in any direction. The stand is constructed of metal, white enameled; the flexible metal shaft can be adjusted in any desired position or height.

Illuminator, Black- (or dark-) ground. An optical instrument in which an opaque surface is introduced behind the object, while illuminating rays are directed around and about it.

Illusion, Visual. A false sensory image. See **Hallucination;** also **Psychology of vision.**

Image. In *optics,* a real or figurative picture of an object produced by reflection or refraction at a surface, or refraction by a lens. A real image is also produced when the rays emitted from an object pass through a small aperture in a dark chamber. It is only a real image that will impress itself upon the photographic plate. The image is said to be *real* when the deviated rays actually pass through its constituent points; whereas, if the deviated rays only *appear* to pass through them, the typical image is said to be *virtual*. Virtual images are situated on the same side of the refracting surface as the object, that is to say in the first medium, whereas real images are situated in the second medium. Real as well as virtual images are produced by a convex lens or a concave mirror; whereas, *concave lenses* and *convex mirrors* produce only *virtual images*. The object and its *inverted real image* are located upon *opposite sides* of a *convex lens,* but on the *same side* of a *concave mirror;* whereas, the object and its *erect virtual image* are on the *same side* of a *convex lens,* and on *opposite sides* of a *concave mirror.* The object and its image, irrespective of their directions from a fixed point, are said to be in the object-space and image-space (q. v.), respectively. The law universally applies that corresponding points of the object and image are conjugate to each other. See *conjugate foci,* under **Focus.**

With reference to an optical instrument, Maxwell's theory is that:

1. A *perfect image* is produced when all of the *emergent rays* corresponding to the rays of a given bundle of *incident rays* proceeding from the object-point intersect in the image-point. When this is not the case, the defect is called *astigmatism.*

2. If the object is a plane surface perpendicular to the axis, the image of any point must also lie in a plane perpendicular to the axis.

When the points of the image lie in a curved surface, the image is said to have the defect of *curvature*.

3. The image of an object on this plane must be similar to the object, whether its linear dimensions are altered or not. When the image is not similar to the object, it is said to be *distorted*. An image that is free from distortion, and which, therefore, is exactly similar to the object in its entire extent, is called *orthoscopic,* or *angle-true,* because straight lines are reproduced as straight lines and homologous angles in the object and image are equal. A lens which projects an orthoscopic image is called a *rectilinear lens.*—(C. F. P.)

Image, Accidental. After-image. See p. 139, Vol. I, of this *Encyclopedia.*

Image, Actual ophthalmoscopic. Indirect image. See **Ophthalmoscope.**

Image, Aerial. See **Aerial images.**

Image, After-. An image perceived by the retina after the exciting stimulus has been withdrawn. When these images are simply continuations of the sensation they are known as *positive* after-images; when they are of a complementary color they are known as *negative* after-images. See p. 139, Vol. I, of this *Encyclopedia.*

Image, Catoptric. One reflected from polished surfaces.

Image, Chiasmal. In *physiologic optics,* a strictly figurative image consisting of that supposititious orderly assemblage of the optic-nerve fibrils, within the cross-sectional and comparatively small area of the optic chiasm, which hypothetically receive their individual stimuli from corresponding points in each retinal image.

Upon this hypothesis its author, Prentice, through the aid of original diagrams and simple mathematics established the law:

In manifest hyperphoria of one prism-dioptry the distance between the chiasmal image-centers is equal to the one-hundredth part of the distance between the nodal point and the retina of the observed eye. See **Chiasmal image.**

Later (*Ophthalmic Record,* July, 1914) both of these images were shown to serve a useful working hypothesis in making a lucid drawing to illustrate the phorias, and as a figure of speech when attempting to differentiate between the ocular images and their corresponding brain-image, also a figure of speech, since it is just as imaginary as its correlative chiasmal image, which, at least figuratively, occupies a more definite location. Moreover, the chiasmal image is quite as conceivable as the all permeant ether through which light is supposed to be propagated, and is fully as justifiable, so long as this figurative image can be shown to serve a useful purpose.

In order to demonstrate the purpose and need of at least one point of orientation, although two different ones will be here jointly applied, let it be supposed that the diagram, **Fig.** 1, represents a horizontal plane, abcd, in which the corresponding sections of the right eye, R, and the left eye, L, are located to view the object, O, upon the median line, MO. It is also assumed that the visual axis of the right eye, R, is faultily directed towards E, as in esophoria, so that its macula, m_2,

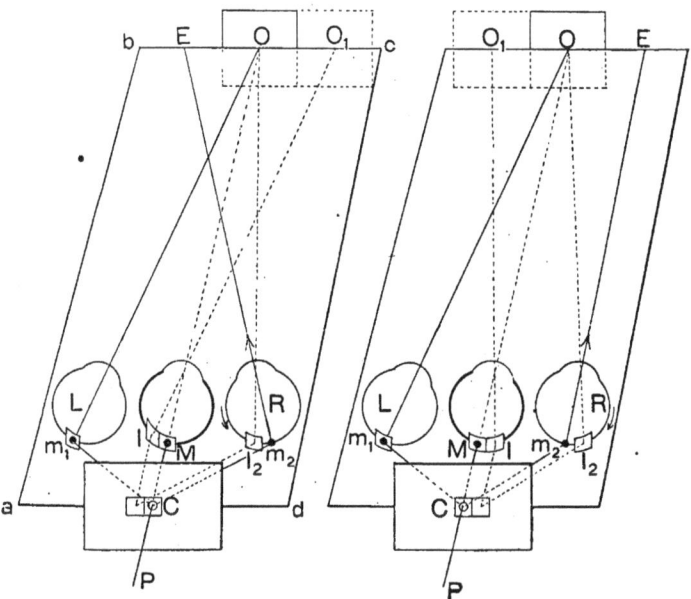

Fig. 1.
Homonymous Projection (Prentice)
Contiguous Mean Cyclopean Images.

Fig. 2.
Heteronymous Projection (Prentice)
derived from Chiasmal Images.

is turned to the right; whereas, the macula m_1, of the left eye, L, retains its normal position with respect to the object, O; and, therefore, also with respect to the center, C, of the chiasmal field and the macula, M, of the mean eye on the median line, and to which points of orientation the macular center, m_2, in the right eye is also projected. Consequently, the macular centers, m_1, and m_2, in both eyes have the same points of orientation, C and M, in common, while the image-center, m_1, of the left eye alone is transmitted to these points.

But, the center of the image I_2, projected from O into the right eye, is situated on the left side of its macula, m_2, and is, therefore, transmitted with equal displacement so as to be located on the left side of the centers of orientation, C and M, in the chiasmal field and mean eye, respectively. Therefore, the displaced image, I_2, in the right eye, is transmitted to and located on the left side of the mean eye as the false cyclopean image, I; and it is this image, belonging to the right eye, that is homonymously projected to O_1, on the right side of and at the same prism-dioptral distance, EO, from the object O.

The points m_1, m_2, C and M are corresponding points with reference to the axis, PCM, of bilateral symmetry within the cranium, which coincides with the median line, MO, in the object-space and is directed to the supposed center, P, of image-perception in the brain.

In Fig. 2, heteronymous projection of the ocular images is illustrated. Both diagrams show that the chiasmal and mean cyclopean images, respectively, are contiguous, because the horizontal diameter of the object is made equal to the prism-dioptral deflection EO, so that the real object, O, and the mentally conceived apparent object, O_1, are also in contact.

The figurative mean cyclopean images, I and M, are graphically projected from their corresponding chiasmal images, so that conjointly they make it possible to pictorially illustrate either homonymous or heteronymous diplopia in a manner not hitherto lucidly accomplished.

In view of the indeterminate psychophysical character of these images, and an effort being made to picture them in a drawing, the delineator will at least need to assume that the center, P, of the so-called brain-image is the center of image-perception; that it is located in the horizontal plane, in juxtaposition to the center, M, of the centered cyclopean image of the object on the median line and, therefore, coincident with the center of the chiasmal image; said line, PCM, within the cranium, being considered the axis of visual orientation, or the directrix of bilateral symmetry of vision in the mind at least of the draftsman.—(C. **F**. P.)

Image confusé. (F.) Flat image.

Image, Cyclopic. G. Ovio (*Archiv. d'Ophtal.*, 1911, Vol. 31, p. 710) means by it seeing only one eye when looking at a plane mirror. The phenomenon results from fixing a point instead of the image itself. It is best seen at 1 meter's distance, though it may be seen at a greater or less distance. Accompanying the cyclopic image is a distortion of the face, which is seen double. See **Cyclopic image.**

Image, Direct. ERECT IMAGE. See **Ophthalmoscope.**

Image, Double. See p. 4006, Vol. VI, of this *Encyclopedia.*

Image, Erect. Upright image.

Image, Extraordinary. See **Double refraction.**

Image, False. See **Diplopia.**

Image, Half-. DEMI-IMAGE. A term applied by **Helmholtz** to one of the two double images cast by the same object, but not seen singly by the two eyes.

Image, Indirect. INVERTED IMAGE. A real, magnified (ophthalmoscopic) image of the fundus of an, eye, in which the emerging rays are focused by means of a convex glass before entering the eye of the observer. See **Examination of the eye;** as well as **Ophthalmoscope.**

Image-line. In *optics,* a straight line situated in the image-space and in an infinitely extended plane in any meridian containing the optical axis of a lens-system. See, also, **Collinear space-systems.**

Image, Negative. See **Image.**

Image, Ordinary. See **Double refraction.**

Image, Orthoscopic. See **Image.**

Image-plane. In *optics,* the real or virtual plane perpendicular to the axis in which are located the constituent points of the real image produced by a lens-system.—(C. F. P.)

Image-point. In *optics,* a point in the plane of the real or virtual image in which are located the vertexes of the effective ray-bundles produced by a lens-system.—(C. F. P.)

Image-rays. In *optics,* the rays that are either actually or virtually directed toward points in the image produced by a lens-system.— (C. F. P.)

Image, Real. An image formed by the convergence of reflected or refracted rays after their emergence from the reflecting source or the refracting medium; so called because actually existing at the spot at which it is seen, and capable of being thrown upon a screen placed at this spot. The images formed by concave mirrors or concave lenses and the inverted ophthalmoscopic image are real. (**Foster.**) See, also, **Image.**

Image renversée. (F.) Inverted image.

Image, Retinal. The image formed upon the retina by rays of light which pass from an external object through the dioptric mechanism of the eye.

Images, Consecutive. Images which follow one another in regular succession.

Images croisées. (F.) Crossed images.

Images, Crossed. Images of objects existing in crossed diplopia, due to divergence of the visual axes.

Images, Diffusion. Images formed by rays of light from an object passing through a lens and falling upon a surface not at the focus.

Images, Homonymous. Those double images occurring on the side corresponding to the eyes; the right image is corresponding to the right eye, and the left image to the left eye. This form of diplopia is caused by convergence of the visual axes.

Images, Incongruous. In certain cases of squint the false projection persists even after the correction of the heterotropia, and the double images in these cases of anomalous diplopia are consequently said to be incongruous.

Image, Size of the. This is a subject of calculation, provided the size of the object and its distance from the nodal point are both known. The size of the image then equals the size of the object multiplied by the distance of the image from the nodal point divided by the distance of the object from the nodal point.

Images, Multiple. See Polyopia.

Images of Purkinje. For the purpose of demonstrating the presence or absence of the crystalline lens and of showing the changes that

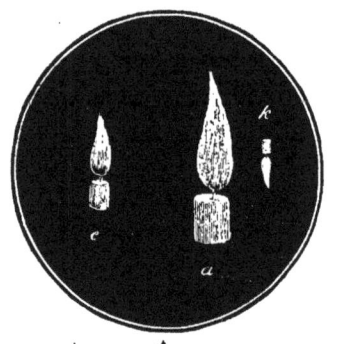 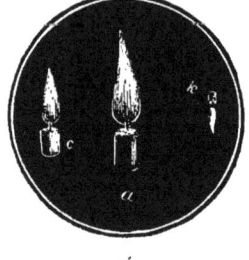

A   **B**

Purkinje-Sanson Images. (Follin-Ball.)

A, In the absence of accommodation, with the pupil dilated. *B*, In accommodation, with the pupil contracted. *c*, Image from the cornea. *a*, From the anterior surface of the lens. *k*, From the posterior surface of the lens.

take place in the pupillary area of the lens during accommodation advantage is taken of the reflexes known as the Purkinje or the Purkinje-Sanson images.. These are catoptric images (i. e., reflected) from the cornea and anterior and posterior surfaces of the lens. They can be understood by a study of the figure. Let light fall on the eye at an angle of 30 degrees. Three images will be seen: the brightest, an erect virtual image, is from the anterior (convex) surface of the cornea; another erect virtual image, larger, but less bright, is from the anterior (convex) surface of the lens; and a small inverted real image is from the (concave) posterior boundary of the lens. The second image is intermediate in position between the other two. If the eye is accommodated for a near point, the corneal image is unchanged. The middle image becomes smaller and approaches the corneal image, showing the curvature of the anterior surface of the lens to be increased. A slight change occurs in the third image.— (J. M. B.)

By means of Tscherning's ophthalmophakometer (*Physiologic Optics,* p. 44), a small telescope supported on a stand, these images may be more thoroughly studied. See, also, p. 1784, Vol. III, of this *Encyclopedia.*

Image-space. In *optics,* the extent of space actually or virtually traversed by the *effective rays* that are directed toward each point of the image produced by an *optical system.* See, also, **Collinear space-systems;** and **Focus.**—(C. F. P.)

Images, Suppression of. When strabismus develops in early life there is no diplopia; it is supposed that the image formed on the retina of the deviating eye is ignored by the perceptive centres in the brain; and this suppression may affect first one eye and then the other.

Image, Stereoscopic. The image produced on the retina of the two eyes by uniting stereoscopically the image of two photographs taken from one and the same negative. This gives an undeniable impression of solidity, although it is simply an optical illusion.

Images, Tipping of. In certain forms of muscle imbalance, when one eye is so rotated that its vertical meridian is no longer exactly perpendicular objects will look as if tipped to one side and in the opposite direction. This condition is seen in both *intorsion* and *extorsion.*

Image, Upright. An enlarged image of the fundus of the eye, seen with the ophthalmoscope (direct method) by aid of the dioptric apparatus of the eye, without the interposition of a bi-convex lens. See **Examination of the eye.**

Image, Virtual. REAL IMAGE. An image formed by the prolongation of reflected or refracted rays back behind the reflecting surface or the refracting medium; so called because not actually existing at the spot at which it appears. The image in a looking-glass, the images formed by concave lenses and convex mirrors, and the ophthalmoscopic image are examples. See, also, **Image.**

Imbalameter, Adams'. A name given to a patented device for detecting and measuring muscular insufficiency or imbalance of the extrinsic ocular muscles at the reading distance.

Imbalance. This term is, in ophthalmology, commonly applied to *heterophoria* and *heterotropia.* See, also, **Muscles, Ocular.**

Imbecility, Ocular relations of. This subject has already been discussed under **Idiocy.** Here it may be said that Pearce, Rankine and Ormond (*British Medical Journal,* July 23, 1910) have reported on the ocular condition of 28 imbeciles, 20 males and 8 females. The average age of death in imbeciles of the Mongolian type is computed by the authors to be between 14 years and 15 years. They point out that nearly 100 per cent. of deaths are due to tuberculosis.

Among their mental characteristics are noted: A strongly marked imitative faculty, and a fondness for music. They are inert and apathetic as a rule. They are very affectionate and fond of being noticed.

Among the physical characteristics the most prominent are: The shortness of stature, due to relative shortness of the extremities. The brachycephalic skull and usually poorly developed occiput. The characteristic facies, broad squat nose, thick lips and usually prominent lower jaw, and interpalpebral fissure sloping up and out. Shortness of and incurving of the little finger. The skin is dry and rough. The voice has a guttural inflection and there is a tendency to "lalling," the patients being unable to pronounce certain consonants properly. The teeth, though not showing any originality in shape, are usually badly formed, loosely set in their sockets and irregular in their position. They are prone to decay. The eruption of the teeth seems to take place at normal periods. The palate is a contracted vault with the sides sloping more steeply in front so that an anterior plateau is formed.

As regards the *ocular conditions* it is known that a large number have some eye defect, either squint, nystagmus, ectropion, or defective vision.

Attention is also drawn to the frequency with which a definite form of cataract is found. In 19 of the 28 cases lens opacities were present, and in 18 of the number the cataract was of a particular type. This form of cataract is seen fully developed in several of the older patients, and is present in what is probably an earlier and less mature form in some of the others.

In the least marked varieties the opacities consist of small dots in the cortical portion of the lens deep to the capsule and nearer the anterior than the posterior surface. These dots are best seen by focal illumination. In the mature cases the opacities consist of two layers enclosing a clear nucleus.

The posterior lamella is concave forwards and corresponds with the curve of the posterior surface of the lens. The anterior lamella is much flatter and is situated about midway between the centre of the nucleus and the anterior surface of the lens. The opacities do not reach the equator in any direction. The lamellæ consist of numerous small discrete dots.

The posterior pole of the cataract which appears to correspond with the posterior pole of the lens is often marked by a star-shaped opacity. The anterior pole of the cataract which does not correspond with the anterior pole of the lens often has a similar opacity to mark its position.

The more fully developed cases might be described as lamellar cataract, the slighter as congenital "dot" cataract.

Very young Mongolian idiots do not exhibit this change. The fact that it is better marked in the older cases suggests that it is a late development.

It remains to be seen whether those cases which now have slight opacities will show an increased number of dots at a later date. It is the author's opinion that the cataract is both partial and progressive, and that it is developed as the result of changes taking place in the lens after its formation.

Though the teeth in these cases are defective they are not of the hypoplastic type.

It was impossible to get any reliable record of the visual acuity in these patients.

The ectropion found in many of these cases is due to a superficial contraction of the skin of the lower lid. The skin of the lid is rough-glazed and dry. Marginal blepharitis is probably in the first instance the result of infection from the hands which are frequently used to rub the eyes, and is kept up by the ectropion, error of refraction, and dirty habits of the patient. The age of the youngest patient examined was 5 years and the oldest 43 years. The youngest patient showing cataract was 9 years of age. The oldest patient has a well-developed cataract of the kind described.

Half of the number of patients examined have the interpalpebral fissure directed upwards and outwards. (J. F. Cunningham, in *Oph. Review,* p. 311, October, 1913.)

Imbedding, Methods of. See **Laboratory methods.**

Immagine capovolta. (It.) Indirect or inverted method of ophthal-moscopic examination.

Immagine diritta. (It.) Direct (ophthalmoscopic) image.

Immagini doppie paradosse. (It.) Paradoxical double images; in-congruous images.

Immature cataract. A term usually applied to the early stages of senile hard cataract. See p. 635, Vol. I, also, p. 1761, Vol. III, of this *Encyclopedia.*

Immersion. In microscopy, the act of immersing the objective in oil, water, or some other liquid for the purpose of preventing total reflection.

Immersion treatment. See **Dam,** p. 3735, Vol. V, of this *Encyclopedia.*

Immigrants, Examination of the eyes of. See **Hygiene** of the eyes; as well as **Trachoma.**

Immunity. See p. 857, Vol. II of this *Encyclopedia.*

Impair. (F.) Uneven; odd (in numbers).

Impetigo contagiosa. This contagious disease may affect the skin of the eyelids and, in rare instances, invade the conjunctiva also. The disease is characterized by the formation of vesicles or pustules which later on are converted into yellowish crusts. As the vesicles and pustules have been found over the lids and on the conjunctiva, it has been thought wise to detail briefly the chief characteristics of the affection in order that ophthalmologists may have at hand a description of the disease.

The disease attacks the face, scalp and other hairy portions of the body, as well as the hands, and occasionally the eyelids, appearing as small vesicles or pustules which enlarge, become purulent and then dry, forming crusts. The lesions are the size of a split-pea and somewhat flattened; the crusts seeming to be "stuck on" in the center, their edges slightly curled up so that they are raised above the skin surface.

The vesicles or pustules may be few or many. They may remain discrete or by the confluence of several, form larger patches, and, rarely, they may form segments or rings or run into serpiginous patches. The patches are superficial and are surrounded by an inflammatory areola. If the vesicle or pustule should happen to break, a thin discharge exudes from the moist, denuded and raw-looking surface; and when the crusts fall off, reddened surfaces remain. The evolution of the eruption requires from two to three days for completion, but the entire disease lasts from three to five weeks.

There are few, if any, subjective symptoms, at most only a slight itching is complained of. But occasionally the lesions present a bullous form, which variety exceptionally occurs in epidemics in institutions and hospitals. In such cases the conjunctival, as well as the nasal and oral mucous membranes are attacked, and in these there may be slight, or even marked, constitutional symptoms.

The lesions are confined to that portion of the skin between the rete and the horny layers with consequent inflammation of the surrounding tissues. The disease is caused undoubtedly, by the activity of the streptococcus, the staphylococcus aureus, and, possibly, the albus, for these organisms are found quite constantly in large numbers in the central portion of the lesions. It is contagious and antoinoculable, and it is usually observed in early life and in children, when it is frequently secondary to pediculosis capitus.

Impetigo contagiosa should be distinguished from other pustular affections of the face, especially acne, pustular eczema and sycosis. Acne, it will be remembered, develops after puberty; it is chronic; it invades the back, chest and shoulders, and black-heads and sebaceous cysts are commonly present. Pustular eczema is essentially chronic, lasting, in some cases, from childhood to adult life; it attacks any portion of the face or body, the pustules sometimes run together to form large patches, which fade off into sound skin. Sycosis is a disease of adult life; it involves the bearded portions of the face, the hair follicles of which are markedly affected.

Impetigo of the eyelids is uncommon. The vesicles or pustules are of the split-pea size. They pursue the same course as that observed in the lesions elsewhere. The subjective symptoms are but slight, usually, and the disease disappears spontaneously in a few weeks. The vesicles closely resemble the phlyctenular, indeed the diagnosis may become obscured by reason of the occurrence of phlyctenules coincidently.

Bullæ may involve the bulbar conjunctiva, as was noted in a case reported by Bayer, in which there were numerous clear vesicles containing cocci at the limbus cornea. But in a case reported by Hansell, each cornea was the seat of a superficial vascular inflammation attended by the formation of ulcers. The circumcorneal tissues were injected, the palpebral conjunctiva inflamed and thickened. The bulbar symptoms arose at the outbreak of the disease and the course of the keratitis, though variable, persisted so long as the disease lasted, both affections reaching their acme at the same time.

The corneal symptoms may be said to have been similar to those of the skin allowing for modifications in the components of the two structures. The centers of the areas occupied the apices of the corneas. White patches were always present, which were densest at the apices, but gradually shaded off into clear cornea before reaching the limbus. They were continuously ulcerated; at one time the necrotic area in the left cornea measured 4 mm. in diameter. The irides were not involved, however, nor were the interiors of the eyes. The usual symptoms of keratitis with photophobia, epiphora and moderate pain were present.

The usual form of impetigo is readily cured, but the bullous type is serious when it is epidemic, and especially so when the mucous membrane of the mouth of nursing infants is affected. The continued presence of bullæ on the conjunctival membrane should cause one to remember the possibility of the affection being pemphigus. But that dread disease rarely attacks children and its course is more protracted and its effects more penetrating than what has been observed in impetigo. (*Vide* **Pemphigus.**)

The treatment should consist in the dabbing of a solution of the bichloride of mercury, 1–4000, on the ruptured areas to prevent the spreading of the virulent discharge, and the coating of the pustules with ammoniated mercury ointment, grains 10 to 20 to the ounce of petrolatum, which should be applied six or more times daily. Precipitated sulphur, and ichthyol lotions, may do well when these simpler methods fail. In the bullous type, saturated solutions of boric acid applied well over the surface to prevent spreading of the disease, and the anointing, with boric acid and bismuth subcarbonate ointment, of the denuded areas left by the rupturing of the bullæ may lead to a speedy cure. When the disease invades the conjunctiva, the lids should be touched with a solution of the nitrate of silver, 10 grains to the ounce, and the edges anointed at night with the yellow oxide of mercury salve. The pupils should be kept dilated and the accommodation paralyzed by atropia. In such cases, as the patient is likely to have been illy-nourished, attention to the diet and hygiene must not be overlooked.—(B. C.)

Impferkrankung des Auges. (G.) Infectious disease of the eye.

Impfgeschwur der Lider. (G.) Infectious ulcer of the lids.

Implantation cysts of the eye. Mention of these tumors has been made under various appropriate captions, e. g., **Cyst of the iris.** In this section reference is confined to a few additional observations. In traumatic cysts of the conjunctiva, which are often implantation cysts, the growths are due to the inclusion of epithelium which subsequently increases but eventually degenerates in the centre and forms a cyst.

Most *cysts of the cornea* are of the implantation variety. These are the result of operations or are due to injuries, some of the superficial epithelium being carried into the corneal stroma. The epithelium proliferates, and forms a cyst which closely resembles pearl tumors of the iris. Subsequently the central cells break down and are absorbed; fluid then collects and a cyst, lined by stratified epithelium, forms in the substantia propria.

Implantation cysts of the iris are described under that heading, as well as on p. 3675, Vol. V, of this *Encyclopedia*.

Implantation cyst of the orbit may follow the entrance of a foreign body or the introduction of epithelium as the result of a punctured wound. The contents of this cyst is usually serous, or sero-sanguinolent, mixed with cell débris, the wall being lined with flat epithelial cells. These cysts are extremely rare. See, also, the various headings under **Cysts**, as well as **Tumors of the eye** and Iris.

Implantation, Delayed. See p. 3808, Vol. V, of this *Encyclopedia;* also, **Enucleation of the eye.**

Implantation of animal eyes. See p. 482, Vol. I, of this *Encyclopedia;* also, **Enucleation of the eye.**

Implantation of artificial vitreous. See **Enucleation of the eye**.

Implantation of fat into the capsule of Tenon. See p. 4445, Vol. VI, of this *Encyclopedia;* as well as **Fat implantation.**

Impolarizable. Not subject to or capable of polarization.

Inaction, Hemiopic pupillary. See **Hemiopia.**

Incandescence. As a body becomes progressively hotter it first becomes visible in the dark as a fog-gray object, then ash-gray, then yellowish-gray, then faintly red, then red hot, orange, yellowish-white, white hot, and lastly bluish or even distinctly blue. Incandescence is usually witnessed in solids; never in liquids; sometimes in gases, as in the hydrogen flame.

Incanescent. Becoming grey.

Incarceration methods. See **Glaucoma.**

Incendie. (F.) **F**ire; conflagration.

Incense tree, The. *Balsamodendron opobalsamum.* The soot and the resin of the incense tree were both employed in the ancient Greco-Roman ophthalmology. Their chief indication would seem to have been injuries of the cornea and in all acute affections attended by copious discharge.—(T. **H**. S.)

Inch system. Lenses were formerly numbered (from their radii of curvature) in Paris inches, or 27.07 mm. Now they are numbered on a metrical basis, the unit being a lens with a focal distance of one metre—a *diopter.*

Incidence, Angle of. See p. 474, Vol. I, of this *Encyclopedia.*

Incident ray. In *optics,* a ray of light that impinges upon a transparent medium or opaque substance at which it suffers either refraction or reflection, respectively.—(C. **F**. P.)

Incipient cataract. IMMATURE CATARACT. The first stages of any cataract, whether hard or soft, cortical or central; the first faint striæ seen at the periphery of a lens or the faint dots seen in the nucleus.

In addition to the matter found on p. 1502, Vol. II, of this *Encyclopedia* Jessop (*Trans. Ophth. Society U.K.,* Vol. XXXIV, p.

151, 1914) believes that non-progressive opacities may be distinguished from the progressive varieties.

He contends that the non-progressive striæ take the form of "thin, fine, generally short, straight lines; dull, dark-grey in color by reflected, and black by transmitted light." "They are situated in the superficial layers of the cortex, and apparently all in the same layer; they are found, as a rule, between the periphery and the equator of the lens, and are often hidden by the iris; in most cases they extend posteriorly, and correspond in position to the anterior striæ." In many individuals over 70 years of age, an appearance, to which Jessop gives the name "arcus senilis lentis," may be found, and is evidently due to senile degeneration. In such cases the opacities form a ring around the lens, and this may be the only change present. At other times, associated with the arcus, there are isolated striæ, which extend towards and across the centre of the lens. It should be noted that these striæ, which show no tendency to coalesce with other striæ, all lie in the same layer of the lens.

Jessop has particulars of fifty instances of the foregoing kind of lental opacity, in patients whose ages have ranged from 50 to 90 years (29 females and 21 males). One of his patients, a male, 88 years of age, had been told thirty years before that he had cataract. The corrected vision is still 6/12 in each eye. Another patient, a female of 55 years, was informed five years before that she suffered from cataract, her vision then being 6/12. Her sight is now 6/6 partly in each eye.

For cases of the kind Jessop suggests that the word "cataract" should be given up, and that some circumlocution, as "senile lenticular opacity," should be employed. Further, he expresses the opinion that a surgeon would be justified in saying that these were not cases of "cataract" if the patient asked the question. See, also, **Cataract, Thompsonian.**

Incisura frontalis. Frontal groove or notch.

Incisura supraorbitalis. The supraorbital notch.

Incisure. A slit-like opening; a notch; a groove.

Inclinometer. This instrument (see the figure) is a patented device for determining the axes of cylinders. Lenses should be placed in the instrument, having the inside of the lens toward the operator. As is shown by the illustration the lens chuck has four points or jaws which engage the lens. The opening of the chuck is accomplished by shifting the finger lever to the left and is closed by releasing it. The lens is securely held in the chuck which is kept closed under spring tension. When the lens is placed in the chuck the horizontal axis of oval centers so as to register with graduation on the dial. The dial is graduated to 5 degrees, reading from 0 degree to 180 degrees. The pendulum, which swings from a central stud, has a series of teeth which engage with the teeth below the surface of the dial. These teeth coincide with the graduations on the same. The graduation of the teeth is arranged so that when the axis of the lens is less than $2\frac{1}{2}$

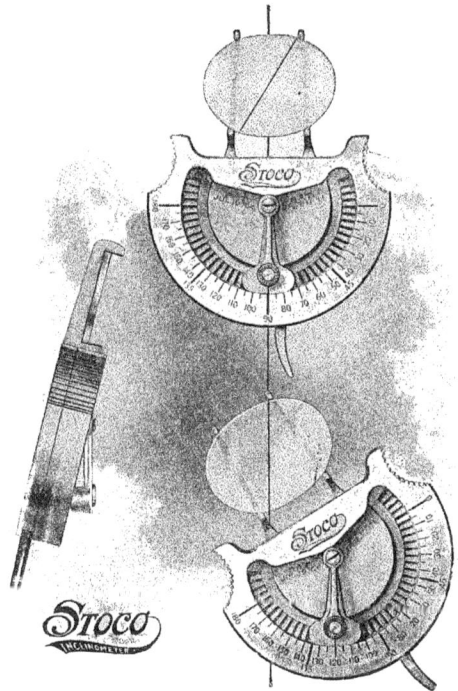

The Inclinometer.

degrees off from the axis specified on the prescription, the instrument registers in favor of the required axis and the lens is not disqualified. If the axis of the lens is more than $2\frac{1}{2}$ degrees off it will register 5 degrees from the required axis.

Cases in which finer readings are desired they can be obtained by reading direct from witness mark without letting the pendulum come in contact with teeth in the groove. When not in use, the pendulum can be locked by pressing the knurled button and turning same to the right. This can also be used to preserve readings obtained.

The name "inclinometer" is also applied to a German instrument for determining by means of retinoscopy the *two principal meridians in astigmatic eyes*. See the cut.

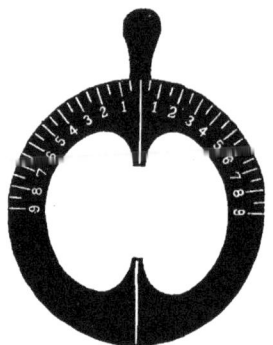

Inclinometer. (Jung.)

Inclusion blennorrhea. INCLUSION CONJUNCTIVITIS. See p. 3111, Vol. V, of this *Encyclopedia*.

Inclusion cells. Cells surrounded by a tissue or covering which separates them from the main body or collection. See **Conjunctivitis, Inclusion**; also, **Trachoma**; as well as **Bacteriology of the eye.**

Inclusion cysts of the orbit. In addition to references to these tumors made under the caption **Cysts of the orbit,** p. 3694, Vol. V, of this *Encyclopedia,* an abstract of the excellent account more specifically given by Parsons (*Pathology of the Eye,* p. 721) is in order. Cysts formed by the inclusion of a portion of the meninges and brain are even rarer in the orbit than in other parts of the skull. They occasionally occur, however, usually at the inner angle, seldom at the outer. When the hernia is composed of the membranes only, enclosing cerebro-spinal fluid, the cyst is a meningocele; if part of the brain substance is also prolapsed, an encephalocele is formed; and if a cerebral ventricle is also involved, a hydro-encephalocele results. These cysts are characterized by greater or less fluctuation and greater or less reducibility under pressure. Reduction may be painful, and followed by convulsions or coma. Respiratory and circulatory pulsations are rare in orbital inclusion cysts, owing to the constriction of the pedicle.

As regards situation, Larger found thirteen at the inner angle, one at the outer angle, seventeen at the root of the nose, in forty-four cases. Those at the inner angle may resemble a distended lachrymal sac, and are not infrequently bilateral. They are also often double in this situation; elsewhere they are usually uni-, rarely multi-locular. They may be as large as a large hen's egg. They are seldom so pedunculated as to allow of free movement.

The invariable greater or less deformation of the skull bones is of diagnostic importance. The hernia generally passes between the ethmoid and the frontal bones, at the expense of the horizontal plate of the ethmoid; the orbital opening is at the junction of the frontal, lachrymal, and nasal process of the superior maxilla. The line of exit follows the line of the first branchial cleft. Others pass through the sphenoidal fissure or optic foramen. The orifice is rounded, with sharp, though smooth, edges; it may be extremely small, or large enough to admit the finger.

Histologically, the outer covering is fibrous, corresponding with the dura mater. This may be adherent to thinned and very vascular skin. The arachnoid and pia mater are so altered as to be scarcely recognizable. The brain substance is edematous and degenerated; in hydroencephalocele it is covered on the inner side with ependyma, which is often well preserved.

Comparatively few of these cysts have been exhaustively examined histologically, so that it is difficult to say which is really the commonest. Probably most, if not all, contain some nerve substance which has undergone cystic degeneration.

Incoloration. Lack of color.

Incolore. (F.) Wanting in color; deficient in coloration.

Incongruenz der Netzhäute. (G.) Incongruous images perceived by the retinæ. See Images, Incongruous.

Incrostazione con piombo. (It.) Incrustation with lead.

Incruciatio nervorum opticorum. (L.) Chiasm.

Indarsol. (G.) This is one of those numerous proprietary organic arsenical compounds intended, like salvarsan and atoxyl, to be used in the treatment of luetic affections. At the request of the proprietors, Birch-Hirschfeld and Inouye (Graefe's *Archiv f: Ophth.*, lxxix, p. 81, 1911) made experiments with the new drug on cats and rabbits. Microscopic study of the tissues showed that indarsol, like atoxyl, is capable of causing considerable injury to the retina, without any objective changes being observable by means of ophthalmoscopic examination or test of pupillary reaction. The most marked changes occurred in the ganglion cell layer of the retina; the internal ganglion layer being affected in lesser degree.

Index, Absolute. The absolute index of refraction is the ratio of the sine of the angle of incidence to the sine of the angle of refraction when the ray passes from a vacuum.

Index, Broca's orbital. As is well-known the size, shape and relations of the base of the orbital cavities vary greatly. For the purpose of definitely measuring these Broca introduced an orbital index which is the ratio of the height to the breadth of the base. In other words, this index equals the height of the orbital base multiplied by 100 and divided by its width. See **Broca's orbital index.**

Index-correction. The correction for the graduation or index error of an instrument.

Index glass. The pivoted reflector of a sextant or similar instrument.

Index myopia. This form of short-sightedness is so-called because it is thought to result from an increase in the refractive index of the aqueous or lens, or decreases in the index of the vitreous humor. An increase of from one to two D. as a result of iritis has been frequently observed, but the exact cause of this refractive change has not yet been discussed. Myopia due to increase in the index of the aqueous in jaundice and in diabetes has also been reported.

Index myopia due to the lenticular changes of advanced life, especially of sclerosis of the lens, has often been observed. Landesberg has reported myopia of all degrees up to 10 D. and in practically all the cases there was incipient cataract. According to Risley and others diabetic myopia is due to an increase in the refractive index of the lens. It is transient in character, appearing in some cases of diabetes on marked increase of sugar in the urine, disappearing when the amount of sugar decreases.

Index of refraction. In *optics,* the ratio between the sine of the angle of incidence (i) and the sine of the angle of refraction (r) for a ray of light passing from one transparent medium into another. It is a *constant* whose value depends on the nature of the two media separated by the refracting surface, *provided* the media have the same properties in all directions and the kind of light is specified. This, *Snell's Law,* established by Willebrod Snellius, is expressed by the equation: $\sin i / \sin r = n$, the index of refraction, or refractive index of a medium exposed to the incident light having a *specified* wave-length. See also **Achromatism.** When the light, before meeting the surface, has been traveling in a vacuum, the constant n is termed the refractive index of the medium in which the refraction occurs. When light is incident in air on a transparent medium, the index of refraction is practically the same as if the light had been incident in a vacuum on the same surface. Thus, the above ratio for a ray passing from air into water is about 4/3, or more exactly, 1.336.

When n is greater than unity, it follows that r is less than i, and the refracted ray makes an angle with the normal which is smaller than the angle of incidence. In fact, the incident rays at the point of impact on the surface may be said to be bent toward the normal within the medium. This deflection generally occurs when light passes from a rarer to a denser medium; so that the latter is called the *optically denser* medium, whatever the mechanical densities of the media may be. Conversely, when light is deflected at the surface of separation of two media so as to be bent away from the normal, the index of refraction is less than unity, and the second medium is said to be *optically rarer,* or less dense, than the first.

When light is incident in a vacuum (or in air), on a transparent surface, it is nearly always deflected toward the normal, so that the refractive indices of nearly all transparent media are greater than unity. Light can penetrate to a small depth into a metal, and in this case it is sometimes bent away from the normal (in the case of sodium, gold, and silver) and sometimes toward the normal (in the case of platinum and iron). Thus, the refractive indices of sodium, gold, and silver are less than unity, whilst those of platinum and iron are greater than unity. See **Indices of refraction.**—(C. F. P.)

A knowledge of the refractive indices of the ocular media is of much importance to the ophthalmologist. Compared with air, 1,000 and water 1.335, the following indices are commonly given:

Aqueous humor 1.3365
Cornea 1.337
Vitreous humor 1.3365
Lens (average) 1.437

The refractive indices of the various forms of glass are as follows:

Crown glass (used for spectacle lenses) 1.525 to 1.534
Quartz .... 1.547 to 1.548
Flint glass .... 1.578 to 1.580

Commenting on the generally received indices of the ocular media Cirincione (*R. Clinica oculistica di Roma,* 1913) believes that the index of refraction of the ocular media in man at the temperature of the living gives a value different from that which is found in the dead, and this is not only by reason of the difference of temperature, but because of the fact that the transparent humors of the eye are altered in their composition and their optic behavior in the dead. The aqueous and the vitreous, because they absorb the products of decomposition from the neighboring tissues, have, in cadavers, high indices. The cementing substance of the lamellæ of the crystalline is liquefied, and to this is due the discovery by several authors of the presence of an albuminous substance at the anterior pole within the capsular sac;

while, in the normal crystalline, the superficial strata are solidly adherent to the capsule.

If the index of the aqueous of the normal eye be 133,325, that of the vitreous is 133,312. These figures show that the index of the aqueous and that of the vitreous are identical in animals and man when the material is equally fresh, but not so in the cornea, which gives for man the value of 13,731. It is probable that this serves to compensate for the lesser refracting power of the human crystalline which, as well in the nucleus as in the cortical strata, has an index less than that of corresponding points in the crystalline of animals, while its antero-posterior diameter is shorter.

The index of the more superficial stratum of the crystalline (capsule with the subcortical superficial stratum) is in the adult 13,883, and in the infant 13,890; the immediately underlying strata gives respectively the value 14,011 and 13,959.

At the posterior pole the superficial cortical stratum and the deep stratum give 14,008 to 14,014; in the aged 13,894, and 13,960 in the infant. The index of the aqueous is in the first 14,080; in the second 14,000.

The curve of the index for the human crystalline shows thus a behavior analogous to that of animals; but is proportionally lower, the difference lying between the cortical and smaller nuclear strata at corresponding distances between these points.

The variation in the value of the index in the different strata of the crystalline with age are in the human eye sufficiently important, in that they show sensible differences throughout the same strata between youth and adult age.

The index grows with the age, and with the growth of the index the consistence of the crystalline increases, without, however, obtaining the resistance of that of animals, and it is for this reason that its lamellæ and its fibers are capable of being modified at a late age or by rupture of its zonular connections.

No marked difference exists in the value of the index of the cortical layers of the two poles of the human crystalline in repose and during strong spasm of accommodation. The albuminous substance, as Heine describes it, is not met with in eyes recently removed.

Index, Opsonic. See **Opsonic Index.**

Index, Orbital. See **Orbital index.**

Index, Phosphatic. J. C. Clemesha (*New York Medical Journal.* March 23, 1912) supports the old idea that asthenopia, or eye-strain, is sometimes due to a lack of nerve energy, rather than always to an imbalance of the ocular muscles, which, by the way, may be symptomatic at times. His idea is to consider the metabolism of the nervous system with certain attempts to measure and regulate nervous, energy produced and exerted at various times, and under varying conditions by the human organism. His conclusions are that the Dowd phosphatic index measures the amount of nervous energy present in the organism. The urine examined should be passed at ten a. m., the second in the morning. The crystals should be examined for size and quality. In any functional disorder or one accompanied by organic lesions, the phosphatic index is of the greatest value as a guide to treatment. In all cases look to assimilation and correct any intestinal putrefaction shown by an excess of indican. A high index will note a condition of irritation or a want of adjustment of the nerve cells. A low index shows a lack of nutrition of the nervous organism, a using up of the reserve, and a condition below par. A high index calls for nerve sedatives, valerian, or bromid of gold and arsenic. A low index calls for food, eggs, etc., and the administration of phosphorus and strychnin.

India ink. INDIAN INK. A dried mixture of fine lamp-black and size or thin glue. In ophthalmic surgery it is exclusively employed in tattooing a leucomatous cornea.

Komoto claims to have made decided improvement in the vision of albinos by the subconjunctival injection of India ink. Galtier found that the operation was followed by no unpleasant results, and that it gave a bluish-white tint to the sclerotic similar to that seen in eyes in which the choroidal color appears through a thin and translucent sclerotic. It is not disfiguring. He proposes, in addition to the coloration of the sclerotic by India ink, to tattoo a peripheral zone of the cornea three or four mm. in width. See, also, **Tattooing.**

Indian dye. See **Hydrastis.**

Indian methods of cataract extraction. See **Cataract, Couching of;** also p. 1507, Vol. III, of this *Encyclopedia.*

Indians, North American, Eye diseases among. Most observers have reported from 50 to 75 per cent. of *trachoma,* and this disease is by far the most frequent and the most common cause of blindness among these aborigines. The Canadian and U. S. Governments have the matter well in hand, and have established stations and appointed surgeons to treat these unfortunates. Emil Krulish (*New York Med. Jour.,* August 22, 1914) has given information regarding the Alaskan Indians. Aside from general diseases and conditions, some 2.8 per cent. of Krulish's examinations discovered eye diseases (trachoma, pterygium, conjunctivitis are common) ; there are 13 per cent. of such sufferers. Twenty per cent. of the trachomatous are blind. In segregated families, the parents are usually completely or partially blind, the older children show advanced scleral changes, while the younger children evidence recent infection. Well-advanced cataracts in natives 35 years old were not uncommon. See, also, **Trachoma**.

India, The native ophthalmology of. See **Hindu ophthalmology**.

Indicanuria, Ocular relations of. Indican is a colorless glucoside, found in the blood and urine of certain animals, including man. It is an oxidation product of indol. Although its estimation in urine is of considerable clinical value in some general conditions, its importance in ophthalmology is at least questionable.

Stuelp (Graefe's *Arch. f. Ophth.,* LXXX, p. 548, 1912) reports examinations for indican in the urine of 511 patients suffering from eye diseases, probably not due to auto-intoxication. Indican was found in thirty-eight. Among fifty-six healthy persons, five had indicanuria; of eighty-two patients suffering from inflammations of the uveal tract only seven showed indican in the urine. Stuelp, therefore, concludes that it must be but rarely associated with these diseases.

von **H**ippel (Graefe's *Archiv f. Ophth.,* Vol. 81, part 1, 1911), on examining 416 cases of ocular disease for indicanuria found positive findings in only sixteen. Only those cases were considered positive in which the blue iron chlorid reaction was unmistakable. The different results obtained by other investigators may possibly be attributable to faulty technic. Thus Colombo found almost 100 per cent. indicanuria in phlyctenular kerato-conjunctivitis. It should be remembered, however, that indican is a constituent of normal urine, although the amount is generally so small that it is seldom difficult to differentiate a physiologic indicanuria.

von **H**ippel concludes that indicanuria in ocular disease, concerning which Elschnig has written extensively, has no etiologic significance.

De Schweinitz (*Arch. of Ophth.,* Vol. XLI, p. 615, 1912) thinks that the presence of indicanuria alone must not be taken as the index of auto-intoxication, as it would be practically valueless in the absence of other findings. **H**is communication is based upon twenty-three cases, carefully studied by exhaustive laboratory methods. No definite toxin that might cause such disease has been isolated. Nevertheless, a strict dietetic régime has been most beneficial to such cases, and departure from it was often followed by relapse.

Indication. (F.) Indication; symptom.

Indice. (F.) Indication; symptom; sign.

Indices. See **Index**.

Indigo. BERLIN BLUE. See p. 939, Vol. II, of this *Encyclopedia*.

Indigometer. An instrument for determining the colorific value of indigo.

Indirect ophthalmoscopy. See **Ophthalmoscopy** and **Examination of the eye.**

Indirect vision. This form of eyesight occurs when the rays from an object fall on the peripheral part of the retina. Indirect vision—although much less acute than direct—is of great assistance in distinguishing many movements, changes, or intermission of visual impressions.

As **H**arold Grimsdale (*Ophthalmoscope*, p. 137, March, 1915) points out, many investigators have attacked the problem of the measurement of indirect vision, but so far there has been evolved no method so simple and exact as to commend itself to clinical workers, and in practice, the sole measurement of the peripheral acuity of vision has hitherto been the examination of the extension of the visual field, and, in some cases, the examination of the intermediate zone for scotomata.

Calderaro (*La Clinica Oculistica*, Oct.-Dec., 1913) finds that a white object on a black ground serves better to determine the condition of the luminous sense and the acuity of the peripheral retina than a black object on a white ground, though he prefers two black squares on a white ground to determine the sense of form. Letters and similar test objects are not well adapted to the researches, because the sense of form is very feebly developed in the peripheral retina. **F**or the examination of the color sense, he makes use of colored squares on a black ground.

The examination of the peripheral retina should be conducted in daylight, if possible. Objects are more readily perceived when they are moved slightly in a sense tangential to the luminous ray which strikes the eye under examination. It is well-known that a movement of any object appears greater in the peripheral than in the central field. On the other hand, a constant stimulus very soon exhausts the peripheral retina.

Calderaro has noted a curious fact concerning indirect vision, viz., that two test objects which at different distances subtend the same angle, do not represent the same acuity of vision in the examination of the peripheral retina; thus, if two squares, having a side of 2 mm. and a distance separating them of 2 mm. are seen separate at a distance of 50 cm. on an oblique axis 30° external to the fixation point, it does not follow that two similar squares having sides 4 mm. will be seen in the same axis at a distance of 100 cm.; probably they will have to be brought to within 80 cm.

Of the two methods of examination hitherto in use, the circular at fixed distance (as in the ordinary perimeter), and the radial at varying distances, Calderaro has selected the latter on account of the facts just mentioned. He makes the examinee sit at an ordinary perimeter, with his head inclined 30° inwards and 10° upwards to avoid the prominences of the nose and eyebrows, and with his back to a north window.

He "fixes" during the examination a letter of Snellen's test type (Sn. 5.0) stuck on the wall at a distance of 5 m. The surface of the wall is uniformly blackened. The eye not under examination is closed with a bandage.

From a spot on the floor corresponding to the position of the eye against the rest of the perimeter are drawn lines which radiate thence in a fan showing every 10°. On each radius are drawn lines marking every 20 cm. Along these radii an assistant moves carrying the test object, and notes at what distance it is recognized by the examinee. In this way he measures for each radius the maximum distance at which the object is seen.

The results given by certain pathological eyes are also recorded by Calderaro who concludes that the test objects best suited to examination of the indirect vision are: (1) for the light sense, a square of white 2 mm. inside, on a black ground; for the color sense, squares of the same size, of blue, red, and green; (2) for the form sense, two squares of black (side 5 mm.), on a white ground, separated by a space of 5 mm. The best method of examination is by means of an object of fixed size and varying distances, not as in ordinary perimetry, at a fixed distance with varying size. The object should be moved centripetally on successive radii towards the eye. To get accurate measurements, repeated testing is necessary, but with this, accurate results can be obtained even in patients of limited intelligence. The point fixed ought to be at least 5 m. away to relax all accommodation. The light sense has the most extended limits in indirect vision, then comes the sense of form, then the limits of blue, of red, and of green in that order. The fields of red and green are very similar in size and shape, and often run together. These limits in the horizontal plane, describe an elongated trapezoidal space which extends a little further on the temporal side. The relation between the central and peripheral vision varies for the various sensations. The decrease is least rapid for blue, more rapid for white, red, form sense, and lastly most rapid for green. The influence of accommodation is to reduce the acuity sensibly in the paracentral regions up to 30°, and to increase it very slightly in the periphery. The limits of indirect vision of hypermetropes are identical with those of emmetropes, but the limits of myopes are distinctly less. The measurements of the peripheral vision may give valuable assistance in the diagnosis and prognosis in doubtful cases of nerve lesion. The alterations of the indirect vision are more early than alterations of the central acuity or of the field taken by the perimeter.

Indischer Hanf. (G.) Cannabis indica.

Indisches Süssholz. (G.) Jequirity.

Indistinctness of image. See **Abbe's measure.**

Indotint. A print made by a form of collotype process.

Industrial injuries to the eye. See Legal relations of ophthalmology; as well as **Conservation of vision; Injuries of the eye** and **Blindness, Prevention of.**

Inequality of pupils. ANISOCORIA. Inequality of the pupils (anisocoria) rarely occurs in health. It is found where one eye is blind, in disease of the teeth, in traumatism producing minute tears in the sphincter of the iris, in tabes, cerebral syphilis, disseminated sclerosis, paretic dementia, epilepsy, and probably in a few other conditions. Inequality alternating from one side to the other (springing or alternating mydriasis) occurs as a premonitory sign of insanity.

The presence of anisocoria suggests the need for a careful examination of the pupillary reflexes. While anisocoria often leads to the detection of important nervous diseases, it is not always pathologic. It is found exceptionally in healthy persons whose eyes differ in refraction (anisometropia).—(J. M. B.) See, also, **Pupil.**

Inequidistant. Not equally distant.

Inequilateral. Having unequal sides.

Infantile dacryocystitis. Mucocele of the new born. This is usually a congenital condition, as Donald Gunn has pointed out. See **Blenorrhea, Lachrymal, of infants.**

Infantile eye diseases. See **Childhood, Eye diseases of;** as well as **Measles; Cerebrospinal meningitis** and allied captions.

Infantile glaucoma. Congenital glaucoma. See **Buphthalmia.**

Infantile paralysis, Ocular relations of. There are few or no eye symptoms significant of this disease, although optic neuritis, hemianopsia, paralysis of the ocular muscles, and, occasionally, nystagmus have been noted. Cases with optic atrophy associated with diplegia have been reported by **F**reund.

Infantile ulceration of the cornea. See **Keratomalacia.**

Infants, Spectacles for. Worth (*Squint*, p. 105) has some very sensible remarks on this subject. **H**e says that spectacles for children of three years and upwards should have flexible curl sides to hook behind the ears; also that infants and very young children should have their

glasses tied on. The sides, in this case, should be straight, should
have a loop at the end and should be very short, only reaching to just
above the ear. About ¾ inch of each side near the loop may be
wrapped with wool. The glasses may be tied on with tapes, or, perhaps better, have rubber tubing over the tape, which is passed through
the loops, behind the child's head. These frames are very comfortable. If the sides are of the usual length the tapes may act as the
end of a long lever, causing pressure above the ear, and perhaps
ulceration of the tender skin of the infant, which should be guarded
against.

It is usually stated that children under three or four years of age
are too young to wear glasses. *No infant is too young to wear glasses
should they be required.* Many of Worth's squinting patients began
to wear spectacles before twelve months of age.

Of course, young children sometimes break their glasses, but
Worth has never known a case in which the eye has been injured
thereby. The lens, being held in the frame, does not break into
splinters, but cracks across, or chips at the edge.

Infarcts, Ocular. Deposits in various ducts, glands and blood-vessels
of the ocular apparatus are not uncommon. For example, see **Conjunctiva, Lithiasis of the,** which is really an infarction of the Meibomian glands and ducts. Coats (*Ophthalmoscope*, Vol. II, p. 708, 1913)
has been able to study a case of infarction of a posterior ciliary artery.
A man, 40 years of age, who had had an attack of iridocyclitis
with increased tension two years previously, lost the same eye from
an infective ulcer of the cornea. Pathologie examination showed a
large, roughly triangular, white area on the nasal side of the nerve
entrance, consisting of a wedge of necrosis in the inner layers of the
sclera, with surrounding inflammatory lesions, and of profound
degenerative changes in the choroid and retina, with but little inflammatory disturbance. The affected areas in the choroid and retina
were larger than in the sclera. The retinal changes elsewhere were
slight, and the choroidal almost none. Except at their edges the
necrotic areas were not at all infiltrated. The lesion was probably
due to sudden occlusion of a ciliary vessel by thrombus or embolus.
See, also, **Embolism of the central retinal artery**; as well as p. 1962,
Vol. III of this *Encyclopedia.*

Infécond. (F.) Barren; sterile.

Infection. See **Bacteriology. Asepsis. After-treatment.**

Infectious diseases, Ocular relations of. This subject is discussed under
such headings as **Diphtheria; Measles; Scarlatina; Smallpox,** etc., as
well as under **General diseases in ophthalmology.**

Inferior cervical ganglion. See p. 4843, Vol. VI, of this *Encyclopedia*.

Inferior oblique muscle. See **Muscles, Ocular;** also **Anatomy of the eye.**

Inferior rectus muscle. See **Muscles, Ocular;** as well **Anatomy of the eye.**

Infiammazione del ottico. (It.) Inflammation of the optic nerve.

Infiltration anesthesia. See p. 443, Vol. I, of this *Encyclopedia.*

Infiltration, Annular. A synonym of ring abscess of the cornea. See p. 3440, Vol. V, of this *Encyclopedia.*

Infiltration, Posterior. A term applied to the deep infiltration accompanying most cases of serpent ulcer of the cornea. See p. 3447, Vol. V, of this *Encyclopedia.*

Infiltration ring. In induced and some other forms of keratitis, where the injury is central, the peripheral opacity may clear from the outside, leaving a dense *annulus* about the central focus. Leber thinks this opacity is produced by a positive chemotaxis.

Infinite rays. Light rays that come from infinite distance—that somewhat indefinite position of an object—are parallel. Practically it is about 20 feet, as the rays emanating from such a point are so slightly divergent as to be regarded as nearly parallel.

Infirmier. (F.) A male or female attendant or nurse for hospital patients.

Inflammatory cataract. (Obs.) A secondary cataract resulting from an intra-ocular inflammation of some kind.

Inflection. DIFFRACTION. INFLEXION. The deviation of a ray of light from the straight path, when it passes over the edge of an opaque body or through a ruled screen.

Inflexoscope. A device for demonstrating diffraction.

Influenza. (L.) LA GRIPPE. THE GRIP. A specific catarrhal inflammation of the mucous membrane of the air-passages with severe constitutional disturbance. The disease is invariable in its essential characteristics, frequently prevailing as an epidemic, attended by lassitude and prostration to an extreme degree, with special and early implication of the naso-laryngo-bronchial mucous membrane [including, often, various infections of the ocular tissues]. Chills occur, and great sensibility to cold exists over the surface of the skin; the eyes become injected, and tend to fill with tears, the nostrils discharge an acrid fluid, and there is an intense pain in the head, mostly frontal, sometimes attended with giddiness. The nights are sleepless, with delirium or lethargy, cough prevails with yellow expectoration, most troublesome at night and tending greatly to increase the headache. Fever attends the disorder, sometimes slight and sometimes severe, and of a type varying in different epidemics and localities. The duration of the fever is from four to eight days. The sense of taste is generally much disordered, and there are great anxiety and oppression in the region of the heart. After the acute symptoms have subsided there is great debility, which often lasts for many months.—(Foster.)

According to Weeks (*Text book,* p. 763) the most common eye affection in influenza is conjunctivitis. A very mild congestion of the conjunctiva accompanies almost all cases of influenza, but an acute muco-purulent conjunctivitis, such as is at times produced primarily by the influenza bacillus, is not common as a complication of the general disease. Ulcer of the cornea with perforation and panophthalmitis; transient paralysis of various muscles, most commonly of the abducens; paresis of accommodation, usually bilateral; optic neuritis, which may be recovered from or may be followed by atrophy; retrobulbar neuritis with central scotoma, usually absolute, transient in the greater number of cases, may occur. Sönderlink (*Receuil d'Opht.,* April, 1905) reports a case of optic neuritis followed by atrophy and blindness. Hemianopsia (*Ophth. Record,* May, 1893) has been observed, probably due to a cortical or subcortical lesion. Intense pain in the eyeballs, at the apices of orbits and over the frontal sinuses, lasting three to five days, is common. It is very probable that many of the paralyses and optic-nerve affections accompanying influenza are due to extension of the inflammation from the frontal, ethmoid, and sphenoid sinuses, and not to the presence of the influenza bacillus in the tissue of the nerves affected. The toxins produced by the bacilli may play a rôle. Many of the numerous affections of the eye that have been observed to accompany influenza (*Berl. klin. Woch.,* No. 27, 1890) are probably due to microörganisms other than the influenza bacillus.

Rosenhauch (*Klin. Monatsbl. f. Augenh.,* Oct., 1908) has reported six cases of ocular disease, due to the influenza bacillus. There were three cases of conjunctivitis in infants aged 2 weeks, 3 weeks, and 3 months. One was a subconjunctival abscess in a girl of 19, and one a superficial keratitis, dendritic in form, in a man of 34. The sixth was a case of orbital abscess. These cases are of especial interest from the care that was taken to determine the cause of the lesion. The influenza bacilli predominated in all cases, though xerosis bacilli and staphylococci when found were tested by inoculation, and proved non-pathogenic.

Jackson (*Ophth. Rec.,* April, p. 198, 1908) reports a case of panophthalmitis in which the bacillus was found in pure culture in the pus from the interior of the eye. The attack began as one of glaucoma.

Spriggs (*Prac. Med. Series, Eye,* p. 197, 1910) gives histories of ten cases of edema of the eyelids occurring during an epidemic of influenza. This symptom, occurring as an early symptom of influenza, was sometimes followed or accompanied by pyrexia and other general symptoms. The usual history in a series of 40 cases was as follows: The patient goes to bed well, but wakes with marked edema. There is no redness, or at most a faint-pinkish tinge. At this stage there are no general symptoms. During the next twenty-four hours a bad headache develops, strictly localized to the supraorbital region. The edema advances till the eyes are completely closed, and may spread downward into the cheeks. In at least half the cases there is deep congestion, often accompanied by edema of the conjunctiva, but there is no discharge. The temperature never rises above 101° **F**. In more than half the cases the above symptoms constitute all the illness; but in a fair proportion, perhaps half, after a few days, as the edema recedes, the ordinary symptoms of influenza set in, and there are pains in the back, legs, etc., and great prostration. The urine is normal.

The great majority of cases occurred in poor patients; there was a large preponderance of females. There is little doubt about the influenzal origin of the edema. The prognosis appears to be excellent. The usual lines of treatment for influenza should be followed; cold compresses, or cold boric eyewashes appear to hasten the subsidence of the edema. See, also, **Conjunctivitis, Influenza, Bacteriology of.**

Infra-obliquus. (L.) The inferior oblique muscle.

Infraorbital canal. A small canal running obliquely through the bony floor of the orbit. It begins behind as a groove, and divides anteriorly into two branches, one of which descends into the anterior wall of the maxillary sinus, while the other terminates in the *infraorbital foramen*. It transmits the infraorbital artery and nerve.

Infraorbital foramen. See **Infraorbital canal.**

Infra-red rays. The red rays which extend beyond the extreme end of the visible red rays of the spectrum. They are of greater wavelength, less refrangible and of higher temperature than the visible red rays. The instruments used for absorbing radiations, and indicating the consequent rise of temperatures produced, are the thermopile, the radio-micrometer and the bolometer (q. v.).—(C. **F**. P.)

In their remarks regarding the effects of various color rays on the eye Verhoeff and Bell (*Ophthalmic Year-Book,* p. 440, 1914) claim that the abiotic action on the cornea and conjunctiva produced by any radiating source follows the law of inverse squares and is directly proportional to the total abiotic radiation directly received. The combined effect of repeated exposures to abiotic radiation is equivalent to that of a continuous exposure of the same total range, provided intermissions are not long enough to establish reparative effects. Destructive action for living tissues is confined to wave lengths shorter than 305 $\mu\mu$, at which length, abiotic effects are evanescent, while for shorter wave lengths they increase with considerable rapidity. The abiotic activity of the rays absorbed by the cornea is eighteen times greater than those which are transmitted by it. The corneal stroma is strongly affected by waves shorter than 295 $\mu\mu$ which it completely absorbs; but, is very slightly affected by the remainder of abiotic radiation.

The histological changes produced by abiotic radiation are radically different from those produced by heat, and the cell changes are best seen in flat preparations of the lens capsule. The characteristic change is the breaking up of the cytoplasm into eosinophilic and basophilic granules. In the normal eye, the lens completely protects the retina from the smallest proportion of feebly abiotic rays, which can penetrate the cornea and vitreous. The cornea and the vitreous bodies adequately protect from injury the retina of the aphakic eye from any exposure possible under any ordinary conditions of life.

Infra-red rays have no specific action on the tissues analogous to that of abiotic rays. Any effect due to them is simply a matter of thermic action, and such rays are in the main absorbed by the media of the eye before reaching the retina. Eclipse blindness, the only thermic effect on the retina of common occurrence, is due to the action of the concentrated heat on the pigment epithelium and choroid, this heat being almost wholly due to radiation of the visible spectrum in which the maximum solar energy lies. Abiotic energy in the solar spectrum is a meager remnant between wave lengths 295 $\mu\mu$ and 305 $\mu\mu$. At high altitudes and in clear air it is sufficient to produce slight abiotic effects such as are noted in snow-blindness and solar erythema. Glass blowers' cataract, often charged to specific radiation, ultra-violet or other, is regarded as probably due to the overheating of the eye as a whole with consequent disturbed nutrition of the lens.

The glass enclosing globes, used with all practical commercial illuminants, are amply sufficient to reduce any abiotic radiation very far below the danger point. The chief usefulness of protective glasses is not so much in their absorption of any specific radiation, as in their reducing the total amount of light to a point where it ceases to be psychologically disagreeable or to be inconveniently dazzling. For protection against abiotic action in experimentation or in snow fields ordinary colored glasses are quite sufficient. Glasses which cut off both ends of the spectrum and transmit chiefly only rays of relatively high illuminosity give the maximum visibility with the minimum reduction of energy.

Infratrochlear nerve, Avulsion of the. In 1883, Badal (*Annales d'Oculist.* 1883, p. 84) recommended stretching of the infratrochlear branch of the nasal nerve to relieve the pain of glaucoma. It was noted that hypotonus frequently followed several weeks after this procedure, but the degree of the hypotonus was less than after iridectomy or sclerotomy, and was probably occasioned by the simultaneous avulsion of the sympathetic root of the ciliary ganglion. Abadie and Indovian (*Arch. d'Ophtalm.*, II, p. 225) operated on several cases after this method, and Angelucci on 13. In all cases, a temporary decrease in pain and hyperemia and intraocular tension followed, but the symptoms reappeared after several days. The procedure has been especially recommended in glaucomatous myopic eyes in which dislocation of the lens was to be feared at the time of operation (*La Clinique Ophtal.*, 1902), also in hemorrhagic glaucoma, and finally Villemonte (*Rec. d'Ophtalm.*, 1906, p. 513) thinks it of service in glaucoma simplex and secondary glaucoma.

Infundibulum lacrimale. (L.) Lachrymal sac.

Ingrain colors are those formed in the actual fiber, either by the union of a dyestuff with a mordant already placed there, or by decomposing a soluble compound which has been soaked into the fibers into an insoluble one that must remain. Such colors are particularly fast in washing. See **Fast colors.**

Ingrassial. (F.) A name applied by G. Saint-Hilaire to the lesser wings of the sphenoid, as a separate bone.

Inguérissable. (F.) Incurable.

Inheritance, Abridged. A term applied by Haeckel to the fusion or omission of certain characteristics in an offspring which were present in the ancestors.

Inheritance, Amphigonous. A term applied by Haeckel, in sexual generation, to the inheritance of character from both father and mother.

Inherited keratitis. See **Keratitis parenchymatosa.**

Inhibition. A preventive or restraining action.

Iniops. (L.) A double syncephalic monster having two bodies, distinct below the umbilicus, but joined above. The head is incompletely double, presenting on one side a complete face (which distinguishes it from the janiceps), the incomplete face having a single eye and one or two ears.

Injection. HYPEREMIA. The name used to indicate congestion of bloodvessels. It is especially necessary to distinguish the hyperemia of conjunctivitis from that which occurs in keratitis and deep-seated ocular diseases, such as iritis, choroiditis, and iridochoroiditis. The former is known as conjunctival, and the latter as ciliary injection. Although in severe forms of inflammation of the anterior ocular segment the two types of congestion are associated, as would be expected from the numerous anastomoses between the posterior conjunctival and the anterior ciliary vessels, yet in many cases they can be readily distinguished. The points of differentiation between these forms of hyperemia are as follows:

CONJUNCTIVAL INJECTION.	CILIARY INJECTION.
1. Comes from the posterior conjunctival vessels.	1. Comes from the anterior ciliary vessels.
2. Is found in conjunctival diseases.	2. Is found in diseases of the iris, ciliary body, and cornea.
3. Is movable with the conjunctiva when pressure is made with the eyelid intervening.	3. Is immovable when the conjunctiva is moved.
4. The greatest redness is posteriorly, in the fornices.	4. Greatest redness is circumcorneal.
5. Redness lessens toward the cornea.	5. Redness lessens toward the fornix.
6. Color is a brick-red.	6. Is of a pink or lilac color.
7. Is composed of coarse, tortuous, superficial vessels whose meshes can be discerned.	7. Is composed of a series of fine, straight vessels radiating from the periphery of the cornea. The individual vessels are not easily recognized.—(J. M. B.)

Injections. See **Hypodermic injections**; also **Subconjunctival injections**; as well as **Intravenous injections**.

Injections, Intracutaneous. See p. 443, Vol. I, of this *Encyclopedia.*

Injections, Intramuscular. See **Intramuscular injections.**

Injections, Intraocular. See **Intraocular injections.**

Injections, Intraorbital. Injections into the orbital space are generally employed for anesthetic or disinfectant purposes. See, for example, p. 3605, Vol. V, and p. 437, Vol. I, of this *Encyclopedia.*

In this connection Weeks (*Diseases of the Eye,* p. 899) believes that intraorbital injections of mercuric chloride as strong as 1:3000— 1000, or solutions of the cyanide of mercury, 1 to 5000, may be employed. When used in cases of orbital cellulitis the injection may be made in two or three places at the same sitting. Bull and Weeks have employed solutions of mercuric chloride in orbital cellulitis with benefit. Valois (*Receuil d'opht.,* 1903) reports satisfactory results from the injection of solutions of the cyanide of mercury in two cases of sympathetic ophthalmia after the classical methods had failed.

Injections, Intravenous. See **Intravenous injections.**

Injections, Subconjunctival. See **Subconjunctival injections.**

Injuries, Obstetric ocular. See **Birth injuries.**

Injuries of the eye. OCULAR TRAUMATISM. Although under this heading the majority of the traumas that affect the visual apparatus will be discussed yet the reader is also referred to such captions as **Blindness, Prevention of**; **Conservation** of vision; **Birth** injuries of **the eye**; **Iris, Injuries of the**; **Cataract, Traumatic**; **Entropion**; **Fulguration**; **Iridodialysis**; **Sympathetic ophthalmia**; **Eclipse ophthalmia**; **Burns of the eyes**; **Military surgery of the eye**; **Electromagnet**; **Visual economics**; **Legal relations of** ophthalmology; etc., where these important subjects (closely related to this major heading) are fully treated.

The present section will be divided into, *Injuries of the ocular apparatus in general*, and, *Injuries mostly confined to particular organs or tissues.*

By injuries of the eye is understood all changes in this organ and its adnexa that may be caused by traumatisms affecting its functions and appearance through mechanical, thermal, chemical, or electrical forces.

Few injuries are confined to one membrane or part of the eye, and injury to one portion may be felt in another, the whole affecting the function or the cosmetics of the organ. Moreover the injury to sight in many instances affects deleteriously the whole organism and its function, as well as the place of the patient in society.

Ocular traumatisms may be divided into several classes: *(a)* Wounds without retention of foreign bodies. *(b)* Wounds with retention of foreign bodies. *(c)* Contusions, concussions, ruptures and dislocations. *(d)* Thermal injuries, including the effects of heat, light, electric and chemical burns. *(e)* The effects of explosions. *(f)* Gunshot injuries. *(g)* Infected wounds. *(h)* Poisons.

A *wound* may be defined as a solution of continuity, occasioned by extraneous force. Simple wounds of the ocular structures occur only to the lids and lachrymal passages, to the conjunctiva and cornea. Wounds of the sclera, of the lens, iris, and ciliary body and deeper structures occur through the cornea and anterior chamber, or through the conjunctiva and sclera.

Complicated wounds of the orbit pass first through the lids or the eyeball to the contents of the orbit, the lachrymal glands, the orbital fat, extra-ocular muscles, Tenon's capsule, the nerves and blood vessels, and the optic nerve; these may be further complicated by simultaneous injury to, and resultant disease of, the bony walls of the orbit, the contiguous sinuses, and the cerebrum.

A clinical classification of wounds of the eye is: Anterior wounds through the cornea, lateral wounds through the ciliary region, and posterior wounds through the conjunctiva and sclera. These wounds are also characterized as non-penetrating and penetrating, depending upon whether the eyeball be opened or not. As to their nature they may be incised, pierced, flapped, lacerated, contused, and infected or poisoned. The entrance of micro-organisms causes infection; bites and claws of animals, beaks and claws or talons of birds may produce special infective disease, and the bites of serpents and stings of insects may give rise to a chemical poisoning. The retention of foreign bodies and the effects of concussion and heat further complicate such injuries.

We may likewise differentiate clean-cut and piercing wounds from those whose edges are lacerated and bruised. To the first group belong the incisions, stabs, and flap wounds; to the second the contused, lacerated, and bite wounds. Firearms and explosions cause both forms of injuries, and in addition to the wound there is concussion and burn as well as retention of foreign bodies. These wounds may or may not be accompanied by a loss of tissue, and may be characterized by the formation of a flap.

Perforating wounds of the eye are those in which the ball is opened, by which the aqueous or vitreous is tapped. Non-perforating wounds are those in which the external tissues are injured, but the eyeball is not penetrated. This differentiation is of importance, as the possibility of infection is greater in a perforating than in a non-perforating wound.

In practice it is necessary to note the length, breadth, and depth of wounds, their form and direction, and if or not accompanied by loss of substance. In shape the wounds may be linear, fork-like, bow-, sickle-, or flap-like; in direction, perpendicular or tangential to the surface of the globe. Their position relative to the pupil and the limbus should be estimated. Their character, whether cleanly-incised, torn, bruised, or infected, and in the case of fine piercing wounds the direction of the canal should be noted.

Foreign bodies are found in the lids, orbit, ocular tissues, and within the ocular globe.

It is of the greatest importance clinically to determine whether or not an injury be complicated by the retention of a foreign body. Until the advent of aseptic surgery the removal of an eyeball so injured was deemed imperative, and eyes in which a foreign body had been retained a long time without causing blindness to the injured eye and sympathetic disease in the other were looked upon as pathologic curiosities.

Until the use of the magnet for the removal of magnetizable objects was taken up it was the rule to enucleate such injured eyes, and until the advent of the X-ray a definite diagnosis was in most cases impossible.

Thus in former years many eyes were sacrificed to the bugbear of sympathetic ophthalmitis, and others were allowed, through ultra-conservatism or through ignorance and neglect, to go on to sympathetic disease and blindness.

Only an aseptic and chemically indifferent body can be retained in the globe without causing irritation and inflammation. Feebly chemical substances, as iron, copper, glass, and stone, may cause but slight local exudation and become encapsulated, but contraction of the new-formed tissue, with further changes in the anatomical relations of the structures, ultimately and in opacities and dislocations, interfering with vision or causing blindness.

It is also possible from the irritation and proliferation of tissue cells that a foreign body may be carried away from its original position of impaction and be spontaneously extruded.

A foreign body to be retained within the globe must have been aseptic and have carried no germs with it in its passage, and tolerance of the tissues must have developed. The choroid and ciliary body most easily become irritated, the vitreous and retina next, but the lens is specially tolerant, for it is derived from epithelium and mostly composed of albumen, tolerating foreign bodies as well as other epithelial structures.

The size and shape of the foreign body have much to do with its retention; small, rounded intruders being tolerated much more readily than large, sharp, or pointed objects. The length of time in which a foreign body has been retained is important; the longer it remains, the greater is the possibility of full tolerance being reached. The chemical nature of the particle is also of importance. Inert substances are not apt to cause irritation.

Chemical effects of metals and glass within the eyeball. Gold and silver within the eye are very slowly acted upon by the tissues, but may ultimately become absorbed. Glass may remain in the anterior chamber for a long time, but becomes dull and the edges rounded, and if in the vitreous it may ultimately cause changes in the nerve elements of the retina.

Iron and steel in the anterior chamber soon become rusty, are covered by fibrin and discolor the tissues. In one case a needle point remained 527 days in the cornea, causing, however, rust and stain in this location. Iron particles are well tolerated in the lens, but color it by rust. Iron particles in the anterior portion of the eye do not cause hypopyon formation. In contradistinction to the effects of iron in the iris and anterior chamber are the severe changes produced in the vitreous and retina, where a hyalitis and shrinking of the vitreous occur from the irritation, with ultimate siderosis, detachment and atrophy of the retina from the formation of an iron carbonate caused by the combination of the albumen of the tissues and the oxide of iron from the rust.

Cases in which the cornea was stained brownish for some distance around a fragment of iron which had been lodged in it for weeks, are common. See **Siderosis.** The change in color of the iris is seen only in cases in which the yellowish-brown dots arranged in the form of a wreath. under the anterior capsule of the lens were present at the same time; both a yellowish-brown and a greenish-brown discoloration have been observed, but the first more frequently. A similar discoloration appears after hemorrhage into the vitreous and sometimes, also, into the anterior chamber. The yellowish-brown discoloration is of greater practical importance. Round, less than a mm. diameter, yellowish-brown spots appear at intervals of a mm. or two, in a circle, in or about the capsule of the lens. There are often spots on the anterior capsule, situated nearer to the anterior pole—the remains of broken posterior synechiæ. The spots behind the capsule are seen only after nearly *ad maximum* dilatation of the pupil. They are repeatedly seen in eyes in which the lens is still transparent and in which the capsule has not been ruptured. In all cases in which they are present iron is found back of the lens.

Among other symptoms of siderosis bulbi are ochre-coloring of adhesions between iris and lens, spontaneous mydriasis, subluxation, torpor of retina, concentric contraction of the visual field and defective color perception.

Copper particles give rise to even more severe chemical reactions. Pieces of copper put into the anterior chamber of rabbits' eyes cause a local purulent exudate so that within twenty-four hours they become fully covered. If removed the eye recovers, so it is not a microbic but a chemical purulent process. After a while the severe inflammatory process ceases, but hypopyon forms, the cornea ulcerates, and the foreign body is extruded, or the particle becomes enveloped by a fibrinous capsule. Copper chips in the lens cause opacity, but are tolerated therein. This difference is due to the copper going into solution in the aqueous and not being absorbed so rapidly when in the lens. Copper in the cornea does not cause reaction as within the globe. Copper particles in the vitreous act like iron, leading to necrosis and detachment of the retina.

Copper in the conjunctiva and outer layers of the eye is not dangerous. Small splinters may be usually seen and readily removed. In the iris the splinter usually sticks into the lens and offers no difficulty in removal.

Copper particles have remained in the lens for months and years without causing full clouding, but a sudden swelling with the formation of cataract later occurs. Removal with the lens is indicated. When in the vitreous copper particles usually cause acute suppuration, seldom chemical irritation, and proliferation of the connective tissues. The eye is usually lost and has to be removed.

In the fundus the changes are due to purulent inflammation as in the vitreous, seldom with connective tissue formation and detachment of the retina.

CONTUSIONS, CONCUSSIONS, RUPTURES AND DISLOCATIONS.

Injuries from large and blunt objects produce contusions, concussions, and ruptures, with dislocation of the ocular structures, in contradistinction to those from sharp or pointed objects which cause wounds. The effect of these may be local, upon one or more tunics or structures, but as a rule they affect several of the tunics or tissues. In wounds the injury is produced directly by the object, but by blunt force the effects are both direct and indirect. In the former the effect is directly upon the structure impinged, in the latter by transmitted force or counter-stroke, due to a rebound of the globe from the orbital tissues or its walls.

Contusions are of three grades. In the lighter forms there is more or less tearing of the perivascular tissues of the finer structures. In the medium forms this is combined with laceration of the inter-cellular substance, and in the severe forms with destruction of tissue and breaking of blood-vessel walls. Pathologically these injuries are expressed by changes in the vessels and tissues; in the lighter forms by changes in the tunics of the vessels, and in severe types by interruption of the contiguity and continuity of the blood vessels and tissues.

Paralysis of the vaso-motor nerves with edema of tissue and transudation from the vessels occurs; in severe cases accompanied by bleeding into the structures, rupture of continuity, and dislocations.

The lighter grades of paralysis of the vaso-motor nerves are followed by edema, as shown in commotio retinæ, and in paralysis of the pupil and accommodation. Various authors have attributed these pathologic conditions to bleeding within the tissues, but the edema about the nerve endings is sufficient to explain the paralysis. The pupil does not fully dilate to atropin or contract to eserin after contusion. Disturbances of the circulation give rise to opacification of the lens after the capsule is broken. Bleeding follows severe contusion; in the lids causing severe ecchymosis or suggulation—the ordinary "black eye;" in the orbit a blood-tumor; under the conjunctiva ecchymosis; and in severe types an hematoma.

Bleeding from the iris or within the anterior chamber is called hyphema. In rare cases the blood extravasates within the corneal lamellæ. From the retina the blood may show in the vitreous or as a subretinal hemorrhage. From the choroid as a subretinal or a subchoroidal hemorrhage, in the latter case producing discoloration of the choroid and retina.

In *concussion* the transmitted force jars the structures, disassociating the connections of the elements. In rupture there is also solution of the continuity of a tissue or structure.

Rupture occurs most often to the ocular capsule, especially the sclera, less often the cornea, then the choroid, iris, and but seldom the ciliary body or zonule. The choroid is often affected alone, but sometimes in connection with the retina. The iris may be torn away from its insertion, producing iridodialysis, or more seldom radial tears, here causing sphincter paralysis and mydriasis. Isolated tears of the retina seldom occur. The optic nerve or its sheath may be thus torn when atrophy results. Rupture of the zonula allows of dislocation of the lens, and here the hyaloid membrane is also usually broken.

Disassociation of the continuity of the intraocular structures occurs, the most common of which is detachment of the retina and partial or complete luxation of the lens. But this form of accident likewise occurs to the choroid, vitreous, and iris. Dislocation of the entire globe occurs only from direct force, as in gouging.

THERMAL INJURIES.

Such traumas are comprised under burns, scalds, chemical and electrical destructions of tissue caused by dry and moist heat, by the effect of chemical irritants or electricity in its various forms, as well as injuries from the sun and lightning.

Most of such injuries affect the skin of the face and lids primarily, with or without the implication of the globe. Those of the skin may be divided into the classical forms of burns: First degree, hyperemia of the skin; second degree, a superficial inflammation resulting in the formation of vesicles; third degree, partial or complete carbonization of the part. We may further classify these forms of injuries under the heading of burns which are caused by substances raised to a high degree of heat, scalds by heated fluids, and cauterizations caused by the entrance of chemical substances within the eye or on the eyelids. These injuries almost invariably involve the face and lids as well as the eye, and vary from trivial burns of the first degree to those causing destruction of tissue with subsequent loss of function and disfigurement.

Burns may be divided into those occurring mainly in domestic life, and which are largely caused by heated fluids, such as boiling water, soap, fat or lard, which are as a rule not serious and confined to the skin of the lids and outer coats of the eye; and industrial accidents occurring in trades. Burns from flame occur largely from furnaces and gas-ranges, and occasionally as the result of an explosion. They are usually only of the first degree, as the patient is able to get away speedily from the cause, although occasionally more serious injuries are met with. The eyelashes, brow and hair are usually involved, but seldom the cornea. The lids close so quickly and thus protect the globe so that few of such cases afford serious burns of the globe. Burns from bursting boilers and steam pipes and hot liquids used in the arts afford more serious cases. Hot blasts of air from furnaces or fires are found both in domestic and professional life.

Besides these casual factors, occurring in domestic life, there are burns from lighted ends of cigars, cigarettes, shreds of tobacco blown from pipes, the ends of sulphur matches, heated curling irons, etc. One might go on to detail a number of cases of superficial injuries from heated water or soup getting into the eyes, but these are inconsequential. Accidents from the blowing up of boilers of steam engines, if they do not kill, sometimes give rise to great disfigurements when the steam comes in contact with the face and eyes. Although we read of such cases constantly in the newspapers, yet the writer has seen but one such case and that some years after the accident, when ectropion and leucoma of the cornea was the most pronounced effect to be observed. As a rule such cases are attended by wounds of the face, eyelids and globe, and are treated under the subject of explosives and wounds. Many such extensive burns of the face, as a rule, are fatal, as they are usually complicated by injury elsewhere.

The *therapy of facial burns* belongs to the general surgeon. Aside from gunpowder explosions it consists of the application of carron oil, or 5 per cent. picric acid, to the burnt skin. Treatment of the eyes is as directed under treatment of burns by acids.

The complications and sequelæ of burns vary from infection, contusions, wounds or injuries to parts of the eye with loss of function, and require operations of various forms on the lids, conjunctiva, cornea, iris and lens which may have to be made for relief of sight or cosmetic injuries.

Injuries to the eyes by glowing metals. Particularly glowing iron, slag, solder and lead, are generally in the shape of masses that have been subjected to great heat during the process of manufacture—i. e., in industrial shops using coal and iron, molten lead, heated pitch or tar.

Surgeons living in a manufacturing community will occasionally be consulted in regard to injuries happening from the splashing of solder in the case of plumbers; from glowing iron and slag in the case of metal workers. At first it would seem that such injuries must necessarily be very severe, taking in conjunction the effect of the foreign body and of the intense heat. But as a rule injuries received from such substances are of moderate severity for the reason that they remain in contact with the parts but a fraction of a second, and during that time there is interposed between the glowing melted metal and the part upon which it falls, a thin stroma of watery vapor which arises from the skin or the eye, and materially protects it by reason of the physical law that "rapid evaporation produces cold."

Burns from iron dross, wrought iron, fused brass and steel, slag and glass, however, whose temperatures are above 1000° C., are ordinarily quite deep and lead to loss of the eye or extensive cicatrization.

In Giessen, during eight years there were 106 persons treated for injuries of the eye produced by glowing metal, which was 0.37 per cent. of the whole number; of these there were 65 by glowing iron; 7 by fluid lead or zinc; 34 by glowing slag. The latter were much more severe than the former, because the glowing slag sticks to the place of impact, retains the heat longer and thus causes a more deeply penetrating combustion and necrosis. Almost all patients could pursue their former occupations, but a considerable number—i. e., 9 of the burns from glowing iron and 12 of those from slag—were totally blinded on the injured side; in only one case was the vision of both eyes much injured. In 33 per cent. of injuries from iron and 45 per cent. of injuries from glowing slag, pterygium, local cicatricial symblepharon, entropion, trichiasis or ankyloblepharon occurred. Quite a number of patients injured from glowing slag had to give up their former work and rely on their accident insurance.

Superficial combustion of the corneal epithelium by hot iron, cigars, etc., may heal without the least impairment of sight, as the nutrient vessels which supply the cornea are not usually injured. It is noted that even if the cornea be not injured a purulent choroiditis may develop when the conjunctiva and sclera are burned as far as the limbus. Very severe burns of the sclera may lead to purulent affections of the uveal tract and vitreous and terminate in panophthalmitis.

Hot chips of iron may have a high temperature when they strike the face or eyes, and as these usually do strike with considerable velocity, there is added to the effect of their burning powers the damage done by the force of the blow, which is usually of more moment than the burn. The fact that the foreign body is a heated one usually makes the injury aseptic, and such wounds go on to more favorable resolution than others where the blow is received from a more or less dirty instrument. Of course, many workmen immediately take their soiled handkerchiefs, upon which they have blown their noses, wiped their hands or polished objects, and apply it to the part and thus infect with naturally deleterious consequences what might otherwise have remained an aseptic wound.

Burns from electric flashes are usually the result of "short circuiting." They are of the same character as ordinary burns and are treated in a similar manner. Electric light flashes may likewise produce a burn of the macula, the light being focused by the refractive media of the eye strongly upon the macula and thereby destroying the retinal elements. These always cause irreparable damage to vision.

Electric discharges from the ordinary commercial current are attended by thermic effects which, if of sufficient severity, burn the lids and hairs, then cause katalytic changes in the albumen of the tissues, later causing changes in the nutrition of the lens and cataract through alterations in the tonicity of the vessels.

These ocular troubles are the result of intense light at a short distance, and not of the short circuit through the patient's body. The absence of progression of the opacities, which are partial cataracts, and mostly confined to the anterior capsule, is noteworthy. The changes consist of linear and punctate spots scattered over the surface, being capsular and non-capsular, the posterior surface being free from opacities.

It is not the ultra-violet rays nor the ill-defined action of the heat, but a special electrolytic action that produces the opacities. The intense irido-ciliary hyperemia set up causes osmotic interchanges between the vitreous and the lens, and the current changes the aqueous so that it is unfit for osmosis. Still another hypothesis is that the current acts traumatically.

Externally, combustions at the places of entrance and exit, edema of the lids, conjunctivitis and chemosis are noticed. In Haab's disease there is a slight milky opacity of the whole macular region and along the upper border of the fovea numerous whitish-yellowish spots of irregular form and various sizes, with corresponding defects of the visual fields. See **Electric ophthalmia.**

The *Roentgen ray* produces an erythematous dermatitis which is to be avoided by current dosage, shields, grounded screens, proper regulation of exposure and state of tube. The dermatitis in some cases is destructive and has produced severe ulceration and cicatrization, ectropion and entropion. No damage to vision has been reported, as well as no damage to the operator from the use of fluorescein screens The action of the rays is cumulative.

The anatomical and histological changes found in the crystalline lens are more or less degeneration of the capsular epithelium and the cortex, which is most marked at the equator and the posterior cortex. Active processes of regeneration in the epithelium of the lens with formation of cell complexes, "pseudo-epithelial strata," and degenerative changes in the new-formed tissue are also seen.

Burns by static machines have been reported.

Conjunctivitis and incipient retinitis may be produced from X-rays. Operators subjcet to long-continued exposures suffer from irritability of the eyes, which may develop into inflammation with sufficiently intense exposure.

The obvious protection for operators using X-rays and finding trouble with their eyes is the same as that employed in phototherapy. The chemical rays are nearly stopped by plain clear white glass, and the physician who does not wear glasses for visual defects can avoid irritation during X-ray work by wearing a pair of large plain glasses without focus.

Treatment of simple burns consists in immediate removal of the foreign bodies, antiseptic washes (preferably of boric acid or weak sublimate solution), holocain, dionin, vaselin or iodoform vaselin, iced compresses at first to subdue the swelling arising from the immediate effects, hot compressing afterwards to stimulate nutrition of the injured parts; atropin may be used in severe injuries to open the pupil, and holocain and dionin for the relief of pain, and general analgesics, such as morphin, may be necessary. The lids must be kept from growing to the eyeball by passing a probe and the interposition of ointment, and sometimes general anesthesia is necessary for this procedure; if such occurs or if cases are seen afterwards, surgical methods may be necessary for the relief of the subsequent deformities and adhesions.

Freezing of the eyes or even of the lids occurs but seldom. The blood supply is so rich and the parts so sensitive that the patient quickly protects them from further exposure. Even Arctic explorers and farmers on the great plains, while reporting freezing of the cheeks, hands and feet, do not seem to have suffered such injury to the eyes, and there are no cases reported in ophthalmic literature.

Injuries to the eyes have been observed *after lightning strokes* which caused superficial burns of the lids and cornea with singeing of the hairs and the face. Cataract is not an infrequent result which has been attributed to electrolytic action similar to that which produces curdling of the milk in a storm. In the case of lightning stroke or severe electric shock some of the injury may be directly due to the severe jarring of the entire body. Cataract from lightning is not due to glaring, but to a mechanical lesion of the lens. Cataract has never been observed from mere glaring by lightning or short circuit. See **Fulguration.**

Injuries from sunlight and electric light exhibit at first a thermic change of the outer portions, later followed by chemical and atrophic changes which destroy the finer structures of the rods and cones of the retina with resultant atrophy, even to the percipient cells of the brain. These cause disturbances of function from opacities of the cornea or media, to destruction of the retinal cells, the fibers of the optic nerves and tracts, and atrophy of the visual centers.

Ultra-violet rays are held responsible for much of the damage done to the eyes by various lights and flames. See **Glaring**; as well as **Dazzling,** and **Glass-blower's cataract**; also **Illumination.**

Woodruff, in speaking of the effect of *tropical light* on the eyes, says: "We have a disease in the tropics similar to snow-blindness, but it is mild, as we never have the great radiance from the ground, such as we receive from the snow. We also have an affection similar to vernal conjunctivitis, which, of course, is merely a mild form of what, in winter, we call snow-blindness. In both extremes of temperature, then, either the arctic cold or tropic heat, it is due to the light, and we can have every conceivable grade of the affection, from simple conjunctivitis to paresis of the optic nerve and retina (nightblindness), or paralysis and atrophy with permanent blindness."

The answer to the question as to the protection of the eyes against the evil effects of short-waved light greatly depends upon the kind of light. If this contains an abundance of intense ultra-violet rays, as the arc lamp, mercurial vapor lamp, etc., globes of euphos glass are recommended, the intensity of the blue and violet rays must be subdued by yellowish-green or frosted globes, or by indirect illumination. If these precautions are not feasible, persons exposed to these lights must wear protective glasses of euphos glass (which for the absorption of violet and blue rays must be made darker), enixanthos or Hallauer glass, which also suffice for tours on glaciers and as protection against snow-blindness. Against light which contains less ultra-violet rays (daylight, sunlight on plains), amethyst, amber or smoke-colored are better than blue glasses for sensitive and diseased eyes.

Snow-blindness. This condition is more particularly an ophthalmia produced by the action of light on the skin of the face, lids, conjunctiva and cornea, though it has been ascribed as well to irritation

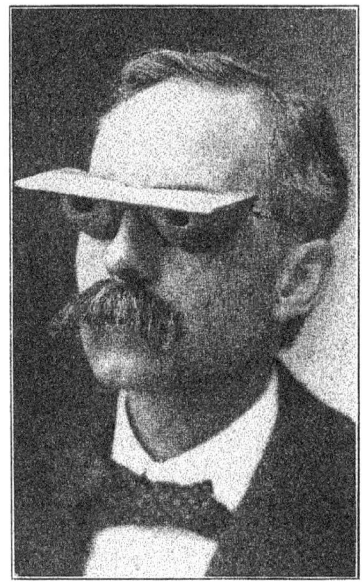

Goggles for Snow Blindness Used by the Native Alaskans.

of the retina from prolonged exposure to light. See p. 1197, Vol. II, of this *Encyclopedia*.

BURNS FROM ACIDS AND ALKALIES.

Burns from acids. Sulphuric, hydrochloric, nitric and acetic are the most common acids that lead to injury to the eyes. The first stage of *corneal* burn from these agents is shown by death of the cellular elements of the cornea, with a swelling of the corneal lamellæ similar to that which is noted in the laboratory when connective tissue is treated with acid. From the earliest hour, therefore, the cornea is deprived of active life, although it retains its shape.

The second stage shows invasion of the cornea, the anterior chamber and the iris by leucocytes, which may also infiltrate the eyelids. The subepithelial layers are especially involved, while the destruction of the epithelium increases with abundant and muco-purulent discharge.

In the third stage corneal perforation occurs, not as in ordinary cases, however, but from destruction of the corneal tissues by the acids. The lips of the ulcer are swollen and infiltrated by leucocytes, while from the limbus there is an advance of rapidly-multiplying epithelial cells. The palpebral epithelium is replaced by epithelium of the pavement type. The subepithelial area is deeply-infiltrated by leucocytes.

In the last stage, or stage of cicatrization and reparation, the corneal opening may be closed by a protruding iris, over which epithelium from adjacent conjunctiva has grown. In other cases the opening may be closed by a union of the lids to the border of the ulcer—i. e., if the latter is peripheral and not too broad. Finally, in advanced cases, or in those in which the tissue loss has been great, the perforation may be closed by a complete union of the palpebral lips to the remains of the eyeball.

Burns with acids are less dangerous than with alkalies. Ammonia is an exception to this rule. One drop of nitric or sulphuric acid is sufficient to destroy the eye. A drop of sulphuric acid with an equal quantity of water causes an indelible cloudiness. Caustic potash has a more powerful action than acids. Diluted with water it still destroys the eye.

If the burn be only of the first degree, speedy resolution may take place, but if the true skin be affected or the cauterization extend deeper, suppuration may take place, and the resultant healing is then attended by great disfigurement from scar tissue which produces severe ectropion, and if the eye be not destroyed, leucoma of the cornea at last, or symblepharon, may result, necessitating plastic operations later for partial restoration of the defects. In some cases there is a complication of the injury from cuts due to breakage or explosion of the vessel containing the acid.

Burns from acids largely affect the skin of the face, lids, conjunctiva, and cornea, and may be so deep as to involve the sclera. Such may be followed, as in the case of lime burns, by leucoma or even destruction of the globe. As a rule more extensive cicatrices form, leading to great cosmetic damage and loss of function from symblepharon, entropion, and ectropion.

Photographers and workers in acids sometimes complain of smarting of the eyes and conjunctiva from the effect of the fumes of acids · used in their trades. These can hardly be classed under the head of injuries, but may be mentioned in passing.

Physicians and chemists have at times burned their eyes by flakes of corrosive sublimate, acids, or other corrosive chemicals getting into their eyes in mixing preparations or in the laboratory.

Of forensic importance are those injuries caused by homicidal intent or to mar the countenance of some lover or hated person. The

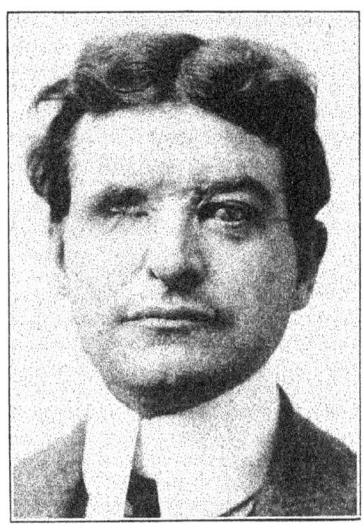

Cicatricial Contraction of Skin, Lids, and Orbit following Sulphuric Acid Burn. (Vail.)

most important of these are injuries from sulphuric (vitriol) or nitric acid, the favorite weapons of the jealous woman against the beauty of her rival. This naturally produces extensive destruction of the soft parts and, when entering the eye, may destroy it. At any rate, disfigurement is always produced, depending upon the amount of acid touching the parts and the length of time it is allowed to remain.

In cases where vitriol was thrown into the face with criminal intent, there may result a moderate degree of disfigurement from ectropion, and partial blindness from leucomata of both corneæ, in others total blindness with great disfigurement of face, and almost total closure of the palpebral tissues has followed. See, also, **Golf-ball injuries.**

In the *treatment* of acid burns, first use water to wash away the excess of acid with neutralization of the remainder by instillations of alkaline solution, bicarbonate of soda or potash, lime-water or milk; iced compresses followed by hot compresses; after this a bland ointment, such as 5 per cent. iodoform in vaselin, or carron-oil (equal parts of linseed oil and lime-water) may be used for dressings and the case treated on general principles. Dionin, 5 to 10 per cent. solutions, at first for pain, later, in powder to assist in the absorption of scar tissue, for which thiosinamin may be used as well in 10 or 20 per cent. ointment or given internally; atropinization to keep the pupil open and prevent iritis.

Alkali burns. The commonest and strongest alkalies are soda and potash lye, and ammonia.

When the vapor of liquor ammoniæ is accidentally forced into the eye, it causes severe pain which soon subsides. The cornea is clouded, wholly or in part, remaining the same for several days, then it gradually becomes more and more opaque until it is chalky-white. The treatment consists in the use of atropin, hot fomentations, subconjunctival injections of salt solution and olive oil by instillation between the lids. In one case that recovered, dionin only was used. The author believes that ammonia causes an occlusion of the canal of Schlemm and the spaces of Fontana. Interchange of fluids into the cornea is sometimes checked, and a dense chalky deposit results.

A burn with caustic potash may produce myopia from general weakening of the tissues.

The *prognosis of alkali burns* depends upon the amount of destruction of tissue, the length of time the alkali was in contact with the eye, the degree of cicatrization of the conjunctiva and lids, which may produce symblepharon, entropion, ectropion or leucoma of the cornea.

If the cornea be injured a diffuse haziness develops or purulent sloughing with perforation, complicated by iritis and hypopyon, sometimes ending in panophthalmitis. A very protracted course is characteristic, and the at first apparently benign prognosis may become very doubtful, as the inflammation of the iris and cornea may set in very late. Therefore, anesthesia and haziness of the cornea are ominous signs.

The treatment of alkali burns is similar to that of acids, except, if seen within a few moments, dilute acetic acid may be first used to neutralize the alkali. Immediate paracentesis of the cornea in ammonia injuries is recommended, as experiments show that soon after the injury ammonia is found in the aqueous.

Injuries from lime are of great importance; contrary to the usual belief, the injury is not caused by the heat of the lime, for the effect of slaked lime is quite as disastrous. It is a chemical burn followed by infiltration of insoluble calcium into the tissues. Such are usually combined with other foreign bodies, as the impaction of sand from the mortar in which it is usually mixed. From the deposit of chalk in the cornea, with resultant leucoma, result the most serious damage to vision.

The whiteness of lime burns in the cornea is due to a chemical compound (calcic albuminate) of the lime with the albumen of the tissues. The burning by unslaked lime is in part due to coagulation of albumen and in part to the imbibition of chalk. Guhman states that the deposit is not calcium hydrate but the chloride of calcium, combined with the phosphate and chloride. While calcium hydrate is a most effective corrosive, yet the last-named salts are not. The chemical change occurs in the lime at the time of its entrance into the tissue. If the lime keeps up its caustic action then perforation of the cornea may occur.

The use of a sugar solution to neutralize the lime was first advised in 1855, but is inadvisable on account of the heat produced. While water assists in the diffusing of the lime into the tissues, yet it is best to remove the lime particles by its mechanical action. It may be well to enter somewhat into the mechanism of burns by lime and its compounds.

Most derivatives of calcium are soluble in water and are dangerous. Calcium carbide, extensively used in the manufacture of acetylene gas, if brought into contact with water, is decomposed into acetylene gas and hydrate of calcium, and if done suddenly the temperature may rise to about 500° C., so that an actual explosion may result.

Oxide of calcium, or unslaked lime, obtained by the burning phosphate of lime, is the chief ingredient of mortar. The process of slaking consists of pouring water over it, by which it is converted into hydrate of calcium.

Hydrate of calcium is much more detrimental to the eye than is the oxide; this is opposed to the general belief. Vienna lime, hyperoxide of calcium, chlorite of lime, chloride of calcium, sulphite, bisulphite, and nitrate of calcium are also very injurious. They are used in plastering, in cement and in hydraulic lime. Solutions of the calcium salts act temporarily and slowly upon the eye, the paste acting strongly and lasting for days, the dry preparations less rapidly, but on the moist eyeball the dry preparations soon assume the actions of the moist.

The *therapy of lime burns* consists of extensive douching with water, the first that comes to hand, picking and wiping out of the lime, later using ammonium chloride solution.

It is only lately that we have been able to remove opacities of the cornea from lime injuries by any method. Ammonium chloride in weak solutions—i. e., 2 per cent. are to be applied for a considerable length of time, followed by stronger solutions, up to 20 per cent. Holocain solution or ointment is probably the best at first dressing, followed by dionin to relieve the pain. The stronger solutions are indicated only after complete cicatrization has taken place and should not be used, on account of the irritant action, while the injury is fresh.

COMBINED OR COMPLICATED INJURIES TO THE EYE.

Explosives cause complicated wounds, with or without retention of foreign bodies, bruising and shock to the tissues, burns and subsequent infections. The main effect of the more serious injuries is from contusion and flying foreign bodies.

Burns and injuries from gunpowder explosions. Independence day accidents involving burns, penetration of the face, eyelids, cornea and conjunctiva by explosions of powder are very common in spite of recent campaigns for a "sane Fourth."

These powder injuries vary from burns of the most superficial character of the eyelids and face, and a slight searing of the conjunctiva and cornea, to complicated injuries of the most serious nature. They are caused as a rule by boys making a "fizzer" out of a cannon cracker or firecracker, by putting loose powder in a can or glass bottle, by the premature or delayed explosions of toy cannon or firecrackers, rockets and other fireworks. Many an American youth has cause to remember the firecracker that "wouldn't go off" until he had raised it to his eyes to find out the reason why. At the very least these injuries from fireworks cause a burn of the first degree of the face, lids, conjunctiva and cornea, with the impaction of grains of powder, which, if not removed, leave lasting tattoo marks and permanent disfigurements.

Hunting accidents may likewise occasion the same character of injury.

The "flare back" from heavy ordnance is not so common in these days of breech-loading cannon, but does sometimes disfigure the faces and blind the eyes of our soldiers and sailors.

Dynamite and various other compounds made from nitro-glycerin used for blasting and in the manufacture of ammunition for large guns contain not only gas producing substances but certain solid bodies, which, together with the flame, the contusion and the chemical action, cause myriad wounds and retention of foreign bodies in the tissues. Thus dynamite contains a clay, the cartridge may be wrapped in papier maché and be encased in a wire gauze and have solid copper or brass ends. Explosions of such substances affecting the eye almost invariably damage other portions of the head or body, and as a rule are either fatal or extremely severe. This subject is dealt with in other sections in this *Encyclopedia*, but in so far as the burning by the flame as one of the immediate results, it is in part treated here.

Farmers clearing land by the blasting of stumps with giant powder, nitro-glycerin and dynamite occasionally find that the fuse does not burn quickly, whereupon examination may result in explosion with loss of life, limb, or sight.

The prognosis in gunpowder and dynamite explosions depends (1) upon the severity of the damage; if the burn be of the first degree and no other injury be done, full restoration of function and appearance may be expected; if of the second degree, partial restoration of function with cosmetic damage; and if of third degree, total loss. If the burn be very extensive, even though but of the second degree, and covers a considerable portion of the head (or one-fourth of the body), death is to be expected.

The prognosis as to sight depends upon the concomitant wounding, loss of tissue and subsequent infections. Maculæ and leucomata of the cornea following will prevent good vision. Iritis and occlusion of the pupil will blind the eye. Perforating injuries, and, in particular, injuries in the ciliary region and retained foreign bodies may cause panophthalmitis, irido-cyclitis, sympathetic ophthalmia, and blindness of one or both eyes.

Treatment of such cases is based upon general surgical principles. Burns of the face of this character are usually of the first degree, i. e., superficial, only involving the epidermis; when its vitality has been destroyed and the true skin or corium cooked by the heat, the burn is then that of the second degree. Application of a mixture of linseed oil and lime-water, picric acid 3 per cent., or 5 per cent. boric acid ointment is the treatment.

The use of a stiff brush with soap and water renders it unnecessary to pick out each individual powder granule or powder stain, for the nitrate of potash becomes absorbed a few hours after the injury, leaving only the carbon of the powder in the wounds. The brushing in severe cases should be done under general anesthesia, as it is extremely painful. The application of hydrogen peroxide, which forces out the stains, the application of papoid, which is a digestant and attacks the injured tissue only, thus aiding in the exfoliation of the dead tissue and with it the carbon stains, are valuable. After-treatment with antiseptic ointment is all that is necessary. Very few cases will thus be left with their faces disfigured by the tattoo marks of the powder explosion.

The eyes should be treated on general surgical principles, the foreign bodies removed by a spud after the use of holocain (not cocain, as cocain diminishes the vitality of the parts), and the application of antiseptic ointment, boric acid washes, and, if ulceration ensues, hot fomentations, preferably applied for twenty minutes every three hours, with the use of dionin, atropin and bandages. Even if the eyeball has been penetrated, if it is only the cornea or only the sclera, sight may be saved; if detachment of the retina has occurred from the force of the explosion, or suppuration ensues, or if the ciliary region has been injured, blindness or even loss of the eyeball may occur. Severe injuries of the skull may lead to death. Enucleation may have to be resorted to, and plastic procedures on the lids for subsequent contraction are at times demanded.

Gunshot injuries may come from large or small arms, from birdshot, bullets, shells, broken parts of firearm, explosives, lead and iron projectiles, metal particles or fragments, wadding, etc., from the cartridge, pieces of stone, sand, iron, earth, wood, bone from the skull, etc. Cannon shells, bombs, rifles and revolvers, shot-guns, the air rifle and sling shot are the usual weapons. The injuries happen either through carelessness in handling at home or in the field, mistakes in aiming or observation of objects, glancing shots and spent balls, attempts at murder and suicide, and during war. See **Military surgery of the eye.**

INJURIES TO THE EYES IN DOMESTIC LIFE.

The objects causing these injuries and the accidents themselves are very numerous. Amongst the common or more important are motes. and objects flying into the eye while on the street or railway cars, injuries from finger nails, pins, needles, hat pins, broken spectacle lenses, pocket knives and scissors, the two latter particularly common to children; also from table utensils, as forks; from carpenter's tools, flying nails or pieces of wood; burning fire-brands, hot cigar ashes or ends; burns by hot irons, curling irons, whitewash, lime, powder burns, gas explosions, acids, etc. Blows during rough sports as boxing, la Savatte, foot-ball, base-ball, la crosse, hockey, and even croquet and tennis are responsible for some injuries to the eyes; blows in fist fights or in falls, contusions from stones, pencils, etc., occasionally destruction of the eye from severe blows, from sharp instruments or gun-shot injuries. Mistakes in eye medicines or applications; even the leech has been known to migrate, during application, to the globe or cornea and cause ulceration. Malpractice of irregulars, also attempted suicides and murders swell the quota of the severe cases. Self-inflicted injuries to escape conscription for military duties, or even to gain damages for alleged accidents, are known. Accidents during, or from ill-performed, surgical operations may occur. See **Conservation of vision.**

INDUSTRIAL OR OCCUPATIONAL INJURIES.

In the so-called dangerous trades, particularly those dealing with the iron and steel industries, workers in machinery, butchering work, and building trades, occur the larger number of ocular injuries. Among these are the miners of iron, copper and coal, the smelters and machine builders. Those that are most subject to flying foreign bodies causing wounds of the eye are foundrymen, stone-cutters, machinists, turners, borers, boiler-makers, fettlers, smiths, and polishers. Workers by fire and heat, puddlers, casters, glass-workers, etc., are burned by fire, ashes, or iron and slag. Contusions of the eyes from falls, blows and thrusts come to all classes. In agricultural pursuits there are many kinds of injuries, especially from foreign bodies. In lands where the ground is tilled largely by hoes, as in the stony country of Switzerland, the breaking of these instruments against rocks causes many such injuries. Wounds from straws, pieces of wood, and instrument handles are common.

In 1,409 cases of accidental injuries to the eyes in farming occupations an extraordinary number of these accidents occur during the hot months, especially in the harvest months. The causes were injuries by straws, by branches in the woods, in working about cattle and by farming implements. There are especially injuries from foreign bodies to the cornea and conjunctiva, perforating wounds, contusions from sharp or pointed objects, injuries from lime or dung, burns and insect stings.

In the *building trades* there are injuries from iron, stone particles, and splinters of wood, and from instruments used in work; in quarries and mine explosions of powder and dynamite. Injuries from lime are common among painters. In laboratory workers foreign bodies, burns and scalds, and splinters of glass; in glass-blowing, burns and the formation of cataract; in cabinet-workers' injuries from the materials they work with, steel, wood, and bone; in turners, injuries from wood, bone, ivory, and stone, blows from sharp knives, etc.

Generally the injury is inflicted by fragments flying off while the mechanic was striking a chisel or piece of metal, or a hatchet with a hammer. The hammer is often a cheap one, and the purchase of hammers of better quality would prevent such accidents to a considerable degree. (See p. 1162 *et seq.*, Vol. II, of this *Encyclopedia.*)

The breaking of water and oil gauges on railroad engines is caused by the vibration of the engine, which subjects that portion of the glass of oil and water gauges which is inserted into the metal caps or holders to constant friction, causing the inequality in the thickness of the glass and rendering it unable to stand the required pressure of 200 pounds to the square inch. In water gauges, the friction of the water alone is sufficient to wear little seams in the glass and render it unsafe, in some instances even after a few days.

Accident may be due to disease caused by noxious influences, connected with certain occupations, as an acute or a chronic affection. Thus, direct lesions by solid or gaseous substances, as in the conjunctivitis of people exposed to the inclemencies of weather, stone impregnation of the cornea in stone-cutters, ribbon-shaped keratitis of hatmakers, masons, steel-grinders, opacities of the cornea from nitronaphthalin and analin, keratitis of oyster openers and caisson laborers, cataract of glassblowers.

A second group is caused by indirect lesion through circulation or direct toxic lesion of the optic nerve from carbosulphide, nitroamido-benzol, lead; and the third consist in neuropathies, as nystagmus of miners, spasms of the orbicularis of watchmakers and spasm of the ocular muscles from military drilling.

By far the most serious eye accidents happen to workers in iron or steel. Particularly in iron manufacturing districts the majority of serious eye accidents occur from chipping iron and steel. See **Blindness, Prevention of.**

Castings of either iron, steel, or brass are the most dangerous to work upon, because the chippings fly about on account of the metal being brittle. It is very dangerous chipping castings in corners or where the chipping strikes the metal and rebounds. Chippings from the castings are about ¼ inch to ¾ inch long and very sharp. When chipping thin plates on the edges, the chippings are sometimes 1, 2 and 3 inches long before they break off. All castings are "fettled" at the foundry, that is, the runners are cut off, and the plates where the metal has run at the joint of the moulding boxes are trimmed off.

The sizes of the splinters spoken of vary from the most minute to those measuring some inches in length, and they may be thick or thin. The injury inflicted differs, of course, in proportion to the size of the missile and the force with which it is projected. Small fragments may be thrown off with such velocity that they penetrate

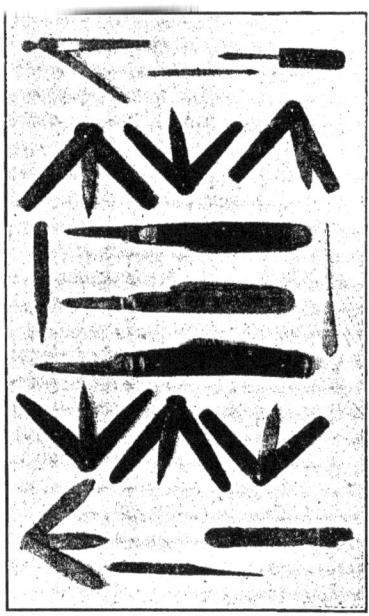

Different Kinds of Workmen's "Mote-Removers."

the eyeball and become imbedded in its interior, in some instances passing through the eye-lid before reaching the globe. The destruction to sight in this way is very extensive.

In a considerable number of the trades in which iron and steel are used the operatives are liable, though to a less degree than the grinder, to get these "motes" into their eyes. Many workmen are skilled in removing "motes" from their comrades' eyes. In all the large works there are men who have a reputation in this way. It is, besides, not an infrequent sight, even in the streets, to see a man with his head pressed against a wall and a fellow workman endeavoring to remove a foreign body from his eye. The number of foreign bodies some of these men remove in the course of a day is very large.

Doubtless, in many instances, these motes are skillfully removed; in others there is a good deal of bungling. The instruments generally used are unsuitable. Not infrequently cases come under observation in which sloughing corneal ulcers have resulted from the efforts made to remove a "mote," followed by infection from a dirty knife-blade or other instrument employed for the purpose.

In the case of *breweries and bottling works,* particularly of bottling aërated water, there is a comparative frequency of accidents from the breaking of the containers. A firm in Sheffield having several different factories employing from 2,500 to 4,200 hands, states that in spite of the most careful enforcement of the use of masks, gauntlets, etc., in one year there were nearly 400 accidents. The number of bottles that burst in one year is very considerable; new bottles or syphons are twice as liable to break as the old ones. About 1 per cent. of both new and old bottles break when filled. Syphons burst less frequently but the explosion and danger are greater; about one in 5,000 break in winter, while the percentage is greater in hot weather. The greatest number of bottles break in the filling machines, but there is practically no work in any part of the factory which may be regarded as free from danger.

Certain forms of injury are more apt to happen to some parts of the eye than others. Cuts and gashes occur mostly upon the anterior portion of the eye and its protecting organs, the lids, globe, cornea, ciliary region. Perforating wounds may go from the cornea and sclera through the bulb into the orbit and the optic nerve. Lacerations, tears, and the wounds from the bites of animals, are upon the more exposed parts, while shot wounds affect all portions of the eye. Flying foreign bodies or motes are usually found under the lids, though they may be impacted in the outer part of the bulb, especially the cornea. These consist of cinders, iron and copper splinters, the latter of which are often imbedded in the anterior, or even go to the posterior, portion of the eye, remaining in the iris, vitreous, or the coats. The cornea most often contains foreign bodies, less often the conjunctiva and sclera. The effect is most apparent upon the outer portions, the lids, brow, and then the bulb. In the eye itself they cause tearing of the retina and choroid, the blow indenting the eye and may push the lens away, causing detachment. Burns and cauterizations, as a rule, affect only the outer structures, the lids, cornea, and conjunctiva. The same may be said of burns from flame, the effect of lightning, electricity and sunlight, which may affect the lens and later the retina.

PROTECTION FROM INJURY AFFORDED BY NATURE.

The ocular globe is suspended and held in place by elastic and muscular bands, and rests upon a cushion of fat. It glides within a slippery capsule and is protected from flying objects, that can be seen, by the rapid reflex closure of the lids and the quick movements of the globe; from large objects by the protection afforded by the bony case of the orbit, by the projections of the brow, cheek and nose on all sides, except outwards and downwards, and by the rapid movements of the head, by which the approach of large objects may be dodged. Thus it is that the myriad of moving objects coming in the direction of the head and eyes in daily life are escaped, and only unforeseen or accidental injuries occur, and this to but a small percentage of the population. Even after the impact of a foreign body the reflex closing of the lids, the copious lachrymation and rolling of the globe assist in some cases in the expulsion of the intruder.

DISPOSITION OF DISEASED AND ABNORMAL EYES TO INJURY.

Weak sight disposes to injury because the individual cannot as well as the clear-sighted escape accidents, or specific injuries, to the eyes.

Diseased and abnormal eyes, as in those suffering from senile degeneration and weakened walls of the blood vessels, are predisposed to bleeding into the tissues from contusions and concussions, and to this condition persons suffering from arterio-sclerosis, glaucoma, diabetes, leukemia, and renal disease are likewise subject.

High grades of myopia—i. e., over 10.00 D.—are subject to retinal detachment, which is estimated to occur in 5 per cent. of the cases. The exciting cause of this may be ascribed to some slight local injury. Rupture of the sclera is predisposed by posterior staphyloma, due to myopia, and rupture of the cornea from anterior staphyloma.

Congenital ectopia lentis may be caused by a weak zonule, and excited by injury to the maternal abdomen before delivery, or by pressure in the maternal tract during delivery.

Scrofula, tuberculosis, and syphilis predispose to weakened tissues and poor resistance to injury as well as to poor restitution. In the case of bruising of the rim of the orbit periostitis, caries and necrosis may follow.

Injury to the cornea in syphilitic subjects may give rise to typical interstitial keratitis, or to inflammation of the iris and ciliary body.

TRAUMATISM AS AN EXCITING CAUSE OF CONSTITUTIONAL EYE DISEASES.

Parenchymatous keratitis can be elicited by traumatism in an individual of hereditary tuberculosis or syphilitic predisposition. The predisposition in tuberculosis and syphilis consists in a circulating metabolic poison, as in other infectious diseases, influenza, malaria, etc. The poison in hereditary lues shows itself in a predilection for establishing its action in the cornea, and more so if the resistance of the latter is weakened by traumatism. The development of parenchymatous keratitis in the other eye in a case under consideration is also explained by a toxic action on the cornea of the second eye, prepared for it by the sympathetic (not in the usual sense) influence of the traumatism affecting the first eye. We know that after injury of one cornea, the pericorneal and other blood vessels of the anterior segment of the second eye are frequently injected, which cannot be without influence on the consistency of the aqueous and the nutrition of the tissues, even if they do not lead to marked inflammation. In hereditary lues it is not the sympathetic irritation as such which produces keratitis in the second eye, but its combination with the enzymatous poison of hereditary lues.

If we knew a poison which had the same bio-chemical relations to the uveal tract as the poison of syphilis must have to the cornea, and were we allowed to suppose that in typical sympathetic ophthalmia it circulated in the body, the understanding of the former would meet with no obstacles, and we would not need to search any longer for bacteria.

Traumatism may be the exciting cause of syphilitic iritis and it is possible that a corneal wound may be the point of entrance for an exogenous infection, or a syphilitic iritis may be superimposed on an iritis from other cause.

Not only may a trauma develop benign growths in the conjunctiva, cornea, and iris, such as granulation tissue and polypi of the conjunctiva, cysts of the cornea and iris, but it may likewise be the exciting cause or point of entrance for tuberculosis and sarcoma, and a differential diagnosis is essential. This may be made by the microscope and bacteriologic cultures.

Wound of the conjunctiva from bites has produced conjunctival tuberculosis and epithelioma of the conjunctiva.

Granuloma of the iris has been observed after abscission of the cornea for staphyloma following a blow on the eye.

Tubercle bacilli may enter the iris after trauma, as has been many times experimentally shown in rabbits for laboratory diagnosis in suspected cases.

Infection seldom occurs from injury to the lids or conjunctiva, but commonly from both perforating and non-perforating wounds of the globe, especially of the cornea, and in perforating wounds of the uvea in the following order: the ciliary region, iris, and choroid.

Infections of the ocular tissues and organs following injury will be mostly described under their appropriate captions, e. g., **Iritis, Traumatic; Panophthalmitis; Corneal ulcer; Iridocyclitis, Traumatic**, etc.

The *diagnosis of injuries to the eye* is made by subjective and objective examination, of which the history, symptomology, and the visual acuity, field, condition of the ocular musculature and the refraction are given their proper consideration.

Objective examination by direct and focal illumination, the ophthalmoscope, diaphanoscope, sideroscope, magnetic attraction and the X-ray offers exact means of diagnosis.

A careful history should be obtained, giving the date and hour of the accident, the character of the work and surroundings, the instrument concerned, object or foreign body causing the lesion, and, in special cases, the names of the witnesses to the accident; also the character of attempts to remove a foreign body, and whether or not the case has been attended by a physician, are facts that should be elicited. Remember that while the interests of the patient are of prime importance, yet we should be guarded in our prognosis, as it depends very largely upon previous injuries and the character of the first dressing. We should never give an opinion reflecting upon the first consultant, or as to the liability of the employer, for these are theories that the lawyers may be allowed to fight about and the courts to decide. The less we have to do with the legalized human parasites who are in the habit of soliciting personal damage suits, the better it is, and we should not furnish information in advance upon which a personal damage or malpractice suit might be based.

Usually an examination may be conducted without a local anesthetic, as cocain or holocain, but such are frequently needed to subdue irritability; adrenalin to lessen congestion, and cocain, homatropin, euphthalmin, or atropin for mydriasis. The visual acuity, and in some cases the visual field, muscle balance, duction and versions, the refraction, etc., should be ascertained. In fact, in medico-legal cases a full examination should always be made, and sketch drawings or water colors may be made, as well as full notes taken. The literature of the subject should be looked up, as then the medical examiner, as a medical witness, will be fully prepared for his own answers in court.

The demeanor, willingness of the patient and actions of his companions should be noted, as thereby hints as to malingering may be obtained. See **Legal relations of ophthalmology.**

Owing to the transparency, translucency, and delicacy of the ocular structures a number of special methods of examination are of help, of which general inspection by direct and reflected light should first be used.

Inspection by direct illumination by day light, electric light or reflecting mirror is first made. The skin, lids, cornea, conjunctiva, puncta lachrymalia, etc., are observed. Then the retro-bulbar folds and under surface of the lids are brought into view by eversion with the fingers, but preferably by pushing down the retrotarsal folds with a smooth instrument, as a small glass rod, handle of an instrument, or cotton-tipped stick, as it is here that most diseases of the conjunctiva are prominent and where foreign bodies may be impacted.

Many small and otherwise almost indistinguishable abrasions of the corneal epithelium, wounds and small foreign bodies in the cornea, may be brought into view by the staining of the tissues by a 2 per cent. fluorescein and 2 per cent. bicarbonate of soda solution. This aniline dye will not stain the intact corneal epithelium, but readily passes into the subjacent parenchyma and abraded epithelial cells, forming a bright-green background upon which foreign bodies may be readily perceived.

Magnification of the eye by a lens, preferably by the Berger or Jackson binocular loupe, is of great value.

Focal illumination in the dark room is ordinarily carried out by focusing the light upon the eye by a large loupe. The use of the diaphanoscope for this purpose gives, however, a much better illumination, as the light is confined to a narrow beam. The author's trans-illuminator is the size of an ordinary fountain pen and is as readily handled. See, also, **Examination of the eye,** and **Diaphanoscopy.**

The *prognosis of ocular injuries* depends upon the part of the eye that is damaged, more especially that having to do with the functions of sight. Of first importance is the central visual acuity; secondly, the visual field; thirdly, the ocular movements; and lastly the light and color sense. To these may be added the cosmetic damage and the ability to use the eyes for work, or the ability to compete; and the sum of them all results in the economic vision. See **Visual economics.**

The prognosis also depends upon the amount of damage; the size and character of the wound; whether penetrating, perforating or non-perforating; whether foreign bodies are carried in; and whether infected or not.

Trauma acting on the parts of the eye necessary for clear vision, as the visual zone of the cornea, the lens, vitreous, macula lutea, does more damage in proportion than to peripheral tissues and organs. Injuries to the optic nerve and visual sphere are usually followed by atrophy and blindness. Injuries of the ciliary region are provocative of sympathetic ophthalmitis and loss of the other eye as well. As a rule clean-cut wounds heal well if not infected. Infection may, as as rule, be successfully combated if seen in the early stages. Retained foreign bodies are always dangerous. Contusions are generally danger-ous, as they lead to secondary degenerative changes and detachment of the retina. Burns of the anterior portion of the globe are always to be feared, lime injuries especially. Electrical injuries result in primary or secondary damage to the lens and retina. Double perfor-ating wounds of the globe, even with retained foreign bodies behind in the orbit, are compatible with comparatively small amount of damage to the function.

Local fractures of the orbital walls are of less moment, *quoad vitam,* than those which extend along the base of the brain.

PROPHYLAXIS OF INJURIES OF THE EYE.

While many eye accidents are unavoidable, yet the large majority are preventable by due care of the patient, parents, fellow-workmen or employers.

In domestic life a large proportion happen to children from ignorance or carelessness in playing with dangerous objects, such as dynamite caps, fireworks, firearms, etc., hot and boiling fluids, water, kitchen products, melted lead, sharp and pointed objects of iron, glass and wood, the throwing of sand, dirt and stones, the shooting of arrows and darts, blows with sticks, etc.; teasing of house animals, as dogs and cats, with resultant bites therefrom, about which frequent warn-ings by parents are necessary.

In agricultural life many accidents occur from carelessness, injuries from baling wire, straw, hooks, branches, splitting wood, horning by cows, kicks from cows, horses, etc., most of which are to be avoided by due care.

Safeguards against accidents to working men have been forced upon the attention of manufacturers, transportation companies and others, not only by legal measures, but by the necessity for conservation of their own goods and machinery, the loss of service and the cost of care and expense in treatment of such working men, as well as protection from damage suits, which give lawyers lots of work. The policy of making factory work safer and more healthful is profitable as well as humane, and it makes the workman more contented. Safety appliances are in use in most dangerous trades and have markedly decreased the proportion of accidents, particularly of the eye. Note the lessened number of blind from accidents within the last ten years, according to the census. The installation of screens for iron chippers and bottle workers, the pneumatic fan at the grinder's wheel and the forced wearing of masks, spectacles or other eye protection where flying chips of metal, glass, stone, etc., are common, have reduced the number of accidents. But though these materially insure the safety of the workman, it is with reluctance that he uses them and will shirk their application unless carefully watched and continuously warned.

This opposition seems hard to overcome, and while a foreman or skilled workman, who has to go to the wheel occasionally to sharpen his tools, takes measures to protect his eyes, the average workman is either too careless and shiftless to take the trouble to keep the lenses of his protective glasses clean.   See **Blindness, Prevention of,** as well **Conservation of vision.**

The conservation of the wounded eye. The treatment of a wounded eye should be conservative from the first, to retain as much vision as possible, to preserve the cosmetics of the organ, and in some cases even to save life, as well as to relieve the agony of the injury. With this maxim in view we must consider first those methods which will give the best results as regards vision, and secondly, as regards the appearance of the globe and its surroundings, bearing in mind always the dread possibilities of sympathetic disease in the other eye, and remembering the operation of enucleation or its substitutes with which to combat this possibility. A most trivial injury may, through neglect, ignorance, or mismanagement, result in total loss of vision in one or both eyes, disfigurement or even death; in all such cases there may be damage to the earning ability, pain and suffering out of all proportion to the same character of injury inflicted upon other structures of the body.

General therapy. As a rule an injury to the eye immediately incapacitates a person from pursuing the employment of the moment, be it business or pleasure, and he may be so blinded as to, in dangerous surroundings, fall into imminent danger of life and limb and so must seek, or be led to, a place of safety. Very few ocular accidents are attended by severe nerve shock as evinced by loss of consciousness. but such as occur are to be treated by fresh air, the dashing of water in the face, chafing the hands and the use of stimulants. Immediate. severe pain may be met by narcotics, especially by hypodermics of morphine; but, as a rule, cases of ocular injury are ambulatory and seek the surgeon in his office or at the hospital clinic.

The public should be taught that the *first aid* to injured eyes is as a rule to let them alone, except to apply a clean cloth bandage and to immediately seek a physician, more especially an oculist; except where large quantities of foreign materials, such as sand, dirt or corrosive substances (lime or chemicals) enter the eye, when the first application should be free douching with clear, clean water. The use of such house remedies as tea, milk, honey, urine, beefsteak, poultices of bread and milk, antiphlogistine, chamomile, sage-tea, or other applications is to be deprecated, for all of these only assist the growth of germs and act as a poultice. The injured eye is in no sense a "boil to be drawn out!"

Asepsis. The therapy of the wounded eye is based upon general surgical principles and from beginning to end the watchword is asepsis. The surgeon's hands should be clean, his dress neat, and while surgical millinery is superfluous in ophthalmic practice for the most of our work, yet the clean shirt, the changing of the street coat for the white dressing coat when handling cases, and the absence of a beard are details of his personality that prevent in some measure the surgeon from infecting his own patients.

When a patient, with an injured eye enters a hospital, as a rule, unless contra-indicated by his class and appearance, or the necessity of preventing jarring of the eye, a full bath is indicated, and, perhaps, a special preparation of the ocular surroundings by soap and water, 1:5,000 sublimate compress and light bandage, unloading of the lower bowel by a saline (a rectal injection if necessary) for general anesthesia and, if the time warrants, such general care as for other surgical cases.

The writer's rules in cases of injury to the ocular apparatus requiring operation are the following:

Head. Shampoo with green soap the night before the operation.

Face. Wash thoroughly with green soap, and after further cleansing with plain water, use a solution of 1:10,000 bichloride the night before the operation.

Nose. Irrigate with warm Seiler's solution the night before the operation and again the morning of the operation.

Eye. Wash the eyelids and eyebrow carefully with green soap, and after rinsing with hot water use a solution of 1:10,000 bichloride. Wash the eye thoroughly with warm boric acid solution and instill argyrol 50 per cent; a bichloride pad 1:10,000 to be placed over the eye and bandaged all night. Repeat this the morning of the operation.

General. Give the patient divided doses of calomel, one-fourth grain at a dose every half-hour for four hours the night before the operation, and follow with one-half ounce of magnesium sulphate in the morning. Do not allow the patient who is to have a general anesthetic any food the morning of the operation.

But, as a rule, injured eyes in ambulatory patients are first seen by the surgeon at his office. They generally come with a more or less clean bandage applied by themselves, by friends or some physician, and the after-treatment in most cases is carried out by the ophthalmic surgeon at his office.

A general rule in this class of cases is not to allow the injured one, or anybody else, to touch the eye or make any applications until the external wound has healed and there is no longer danger of infection.

Surgical technique of the wound. In general we do five things. (1) Render the conjunctival cul-de-sac, the lachrymal passages and the nose, as well as the lids and skin surrounding the eye, as free from germs as possible. (2) Replace or cut away prolapsed structures. (3) Sew up the wound or coapt its edges in other ways. (4) Use after-treatment by some antiseptic that will prevent the entrance and development of microörganisms. (5) Keep the wound quiet and occluded by bandaging, the ciliary body at rest, and the pupil dilated by cycloplegics.

The cleansing of the cul-de-sac is, of course, more difficult and has to be accomplished as an emergency procedure more generally in ocular injuries than in cases that are to be prepared for an operation. This should be done with chemically indifferent solutions, as douching with normal salt solution or 3 per cent. boric acid. These are best injected into the eye by the syphon bottle of Elwood or Todd, or the undine, which keep the solution from contact with the air and prevent its contamination. The rubber bulb, glass-ended syringe, or other forms of the eye douche, or even a sterile medicine dropper (in emergencies) are also quite useful irrigators.

In America there has been advocacy of a specially prepared 1:3,000 sublimate in petrolatum. The writer prefers this only as an application to the eyelashes or for after-treatment. Other solutions of value for this purpose are mercury oxycyanide, 1:3,000; chinosol, 1:1,000; hydrogen peroxide, 1:15.

It has been shown that it is impossible to entirely free the conjunctival sac from germs, yet by such means as mentioned their number is so reduced and their possibilities of reproduction so hindered that the eye may be made practically free from danger of infection.

The removal of catarrhal nasal secretion by douching, before an operation or surgical treatment of ocular wounds of any gravity, with mild saline, antiseptic solutions as Seiler's, Dobell's or other formulæ is indicated. For this the rubber bulb syringe or glass nasal douche is used, the solution being injected without force and the nose gently blown clear of secretion by the patient.

If upon inspection and manipulation the tear sac is found free from pus, evinced by pressure inwards and downwards with the finger tip, it may be left alone. If suspicious, a weak argyrol or fluorescein solution may be injected by way of the canaliculus to the nose, when upon gentle use of a handkerchief the stain will be found if the passages are patent.

If the tear sac be infected our troubles begin, for here we have the nidus of the pneumococcus, the staphylococcus and the streptococcus. Long previous treatment, advised in similar complications of cataract extraction is not possible in ocular injuries. The canaliculi may be temporarily occluded by passing a needle under the lower tube, coming out above the upper and tying the same.

The puncta may be temporarily obliterated by the galvano-cautery, or a radical extirpation of the lachrymal sac may be done in infected lachrymal passages prior to operations for injury to the eye, at any rate the puncta should be slit, the lachrymal sac thoroughly syringed with antiseptic solution, and the inner canthus strewed with powdered iodoform (or other less objectionable antiseptic powder), leaving the radical operation to be done later.

Surgical treatment of ocular wounds. This should be carefully done by mopping the parts with cotton, wet with a mild antiseptic solution. All foreign bodies should be removed, a prolapsed iris or portions of the ciliary body cut off, the wound edges coapted—if small, without sutures. Scleral wounds may be covered by sliding conjunctival flaps; if large, additional sutures are taken in the sclera itself. Perforating corneal wounds are best covered at once by the Kuhnt method (q. v.) by which many eyes have been saved. It is not only difficult but often impossible to suture corneal wounds on account of the necessary handling causing prolapse and loss of the ocular contents.

Antisepsis of the wound is best achieved with 50 per cent. freshly-prepared argyrol solution, with which the eye is flooded upon completion of its toilet. In suspected infection one may inject a few drops of this solution into the anterior chamber. This causes no irritation and saves infection. The method of inserting an iodoform rod into the anterior chamber has not been generally adopted. In former years powdered iodoform was liberally strewn on wounds of the eye, but recently it has been shown that the antiseptic qualities of the chemical are poor and its disagreeable odor and irritative action have caused it to pass into disuse.

Should the *wound be infected,* after due cleaning a solution of argyrol (50 per cent.) should be freely instilled. If hypopyon ulcer has formed, a free cauterization should be made and the eye filled with argyrol solution, or 1:3,000 sublimate ointment, and bandaged; or the open treatment by hot applications one-half hour every three hours, with frequent instillations of argyrol and sublimate 1:10,000 douching may be substituted.

Subconjunctival injections (q. v.) of 1:5,000 mercuric chloride or cyanide are advocated for intra-ocular suppuration, and even normal salt solution has been efficacious in saving many eyes. See **Subconjunctival injections.**

After-treatment. The after-treatment consists in: 1. An occlusive but *not* a pressure bandage. We know that the secretions of the eye which may contain microörganisms are carried by the lid movements through the tear passages to the nose, and that the ocular secretions are feebly antiseptic. We should not impede these natural safeguards by a pressure bandage; it is sufficient to protect the wound from actual contact with the fingers of the patient and the outer air. See **After-treatment.**

Tendencies in surgery are in the direction of conservatism, and in ophthalmic surgery also we should adopt the same principles, especially in regard to enucleation of the eyeball. We are now able to save many eyes which in earlier times would have been removed. This is due partly to the progress made in the treatment of diseases of the eyes, partly to operative methods adopted as substitutes for enucleation.

Although enucleation (or its substitutes) is the most radical operation, yet there are a number by which the form of the globe is saved, among which are abscission of staphyloma; iridectomy for iris prolapse; removal of the lens for traumatic cataract; operations for reattachment of the retina and others by which though a portion of the organ is removed, sight may be saved; which may then, together with enucleation and its substitutes, be briefly considered. See **Enucleation and its substitutes.**

Blasting and dynamite explosions may cause the impaction of a large number of foreign bodies in the conjunctiva, as well as in the cornea, and here it is not only advisable to pick out each individual foreign body from the conjunctiva with the spud, but to seize the membrane and excise by forceps and scissors the carbon stains that are left.

FOREIGN BODIES IN THE OCULAR STRUCTURES.

Foreign bodies in the ocular tissues and organs. This important subject is fully treated under such captions as **Cornea, Foreign bodies in the; Orbit, Foreign bodies in the; Electromagnet; Examination of the eye,** etc. To the material there assembled will be added some further observations.

A large proportion of the cases brought to the ophthalmologist are of traumatic nature, and, in manufacturing communities, injuries attended by the entrance of foreign bodies are extremely common.

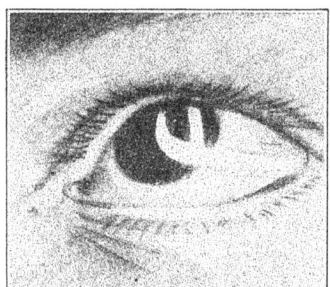

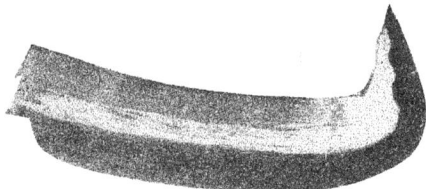

Extensive Laceration of the Eyeball from a piece of Hot Horseshoe. Recovery with $V = 20/\text{xl}$. (Eaton.)

Simeon Snell says that very few persons working at the iron and steel trades escape injury in the course of two years, and there are many more accidents to the eye in the course of this time than the number of men employed.

Clinically we may divide these cases into non-penetrating injuries, with or without impaction of foreign bodies, and these are mostly due to scale or emery, or iron splinters in the cornea; and also foreign bodies which penetrate the eyeball. The large majority of the latter are retained within the ball, but some may pass through the globe and become impacted within the orbit, or, in the case of bullet wounds, pass entirely through.

All these injuries may be infected or non-infected.

Foreign bodies that can be removed from the eye may be classed in two groups: First, those arising from iron splinters, which comprise about 75 per cent. of all injuries or cuts by foreign bodies penetrating deeply, and the balance, of copper, stone, wood and glass particles, which, as a rule, enter the eye more rarely and remain lodged in the anterior portion more often than deeper. Copper particles, however, may enter with exceeding force, as when resulting from explosions and firearms.

An eye in which a piece of iron, steel, or copper is buried invariably deteriorates, and ultimately becomes blind (siderosis bulbi), if the foreign body is not removed, unless it becomes completely encapsulated. In many cases this degeneration is preceded by the symptoms of hemepalopia.

We may thus anatomically, and with respect to prognosis, differentiate these penetrating bodies into two clases, one in the anterior and one in the posterior segment.

It is universally recognized that *when the foreign body is in the anterior segment of the eye,* the injury is much less serious than when it has passed on through the lens into the posterior segment, or has entered the vitreous chamber through the ciliary region or the sclera.

Foreign bodies in the cornea are sometimes difficult of removal, being so firmly imbedded that free incision of the corneal tissue about them is required to loosen them before they can be removed. When the anterior chamber is opened, care must be taken not to push the foreign body decper. Here the large magnet may be useful after the splinter has been partially loosened. When a chip of iron or steel is firmly imbedded the large magnet has no effect whatever.

(Operations for removal of foreign bodies from the external coats of the eye are specifically discussed under their appropriate anatomic headings.)

Foreign bodies in the anterior chamber are usually easy of removal. If they are of iron a small peripheral incision, if the original wound be closed, and a Hirschberg magnet will readily accomplish the result; but even a piece of steel thus situated may resist removal and lead to blindness. The particle may fall into the angle of the anterior chamber or pass through the pupil into the posterior chamber, when, if not iron, it may be difficult of removal and may set up an irido-cyclitis with all its dangers.

Foreign bodies within the globe. A foreign body in the *iris* demands prompt removal, for usually, if allowed to remain, it may set up a severe iritis. If the magnet will not remove it, forceps must, of course, be used. If it cannot readily be disentangled from the iris, we may succeed by drawing the portion of the iris containing the foreign body through the wound, so that we can more readily have access to it, and then after its removal replace the iris. Should these measures fail, it might be necessary to perform an iridectomy, removing the portion of the iris containing the foreign body.

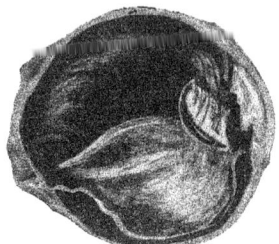

Chip of Iron in the Ciliary Body.
Nearly complete absorption of lens. (Würdemann.)

A foreign body in the lens is less liable to produce injurious symptoms or sympathetic inflammation than when located in other parts of the eye. On the other hand, these injuries sometimes result very disastrously. If the foreign body be in the lens, there is not the same necessity for immediate operation for removal as exists when it is in

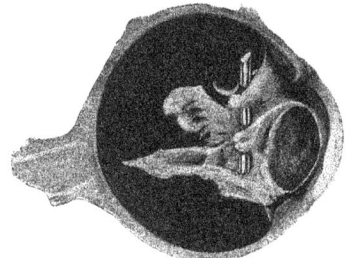

Brass Wire in the Vitreous.

Extensive chemical reaction with organized exudates. Enucleation one week after injury. (Würdemann.)

any other portion of the eye. If the foreign body be allowed to remain in the lens, the opacity is almost sure to increase until the entire lens becomes opaque. If the lens has been only slightly wounded, the cut in the capsule may close up at once so that the aqueous cannot get to the lens. Mydriatics, by keeping the lens absolutely quiet and so preventing the wounded fibers from rubbing against one another, or other fibers, in the varying changes known to be incident to efforts of accommodation, may prevent the increase of the opacity.

It is to be remembered that intraocular *corpora aliena* do in most cases irreparably damage the eye and that even when a foreign body is successfully extracted the eye may be blinded by later detachment of the retina, subsequent irido-cyclitis or the formation of opacities within the vitreous and lens.

These cases are usually seen shortly after the accident, but there are some in which the foreign body has been retained for many years.

FOREIGN BODIES IN THE POSTERIOR SEGMENT OF THE EYE.

A grave history of the dangers, damages and results must be told about foreign bodies in the posterior segment of the eye, for as a rule these have flown with much force, have already wounded the anterior

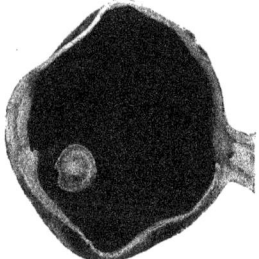

B. B. Shot in the Vitreous.

Eye Filled by Blood clot.   Enucleation twenty-four hours after injury. (Würdemann.)

structures in their course, and if allowed to remain in the eye not only destroy the sight and cause atrophy of the globe, but may result in sympathetic ophthalmitis.

The results of removal are certainly not as good as in the preceding class, for it may be safely said that if the ultimate statistics of cases in which foreign bodies have been removed from the posterior segment by magnet or otherwise could be obtained, far more than one-half would show blindness from irido-cyclitis, atrophy, detached retina, etc., and in a large proportion enucleation ultimately had to be done.

Immediate treatment is the essential point, as in this way many eyes are saved from sepsis, and the foreign body is more readily extracted before clots and connective tissue enclose it. The shorter the time the magnet is used after the lodgment of a piece of steel in the interior of the eye the better.

Every effort must be promptly made to free an eye from a foreign body, because some time or other retinal detachment or destructive inflammation will probably call for enucleation. Permanent toleration is so exceptional that it should not be considered. The presence of foreign bodies (not iron) in the sinus of the anterior chamber is sometimes very difficult to ascertain, especially when associated with hypopyon or granulation tissue in the iris. Then the Roentgen photograph is of inestimable value.

In a critical case where it is questionable if the foreign body be inside or outside the posterior scleral wall, the size of the eyeball should be carefully considered. Eyes vary in their size where high refractive errors exist and are sometimes larger in people who have very large heads.

The diagnosis is of paramount importance, as well as the early removal of a foreign body, especially in recent cases, in which postponement of the operation even to the next morning may mean the loss of an eye. Both Roentgen photograph and sideroscope are necessary in any doubtful case. The sideroscope hardly ever disappointed Hirschberg.

The time intervening between the accident and the operation for the removal is a most important factor, the best results being obtained in those cases which are operated on within the first twenty-four hours following the accident. A body imbedded in the depths of the eye becomes surrounded by a plastic exudate which, though quite soft, appears to hold it firmly and offers great resistance to its removal. When the piece of metal or other foreign body has been in the eye some days or weeks, the amount of force necessary to withdraw it drags so much on the neighboring tissues that the subsequent inflammatory reaction, together with that resulting from the original trauma, reduces the possibility of a satisfactory result and undoubtedly, in some cases, brings on a marked irido-cyclitis, with early shrinking of the globe.

The situation of the wound of entry is of considerable interest and importance. In corneal wounds the ultimate result depends on the final position of the metal; in the lens the results are excellent; when the metal passes through the lens into the vitreous or is imbedded in the coats of the eye beyond, the results are disastrous.

In wounds of the ciliary body, or farther back in the sclera, the results are not usually good and enucleation may be necessary. The danger of sympathetic ophthalmitis is ever present in eyes retained after such accidents, even though the foreign body be successfully removed. Perhaps surgeons are nowadays too conservative in such accidents and some eyes are retained that might better have been immediately enucleated. Such patients should be kept under observation for several years after apparent recovery.

Regarding the size and shape of the piece of metal the spicules of iron or steel are easiest to withdraw, due to the fact that the poles produced on the metal by the magnet are more apart in the long, narrow pieces of metal, while in the small rounded bits of metal the poles are, of course, close together.

Concerning the septicity of the wound, all chips of metal entering an eye may be considered as free from organisms, the septic inflammations being produced by the subsequent entry of organisms either through the tract of the wound or during the operation for removal.

REMOVAL FROM THE EYE OF NON-MAGNETIZABLE BODIES.

The removal of copper, brass, stone, wood, glass, and lead particles from the interior of the eye. Fragments of objects included in the foregoing list are very much more difficult to remove than steel or iron, but fortunately injuries with such particles do not occur at all as frequently, nor is their prolonged sojourn in the eye nearly so apt to damage it as a visual organ. With regard to such particles (not of iron or steel) it is often more advisable to leave them in the eye (unless, of course, they can be seen somewhere in the anterior segment of the globe where they are accessible), than to open up the vitreous and probe around, as it were, in the dark, with forceps and other instruments in search of the foreign body. To endeavor to remove such oftentimes damages the eye more than to leave it untouched.

Fragments of stone, wood and glass enter the eye more rarely than in the case of iron, but they are apt to remain lodged in the front portion thereof. Copper and brass splinters are as a rule projected with much more force, but since the days of the percussion cap are over, they are less frequently met with. We occasionally find copper splinters that enter the eye in the case of brass workers and copper miners, and from the effect of explosions of powder and dynamite caps and shells.

The diagnosis is obtained by the history of the accident, by the ophthalmoscope, diaphanoscope, focal illumination and the X-ray. In recent cases ophthalmoscopy may show a red or yellowish foreign body, or in older ones cyclitis or irido-cyclitis. Before or after an operation for removal, a considerable brownish-red opacity of the vitreous and iris may be seen, and very fine deposits on the lens capsule, where there are symptoms of chalkosis, to be followed by siderosis, which never disappears.

Injuries of the deeper portions of the eye by copper are considered to be of evil prognosis. Leber shows that copper is very apt to arouse suppuration in the vascular parts of the eye even without the introduction of bacteria. On the other hand, copper imbedded in the avascular parts, e. g., the lens, may be well borne. Especially unfavorable are those cases in which the foreign body penetrates into the vitreous, as its extraction may be very difficult or impossible.

Notwithstanding the well-known tendency of copper to produce suppuration, cases of this sort may recover after having harbored a piece of copper for a whole year or more.

Explosion accidents with copper penetration of the eye have been invariably fatal to the preservation of vision and the eye has in some instances come to enucleation.

The prognosis of copper injuries involving the anterior segment of the eye is not unfavorable, provided the metal contains no virulent germs and is removed early; neither a mydriatic nor a miotic should be used, lest the position of the foreign body shift and be lost to view in the anterior chamber. For the same reason attempts at extraction without an anesthetic are dangerous.

If it be decided to attempt removal by either the original wound or a new incision, Desmarres' forceps should be introduced and the object seized and, if possible, withdrawn, followed by antiseptic treatment and bandage. It is exceedingly difficult to grasp such splinters.

Particles of glass, stone and coal penetrating the eye and remaining in the vitreous, if aseptic and in a position difficult of removal, may be allowed to remain in hopes of retention without further damage, as they do not cause chemical changes as in the case of iron and copper, or if the wound is not in the ciliary region, causing fear of sympathetic ophthalmia.

The diagnosis is made as in the case of copper and iron fragments, by the history, focal and ophthalmoscopic examination, and the X-ray, and by careful probing.

Attempted removal should be either through the wound or a new incision by aid of forceps.

Grains of lead are practically only found from shotgun injuries. These are dealt with under the subject of shot and bullet wounds.

For the removal of *magnetizable foreign bodies* from the interior of the eye by the electromagnet, see **Electromagnet;** as well as **Haab's magnet** and **Giant magnet;** also, **Electricity in ophthalmology.**

So far as the subject will permit, a discussion of injuries confined, or mostly confined, to some particular ocular tissue or organ will now be taken up.

INJURIES OF THE CONJUNCTIVA.

These traumatisms are usually combined with injuries of the lids and cornea, or sclera, and, in penetrating wounds, of other parts of the eye. When the conjunctiva alone is affected, with the exception of burns, these injuries are trivial accidents.

Abrasions and cuts of the conjunotiva are of comparatively infrequent occurrence, as this membrane gives before the impact of the instrument, sliding over the ball, and is therefore less apt to be abraded or cut than the cornea. Cuts of the ocular conjunctiva are not painful, soon heal, and seldom become infected. Abrasions are more painful, as they usually occupy larger areas.

The utility of the conjunctiva is well shown in the many operations that may be done upon or through this membrane; thus it may be incised, transplanted or slid to almost any location and stretched or mal-treated in many instances without permanent injury or interference with the functions of the eyeball.

Isolated cuts are rare and harmless; they gape, the space fills with blood and the edges are reddened. They soon come together whether or not sutures be applied, and heal by primary union.

Traumatic conjunctivitis is due to irritation by germs, dust or chemical laden air; to the entrance of small foreign bodies, or to the abrasion of epithelium accompanying wounds and contusions. In the first instance true conjunctival infection, producing the characteristic forms of conjunctivitis, arises; dust and chemicals give rise to occupational conjunctivitis, shown in the form of a chronic conjunctival catarrh, especially of the follicular type; the irritation attending abrasions and wounds soon passes away. Small foreign bodies entering the conjunctiva usually cause a local irritation and congestion.

Motes in the eye. Foreign bodies on or in the conjunctiva or under the lids are of frequent occurrence and happen to every person. These foreign bodies completely though temporarily produce economic blindness, as such patients are unable to go on with their vocations until the offenders are removed. Most foreign bodies are speedily removed by the tears or by the patient himself.

The amount of irritation caused by a foreign body depends upon the position of its impaction. If it penetrates the sclero-conjunctiva, especially to the nasal or temporal side, the irritation may be very slight and after a short time it may completely cease, the body becoming impacted and remaining there for a long time without causing annoyance. The same may be said of the lower portion of the cornea, which is not completely covered by the upper lid in the act of winking. Particles of emery, of iron spiculæ or of stone, in the case of iron and stone workers, have become impacted beneath the ocular conjunctiva and even in the cornea, and have remained for weeks without causing trouble after the first few hours had passed away. The retrotarsal fold will often accommodate foreign bodies of a large size, which remain for a long time without causing much discomfort. This is readily seen in the case of so called eye-stones, flax-seeds and other objects which may have been put in the eye by some self-appointed helper from the laity; or particles of wheat husks, canary seed, corn, beads, etc., all of which the writer has removed from patients that were unsuspicious of their retention. Their symptoms were very slight compared to the

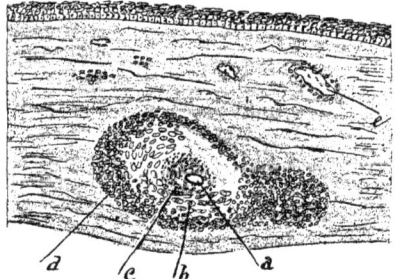

Section of Conjunctiva in Ophthalmia Nodosa. (Hanke.)

a. Section of caterpillar hair.   b-c-d. Cellular proliferation.

excessive irritation caused by gritty particles on the cornea or inner surface of the upper lid. The lodgment of a foreign body in the conjunctiva lining the upper lid, especially that part of it covering the cornea, and on the upper portion of the cornea, produces, on account of the winking, most painful symptoms.

The instant a hard body is deposited upon the eye, the lachrymal branch of the fifth nerve is stimulated, the tears flow, and if the foreign body be free it is washed to the inner canthus, where it will be often found unless it struck with sufficient force to imbed itself in the ocular tunics; this removal would nearly always occur except that the instant a person feels something fly into the eye, the inclination is to rub the part and thereby the particle is pressed into the cornea, or in the conjunctiva usually of the upper lid.

There is burning pain, copious flow of tears and more or less momentary blindness which accompanies the receipt of even a small particle of grit in the eye. The patient involuntarily puts his hand, generally with his handkerchief, to his eye and rubs the upper lid over the cornea, with the result above mentioned. The gush of tears in most cases washes away the intruder; to persons who know the procedure the upper lid is seized by its lashes, pulled down over the lower lid, the lashes of which may brush the foreign body away; in other cases, the end of a handkerchief may have been used, rolled into a cone and passed between the lids. If the foreign body abrades or sticks in the cornea, the symptoms continue and the patient is usually disabled from pursuing his vocation until the particle be removed; if in the conjunctival cul-de-sac, the intruder may remain for a long time.

On account of the eye being constantly bathed in a current composed of the lachrymal secretions, whose direction is from above outwards, down and inwards, foreign bodies are usually carried over its surface. Some of these lodge in the cornea, while others are

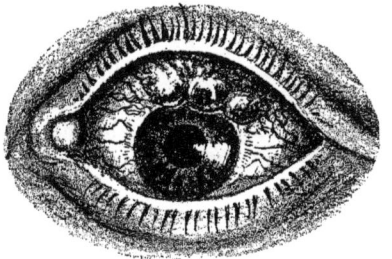

Ophthalmia Nodosa from Grasshopper Leg.

carried down to the tear passages toward the inner canthus, passing out of the eye upon the face, through or into the lachrymal passages, or lodging on the caruncle. The lachrymal puncta should always be carefully examined for fine hairs, such as cilia, hair clippings, grain beards or caterpillar hairs which may lodge therein.

The manner in which small foreign bodies are carried to and impacted in the conjunctiva and cornea is as manifold as their characters. Suffice it to say that motes in the eye come from all manner of domestic and industrial occupations and under all kinds of circumstances. Cinders, chaff, lint, insects, ashes, etc., are mostly met with in domestic injuries, while in industrial life the foreign bodies are particles of the objects being worked in or upon; particles of iron, copper and metals are rare for the average patient, while stone is more common. Particles of oyster shell produce a peculiar ulceration of the conjunctiva and cornea. Hairs of caterpillars, spicules from the legs of grasshoppers, and bee-stings, produce the peculiar ophthalmia nodosa.

Small shot has been found free in the conjunctival cul-de-sac after fowling-piece shot wounds.

The diagnosis is simple and a careful examination will usually reveal the presence of the intruder, but it must be remembered that the symptoms often persist for a time after its removal.

The prognosis is always good if the foreign body has not remained too long and severe inflammation and infection has not occurred.

For methods of examining the conjunctiva for foreign bodies, see **Examination of the eye.**

In the *treatment of conjunctival foreign bodies,* it must not be forgotten that those particles too small or too transparent to be observed by the naked eye may be brushed away by a cotton brush and the eye washed out with weak boric acid or salt solution. Oblique illumination should always be made. It is often difficult to detect a fine piece of steel, emery, glass or any minute shining substance when impacted on the cornea. These may be better seen in a darkened room, examining the surface by oblique illumination and with the ophthalmoscope with $+ 15.00$ to $+ 20.00$ D. for magnification; foreign bodies on the cornea then appear as dark objects. If found or not, the eye should be rendered insensitive by the use of 5 per cent. cocain, or preferably 1 per cent. holocain solution, when it may be more readily examined.

A large majority of cases of foreign bodies seen within a few moments, or within a few hours, after entrance, may be brushed away by using a hard-rolled, small, cotton pledget; in other cases a sharpened toothpick or match stick; while in still others, particularly those of accidents occurring in trades where particles of stone, emery or metal have been driven with considerable force into the membrane, it is necessary to use instrumental means and to dig out the foreign body either with a sharp spud, the cutting needle or a gouge. Particles of coal, such as cinders, and pieces of vegetable matter, rarely need instrumental means for their removal.

Bruising of the conjunctiva occurs with most wounds, but as a rule is not extensive on account of the great elasticity and movability of the membrane.

Conjunctival ecchymosis (effusion of blood beneath the ocular conjunctiva) is characterized by a patch or deep-red ring more or less surrounding the cornea or occupying the whole of the conjunctiva, which gives to the eye an alarming appearance, although it is not in itself a dangerous occurrence, and yet may be significant of arterio-sclerosis or follow a serious injury to the skull. The ecchymosis may be of such extent as to form a blood tumor under the conjunctiva, particularly on the inter-tarsal folds, when it extrudes from the eye in a large mass.

This condition is usually produced by operations on the ocular conjunctiva, blows, lifting heavy weights, vomiting (particularly the strain from the vomiting of whooping cough), cohabitation, the impact of wind on the eyes in bicycling, automobiling, or engine riding, etc.

The predisposing causes are degenerative conditions of the blood vessels, arterio-sclerosis, Bright's disease, diabetes, scurvy, etc.

As with suggulation of the lids (or ordinary black-eye) absorption of the blood is slow, occupying two or three weeks.

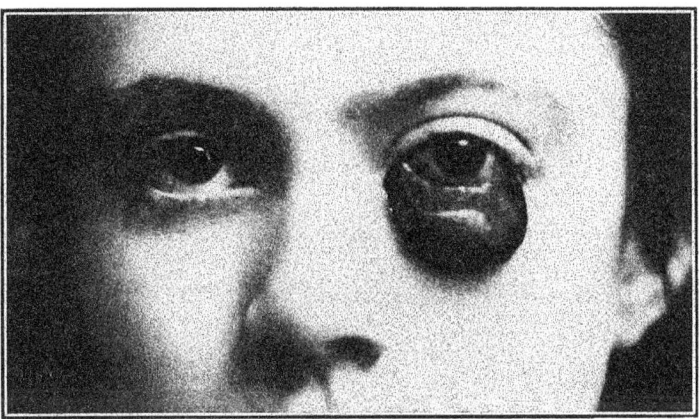

Edema of the Conjunctiva. (Becker.)

The blood usually gravitates to the lower part of the sac, and as a hematoma makes a decided swelling in the lower fornix. The blood is usually resorbed in two or three weeks and changes in color from red to brown and greenish-yellow.

Immediately after the accident ice compresses may hinder further extravasation of blood, afterwards hot compresses and 5-10 per cent. dionine solution will hasten its absorption. Lead water and opium applications are of benefit. See, also, **Hematoma.**

Pigmentation of the conjunctiva. Blue stains of the conjunctiva from methyl violet ink or blue pencil have been reported in a number of instances. If the cornea be not affected thereby, causing chemical cauterization, the stain remains for a few days and then disappears.

Siderosis of the conjunctiva is a yellowish pigmentation due to long-continued internal use of the sulphate of iron, or to the retention of impacted iron particles or scales in the conjunctiva.

Blood-pigment may stain the conjunctiva for a long time as the result of injuries. A number of diseases, such as jaundice or gout, may cause changes in the conjunctiva, but are hardly to be classed under the name of injuries.

Extensive tattooing from powder explosions often results from careless handling of fireworks, firearms and explosives.

Nitrate of silver, argyrol, protargol, or other preparations of silver applied for a long time, particularly if given into the hands of the patient for home treatment, may cause a dirty, permanent, gray, slate color, or brownish discoloration of the conjunctiva. The discoloration is permanent, but a 2 per cent. to 5 per cent. solution of hyposulphite of soda, used for a long time, materially clears the discoloration. See **Argyrosis.**

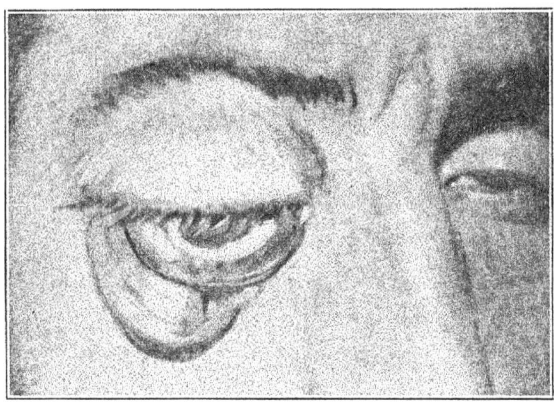

Chemosis of Conjunctiva and Lids following Infected Wound of the Globe.

Burns and cauterizations of the conjunctiva have been dealt with quite fully in connection with the general subject of burns and cauterizations. They occur in all grades, from the burn of sun-blindness and that of the electric light, to extensive destruction of tissue from chemicals and molten iron, which usually involve the lids and cornea as well.

People who work in excessive heat or light, as firemen, glass-blowers, and electric arc workers are subject to an irritative chronic conjunctivitis caused by thermal injuries.

In simple burns of the conjunctiva the burned or cauterized area appears as a grayish-white plaque; if from lime, white from the lime contained in the tissue. The edges of the burn are reddened. There is lachrymation, photophobia, and smarting pain. The wounds granulate, being replaced by scar-tissue, which, however, in this situation is difficult to distinguish from the conjunctiva. Shrinking of the conjunctiva may occur.

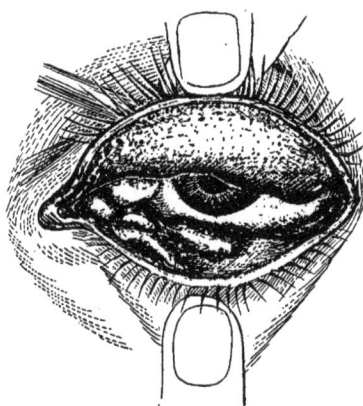

Extensive Burn of the Conjunctiva of the Lids from Hot Fluid Jelly.

Immediate treatment is by a bland antiseptic analgesic ointment, as iodoform 5 per cent., dionin 5 per cent. and iced compresses.

The great danger is from cicatricial union of the lids to the globe, symblepharon, which is to be guarded against, freely separating the

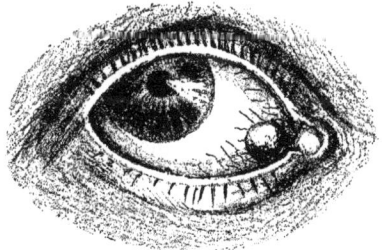

Polyp of the Conjunctiva Following Injury.

lids by daily probing, conjunctival plastics, use of egg film, etc., to keep the two surfaces apart. When severe the shrinking may cause entropion, trichiasis, lagophthalmus, pterygium, symblepharon, ankyloblepharon, shrinking, etc., which must be dealt with by subsequent operations.

Excessive cicatricial formation from treatment of trachoma by such cauterants as nitrate of silver and sulphate of copper has often been observed.

Polypus of the conjunctiva is the main tumor formation from wounds or injuries, especially from those that do not heal by first intention. Granulation tissue proliferates and forms polypi; which should be removed by forceps and scissors. No authentic case of sarcoma of the conjunctiva has yet been ascribed to trauma.

The *impaction of powder grains in and under the conjunctiva* is an accident comparatively often seen, either as the result of powder and firework explosions, and from imperfect breech or back-fires in guns. These powder grains are not to be picked out. It is necessary here to remove a small piece of the conjunctiva and subconjunctival tissue, together with the powder stain or grain, with or without a subsequent suture.

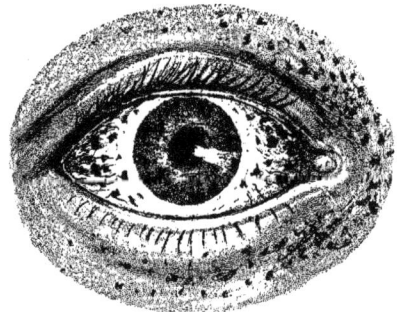

Pigmentation of Conjunctiva and Lids from Powder Burn.

INJURIES OF THE SCLERA AND CORNEO-SCLERAL MARGIN.

Non-perforating wounds. These traumata generally occur in the form of scratches and abrasions, the conjunctiva usually receiving the brunt of the injury. All the writer has seen have been from pencil and hat-pin points, and scratches from claws of dogs and cats, beaks of birds and even bites of animals.

The irritation and pain are much less than in similar injuries to the cornea. As a rule there is some lachrymation and feeling as of a foreign body. Examination shows solution of continuity of the conjunctiva and outer layers of the sclera, with congestion of the episcleral blood vessels and tumefaction of the conjunctiva. If the edges of the wound in the latter are closed perhaps some foreign body may be found lying under the membrane. If the sclera be nearly divided the bluish color of the uvea may show through.

Inspection and the fact that the intraocular pressure is normal will differentiate non-perforating from perforating wounds.

Superficial, non-perforating wounds of the sclera are of little moment and heal kindly if the conjunctival wound be closed over them, hence a simple stitch or two, bringing the edges of the conjunctiva together, insures good healing.

Asepsis and antisepsis of the conjunctival cul-de-sac and application of a bandage usually results in closure of the small wound and restitution within a few days.

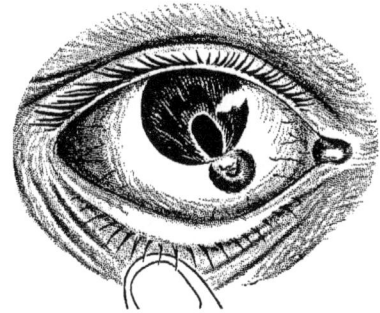

Perforating Wound, Corneal Limbus. Prolapse of iris.

Perforating wounds. Only at the corneo-scleral margin can perforating wounds occur without involving either the conjunctiva, uvea or retina, as well as the vitreous, or the cornea, iris and lens. As a rule such scleral wounds are complicated by injuries to these structures with loss of aqueous or vitreous and prolapse of the interior tunics.

The causes are the same as those which produce perforating corneal wounds, especially blows, bodies flying with force, and knife or scissor wounds.

The irritation and pain are less than in purely scleral injuries when complicated by injury to the ciliary body and cornea. In the latter cases we find swelling of the lids, chemosis of the conjunctiva, bleeding under the conjunctiva and perhaps a hyphema, ciliary injection, and congestion of the conjunctival vessels in the neighborhood of the wound. The wounds may be linear, curved or angular, but are seldom in the form of a flap. They are usually in a direction perpendicular or at an angle to the limbus and are seldom parallel. Small perforating wounds are difficult to see and are marked by small extravasations of blood.

Most penetrating and perforating wounds of the sclera likewise involve the ciliary body and open both the vitreous and the anterior chambers, the iris prolapsing and becoming impacted in the wound. Where the opening in the sclera is great, prolapse of the vitreous occurs and the ciliary body and choroid may be seen in the wound. If the hyaloid membrane is not broken or cut the vitreous may protrude as a clear bead from the wound. In large wounds the lips separate and between them is seen the injured iris and lens matter. Where the ciliary body and choroid protrude the edges of the wound are stained a brownish color. The vitreous extrudes more and more with each movement of the globe and from pressure of the lids. In very large wounds almost the entire contents of the globe may extrude. If the lids be injured at the same time the wound may be seen directly.

If the wound be posterior to the zonula the anterior chamber will be intact; if anterior or combined with perforating injury to the cornea the anterior chamber may be abolished until closed by prolapse of the iris in the minor cases, when it is again restored.

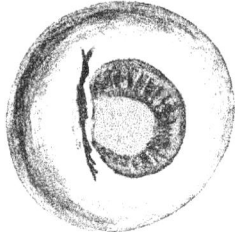

Lacerated Wound of the Ciliary Region.

The intraocular tension is always diminished, even to a flabbiness of the globe.

In favorable cases healing occurs with the formation of a flat scar. The choroid and the retina in the neighborhood of the wound becomes atrophic, ophthalmoscopic examination showing the white sclera at the spot of the injury. Atrophy of the optic nerve fibers corresponding to the portion of the retina injured, with lowered visual acuity and angular defect in the visual field, follows. The conjunctiva is usually attached by cicatricial bands, in a radial form, to the scar and a black or brown pigment deposit forms and persists indefinitely.

In cases where the wound is small, as in piercing injuries, the scar may become thin so that the color of the uvea is observed through it. This may be due to a small prolapse and impaction of the choroid into the wound.

In large, healed wounds cicatricial contraction may follow so that the globe becomes indented.

The healing of scleral wounds is more rapid the sooner the edges are brought together. They generally unite by second intention, that is by new deposits of connective tissue from the conjunctiva and choroid, and from which also vitreal bands are produced. Through subsequent contraction of the scar tissue the choroid and retina may be pulled away from the sclera, and detachment occurs.

Complications. Iris and ciliary body prolapse are most frequent; injury to the zonula causes entire or partial dislocation of the lens; trauma of lens and capsule and body causes traumatic capsular and lenticular cataract. The lens may escape through the wound, in the case of large wounds, together with some or most of the vitreous.

After resorption of the lens the contraction of the lens capsule and thickening of the zonular fasiculæ may drag on the ciliary body and cause sympathetic irritation.

So much of the vitreous may be lost that the eye goes on to phthisis bulbi. How much may be lost with retention of function has not been established, but it is safe to say that if over one-fifth be extruded no vision may be expected. It is doubtful whether the vitreous ever regenerates. Experiments now in progress may settle the contention.

Bleeding into the vitreous usually occurs and may be seen for a long time by the ophthalmoscope, either as blood, blood pigment or membranous opacities.

Loss of a portion of the uvea and retina, as well as impaction thereof and injury to the lens, is an unfavorable sign, as the cicatricial contraction ultimately leads to disturbances of contiguity, while the formation of a thin scar leads to staphyloma from inability of the weak, new-formed membrane to resist the intraocular pressure.

Small perforating wounds of the corneo-scleral margin may heal with the formation of a cystoid cicatrix, caused by lining of the wound canal by the iris or by the lens capsule. The conjunctiva grows over the projection, but the wound canal persists and the aqueous fills it, forming a projecting bead. This condition occurs less often after injuries than from cataract extraction and iridectomy, when the iris or lenticular capsule has not been fully replaced; or in secondary iris prolapse after such operations. Secondary glaucoma or infection is apt to occur.

Scleral staphyloma follows more commonly in case of rupture than in perforating wounds. Ectasia of all kinds predisposes to secondary glaucoma and blindness. Cysts of the iris have been often seen after corneo-scleral wounds.

The future of the eye depends upon the changes in the vitreous, and especially the amount of contraction of the exudation, which we cannot see distinctly in such eyes, but which we recognize by steadily diminishing sight, due to implication of the retina, and gradually increasing softness of the globe.

We should repeatedly test the acuity of vision and the light perception, and when we find perception of light has been lost it is well to enucleate if at the same time the eye has become soft. The observable changes in the anterior portion of the eye are a plastic irido-cylitis, but are not so much to be depended upon as enucleation indications (aside from the infective signs), as those relating to the gradual loss of sight and tonicity of the globe.

Conservative treatment is included under asepsis, antisepsis and surgical procedures. Of special importance is the removal of prolapses

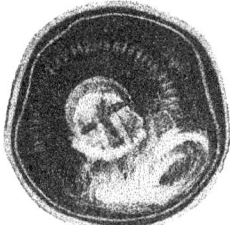

Recent Wound of Lens and Ciliary Body, showing fresh Exudate in the Vitreous.

of the interior tissues; the iris, by iridectomy; the choroid and vitreous, by cautery; with careful suturing of the scleral wound, followed by conjunctival covering.

The writer believes he has saved many eyes from infection by the instillation of 50 per cent. argyrol solution into the conjunctival cul-de-sac, as a routine dressing for injuries and operative wounds, and especially by the injection of a 50 per cent. argyrol solution into the anterior chamber through the accidental wound, even when evidences of infection, as iritis and hypopyon, were already evident. The 1:3000 bichloride ointment as a dressing for the edges of the eyelids prevents entrance of micro-organisms and kills off the streptococcus endemic to the tarsus.

As to *diagnosis*, loss of tension bespeaks an opening of the eyeball. If the wound be posterior to the corneo-scleral margin it will probably remain open, vitreous will be extruded and the tension be greatly diminished. If anterior and followed by prolapse of iris, the latter may clog the wound and the tension be re-established. Careful examination with the loupe by direct and oblique illumination, and by the ophthalmoscope and diaphanoscope, should reveal the condition.

The *prognosis* as regards retention of the globe, barring the possibility of sympathetic disease, is now-a-days very good. In former times most of such eyes came to immediate enucleation. See **Sympathetic ophthalmia**. But even the smallest prick of a needle, if septic, may cause loss of the eye through infection, and as we never know until several days have elapsed as to this probability, the prognosis should be withheld. As regards sight, the prognosis is never good, for the subsequent cicatricial contraction changes the relation of the parts and may give rise to a chronic iridocyclitis, and ultimate atrophy of the globe.

Therapy. We have here to choose between the radical removal of a badly injured eye (that would otherwise prevent the patient from

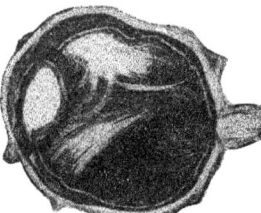

Organized Exudate in the Vitreous from Wound of the Ciliary Region and Vitreous, with Membrane Formation.

working for a long period of time) or make conservative efforts to preserve the globe with more or less sight.

Immediate enucleation, or one of its substitutes, should be done in all badly-lacerated injuries of the ciliary region, particularly if infected or if over 20 per cent. of the vitreous has been lost. Immediate enucleation should be done in badly injured globes where little or no sight can be expected, in the case of working men who cannot afford the loss of time or expense ensuant upon conservative handling. If in spite of conservative treatment inflammation occurs and progresses, we should enucleate as soon as we see that the sight cannot be saved.

The future of the eye depends upon the changes in the vitreous and especially the amount of contraction of the exudation, which we cannot see distinctly in such eyes, but which we recognize by steadily diminishing sight, due to implication of the retina, and gradually increasing softness of the globe.

We repeatedly test the acuity of vision, the light perception, and when we find perception of light has been lost it is well to enucleate if at the same time the eye has become soft.

The next indication is the iridectomy for prolapsed iris. It is generally useless to attempt to replace a prolapse; it only recurs, because impacted, and results in a cystoid cicatrix with its resultant dangers. Eserin likewise is a failure in the attempt to produce union, and retraction of the iris from the wound. Indeed, neither atropin nor eserin exercises any effect upon the position of the pupil if the anterior chamber be open. It is good, then, to seize the prolapse with delicate forceps and by gentle traction draw it out a little, immediately snip it off, and complete the toilet of the wound.

Protruding portions of the ciliary body and choroid should not be excised, on account of possibility of loss of vitreous and infection of the interior of the globe. Prolapses of the vitreous should be excised. If the lens be injured it is best, as a rule, to wait a number of days before sewing up the wound, or weeks, before attempting removal of the traumautic cataract by discission or linear extraction.

Penetrating wounds of the posterior part of the eyeball pass through the conjunctiva and sclera, and involve prolapse of the intraocular contents. These wounds are most successfully treated by the conjunctival flap method, with or without scleral stitches.

Foreign bodies in the sclera occur about 200 times less frequently than in the cornea, the cause being the more efficient protection by the brows and lids; its resiliency from being of a greater radius than the cornea, and foreign bodies rebounding therefrom or boring through into the interior of the eye rather than remaining in the scleral tissues. In very few cases does the foreign body remain in the sclera or scleroconjunctiva. Of these, powder grains, sand, etc., the result of explosions, are most common. Surgical accidents, like the breaking off of needle points in advancement operations, or the point of a cataract knife in corneal incisions, doubtless happen to all operators.

The writer has seen no case of iron particles in the sclera, but has observed several glass, stone and powder splinters, and shot grains. Others have reported lead, brass, and wood splinters.

A hemorrhagic spot is usually seen at the wound of entrance and the conjunctiva may be moved over the foreign body, the latter membrane may have been more or less torn by its entrance and stained by particles of the same substance. Small, glowing foreign bodies may burn deeply into the sclera and remain there, as hot sand, particles of metal, etc. After powder and dynamite explosions many grains of powder, sand, etc., may be found in the skin of the lids, in the corneo-scleral conjunctiva and sclera occupying in the eye the opening of the lids. As a rule the further course is attended by swelling and injection of the conjunctiva. There is not much pain and small aseptic foreign bodies, as powder grains, sand, etc., may heal into the tissues without causing irritation. Large foreign bodies may remain in the sclera or penetrate into the capsule, ultimately causing loss of the globe by infection.

Small foreign bodies lodged in the sclera may not be visible on first inspection on account of the conjunctiva being stretched over them, their imbedment and blood clots disguising their nature. So days and even weeks may pass without their presence being known. However, most of them may be seen in the eye, or felt by means of a probe passed over the surface of the wound.

The *prognosis* is generally good, as small foreign bodies may heal in the tissue of the sclera without much irritation and at any rate when diagnosed they may be readily removed, except when perforating.

Medium-sized foreign bodies sticking into the sclera, may, after cocainization of the eye, be seized by the forceps and pulled out. Others have to be cut around by the scissors points, gouged or cut out by the gouge and knife, care being taken not to push the foreign body through into the interior of the eye. In the case of iron the magnet may be first tried. If the foreign body cannot be removed, in a first attempt, without too much discission, it is better to wait a few days and then to try again. Powder grains and stains, and particles of stone or sand, may be cut and scraped away after incising the conjunctiva.

Bursting of the sclera may be either direct or indirect. It usually involves all the layers but in rare instances may be partial. It generally occurs within 3 mm. of the corneo-scleral margin, that being the weakest portion, but may in exceptional cases be posterior.

Direct rupture results from a blow with a blunt object, striking the eye directly, and is of less frequent occurrence than indirect rupture of either the sclera or cornea.

Indirect rupture results from the globe being driven against the walls of the orbit and suddenly put in a condition of increased tension, and thus bursts between the nether and the impinging body. As a rule such a blunt body as a cow's horn enters between the eyeball and one wall of the orbit, although sudden, even compression, as from the blow of a fist, may do the same injury.

Sachs, in 97 cases gives the causes as follows: 23 from cow's horns; 19 by falls against ordinary household furniture, as tables, bureaus, beds; 14 from ends of wood or iron objects as sticks, wagon-shafts, gas-jets, gun-barrels, etc.; 8 from fisticuffs; 6 from finger ends; 1 from the outstretched hand; 9 from flying pieces of wood; 3 from thrown pieces of stone or chunks of earth; 4 from hoofs; 3 from whiplashes; 2 from falling against a door; one each from a blow by a hammer, quoit, rapier or rod. In Müller's cases 14 were due to a cow's horn, 22 to other blunt, and 5 to sharp-ended objects.

It is remarkable that indirect rupture has not been reported from gunshot injuries. Older eyes are more subject to scleral; younger to corneal rupture.

Not only may normal eyes be injured but diseased organs with staphyloma, both anterior and posterior, high grades of myopia and buphthalmos, are physically predisposed to such a break in their walls.

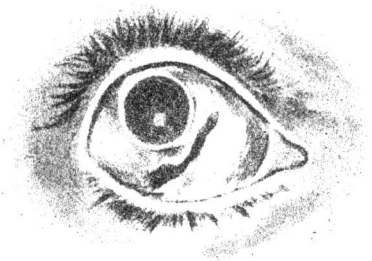

Rupture of the Eyeball at the Limbus.

Eyes blind from glaucoma have already heightened intraocular tension and are predisposed to bursting. Blind or poor-sighted eyes from other causes are more liable to acquire injury from not seeing objects and being able to dodge their approach.

The *mechanism* of direct scleral rupture is the same as that of direct corneal rupture. The portion of the eye impinged upon by the force gives way and the eye bursts at that point.

Indirect scleral rupture is due to bursting of the globe where it has no cushion of fat to afford it resiliency and to absorb the shock in the weakest place. The strongest place in the sclera is just behind the insertion of the extraocular muscle tendons, for this is protected by the orbital fat and the globe never bursts here, but in the zone between the insertion of the muscles and the limbus. The rupture takes place from within outwards, in the region of Schlemm's canal, which is the weakest place, for here the tough inner layers of the sclera are transformed into the delicate lamellæ of the ligamentum pectinatum and its resistance diminishes at this point.

Most scleral ruptures start from a point situated upwards and inwards, where the trochlea forms a bony prominence, at the upper and inner angle of the orbit, and when the eye is forced against it by a blow coming, as most do, from below and outwards, the trochlear prominence presses into the sclera and causes the rupture to begin in this meridian. The rupture is in the so-called meridian of expansion about 2.5 mm. behind and concentric to the limbus.

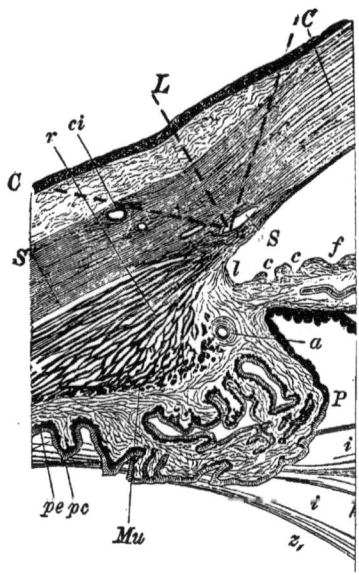

Course of a Limbal Scleral Rupture. (Modified from Fuchs.)

It varies in length from 3 to 12 mm., being commonly ⅓ to ½ the corneal circumference, and sometimes much larger than the ordinary cataract extraction wound. At either end the rupture does not usually go through all of the lamellæ. The wound usually gapes and the vitreous extrudes, however in some cases in not a sufficient quantity to ruin the eye.

In 29 cases, 22 were out and above, 3 in and down, 2 down, and 2 out and down.

In 17 cases of the 29 the distance of the middle of the rupture from the point of impact was 90°; in 3 cases less and 5 greater. In one case the point of the cow horn had bored between the bulb and the orbital wall. In statistics of 20 cases, 11 times the foreign body had passed between the globe and the orbital walls.

Ruptures of the sclera are such serious injuries because a force sufficient to burst the eye causes injuries in more than one place. The eye is immediately blinded, the fluids run out, lachrymation and pain with occasionally great nervous shock are the immediate symptoms.

The iris is almost always torn away from its insertion at a point corresponding to the extent of the scleral rupture, causing irido-dialysis; it either protrudes or is incarcerated under the conjunctiva, the eye presenting a coloboma. The portion of the iris remaining in the eye retracts or infolds in itself (inversion), or shrinks so that but little of the structure can be seen (irideremia), or the whole iris may be extruded (aniridia). However, the iris may continue intact and the pupil remain round, especially in cases where the lens is luxated under the conjunctiva, for here the aqueous does not flow out and force the iris into the wound.

The ciliary body in many cases is injured and severe bleeding into the anterior chamber and vitreous results, so that at first the internal conditions are not visible. Where the iris is inverted the ciliary processes can not be seen, but when a dialysis or aniridia is produced they are ultimately visible.

In but few cases does the lens remain in position, being usually extruded from the wound as the pit from a cherry, or it may lodge under the conjunctiva, provided the latter be not ruptured. The lens usually comes away in its capsule, the latter seldom remaining in the eye. It may also be dislocated into the vitreous. The vitreous extrudes and is lost to a greater or less extent, even to total loss. Bleeding is usually extensive into the vitreous. The tension is always diminished; the anterior chamber is deepened; hyphemia usually occurs. The retina and choroid may remain intact but are frequently torn or detached by sub-choroidal hemorrhage. Where the visual acuity is restored they cannot have been injured.

In very favorable cases, where the iris, ciliary body or lens are not affected, the eye heals in 4 to 6 weeks. The hemorrhage is resorbed; the wound is filled in by scar tissue. Even where the lens has been extruded, vision may remain.

Since to the severity of such lesions as above described there is added the danger of subsequent infection of the wound, traumatic irido-cyclitis, formation of membranes in the vitreous, scleral staphyl-oma, phthisis bulbi and sympathetic ophthalmitis, it is little to be wóndered that most such eyes go on to destruction, or are early enucleated to avoid these disastrous sequelæ.

A few of the rarest complications are concomitant dislocation of the bulb, fracture of the orbital walls and traumatic tetanus.

The character of the injury, its position, the usual loss of the lens and scleral impaction of the iris, loss of vitreous and diminished ten-sion, tell the tale of a ruptured sclera.

It is difficult to distinguish a direct rupture from an indirect, but in the former the area around the rupture shows evidence of bruising, laceration and loss of epithelium. The bleeding into the anterior chamber, in the wound, and under the conjunctiva prevents all the injury from being immediately seen, but this clears up in a few days when the injured parts can be thoroughly examined.

The *diagnosis* is helped by transillumination which shows up the interior blood clots, the iris, ciliary body and lens, if the last remain. If the Purkinje-Sanson reflexes, antero-posterior surfaces of the lens, be absent, diagnosis of aphakia may be substantiated, or if present and misplaced, of dislocation of the lens. A tremulous iris bespeaks aphakia or total dislocation; an iris that is pushed forwards in one part, the opposite being tremulous and the anterior chamber deeper, tells of a partial dislocation. Sooner or later such lenses become cataractous and are then readily seen.

The *prognosis* is usually unfavorable, except where the iris, ciliary body or lens are not affected, or the eye remains free from infection. As a rule traumatic irido-cyclitis sets in and the eye goes on to atrophy. Müller had 12 favorable outcomes in 35 cases.

Therapy. The first duty is to cleanse the injured eye; bandage both to keep them still and prevent further loss of vitreous, and in about 48 hours to remove the iris prolapse, put in scleral sutures and sew over the wound a bipedunculated conjunctival flap. Next, con-trol the hemorrhage by the application of cold, and instil antiseptics in the conjunctival cul-de-sac. Both eyes should be kept lightly bandaged and the patient in bed. The after-treatment is that of per-forating wounds of the sclera and sclero-corneal margin.

The lens should be removed if under the conjunctiva. Cataract may be later dealt with by the usual method if there is enough vision left to warrant the operation.

Cystoid cicatrices may be ablated by the cautery, or various opera-tions done upon the staphyloma, but the treatment of sequelæ fre-quently sums itself up in enucleation, or one of its substitutes.

The writer has taken out nearly all eyes that have come with rupture of the sclera, so great is one's dread of sympathetic disease. However, in several in which a scleral rupture had occurred the remarkable efforts of Nature conserved the eye with some vision.

Rebounding missiles of small size, such as spent balls from firearms, have caused *posterior, indirect ruptures of the sclera*, which are usually concentric to the papilla. (Posterior direct ruptures from double penetrating wounds by missiles will be discussed under **Military surgery.**)

Rupture of the canal of Schlemm. The rupture of the sclera may be slight and not proceed beyond the canal of Schlemm, where, as has been noted, all anterior indirect ruptures begin.

Contusions at the limbus, more particularly from small, semi-rounded objects as pencil ends, flying foreign bodies of small size and some weight, as spent shot, pieces of metal, small projectiles from play things, as beans, peas, etc., may strike the eye at the corneo-scleral margin directly, or force be communicated through the lid and break the *sinus venosus sclerœ*, causing a direct rupture, with bleeding, into the anterior chamber.

Indirect bursting of the canal of Schlemm alone is due to an incomplete rupture of the sclera at this point where only the inner wall bursts.

In both these forms of injury bleeding rapidly occurs and is seen as a bright-red hyphema. Later, diffuse dullness and fine dark or reddish lines, extending inwards from the limbus, appear in the cornea. The lines appear against the opacity, in examination by focal illumination, as a glass rod does in water. They lie in the posterior layers of the cornea and are probably due to folds in Descemet's membrane, or perhaps to tears in the same with imbibition of the aqueous and blood. The pupil is temporarily dilated but returns to normal after a few days.

The subjective symptoms are slight pain and temporary loss of vision from the hyphema, which resorbs in a few days. The vision remains affected until the corneal dullness disappears and if there has been no rupture of the iris, ciliary body or zonule *restitutio ad integram* occurs.

The diagnosis is from the hyphema unaccompanied by damage to the iris, and by the mydriasis disappearing.

The prognosis is good, recovery ensuing in a few days.

The therapy is atropin and occlusion of the eye.

Burns of the sclera proper are always complicated injuries; not alone the sclero-conjunctiva and scleral tissue may be burned, but in severe cases the true sclera, even to its entire thickness, from which a defect occurs with prolapse of vitreous and uvea.

Deep burns occur from glowing or fluid metals or slag, the more superficial ones from chemicals, as acids and alkalies, especially lime, the latter of which may remain for a long time in contact with the tissues.

Symptoms, course, and complications are such as belong to severe burns. In addition there is the danger of infection, which in perforating injuries usually leads to panophthalmitis. More particular is the danger to the nutrient vessels of the cornea in burns involving the sclero-cornea, by which its nutrition is cut off and necrosis ensues.

The *therapy* is that of thermal injuries to the conjunctiva, cornea, and burns in general.

Scleral injuries from firearms are, in civil life, due to fire-works, gunpowder and dynamite explosions and the air-rifle in the hands of boys. Others occur from hunting accidents. A few bullet wounds occur as the result of attempted suicide or murder; in war the small shot is eliminated and the wounds are from bullets or particles of shells or their surroundings.

Tangential and glancing wounds of the sclera occur in conjunction with those of the conjunctiva and cornea. They either cut through only the overlying areas or the entire thickness. Shot pellets may be retained between the conjunctiva and sclera without opening the globe. It is often difficult to find the opening in the sclera of penetrating shot wounds, and still harder to see the wound of exit in double-penetrating cases. Bullet wounds make a larger opening and usually pass entirely through the ball, lodging in the orbit or cranial cavity. Small shot wounds are usually round, seldom irregular or flap-like, the latter occurring when the shot does not strike perpendicular to the surface of the globe, nor in a tangential direction. In the neighborhood of the wound the conjunctiva is suffused with blood, the ciliary body, retina and choroid may be seen impacted in the opening. In the case of perforating wounds at the limbus the iris prolapses and the anterior chamber is deeper than normal. The anterior chamber and vitreous fill with blood. The lens may likewise be broken up by the passage of a pellet.

Shot pellets and even portions of bullets may remain in the conjunctiva, under it and in the sclera. A grain may pass into the eye and be impacted in the posterior wall of the sclera, and in this case, if not much damage be done by the trauma after the bleeding is resorbed, it may be seen by the ophthalmoscope. A spent shot may strike the sclero-conjunctiva and produce thereby only a bruise, or the blow itself may be sufficiently severe to injure the choroid and retina, producing sub-retinal or sub-choroidal hemorrhage, or later retinal detachment.

Direct ruptures of the sclera are common in injuries to the eye from bullet wounds, and such are reported in statistics relating to war. See **Military surgery of the eye.**

Therapy. Excepting the most trivial wounds from shot grains, cases usually come to enucleation, on account of the great damage done by the trauma.

The scleral suture. All scleral wounds over 0 mm. in length are apt to gape and allow extrusion of the intraocular contents. Interrupted sutures, in the shape of the finest catgut, kangaroo or rat-tail

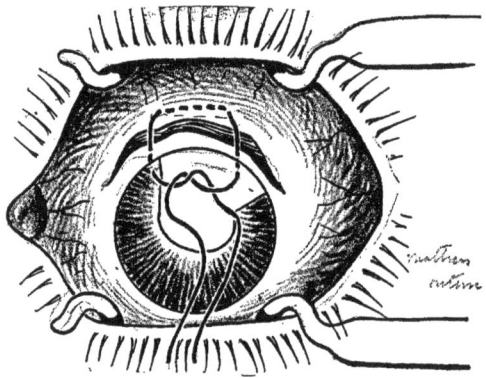

Mattress Suture in Scleral Wounds.　(Würdemann.)

tendon, threaded on very sharp, moderately-curved needles, may be passed through the lips of the scleral wound and coapted thereby, care being taken not to lose more vitreous; the lips of the wound may be seized by toothed forceps and, with needles sufficiently sharp, the central suture is taken first and loosely tied. The stitches are snipped close to the knots and a flap of the conjunctiva dissected up and sutured in place by interrupted, iron-dyed silk sutures, the line of the conjunctival stitches passing outside of the sclera, the stitches in the latter being buried and allowed to absorb, those in the conjunctiva being removed about the fifth day.

The scleral suture protects the interior of the eye from infection; hinders the further loss of vitreous; prevents the formation of fistula, cystoid cicatrix and staphyloma; causes the formation of a much more regular and flat cicatrix, and the probability of secondary retinal detachment is less. It also shortens the healing period.

The following are contra-indications for the scleral suture: 1. In severe, and especially deeply-penetrating wounds with extensive loss of vitreous, threatening entire loss of the intra-ocular contents, extensive bleeding into the vitreous cavity, and when the eye is so severely damaged that its removal is immediately indicated. 2. When a foreign body remains which cannot be removed from the globe. 3. When appearances or course point to inflammation of the globe.

The needle and suture operation is made as in the case of corneal suture under local or general narcosis, the edges of the wound being held by fine forceps or by a fine hook. If the conjunctiva be torn or

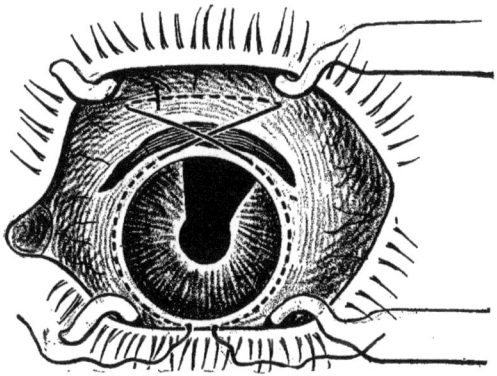

Nuel's Suture in Scleral Wounds.

wounded at the same place the needles and threads may pass through the conjunctiva or episclera, when silk sutures may be used. If the conjunctival wound is at another place the sutures should be of catgut or tendon and the conjunctival suture of silk.

The various forms of *conjunctivoplasty* for the protection of scleral and other traumas are fully described on p. 3508, Vol. V, of this *Encyclopedia*. Here it may be added that in some cases the writer uses his so-called mattress suture, made by passing the first needle of the double-armed suture from without towards the lower lip of the wound, through the corneal or episcleral substance, then across the wound, again into the episclera of the lip of the wound, crossing over, entering the scleral tissue again behind the lower lip of the wound. The wound then being approximated by forceps the knot is tied on the surface of the cornea. See the figure.

Another kind of retaining or tension suture has been made by Nuel for corneo-scleral rupture. A double-armed suture about 2 cm. long is passed under the conjunctiva behind the wound about the equator of the globe, then crossed over the wound to the inner side, being tied below. These sutures may be removed about the fifth day, when the wound will be found to have sufficiently coapted.

INJURIES OF THE CORNEA.

Injuries of the cornea are of daily occurrence, not only in the practice of the ophthalmologist, but are frequently seen by the general practitioner. Indeed, most of the so-called trivial injuries, abrasions, motes in the eye and smaller wounds are first attended by the latter. These injuries run the gamut of all the forms of trauma that occur to the external tunics of the eye. In many instances they are uncomplicated by injuries of the other structures and generally heal kindly, · leaving, however, in all instances where the true corneal tissue is affected, more or less cicatricial tissue which may or may not affect the visual acuity, depending upon the position of the wound. Restoration of the external epithelium, however, may be perfect without scar-formation.

Erosions or abrasions of the cornea. These injuries consist in a solution of continuity of the anterior layer of epithelium in which the anterior elastic layer is laid bare, exposing the sensory nerves, and are accompanied by distressing symptoms. As a rule they do not involve Bowman's layer or the substantia propria, and heal most quickly, even in almost complete exfoliation. ·

Direct erosions occur from impact of substances striking with slight force, as finger nails, pencils, broom straws, clothing, as well as small utensils used in domestic life; impact of twigs, straws, etc., in country life, and the same character of objects met with in industrial pursuits. Spatters of hot fluids, water, grease, etc., are likewise responsible. To these causes must be added the effect of strong medicinal applications, as copper sulphate, silver nitrate, and especially the applications of strong cocain solutions, which, however, the profession has learned to use sparingly and not to give into the hands of patients.

Snow blindness is largely due to corneal erosions, which are readily stained by fluorescein. See **Blindness, Snow.**

In this disease the corneal epithelium regenerates so quickly that in many cases within twenty-four hours after an injury the continuity has been restored. Septic infection, however, is not uncommon. Examples of the rapid restoration of the corneal epithelium may be seen after cocain in strong solutions has been applied and the eyelids kept open by the speculum, as happens occasionally from imperfect technic in operations for squint and others in which the lids are kept apart for a considerable length of time.

After operations upon the sympathetic a disturbance of the trophic

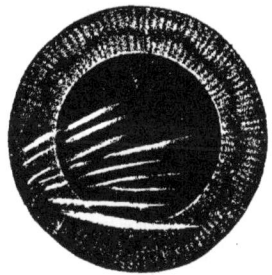

Scratches of the Cornea from Broom Straw.

nerves results in neuroparalytic keratitis similar to that observed in corneal disease following facial paralysis.

Indirect erosions are of common occurrence from motes in the eye, the particle getting under the upper lid, and the eye by being rubbed by the patient, thereby scratching the anterior surface of the cornea.

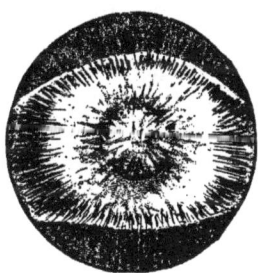

Erosion of the Cornea.

Edema and desquamation of corneal epithelium from prolonged cocain instillation.

Traumatic defects in the continuity of the corneal epithelium is observed either by direct or focal illumination. The surface is clear and not opaque, as in the case of an ulcer. The form depends upon the character of the injury, the smaller erosions are usually due to the scratching of a foreign body, larger ones to finger nail injuries; scratches to medium sharp small objects, as broom straws, hair brushes, wire, glass, etc.

The subjective symptoms are typically severe pain, photophobia and lachrymation, and feeling of a foreign body. The pain occurs immediately upon the receipt of the injury, is piercing, pressing or burning, and feels as if the whole of the eye was hurt. It is increased by movement of the globe and opening and shutting the lids. Hot tears flow over the cheeks. The patient holds his hand and handkerchief to the eye to keep down the movements of the lids. The other eye tearfully sympathizes and is kept partly closed. The great pain is caused by exposure of the corneal sensory nerves in a mass. Clean out wounds do not give as much pain. In very nervous individuals clonic cramp of the side of the face is seen.

The *diagnosis* under inspection is difficult in very small erosions. Small and otherwise almost indistinguishable abrasions of the corneal epithelium, wounds and small foreign bodies in the cornea, may be brought into view by the staining of the tissues by a 2 per cent. fluorescein and 2 per cent. bicarbonate soda solution. Focal illumination and magnification of the eye by a lens, preferably by the Berger binocular loupe, is of great value.

As a rule the *prognosis* is good. Small defects heal in 24 hours without a scar. All cases where a facet or cicatrices follow have had more than an erosion, and the solution of continuity has gone through Bowman's membrane into the corneal tissue proper. Septic infection, however, in some cases leads to corneal ulcerations, abscesses and even to panophthalmitis. The sepsis is not always carried by the foreign body but is frequently brought into the eye after the injury by the patient himself from rubbing the eye with his fingers, a dirty pocket handkerchief, or by the use of home remedies or even by exposure of the injured parts to the air, which, as we all know, contains septic germs. Examples are of frequent occurrence in large dispensary or private practice.

The presence of a lachrymal sac suppuration of course predisposes to such infection. There is a special disposition to infection of corneal erosions in childbirth and during nursing, especially when these conditions are complicated by diabetes and albuminuria or other constitutional derangements.

An unpleasant sequel is the formation of cicatrix dolorosa, which is either due to a microscopic neuroma or to hysterical keratalgia or to wound infection by bacteria or the aspergillus.

Recurrent corneal erosions. In a very few cases the erosion, especially in the morning, may be seen for weeks or months afterwards. The newly-formed epithelium adheres to the conjunctiva of the lids when they are closed, and so is stripped away anew each day. The regenerated epithelium is not firmly adherent to its bed and under the action of some injudicious cause is separated and cast off. This separation takes place in the form of a vesicle which, however, ruptures so quickly that we do not see it, but only the consequence of the loss of epithelium. Cases are seen where subsequent attacks occurred several times a year after the primary injury.

Treatment of uncomplicated corneal abrasions, or cases which do not perforate through its entire thickness, is antiseptic washing by 3 per cent. boric acid solution, 1:10,000 sublimate or 1:1,000 chinosol solution, or normal salt solution preceded by instillation of cocain or holocain to allow of inspection and to relieve the pain, and argyrol, dionin and application of aseptic bandage. Five per cent. iodoform ointment or the White bichlorid ointment, makes a good antiseptic application. A bandage should be left on for 24 hours and removed by the surgeon himself. If the parts have healed, which is readily seen by the instillation of 2 per cent. flourescein solution, which colors the denuded area green, then a light bandage or not may be put on, as may seem best.

If there is not complete healing, atropin should be used to dilate the pupil and get the edge of the iris away from the lens so that a subsequent iritis may not cause posterior synechia. A bandage is essential to keep the lids closed. If pain be severe, 5 per cent. dionin solution applied once in 6 to 24 hours may be dropped in the eye, but all meddlesome handling, especially with hands unprepared as for surgical operation, should be discouraged; if complications of sepsis have set in the wound may be immediately cauterized by 95 per cent. phenol, or with the galvano-cautery. The cautery is used too little; the scar from its use is less than that following the ulceration which is present or will ensue.

The writer protests against the use of cocain solutions in the patient's hands; they should only be used by the surgeon, and only for surgical operations or to facilitate examination, as cocain interferes with the healing process by cutting off nutrition; the same may be said of suprarenal extract and its active principle, adrenalin, after injuries to the eyes. See, also, **Recurrent erosion of the cornea**; as well as **Cornea, Erosion of the.**

Cicatrix dolorosa should be curetted or cauterized. Complications of keratitis or ulceration are to be treated as advised under these headings.

NON-PERFORATING WOUNDS OF THE CORNEA.

In these the solution of continuity goes through the lamina elastica anterior into the substantia propria, and in some cases as deeply as the lamina elastica posterior, but in which the anterior chamber may not be opened. Incised, punctured and gashed wounds are more common than lacerating or flap wounds. They occur from flying foreign bodies of iron or other metal; glass and stone which fall away after impact or grazing of the cornea; from sharp instruments, as knives (pointed ones), pins, needles, shears; and from such other sharp-pointed objects such as wire, sharp splinters of wood or bone, etc. Flap wounds are usually finger nail accidents.

Soon after the injury the margins of the wound become cloudy and swollen from imbibition of fluid, and in irregular lacerated wounds the cornea may become opaque over a large area. As the wound heals the

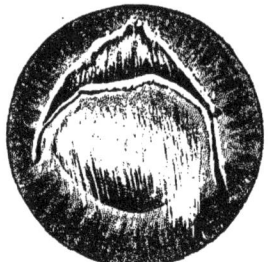

Large Superficial Flap Wound of Cornea made by Finger Nail.

cloudiness disappears, although sometimes a dense opacity remains around the wound area. This opacity is often associated with irregular bulging of the cornea and irregular astigmatism.

The symptoms are much the same as just outlined, except in the case of clean cuts. Here the pain is not at all great and if the wound be in the part of the cornea not covered by the lids but little irritation may be felt. There is some lachrymation and redness but in many cases the patient may not consult his physician until the day's work is done, or perhaps not for several days, during which period there is ample time for infection.

Where, however, the wound is extensive, lacerated or a flap has formed, the symptoms are more severe. The results depend upon the amount of opacity produced and the astigmatism which always follows wound healing.

The examination is to be conducted under cocain, in some cases with use of fluorescein, direct and focal illumination, the magnifier and other aids.

The *prognosis* is in doubt, even in seemingly trivial injuries, until the presence of infection can be excluded. Clean cut wounds heal well and speedily. Quick repair of the corneal tissue proper is a daily observation with eye surgeons, as the lips of the wound after cataract extraction are usually gummed together within a few hours after the operation. But even slight injuries infected by unclean instruments, or subjected to secondary infection, may be followed by severe inflammation, ending in loss of sight or even of the eyeball. Of these septic agents, unclean instruments, the finger nail, hairpin, hatpin, pocket-knife or scissors, are perhaps the most dangerous. Wounds of the cornea which do not penetrate into the anterior chamber, which are characterized by the formation of a flap, are perhaps the most dangerous if caused by septic instruments. The reason for this lies in the fact that the flap may almost immediately fall back into place, becoming gummed at the edges and retaining in the cornea a nidus of septic material.

PERFORATING WOUNDS OF THE CORNEA.

Perforating wounds of the cornea may be defined as those which completely penetrate all its layers without the retention of a foreign body therein or within the eyeball. They are often complicated by prolapse of the iris and if the cut extends sufficiently deep, as it commonly does, injury to the lens capsule or lens, or often of deeper structures, complicates the trauma. If septic, to the dangers of the wound itself may be added hypopyon keratitis, iritis, infection of the other portions of the eye and panophthalmitis. Wounds of the sclero-corneal margin are especially dangerous on account of injury to the ciliary body, and subsequent sympathetic irritation or inflammation in the other eye, and of the tendency of the iris to prolapse, with subsequent posterior synechia. It is safe to say that wounds of the cornea, per se, and limited to this structure, seldom give rise to sympathetic inflammation or irritation.

Incised and punctured wounds are most often seen; lacerated and contused wounds more seldom, most of such cases being complicated by injury to the iris, lens, and ciliary body.

As a rule the eye has had ample opportunity to become infected before examination by the eye surgeon and where such occurs the infection is almost invariably communicated by the working man from his finger nails or dirty handkerchief, or by ill-considered operative procedures by fellow-workmen in the factory, or even by physicians.

The objects producing such injuries are manifold and at times bizarre. Perhaps little children are the most common patients, having injured themselves by pen-knives, forks, needles and hat pins. On farms the act of splitting fire wood; and in the trades, wire, nails, breaking bottles and water gauges. Shot grain wounds generally penetrate.

In perforating wounds of the cornea prolapse of the iris into the wound is an attempt by Nature to avoid infection; but the effort on the part of the iris is a suicidal attempt, for this structure becomes pinched and sooner or later gives rise to irritation, causing irido-cyclitis and sympathetic ophthalmitis.

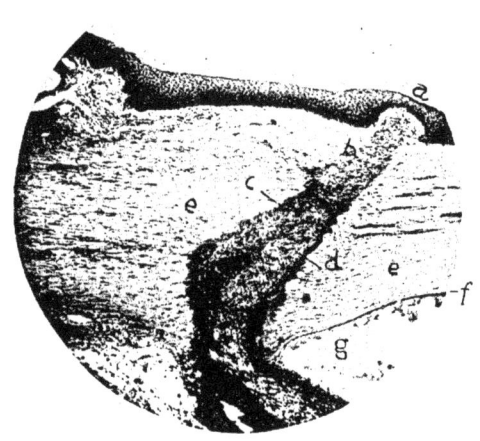

Prolapse of the Iris into the Corneal wound, Filling the Perforation.

a—Regeneration of corneal epithelium over point of perforation. b—Scar tissue. c—Infiltrated iris with scattered pigment cells. d—Blood vessel in iris. e—Clear substantia propria. f—Rupture of Descemet's membrane. g—Absence of pus in anterior chamber. (Tooke.)

It cannot be denied that many lamentable results are avoidable by performing an iridectomy, or by releasing the anterior synechia. The writer does not contend that Nature's method is superior to surgical interference, but presents it as the means Nature adopts for closing an infected hole in the cornea in a most effectual manner.

As a rule perforating injuries cause severe pain, burning, lachryma-tion, photophobia and immediate blindness. There is ciliary conges-tion, and commonly edema of the lids and conjunctiva. Examination shows a more or less wide-open wound involving all the corneal layers;

if existent more than a day, its edges are macerated, the anterior chamber empty, the iris prolapsed and perhaps impacted in the wound, the
pupil drawn to one side, and if the lens be injured, it is whitish and
does not allow an examination of the fundus by the ophthalmoscope.
It is well to ascertain not only the apparent character of the wound
but the instrument causing it, and the direction from which the cut or
wound came in order to judge of its depth and the amount of injury
to the deeper structures of the eye, for it is almost needless to observe
that probing of ocular wounds is, as a rule, to be discouraged.

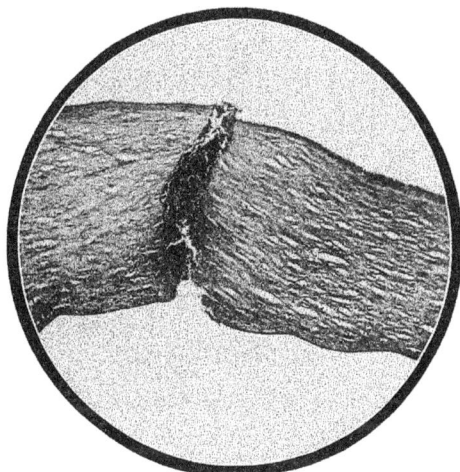

Septic Wound of the Cornea.

Space between lips of wound occupied by pus. No effort at repair of corneal
cells. Contortion of corneal cells. Dilatation of intercellular spaces filled with
leucocytes. (Tooke.)

The edges of cuts, gashes, and lacerations are at first sharply-defined,
but later the lips become swollen and the edges rounded. Proceeding
from the wound into the cornea fine, grayish stripes are seen. The
various layers may be separated so as to be readily distinguished.
Sometimes the lips of the wound over-ride, but as a rule they gape.

Simple uncomplicated injuries heal very rapidly, the cornea being
soft and pliable and accommodating itself readily to the altereu condition, the lips of the wound usually coming quickly together, union
taking place within a few hours.

Whiplash injuries often look like incised wounds. Punctures from
needles, etc., are often so fine that they are with difficulty observed;

under magnification the grayish canal of penetration will be seen in the cornea. Knife and scissor wounds, and those made by other metal objects, are often large and flap-like, so much so that often the lens escapes at the time of the accident, and vitreous is lost. In small wounds the iris comes forwards and attaches to the posterior surface; in larger ones it prolapses.

Vision varies from the normal in small lateral punctures of the cornea, with no loss of aqueous and no injury of other parts of the eye, to complete loss of light perception in cases with great tissue destruction.

All considerations regarding kind, size, location, complications, whether or not infected, nature of the wound, obtain in the course of previous discussions of corneal abrasions and non-penetrating wounds.

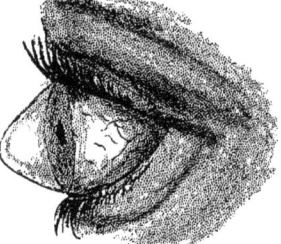

Keratoconus following Central Punctate Injury of the Cornea.

If a clean-out penetrating wound of the eye has occurred without any prolapse, by a clean and sharp instrument, the prognosis is generally good; such is the case in wounds involving incision of the cornea as for iridectomy, cataract extraction, and of the sclera for glaucoma. The edges of the wound usually coapt; there is some redness in the neighborhood, and under protection from the outer atmosphere the wound heals and the shape of the globe, together with the function of the organ, is usually preserved or restored; if the wound remains open, such as from delayed healing in cataract extraction, the chances for the entrance of pathogenic germs and consequent inflammation are greater.

The opened eyeball; the lowered tension; the shallowness of the anterior chamber; the marked extrusion of a portion of the iris; together with the history and symptoms; all these plainly indicate the character of the injury. The determination as to whether or not a foreign body has passed through and still remains in the eyeball should always be made, as discussed elsewhere in this section.

The *prognosis* depends upon the size and seat of the injury. In seriousness these injuries range from the smallest perforation by an aseptic needle, producing no destruction of tissue, without complications, and which permanently heal in a few hours, to those of great tissue destruction and injury of many parts of the eye, with immediate and permanent destruction of function. Also the small and innocent-looking puncture of the cornea with few immediate symptoms may be the channel through which a foreign body has entered, carrying with it the germs of a destructive inflammation; hence no penetrating wound of the cornea should be considered an insignificant affair, nor should an immediate favorable prognosis be given in any case. The condition of the wound union soon after the accident should not be used as a positive guide in prognosis. The larger the wound the more the consequent cicatricial opacity and distortion of the shape of the globe, following the healing, and the worse the resultant vision.

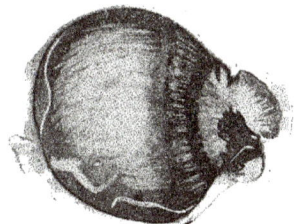

Anterior Staphyloma of the Cornea.

Five years after perforating injury from a splinter of wood; ulceration and prolapse of iris followed. Enucleated for prothesis.

Complications of penetrating wounds of the cornea are many. Aside from injuries to the iris, lens, ciliary body and deeper structures of the eye, and the entrance of infection with its consequences, others occur in the course of the healing.

Iritis with posterior synechiæ is unfavorable. Tetanus with meningitis, followed by death, has been observed.

Corneal staphyloma is common following large wounds. Most of these may be prevented by the Kuhnt conjunctival flaps.

The writer has seen almost perfect conical cornea with corneal maculæ follow a central punctate injury of the cornea; also a most peculiar, clear projection of the cornea from a hat-pin injury.

Fistula of the cornea is not uncommon. One such was observed in a negro woman following a perforating, and later infected, needle injury. This healed under conical incision, antiseptics and bandage.

The Kuhnt method of keratoplasty by conjunctival flap is a more modern method of treatment.

Astigmia follows iridectomy and ,cataract operations, generally against the rule, viz., axis 180°, the greater the more the wound is made in the cornea. It is usually 5-6 D. shortly after an operation, gradually diminishing in amount until in six months it is only about 1.50 D. Cases of 6-10 D. are not rare. Where the cut is in the sclero-cornea and with a conjunctival flap, the astigmia is less and excessive cases are not found. Clean, incised, injury wounds may also be followed by regular astigmia. Dolganoff ascribes regular astigmia following wounds to the effect of muscular contraction and intra-ocular pressure.

Irregular astigmia is the consequence of irregular healing, and greatly diminishes the vision. It is usually combined with extensive scarring and leucoma of the cornea.

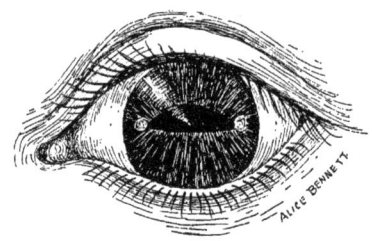

Transfixion of the Cornea by a Hatpin. (Bennett.)

Re-opening of the cicatrix is a very unpleasant after-complication of corneal wounds.

In treating these cases the first and probably most important point is to clean not only the wound, but also the entire conjunctival membrane, along with the lids and adjacent tissues. Strong antiseptic solutions are not advisable for the conjunctival surface, as they usually increase the pain, redness and swelling. Better is thorough irrigation of these parts with a liberal amount of sterile water, or a solution of boric acid, using soap externally if necessary to cleanse the skin.

Fifty per cent. argyrol solutions, even injected into the antèrior chamber, have saved many cases, although apparently already infected. The writer almost invariably uses this as a dressing after injuries and operations. 1:3,000 sublimate ointment is applied to the lids and then an occlusive bandage, which must not be tight enough to press on and interfere with coaptation of the lips of the wound.

The use of local or general anesthesia not only furnishes an opportunity for thorough cleansing, but also for any surgical procedure that may be necessary, such as the removal of any accessible foreign body, replacing or excising prolapsed iris, removal of shreds of tissue, and trimming the edges of the corneal wound when very rough and irregular. In small, fresh wounds attempts may be made to replace the iris by a fine probe or Daviel's spoon. Atropin is indicated in perforating wounds, for while eserin in marginal corneal wounds may be theoretically indicated, practically it has not fulfilled expectations. Very small, point-like prolapses of the iris may be cauterized. After completing the toilet of the conjunctiva, iris and cornea, any wound of the lids should be sutured or otherwise treated as indicated.

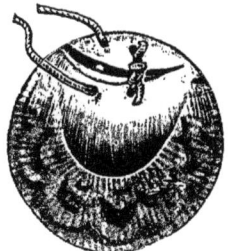

Corneal Suture.

In *treatment of recent complicated penetrating injuries of the cornea*, iridectomy as a first step is advised, especially if the lenticular substance shows a tendency to swell, as in larger injuries of the cornea, iris, lens, vitreous, especially if centrally located and if a primary reunion is not probable, and in large perforated central ulcers. Iridectomy acts here as a safety valve, so to speak, for the following reasons: extraction of a traumatic cataract later on generally requires iridectomy; lens matter is better absorbed, if it is not retained in the posterior chamber but can freely enter the anterior chamber; after iridectomy the -pressure of lens matter on the iris will be less and thus the causes for synechiæ will be removed; the eye becomes quiet sooner; the wound of the cornea is more readily and better agglutinated if tension is diminished through iridectomy; it gives better access to the lens, in case a speedy operation should be required.

Corneal suture in penetrating wounds. The needle and suture are carefully entered through the external layers of the cornea only, about 0.5 mm. from the margin. After pulling the edges of the wound together a square knot retains them in place for five to seven days, when the suture is snipped by the scissors and removed with forceps. As a rule corneal sutures are well borne and have been used many times with good results.

Two sides of a triangle of conjunctiva may be excised at one side of the wound and a flap drawn over the surface of this side by one· of the sutures. An oblong piece may be pulled over the wound and fastened by sutures to the limbus, or the flap may be left adherent at either end. The single or double pedunculated flap of Kuhnt may also be used.

Dissection of the entire margin of the conjunctiva, which is drawn up in a purse-string suture over the entire cornea, may be made in

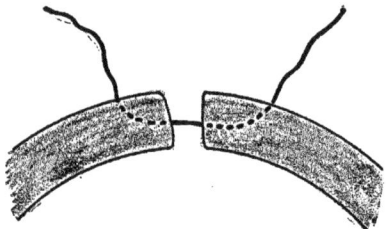

Corneal Suture in Penetrating Injury of the Eye.

extreme wounds. The suture either pulls through or is cut in about 5 days, when the cornea will be found to have coapted under it. The cut edge of the conjunctiva is soon reattached at the limbus and after some weeks cannot be recognized to have been detached.

FOREIGN BODIES IN THE CORNEA.

The larger percentage of foreign bodies on and in the cornea come under the heading of motes in the eye. They may be found lying on the cornea, not firmly attached; or buried in the cornea, as cinders, sparks, emery or metal chips, stone, etc.

Foreign bodies on or in the cornea are most common accidents. Some, as particles of chaff, wheat, husks, rhizomes of plants, etc., simply adhere to its surface. Others cause solution of continuity of the epithelium, as in the case of cinders and ordinary motes in the eye; others penetrate the true corneal tissue and remain impacted, as particles of emery, stone, metal chips, etc.; and others pass entirely through and usually wound the iris, lens or deeper structures, as shot grains, iron and copper chips, etc.

Besides the ordinary run of foreign bodies, thorns, fingernail clippings, insect stings, caterpillar hairs, etc., enter and cause ulceration or perforation of the cornea. Cilia and other foreign bodies may be carried into a wound, rarely remaining inert, usually setting up inflammatory reaction, shown by development of giant cells.

The air-gun gives rise to many of these avoidable injuries, and its use should certainly be prohibited.

The subjective symptoms are usually those of great smarting, or piercing pain, and copious flow of tears immediately following the accident, which is usually reported by the patient to the minute or hour. In sensitive individuals the pain may be great and there may be blepharospasm. Cramp of the face often occurs. The face is congested and the patient holds his hand or handkerchief to the eye to keep the lid from rubbing. But his attempts at removal as a rule only succeed in further impact of the foreign body, which often, in the case of cinders, has at first only lodged beneath the lids. Attempts

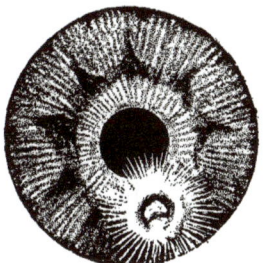

Ulcer of the Cornea with Retained Iron Chip.

at removal are frequently made, particularly in the shops by "mote removers" as hereinbefore described. These persons as a rule succeed in removing such motes, and in some instances quite skilfully. In others the patient may appear to the physician with the cornea pretty well scratched and gouged from a successful or unsuccessful attempt at such removal.

The severity of irritative symptoms depends upon the part of the cornea in which a foreign body lodges, as well as the amount of damage done. As a rule immediate stoppage of work is necessary and the patient is incapacitated until the foreign body is removed and the solution of continuity healed. If the lid edges rub against the mote in the act of winking the irritation is severe, but in some cases where the particle is small and lodged between the lid aperture the patient may not even know that there is a foreign body present, having perhaps forgotten the trivial accident of a few days, or even weeks, before. This often happens in the case of emery.

Sometimes a small foreign body may be driven against the cornea so forcibly that it lodges under the epithelium and at first gives rise to but little inconvenience, as, being covered, it offers no sharp surface to grate against the lid; after a while it projects slightly and the epithelium gives way, then occasioning all the painful symptoms of a foreign body. It frequently happens that patients carry such foreign bodies for many days, and sometimes attribute their sufferings to other causes, and many instances have been seen of improperly diagnosed cases treated for days, weeks, or even months by physicians whose prescription pads are more facile than their eyes and fingers.

The result on vision depends upon the position of the foreign body. If in the optical zone sight may be greatly diminished and the patient see a spot before the eye. Old grinders and workers at the emery wheel may have their corneæ full of many old, impacted, and healed-in pieces of emery, etc., and many small scars of previous accidents. The sight is, as a rule, found to be diminished.

Examination under direct and focal illumination, especially by the aid of the loupe, will usually reveal the presence of a foreign body. Staining of the injured area by fluorescein makes a green background in which the object appears more distinctly, especially if the mote has been in some days, when the edges of the wound are macerated and the fluorescein stains more deeply. All ulcers should be subjected to close examination for the presence of a foreign body, which may lie deeply and have been the original exciting cause.

Adherent husks of seeds, sawdust, fly wings, etc., are usually found at the limbus; other particles may be anywhere on the corneal surface. Penetrating objects are usually emery, sand, stone, particles of iron or other metal, glass, thorns, caterpillar hairs, etc. The majority of objects look dark-brown against the iris and light against the background of the pupil under direct and focal illumination. By the ophthalmoscope even glass chips appear black against the background of the fundus. Under diaphanoscopy the objects likewise appear black.

If the object is retained long on the surface of the cornea it is usually surrounded by mucous secretion; if in the tissue it may heal thereon or the edges infiltrate and ulceration occur. Particles of iron rust cause siderosis of a small or large portion of the cornea if they remain, while recent cases appear glistening gray, and older ones are brown from the rusting. Particles of copper appear reddish-brown and may get greenish from a deposit of verdigris.

On removal of the mote and the use of an antiseptic dressing, healing usually sets in with formation of a more or less minute scar. If infection results it may run the gamut of the various forms of ulceration and even cause traumatic interstitial keratitis in syphilitic subjects. Even the most trivial injuries may prove very serious.

Iritis is often observed, usually accompanied by corneal infection and hypopyon keratitis or onyx.

The *diagnosis* is made by the history and results of careful examination under direct and oblique illumination, usually by the aid of the magnifier, and the area of the wound stained, if necessary, in the case of very small motes, by fluorescein.

Acute inflammations of the eye always call for examination as to the possibility of a foreign body being lodged therein.

The *prognosis*, in nearly all trivial cases, is good. It depends largely upon infection rather than the size or site of the foreign body and amount of immediate damage to the tissues. Long remaining foreign bodies may cause ulceration. Resultant central scars always reduce the visual acuity.

The *treatment* consists of speedy removal of the foreign body, sterilization of the wound, antiseptics if necessary, and a bandage. Motes, such as insect wings, husks of seeds, pieces of leaf, sawdust, and some other foreign bodies that simply adhere to the surface of the cornea by atmospheric pressure may be wiped away by a cotton-tipped pledget. For others where instrumental means are necessary local anesthesia should be obtained by solutions of cocain 5 per cent., holocain 1 per cent., eucain 2 per cent., alypin 2 per cent., which may be freshly prepared from tablets or the stock solutions sterilized by heating from time to time. When cocain is used the eyes should be kept closed, so that one may anticipate any dryness of the cornea and a tendency to erosion of the epithelium. Holocain is more irritating and causes conjunctival congestion, which may be prevented by instillation of 1:10,000 adrin, adrenalin, suprarenalin or other of the suprarenin products.

The removal of foreign bodies under such local anesthesia is entirely painless, and no ill-effects should be observed if the drugs are not used too freely. It should, however, be remembered that idiosyncrasy to their use has been observed, and that minute amounts of cocain and holocain have produced general toxic disturbances. Such, however, should not be confused with hysteric fainting, which is often observed in physicians' offices from the mental effect of any procedure that approaches the nature of an operation.

For the removal of foreign bodies on and in the cornea, the patient is seated in a good light facing the source of illumination, or having it reflected upon the eye by a head mirror, or focused by oblique illumination through a lens held by an assistant, or by the patient

himself, or by the ocular illuminator of the writer. The binocular
loupe aids in the recognition of the object, which is brought into view
by a 2 per cent. sodium bicarbonate fluorescein solution.

The surgeon may stand in front of or behind the patient, as he
prefers. The latter should be seated with his head in a rest, or, in
an emergency, backed against a wall. In quiet patients, superficially lying foreign bodies may be brushed away by a cotton-tipped
stick or toothpick, without a local anesthetic. In most cases, however,

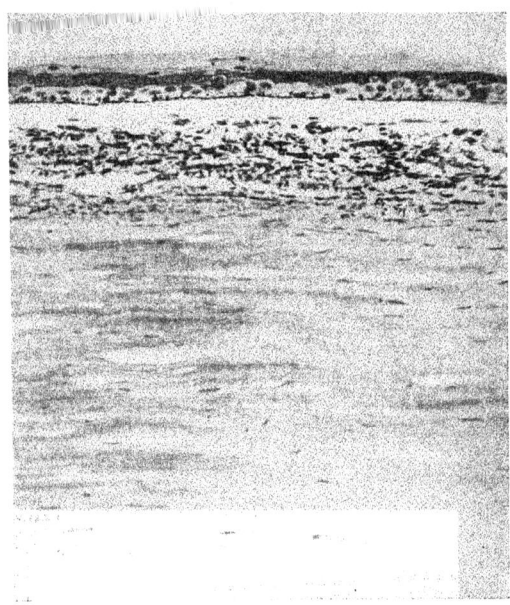

Blood-staining of the Cornea Following Injury.

numbing the tissues by cocain 5 per cent., alypin 2 per cent., or holocain 1 per cent., is advisable. Even dropping sterile, cold water into
the eye will afford a slight anesthesia sufficient to allow of a foreign
body being brushed away.

In shops of the iron and steel trades where many trivial accidents
happen to the eyes daily, "in the proportion of one accident to one
workman a year," the workmen should be instructed to use a wisp of
cotton rolled on a toothpick, to dispense with the usual pin, knife
blade, horse-shoe nail, etc., or instruments of any kind, and content
themselves with simple efforts to remove the foreign body with the
cotton twisted on a stick, which can do little or no damage, and to let

the oculist attend to those cases in which the foreign body is not thus immediately removed. Even the general practitioner would be wise to do little more when the services of an oculist are available, for the usual history of cases reaching the oculist is that some of the mechanics at the shops have first tried to remove the foreign body, with not infrequent infection from unsterilized instruments, and further abrasion of the corneal epithelium.

In undertaking the removal of objects impacted or burned into the cornea, in but few cases is the foreign body so loosely held by the tissues as to be removed by brushing. The patient's eye is then prepared, the head placed in the position just described, while the lids are held apart by the operator's fingers or those of an assistant. If the foreign body be deeply buried in the corneal tissue, it is sometimes advisable to attempt to pick it out, as attempts to reach it from the surface may end by pushing it into the anterior chamber; therefore, after anesthetizing the cornea, a broad needle may be passed into but not through the cornea, inserting it by the side of the foreign body, traversing the corneal lamellæ until the broad part of the blade is behind the foreign body, when another needle may be used to pick from the surface until it reaches the object, when it can be lifted away.

Should the foreign body have so deeply penetrated that it is feared any attempt to reach it from the surface may end in pushing it into the anterior chamber, a keratome, or broad needle, may be passed into the anterior chamber, pressed against the inner surface of the cornea immediately behind the foreign body and the surgeon can then cut through the cornea layer after layer until he reaches the foreign body, removing it by the spud or by forceps if large enough. The latter cases come under the heading of more serious injuries and are usually best treated in a hospital with subsequent rest in bed. When the foreign body has remained in the cornea for a number of days it is apt to be surrounded by a halo of inflammation, which may extend over the whole of the cornea, its epithelium becoming whitish and swollen, the foreign body ulcerating out, if not too deep, and it is then washed away, leaving the cornea in a condition of ulceration, and when cured leaving behind it opacities which impair the vision. Such cases require subsequent treatment by antiseptics and continuous bandaging, until cicatrization of the wound occurs.

Powder and dynamite explosions may lead to the impaction of particles of lead, small shot, sand, stone, or other small foreign bodies in the cornea, which may be picked out as in the foregoing.

In a large majority of these minor injuries the patient does not return to be seen by the surgeon. After removing the foreign body and cleansing the eye regeneration usually takes place within 24 hours. The patient should be instructed to keep the bandage on for that time and to return if the eye be at all irritable. See, also, p. 3369, Vol. V, of this *Encyclopedia*.

INJURIES OF THE CORNEA FROM BLUNT OBJECTS—CONTUSIONS AND RUPTURE.

Contusions   Round, blunt, foreign bodies, usually of some size, as handles of mechanics' tools, stones, balls, etc., as well as shot and bullets coming with slight force (spent balls) may fly against the cornea directly, or the force is communicated through the lids, usually causing bruising, perhaps with erosion of the anterior epithelium. There

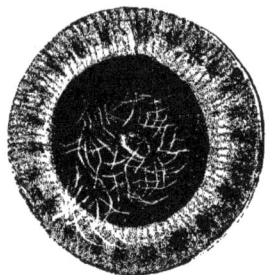

Lattice-like Keratitis from Contusion.

often results an extensive opacity of the central portions, lattice or panel-like keratitis, which under the magnifier is seen to be composed of delicate gray striæ interlacing in different directions, dependent upon reduction of the intraocular pressure. If the force has been more severe, causing dimpling of the cornea, the striae may be more diffuse and dense and is here due to a loosening of the true corneal tissue. In still greater injuries the cornea may be infracted or dented in and remain so, as happens occasionally after small stone or shot, non-penetrating injuries.

In contusion opacities of the cornea the cloudy, deep, opacity is chiefly due to an edema and must be considered a swelling phenomenon of which lesions of the endothelium are perhaps the chief cause.

In these cases the tension of the globe is lowered, the ciliary vessels injected. There is tenderness but not much pain, the absence of the latter due to bruising and consequent destruction of the sensitive nerve endings. The sight is always reduced and if accompanied by hemorrhage blindness occurs.

The cornea eventually clears; if it does not do so a grayish opacity remains. If the blow be very severe chronic irido-cyclitis, degeneration and blindness may result.

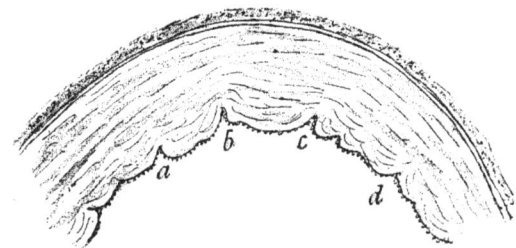

Section of Cornea showing Foldings of Membrane of Descemet in Panel-like Opacity of the Cornea, following Contusion.

The *diagnosis* is obtained by the history and subjective and objective symptoms, particularly loss of vision and hypotension.

The *prognosis* is not good, and extensive secondary changes, even to atrophy of the globe, may occur.

The *therapy* is rest, atropin and symptomatic treatment.

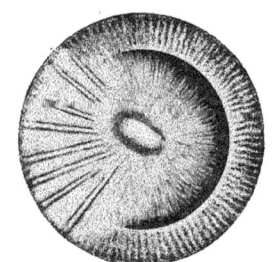

Wrinkling or Rupture of Descemet's Membrane with Blood Pigment in the Cornea, resulting from Rupture of the Canal of Schlemm. (Redrawn from sketch by Swan Burnett.)

Rupture of the cornea is seldom observed, only a few instances having been reported in the literature. The same causes that produce scleral ruptures, which are common, prevail here. Blows from the fist and such other large blunt objects as cow-horns, meat-hooks and wagon-shafts are the most common.

The *mechanism* of direct corneal rupture is the same as in direct scleral rupture. The rupture is due to the action of the impinging body being in such a direction and pushing with such force that there is no place for the globe to go. Hence that portion of the capsule which is impinged on by the foreign body is pushed in quickly into the globe, and bursts, just as the skin of the head breaks under a blow from a cane against the skull. The cornea or sclera is between the foreign body and the ocular contents, which are then under great pressure, and the tunic has to give way at this place and burst inwards.

In *indirect corneal rupture* the cushion of fat of the orbit protects the globe as far as it is encompassed by it and thus the whole of the posterior portion of the eye is protected so that under the pressure that portion of the sclera not so covered, or the cornea, has to give way, and it is usually the cornea, for the resiliency of the sclera is much greater. and the cornea being stiffer is more apt to burst under extraneous force.

Corneæ the subject of cicatrix from previous ulceration are more liable to rupture from a blow directly, or from a jar indirectly, and the rupture may extend from the region of the scar. The limbus is most generally detached, but otherwise there is no typical form in which they occur. In most cases the wounds are straight, but they are sometimes ragged or flap-shaped.

The *differential diagnosis* between lacerated wounds and direct rupture is difficult except upon determination of the object producing the injury. Balls, large handles of instruments, etc., are most apt to cause rupture, while sharp instruments, teeth and claws of animals, beaks of birds, cause jagged wounds.

The *prognosis* is better than in scleral rupture. Infection is the main danger. See *rupture of the sclera* in this section.

The *prognosis* is, as a rule, favorable. It very rarely happens that a rupture is followed by infection of the interior of the eye.

Therapy consists of an excision of the prolapsed iris and the mattress or Nuel suture. If the iris is not excised, vision becomes impaired by the irregular curvature of the cornea and the development of a higher degree of irregular astigmatism; the scar later becomes ectatic and produces an increased tension which may lead to blindness. See, also, p. 3442, Vol. V, of this *Encyclopedia*.

BURNS AND CAUTERIZATIONS OF THE CORNEA.

As a rule not only the cornea but the conjunctiva and frequently the lids and facial skin are at the same time injured by these accidents. In simple corneal burns, there is always photophobia, great pain from the injury and exposure of the ends of the sensitive nerves, lachrymation, considerable conjunctival secretion and usually swelling of the lids and chemosis of the conjunctiva, especially about the limbus. As a rule superficial burns are similar in appearance to erosions, though more painful. Depending upon the form of the injury they cause striped, spotted, large or small grayish opaque solutions of continuity of the epithelium and interlayers of the cornea. If superficial the epithelium is eroded, cast off and replaced within one to two days and full healing results. In deeper burns the cornea becomes more opaque and looks like ground glass; the sensibility remains but is diminished. In the very severe injuries the cornea looks like porcelain, and its nerves being destroyed the feeling is totally lost. In the deeper burns a line of demarcation forms, and the necrotic area is cast off, leaving a corneal ulcer. The vessels are engorged, and healing ulti-

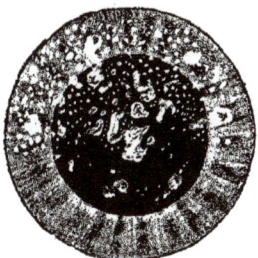

Nodular Opacity of the Cornea from Injury.

mately terminates in cicatricial formations, which may later result in ectasia and corneal staphyloma. All burns of the cornea, except the most superficial, are serious on account of the hindrance to vision. If the circumcorneal zone be injured the nutrient blood vessels are cut off and the whole cornea may come away in a mass.

In the course of healing of superficial and moderate burns vesicles may form which rupture from time to time, with recurrence of pain and other symptoms, described above under recurrent erosion of the cornea.

Sulphuric acid burns of moderate severity are characterized by the formation of phlyctenulæ, especially about the limbus. Lye, ammonia, lime, and other chemical burns have been sufficiently described under the general heading.

A peculiarity in the course of the primary opacity caused by acids is due to their action on the mucoid substance of the cornea. Mucoid is at first coagulated by the acids, and then dissolved. The acids destroy the endothelium of Descemet's membrane, followed by edema of the cornea, which produces the secondary opacities that may lead to ectasia of the cornea and keratoglobus.

Baths of ½ per cent. solutions of hydrate of potash remove the mucoid sediments, and the further course is greatly influenced by the neutralization of the acids by the same agent.

From intense burning, with ulcer formation, secondary iritis with synechiæ results. After the necrosed tissue is thrown off perforation with iris prolapse, formation of cataract, irido-cyclitis, ectasia, or phthisis bulbi, or, in the case of infection, panophthalmitis may result.

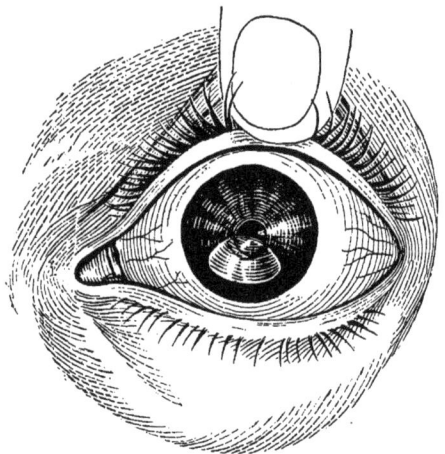

Corneal Ectasia from Injury.

When the chemotic conjunctiva at the limbus comes in contact with a small ulceration of the cornea it may grow fast and be the starting point for a pterygium. Symblepharon occurs in all forms, primarily from the adherence of raw surfaces on the globe and lids, and secondarily from cicatricial contractions. Ankyloblepharon ensues when the lids grow together. In perforation, *leucoma adherens* results. Staphyloma corneæ, with or without complication with the iris, occurs when the structure is so weakened that the intraocular pressure forces the tissue forward. More or less blindness occurs, depending upon the amount of tissue destruction and the resultant leucoma.

The *diagnosis* is to be made from the history of the injury, the finding of particles of lime, molten metal, etc. Heated fluids as a rule affect the conjunctival surfaces more, and particularly the lower part of the globe and the conjunctival surface of the lower eyelid. Fluorescein will determine the extent of the damaged surface.

The *prognosis* depends upon the grade of the injury and the resultant scar tissue formation. As noted, burning of the limbus is particularly unfavorable, as damage to the nutrient vessels results in necrosis of the cornea.

Epithelial burns are trivial and heal in a few hours. The burn from molten lead is as a rule lighter than that from other molten metals. Burns from molten glass or slag are particularly dangerous, as well as those from melted candy, syrup or preserves.

The determination of the sensitiveness of the cornea to touch is a particularly fine point in diagnosis. In trivial injuries the cornea remains hyper-sensitive, in moderate burns it is diminished, and in very dangerous ones that are apt to be followed by necrosis of all the tissue the nerves are destroyed and the cornea is insensitive to touch.

The treatment has already been fully detailed elsewhere. Especially, it is reiterated, is the physician to be warned against the use of cocain and the suprarenin products, for these diminish the vitality of the tissues and prevent nutrition. Removal of the foreign bodies, the use of holocain for anesthesia, dionin for analgesia, atropin, ointments, and mild antiseptics, cold application at first and then heat, are the indications. The formation of symblepharon is to be guarded against by the use of ointment, the passing of probes between the globe and lids, Thiersch grafts, egg membranes, lead, gold, aluminum plates, etc.

The treatment of the resultant leucoma is by massage with ung. hydrarg. oxid. flav., the Bellarminow masseur, dionin in solution or powder, thiosinamin locally and internally.

For the treatment of the symblepharon and the formation of a new pupil behind a clear space of the cornea, and similar operations, see the proper captions. Staphylomata may have to be abscised, and lastly the eye may look so badly that for cosmetic and business reasons enucleation and proper prothesis may be preferable.

GUN SHOT INJURIES OF THE CORNEA.

Gun shot injuries are seldom limited to the cornea. Contusions may occur from air rifles, spent shot, particles of lead from bullets which have struck targets or surrounding objects. Pieces of stone, wood, earth, etc., may be carried by the impact of the projectile, especially from cannon shot and bursting shells, and cause such contusions, as well as the other forms of injury noted below.

Perforating wounds of this nature are more common and are always complicated by injuries to other structures.

Ruptures of the cornea and sclera have been reported from shell injury. Foreign bodies, as powder grains and burns, are often seen from gunpowder explosions, flarebacks of small arms and artillery pieces. Particles of lead from the spattering of bullets on a target have been picked out of the eyes. In the case of larger-sized, high-power rifles, on impact with the iron target, the heat evolved is so

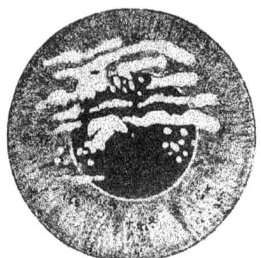

Lead Opacities in the Cornea.

great that most of the lead bullet melts, only a "button" usually being picked up.

Shot wounds of the cornea during war are all complicated and are dealt with under **Military surgery of the eye.**

Changes in the corneal tissues following injuries are also to be studied under **Corneal ulcer; Cornea, Opacities of the; Cornea, Lead incrustation of the; Cornea, Ectasia of the; Cornea, Staphyloma of the; Conical cornea; Ankyloblepharon; Symblepharon;** and under the various **Keratitis** captions.

INJURIES OF THE IRIS.

Wounds of the iris are complicated by perforating wounds of the eyeball, of the cornea or sclero-corneal limbus, and usually by injuries to the lens. Such injuries occur most frequently through wounds of the cornea, then of the sclero-corneal limbus or sclera. The causes are those of penetrating wounds of the eyeball generally, especially sharp and pointed objects, such as knives, glass splinters and iron particles.

The patient complains of pain of slight degree, as is usual after an iridectomy. If inflammation occurs the pain may be severe, especially over the brow; also piercing pain in the eye and headache, worse in the early hours of the morning or after lying down for several hours;

photophobia, loss of vision and lachrymation are the common symptoms of a traumatic iritis.

Wounds of the iris do not close; the margins separate and a coloboma remains. The edges of the wound may then heal to the cornea, causing anterior synechia and adherent leucoma, or to the capsule of the lens—posterior synechia.

If the wound be not immediately obscured by a hyphema it may be seen in the iris as an opening in this membrane, in the depths of which a small blood-clot is observed. The anterior chamber generally has a small hyphema and a little blood may be seen in the wound of the iris, which opens widely.

Prognosis is good, as injuries to the iris without implication of the lens do not materially affect the vision unless iritis occurs.

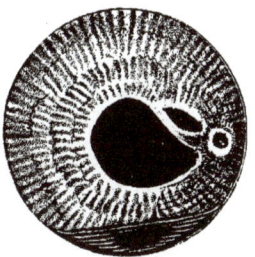

Wound of the Iris.
Anterior synechia; hyphema.

By the use of atropin, and carrying out asepsis, healing usually occurs with posterior synechia, but with a good eye if the other structures be not too seriously wounded. Iced applications, as well as eserin, are recommended by Praun, the latter in peripheral wounds. The writer has never seen any good effects from the latter, as wounds of the iris never coapt and atropin is the one drug indicated to keep the eye quiet, to prevent anterior and posterior synechia, with their subsequent dangers of glaucoma. Asepsis, argyrol and a light bandage are indicated for the accompanying corneal wound.

Prolapse and incarceration of the iris. If the anterior chamber be opened the escape of the aqueous humor drives the iris forward as far as the cornea, and if the wound is sufficiently open a portion of this membrane blocks the opening of the wound, causing incarceration. In this way the anterior chamber may be restored in a very short time.

The extent of the prolapse is proportioned to the size of the opening, and where the corneal tissue has been lost through suppurative necrosis it may occupy the whole extent of the cornea, constituting total prolapse of the iris. If the patient strains hard during the prolapse the protrusion may take place with great force and be large, or if he is restless afterwards a relatively larger portion of the iris will extrude. The relation of the healing of an iris prolapse into the corneal wound is also discussed under **Cornea, Serpent ulcer of the.**

The pupil loses its round shape and is drawn to the wound, the portion of the iris impacted depending upon the position of the wound. If in the ciliary portion the ciliary zone of the iris becomes impacted and the pupil has the shape of a pear, if near the center of the cornea the pupillary edge engages and the pupil is not so distorted—it may be nearly round.

As in other traumas the prolapse is synchronous with the injury; the symptoms are those of a wound. When, however, a wound second-

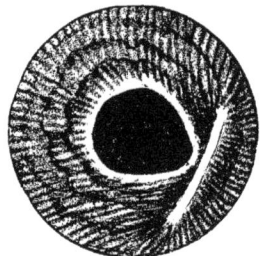

Incarceration of the Iris after Simple Linear Extraction without Iridectomy.

arily opens, or an ulcer bursts, the patient feels the gush of the aqueous and a sharp pain, which may disappear in a few minutes or persist as a dull ache until reposition or operation for its removal.

Prolapse of the iris is manifested differently according to the extent of protrusion. If the iris has pushed through to the outside it is visible as a dark swelling, or nodule, in the wound, in the middle of the section or at the sides. When the iris does not protrude but is merely jammed between the lips, of the wound the pupil is merely displaced. If an iridectomy has been made the corresponding pillar of the iris is shortened and the angle of the sphincter drawn up even so that it may not be visible.

Inclusion of the iris in a wound interferes with the healing of such wound. The cicatrix is less solid, is irregular and even when formed may ultimately give rise to increased intra-ocular tension, inflammation and sympathetic disease. See **Cornea, Ulcer of the.**

Tooke, writing on the protective influence exerted by the iris in perforated wounds of the cornea, says the wound of the cornea is frequently of an infective nature, be it a perforated ulcer or a perforation due to the entrance of a foreign body. By walling off the infected sides of the incision, an effort is made to ward off the entrance of bacteria into the anterior chamber and to avoid subsequent panophthalmitis. Beyond this purely mechanical action the blood vessels of the iris assist in carrying off the localized infection to the general circulation, thus preventing subsequent necrosis of the cornea. A second feature, noted by the presentation of the iris, is that the process of actual healing, or of granulation tissue formation, is materially assisted; that after draining away the infective agencies the number of leucocytes supplied by the blood vessels of the iris readily assists in the formation of new connective tissue elements. This tends to permanently close the per-

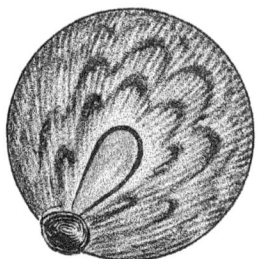

Small Peripheral Prolapse of the Iris.

foration, and allows the reformation of the protective epithelial strata of the cornea. Besides completely filling the gap in the cornea and preventing any escape of the aqueous humor, the anterior chamber is restored and the intraocular circulation re-established.

It cannot be denied that many lamentable results are avoidable by performing an iridectomy or by releasing the anterior synechia.

Prolapse of the iris is common in operations involving opening of the anterior chamber as well as in perforating injuries. Therefore every attempt should be made to avert these results, and the wound carefully freed from all bits of iris tissue, usually by abscission. In but few cases will the iris retract under eserin myosis, which usually proves disappointing. The spatula or a blunt hook may be used either through the wound opening or through a cut in the cornea made some distance away, the second opening equalizing the outflow of aqueous and permitting the pupil to resume its circular form, but iridectomy is the only safe procedure, as a prolapse is with difficulty retained within the anterior chamber. See **Cataract, Senile;** as well as **After-treatment of ophthalmic operations.**

Foreign bodies in the iris, the anterior and posterior chambers. Injuries occurring in trades from flying particles of iron, stone, copper or brass, more seldom wood and glass, shot and powder grains and occasionally other metals, cause the larger proportion of such cases. In addition to these comes that class of cases where cilia get into the anterior chamber, either through perforating wounds or by operations. An iritis nodosa is produced by the entrance of caterpillar hairs into the eye.

These foreign bodies usually enter by way of corneal wounds, less often by the sclero-cornea. In the case of gun-shot injuries the shot or particles of other foreign substances, cilia or other hairs may be carried in first through the lids and then into the eye by the corneal

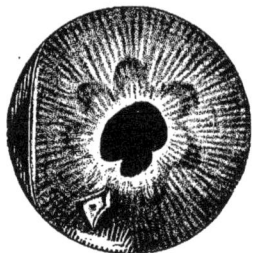

Steel Chip in the Iris.
Wound of cornea; small hyphema; posterior synechia.

route. In a few cases the foreign body may have entered the eye through the sclera, lodging in the lens or zonula and then migrating into the anterior chamber, or in the case of absorption of a traumatic cataract the body causing the lens opacity may drop into the posterior or anterior chamber or become impacted in the iris.

Severe rubbing of the cornea in which a sharp foreign body is impacted, or ill-considered operative attempts at removal, are responsible for quite a number of cases of foreign bodies in the anterior chamber or iris.

The iris is more usually the recipient of a foreign body than the anterior chamber, and the object is very rarely found in the posterior chamber. Those particles which penetrate the iris and go into the lens are not here considered.

The *subjective symptoms* are usually more or less irritation, but occasionally cases appear where the accident has been forgotten until the occurrence of an iritis. The iris is very tolerant of foreign bodies, but their presence near the lens is a source of danger and such patients should be under skilled observation.

Foreign bodies in the anterior chamber are usually in the lower part and difficult to see; larger objects may be anywhere, those in the iris may be in the anterior layers or penetrate the membrane. Long, sharp objects may remain, transfixing the cornea, iris and lens. In most cases of foreign bodies in the iris the capsule of the lens is likewise injured.

In recent cases the anterior chamber is found open and shallow and the tension is diminished; the iris may have prolapsed, but as the foreign body is usually small the wound of the cornea or sclero-cornea is usually too small to allow of prolapse and in these cases the lips of the wound come together very soon and the anterior chamber is speedily restored. If the iris is wounded a small hyphema may be seen, or a flake of blood in the iris about the foreign body. Where the foreign body is large the iris may be so severely wounded as to cause much bleeding and the anterior chamber may thus be full of blood.

The further course of the case depends upon whether or not infection takes place, and upon the chemical character of the foreign body. Indifferent objects, such as gold, silver, splinters of glass, porcelain, stone and wood, powder, lead and shot pellets and cilia may remain for a long time without causing reaction.

If *siderosis of the iris* is lacking in a cataract with yellow dots on the anterior surface of the lens we are justified in inferring a piece of iron in the lens, whereas, siderosis of the iris and cataract with yellow dots on the surface of the lens point to the seat of iron in the vitreous or retina. If the foreign body remains in the eye, the siderosis of the iris may disappear after a few years, but the iris may still give iron reaction. Iron particles usually cause siderosis after some weeks, copper and brass cause a destructive chemical reaction within a few days and destroy the eye. Silver wire, glass, porcelain, stone, iron, copper and other commoner substances have been removed from the iris by ophthalmic surgeons.

Powder grains and shot pellets may be retained within the anterior chamber and iris for months without causing reaction. These occur from powder and dynamite explosion, and from fire arms.

Myiasis of the eye is most frequently observed in children and persons who sleep out of doors. The flies deposit their eggs or larvæ on the lids or into the palpebral fissure at the inner canthus, and the larvæ penetrate from the conjunctival sac into the orbit, eating through lymphatics and veins, causing sometimes a severe general infection.

Cilia in the anterior chamber following accident or operation are rare. Cilia which entered the eye by traumatism are generally tolerated for years without causing the least symptoms. They may, however, give rise to infection, or, more or less early, to irritation, ciliary injection, photophobia, lachrymation, pain, or to the development of epidermoidal tumors of the iris, cysts, with subsequent glaucoma, blindness or loss of the eye. Therefore their early removal is indicated, although even then tumors may develop from simultaneously introduced epidermoidal particles. Each case must be individualized. See p. 2214, Vol. III of this Encyclopedia.

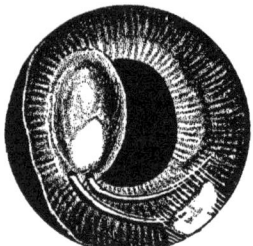

Cilia in the Anterior Chamber carried Through a Wound of the Cornea.

Showing scar, irido-dialysis and cyst of iris.

In the *diagnosis* of foreign bodies in the anterior chamber and iris, in those cases in which the foreign body is lengthy and one end remains in the cornea or sticks out through the iris the problem is an easy one. Recent cases may likewise be readily diagnosed if there has been but little hemorrhage into the anterior chamber, or if there has been no prolapse of the iris or lens mass hiding the object. However, even very small bodies in such cases may be seen by transillumination, and if invisible by these means are shown by the skiascopie plate. The probe may be carefully used to sound within the corneal wound only, but its use is to be deprecated for deeper investigation. When the anterior chamber is free from hyphemia the ophthalmoscope and direct examination by the magnifier will often reveal the intruder. But in older cases where the foreign body has caused irritation and become covered by inflammatory exudate it may not be directly visible. Here the diaphanoscope and the Roentgen ray give us our best means for objective examination. Diagnosis by magnetic attraction may be carefully used.

Free-lying, foreign bodies in the anterior chamber may come into view when the patient stoops forward or lies on one side. Those in the posterior chamber can only be seen after full dilation of the pupil, and are usually incidentally discovered in ophthalmoscopic examination.

The *prognosis* is usually only favorable when the foreign body is early removed from the eye, for despite the curious and rare instances of such intruders being tolerated without damage for months or years, they almost invariably lead to loss of sight and of the eye, and may cause sympathetic disease and blindness in the other. Plastic iritis is usually the first step, then comes closure of the pupil, cataracta accreta, irido-cyclitis, and then the other eye begins to inflame.

Therapy. Extraction of the foreign body is the main procedure, aside from the regular care of the wound and atropinization. The only exceptions to this rule are those cases where, upon examination, a foreign body is found which has been in the eye for a long time, months or years, without causing inflammation. In such cases it is generally safer not to disturb the status quo. In these it is wise to warn the patient of the necessity for operation upon the slightest sign of irritation.

Foreign bodies on the iris demand prompt removal, for usually, if allowed to remain they will speedily set up a severe iritis. An exception, however, sometimes is found, as in a case of the writer's, in which a particle of steel had been resting on the iris for five years.

If the magnet will not remove the steel forceps must be used. If it cannot be readily disentangled from the tissue, we may succeed in so doing by drawing the portion of the iris containing it through the wound, so that we can more readily have access to it, and then after its removal replace the iris. Should these measures fail, it might be necessary to perform an iridectomy, removing the portion of the iris containing the foreign body.

The extraction of a foreign body impacted in the iridic tissues should be done as early as possible after the accident, where its location is not disguised by pus or blood in the anterior chamber. If allowed to remain it may speedily set up a severe iritis. Local anesthesia by cocain is applicable for adults, general narcosis for children. The field of operation should be highly illuminated, preferably by the head lamp, of which the Stucky or Kierstein models are preferred. The former has the advantage of using the 110 volt current with a 6 to 16 c. p. lamp. The latter has miniature lamps, the current being reduced to 6 volts resistance. To the latter an ophthalmoscopic mirror may be attached, useful in magnet and other operations for removal of foreign bodies from the posterior portion of the globe, and, with a combination of the Berger binocular loupe, for operations on the anterior portion of the globe. See **Head light.**

A hand electric lamp held by an assistant is used by many surgeons, particularly abroad, where assistants are plentiful. The instillation of atropin is not always advisable, for the foreign body may be drawn thereby under the pupil, closer in apposition to the lens capsule and cause damage, or it may draw the foreign body out of view behind the limbus or iris. Eserin, however, prevents the foreign body from going against the lens capsule or falling into the posterior chamber. An iris prolapse may thus be reduced and in the extraction of the intruder from the anterior chamber by the interposition of the iris between it and the lens, the capsule is in a measure protected from further injury.

When a foreign body is loose in the anterior chamber, or is not fixed in the iris, the operator should endeavor to let it come out with the flow of aqueous upon the completion of the corneal incision, although this is seldom accomplished.

By depressing the keratome a little on one edge, and bringing its point up to the posterior surface of the cornea, the aqueous comes out more freely, but the point of the keratome is apt to wound the anterior capsule of the lens and thus produce an operative traumatic cataract, as occasionally occurs in operations for the removal of foreign bodies from the anterior chamber and iridectomy for glaucoma. On account of this danger from the keratome many operators habitually use the Graefe knife, whose point, after the counter puncture, is kept away from the globe.

The foreign body may at times be extracted through the wound of entrance, but in most cases this has to be enlarged by the blunt-ended knife or scissors, or if the anterior chamber has been restored a linear incision into the cornea near, and peripherally to, the wound area may be made so that room is obtained for proper manipulation of the instruments and for egress of the foreign body.

Extraction of a foreign body without iridectomy can usually only be made in free-lying objects or those but slightly impacted into the iris. The **H**irschberg magnet, or the extended flexible arm of the Victor magnet with its small tips, here finds its greatest use for removal of small magnetizable pieces of metal after the corneal incision. A magnetized keratome, forceps or steel spud is sometimes here useful. The writer generally prefers the giant magnet, used after the manner of Haab. See **Electromagnet.**

Iridectomy as a rule has to be made either on account of irreducible prolapse of the iris, danger of anterior synechia, or because the foreign body is so entangled with the iris that it cannot be withdrawn without the iris coming with it. At times it may be possible to excise only a portion of the peripheral border of the iris, thus leaving the pupil round and movable without the deformity of a coloboma, such as is produced by the usual iridectomy.

Small particles of iron and steel impacted into the angle of the anterior chamber, or between the sclera and ciliary body, can only be removed by entering the eye with the tip of the magnet, as the power of the giant magnet cannot be applied in such a direction without danger of drawing the chip of metal against, and thus injuring, the lens.

The iris forceps, blunt hook or curette is of use in dislodging such impacted foreign bodies so that the subsequent steps of the operation may be completed by the aid of the magnet. Round foreign bodies may be assisted in delivery by the Daviel or Pagenstecher spoons.

If the foreign body lie in the posterior chamber and be magnetic the giant magnet may be used to draw it into the anterior chamber, and then be extracted as above described. If non-magnetic, as stone, copper, glass, wood, etc., extraction may be attempted by the forceps, blunt hook or curette.

Pieces of stone in the iris are not always followed by identical reactions. Some may rest there quietly for a great many years; others may cause such violent pain that an immediate operation is required. This may be due to the chemical or physical nature of the foreign body, to pathogenic germs or a special predisposition of the injured organ.

Traumatic iritis, while due to traumatisms of all kinds, especially if perforation of the eyeball has taken place, is especially apt to occur if a foreign body be left in the eye. The exciting causes are either those due to mechanical injury from contusion, traction, or pressure, as from the injury, or swollen cataractous lens masses; chemical irritation from decomposition of the foreign body, as from copper particles; or infection, the last cause being most frequent.

Operations on the eye are traumatisms, and of these the most apt to produce iritis and irido-cyclitis are cataract operations.

The *hairs of caterpillars,* spines of grasshopper legs, and portions of other insects, bee stings, etc., not only produce an ophthalmia nodosa of the conjunctiva, but also some weeks or months after their entrance violent inflammation may appear in the iris with development of nodules therein, causing iritis and even loss of the eye. The nodular portion of the iris should be excised by iridectomy. See, also, p. 3123, Vol. IV, as well as p. 1781, Vol. III, of this *Encyclopedia.*

Certain *tumors of the iris* may result from trauma, among them
cysts. As there are no glands nor epithelium in the iris no retention
cysts occur. Those that develop are epithelial in type. Serous cysts
occur in the iris, after penetrating wounds, as a very rare affection.
Pearl cysts are distinguished from serous cysts by their contents,
which are pultaceous or tallowy and composed of epithelial cells constantly thrown off from the inner surface, which undergo fatty degeneration.

Wounds of the cornea heal by the epithelium growing rapidly down
into the deeper parts, sometimes it extends beyond the inner aspect
of the wound, growing into the center of the anterior chamber along
its walls, covering the posterior surface of the cornea and the anterior
surface of the iris, forming an anterior chamber cyst. If the iris be
in contact with the wound the epithelium pushes into it, pushing the
layers of the iris apart, thus forming an iris cyst, its walls being composed of rarefied iris tissue. The site is usually in the iris itself, seldom in the ciliary body. The epithelium is usually transparent and
can only be demonstrated after removal by staining and the microscope.
It is very destructive to the eye, as it leads to increase of tension
because the epithelial lining hinders filtration through the sinus of the
anterior chamber.

Pseudo-cysts occur from portions of the iris and cornea, or lens,
dilating from accumulation of fluid between these structures.

As a rule no irritative symptoms are apparent until the cyst fills
the half of the anterior chamber, when glaucoma sets in. Serous cysts
appear as grayish, transparent vesicles whose anterior wall shows some
pigment and remains of rarefied iris tissue. When they reach the
posterior surface of the cornea they flatten and the cornea becomes
cloudy from proliferation of the endothelium. It then pushes into
the pupil, which becomes kidney-shaped or even reduced to a slit.
Dislocation and opacity of the lens occur from its growth backward.
Disturbances of vision, elevation of tension and glaucoma cause blindness.

The *diagnosis* is made by inspection. The cyst is translucent and
the red glow of the fundus may be seen through it by the ophthalmoscope.

The *prognosis* is good upon early and complete removal, otherwise
the sight may be lost from glaucoma.

The *therapy* is operative, being early removal of the cyst by marginal incision of the cornea at the point corresponding to the cyst,
entering the forceps, withdrawing it together with the iris and excising
it completely, without rupture or damage to the walls of the anterior

chamber, as, if any epithelium be left in the eye, another implantation cyst will grow. Often complete removal is not possible at one operation, hence a recurrence is to be expected, when another operation may cure the case.

Granulation tumors of the iris are rare, but wounds of the iris may granulate so freely as to form a new-growth which must be differentiated from syphiloma, sarcoma, and tuberculosis. These have occurred from ablations of staphylomata of the cornea in which all the iris has not been removed and some of its tissue becomes entangled in the wound and resultant cicatrix.

Tuberculosis of the iris may follow injury, but it is secondary to tuberculous disease in some other part of the body. See **Iritis, Tubercular**.

Hyphema. Although this subject is treated elsewhere under its proper caption, yet it seems well to say here that blows of all characters, especially from rebounding foreign bodies of metal, wood and stone, blows from fisticuffs and blunt objects, as well as actual wounds and the passage of foreign bodies through the parts may cause hyphema, or bleeding into the anterior chamber, from injuries to the iris structure, as in traumatic iridodialysis, or irideremia, sphincter rupture, radial and circular tears and, very seldom, isolated ruptures of the bloodvessels. Bleeding from rupture of the canal of Schlemm has already been described. Bleeding from the canal of Petit is pictured by Jäeger, but it must be a very seldom event; concentric red streaks near the periphery of the lens are then seen. If the zonula be torn the anterior chamber may fill with blood from injuries to the choroid and ciliary processes.

In small injuries the blood flows out of the ruptured vessel and spreads over the iris as a diffuse red-brown flake, which gradually grows smaller and in a few days is entirely absorbed.

In more severe tears the blood may partially or completely fill the anterior chamber. In a few days it sinks to the bottom of the anterior chamber, becoming fully absorbed in the course of three to seven days. Small quantities may disappear in the course of 24 hours. When it occurs in a diseased eye the absorption may be very slow, even taking two to three weeks, and then leaving a residue.

Blood clots in both the anterior chamber and the vitreous, after an injury, may suddenly have the coloring matter dissolved in the ocular fluids and diffuse all through the eye, the aqueous humor, too, becoming colored red so that the iris looks as if seen through ruby glass.

When there is much blood in the anterior chamber, especially if the eye be otherwise diseased, it may remain a long time, even months, becoming darker in color; and thus where repeated hemorrhages have occurred a hyphema may be composed of several different colored strata, the lowest and darkest being the primary hemorrhage. Very old and incompletely absorbed hyphema may become brown or dirty-green in color, the cornea or the iris may become tinged, the latter also from the hemorrhage into the vitreous.

If the blood remains for a long time in the anterior chamber and the eye is also inflamed the colored exudate may become organized and form a permanent membrane, occluding the pupil and negativing the result of operations for clearing the pupil.

Eyes that have an excessive intra-ocular tension, as in glaucomatous states, or where vessel walls are weak from arterio-sclerosis, are predisposed to intra-ocular hemorrhage from injury or otherwise. Changes in the character of the blood, as after inhalations of nitrous oxide or carbonic acid gas, or in anemia or scurvy, likewise predispose to such accidents. The subjective symptoms are those of sudden loss of sight, from the pupil being obscured by blood, and a feeling of fullness in the eye.

The *prognosis* is generally good, the blood speedily resorbing, except in otherwise diseased eyes where organization of the clot may take place. Iritis seldom occurs unless the globe has been penetrated.

The *therapy of hyphema* is usually that of the wound or contusion; atropin, asepsis and rest. However, iced compresses may prevent further hemorrhage; ergot by hypodermic or by the mouth may contract the vessels. Calcium chloride is indicated internally. Hot compresses and dionin locally aid in the resorption of the blood clots, and atropin keeps the pupil free so that the contracting sphincter may not force the possible irido-dialysis wider open. If radial tears are seen then atropin is contraindicated and eserin should be used to contract the pupil and draw the tears closer together. See, also, **Hyphemia.**

Iridodialysis, or tearing away of the iris from its connection with the ciliary body at an angle of the anterior chamber is an interesting clinical event of not uncommon occurrence. Blows striking the sclera near the root of the iris, especially rebounding objects, as particles of coal, stone, wood or metal, corks from charged beverages, ends of canes, spent shot pellets and whip lashes, are the objects that usually produce such an injury.

Direct iridodialysis is sometimes unintentionally produced in the course of operations on the iris if the eye makes a sudden movement at the moment when the operator grasps the iris with the forceps. The iris may be thus separated from its insertion to a varying extent, or even torn out of the eye. In iridectomy for occlusion of the pupil, when the pupillary edge is not first set free from the occluding membrane, the latter pulls with the traction on the opposite side, tearing away the iris at its insertion. Hence the iris should always be released from the occluding membrane by lateral movements of the forceps, before drawing it out of the wound. Iridodialysis may also be produced spontaneously when atrophy has occurred in spots, and by the forward growth of neoplasms of the ciliary body, pushing the iris away from its insertion.

Indirect iridodialysis is produced by a variety of conditions. One of these is flattening of the cornea during trauma, from which its circumference and the circle of insertion of the iris become larger. If this enlargement takes place suddenly the iris can not adapt itself and tears away from its insertion in one or more places. The aqueous may be pushed back through the pupil by the flattening of the cornea,

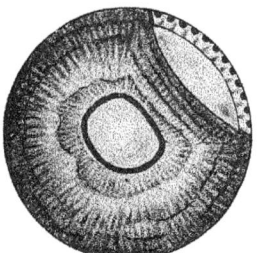

Iridodialysis.

deepening and increasing the pressure on the posterior chamber, the force being exerted mostly at its deepest portion at the base of the iris. This is ballooned forward and gives way at the insertion if a radial tear does not first result. Blows on the edge of the sclera dent in the globe, may also push the vitreous against the ciliary body and root of the iris, which gives way at this point.

If the immediate hyphema is not too great we will find on one side, at the ciliary margin of the iris, a black crescent which is formed by the separation of the iris from its insertion, and then, or after absorption of the blood, we can look through into the interior of the eye. When the separation is considerable we will see the edge of the lens, the ciliary processes and the fibers of the zonula in the gap if oblique or focal illumination is used. The pupil is flattened to the side of the dialysis, being stretched into a straight line by the contraction of the sphincter, occupying a chord of the arc of the rounded pupillary margin. The pupillary margin is drawn inwards, the ciliary insertion drawn away so that it can never heal again to its root.

The extent of rupture may be small, or very great so that an irideremia is produced; in the latter case the iris contracting, rolling up into a little ball, atrophying and sinking down to the bottom of the anterior chamber.

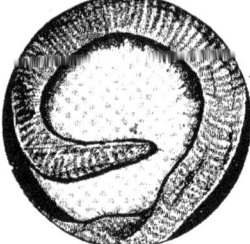

Rupture of the Iris.
Iridodialysis; partial inversion; traumatic cataract.

From the hyphema the eye is temporarily blinded, but vision returns upon resorption.· The sight is but little affected by irido-dialysis; the only thing being that if the eye is not accurately focused, through the formation of another image upon the retina through the peripheral opening, monocular diplopia and confusion occur.

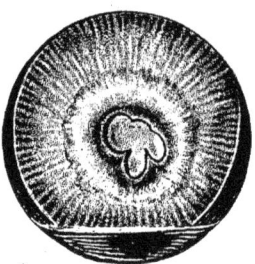

Iridodialysis, nearly Complete, in Iris Bombé with Hyphema.

After resorption of the blood in the anterior chamber the sight returns and the extent of the damage is seen. It may be that some reattachment of the edges of the dialysis occurs if atropin be instilled, but it is doubtful, as we know that the cut or wounded iris does not heal but the wound remains open with no effort of Nature at repair. The pupil remains irregular and there is another permanent opening at the periphery of the iris.

In iridodialysis hyphema always coexists, with radiating tears of the iris structure or margin. Rupture of the ciliary body and choroid, with or without detachment of the retina, may also occur.

After the hyphema is absorbed, or if it is not great, the additional opening may be seen on inspection. If the dialysis be small it will be best seen by the ophthalmoscope. The contour of the pupil gives a hint as to another opening at one side.

The *prognosis* is not unfavorable as to vision if there be no other damage. In mild cases the acuity and accommodation may remain normal, in others this function is lowered on account of complications.

The *therapy* is atropin, iced compresses for two days, then hot compresses and dionin to secure resorption of the blood. Iridotomy and iridectomy may be made to relieve the monocular diplopia. Operative procedures have been undertaken (see **Iridenkleisis**) for their cosmetic effects. See, also, **Iridodialysis.**

Traumatic aniridia, or irideremia. If the irido-dialysis be of such extent that the iris becomes fully torn from its ciliary attachment, it may fall down in the bottom of the anterior chamber and later shrink into an inconspicuous gray mass. If rupture of the sclera in the ciliary region be produced at the same time the iris may extrude or be expelled from the eye.

All very heavy blows upon the globe, especially those which produce scleral rupture, may cause irideremia. It seldom occurs without opening of the globe. The iris has been known to have been entirely torn out of the eye during an operation for iridectomy.

The occurrence of irideremia from contusion without a bursting of the sclera is of different character than when the globe is opened. In the first instance the mechanism is the same, only greater in degree, as that of iridodialysis. The lens remains, although it may be dislocated at the same time; in the second case the iris extrudes from the wound, usually with the lens. The force of the blow must have first caused the complete loosening of the iris at its attachments to the ciliary body and the outflow of aqueous through the wound forces it out of the eye.

After resorption of the hyphema, which is usually great, the whole corneal space is black and by the ophthalmoscope is seen to be all pupil. The remains of the iris, where there has been no opening of the globe, are to be found in the depths of the anterior chamber as a little black ball which may vary in its location with the movement of the globe. The retina may be detached; the lens usually is dislocated from rupture of the zonula.

In cases where aphakia coexists there is a flattening of the limbus so that the globe becomes somewhat conical. In this condition the whole interior of the eyeball becomes one chamber and the pressure of the extrinsic muscles lengthens the globe to an ovoid.

Hemorrhages occur in the vitreous, showing a dark-red reflex. If the media be clear, streaks of blood in the vitreous, the glare of the fundus and the ciliary processes may be seen on direct examination. In a few cases a portion of the iris may remain attached to its insertion and the remainder of the iris hang from it on a pedicle. In several instances the iris has been completely detached, expelled from the anterior chamber through the scleral opening, with or without the lens, and remained impacted under the conjunctiva. If any vision remains the symptoms are of asthenopia due to glare, the protecting iris being removed, and total loss of accommodation. If the lens be extruded 10 D., or more, of hyperopia is produced.

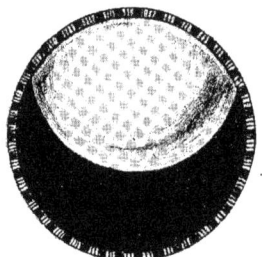

Traumatic Irideremia with Dislocation of the Lens Upwards.

The *differential diagnosis* is to be made between aniridia and total inversion of the iris. The latter is very rare and in the former the ciliary processes are to be seen, while in the latter they are covered by the iris.

Prognosis. These eyes are usually blinded, but in some cases sufficient vision remains to allow the patient to get about.

Therapy. The immediate treatment is that of the contusion with hyphema, or of scleral rupture. Increased tension is to be combated with eserin or paracentesis of the cornea. Sphero-cylindric lenses help the vision when the retina yet functionates. The theoretically advised stenopaic glasses do not seem to be of much use and are generally worn by patients for but a short time.

See, also, p. 483, Vol. I, of this *Encyclopedia;* as well as **Irideremia.**

Inversion or retroflexion of the iris. Inversion of the iris consists in its being pushed back so as to lie upon the surface of the ciliary body and looking as if it were absent. Partial dislocation is frequently observed and here the iris seems to be wanting, a coloboma appearing to exist. Total inversion is very rare.

This form of injury results from contusions of moderate severity, the other factors in the causation of this injury being due to the cornea being flattened, which pushes the aqueous backward against the posterior wall of the anterior chamber, in which the area of the pupil is formed by the lens and in the rest of its extent by the iris. The latter when pushed backward finds its support in the lens, except in the marginal portion of the iris where the posterior chamber is deepest and, therefore, the periphery forms the most yielding spot and is the first to give way before pressure; this forces the iris back as far as the zonula or even into the vitreous, causing inversion of the iris.

In but few cases is the iris entirely inverted, usually only a fourth or half gets into this position. If all be inverted a maximal mydriasis

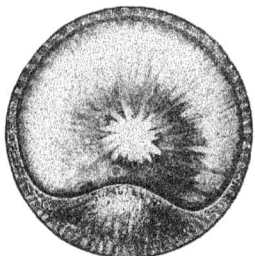

Nearly Complete Inversion of the Iris; Traumatic Cataract.

is accomplished, usually without luxation of the lens into the anterior chamber, which, however, may accompany the disassociation of relation. If a portion of the iris suffer this posterior prolapse a more or less large coloboma will be apparent, the base of the iris, however, not being involved and frequently only the pupillary edge being folded over. In contra-distinction to irideremia, the ciliary processes are covered over by the enfolding iris and are not to be seen in the coloboma. Atropin has no effect in retroverting the iris, as the pupillary edge becomes attached to the ciliary body by adhesions. There are no special subjective symptoms except from the contusion. Dazzling from the wide-open pupil may be noticed.

Maximal mydriasis and a coloboma with the base of the iris remaining, and the folding over of the edges of the iris, should be observed. If the lens be partially dislocated the coloboma pillars will not be in the same plane as the rest of the iris.

In uncomplicated cases there is nothing to be said about prognosis or therapy. The iris remains in the new location without causing any particular disturbance.

Laceration of the sphincter pupillæ. Sphincter rhexis; marginal tears of the iris. Lacerations of the iris usually start from the pupil and may extend to the ciliary margin so that the pupil appears to be pear-shaped; or the laceration may be in the form of a pointed Gothic arch, or the pupillary margin may be torn but little and the gaping can only be discovered by careful examination.

Such lacerations are the most frequent cause of dilatation of the pupil occurring after contusions (mydriasis traumatica), as they cause weakening or paralysis of the sphincter, due to laceration of its fibers; they frequently accompany simple cataract extraction (without iridectomy) and are caused by tearing of the iris in the efforts to remove the cataractous lens through an unyielding pupil. The ciliary muscle may also be paralyzed by contusion so that accommodation is affected.

There may be one or more tears at the same time. The edge of the pupil remains passive over the convex surface of the lens during the trauma and has to give way by a rupture. At the moment of trauma a spastic contraction of the sphincter exists, while the corneo-scleral ring is enlarged, and if this does not give way, producing a dialysis, the pupillary tear occurs. The indentation of the cornea by the object producing the injury presses the iris on the lens and holds it fast so that the aqueous goes on either side and exerts a force sideways, thus tearing the iris apart.

The sphincter tear may go entirely through the membrane or only the muscle may be torn. In the former case the objective damage is apparent on direct examination, in the latter only by diaphanoscopy. Small tears are more common, extending 1-2 mm. from the pupillary edge. The edges of the tear separate so that a triangular enlargement of the pupil is seen. As a rule the bleeding is slight, only causing a hyphema of a couple of mm. in height. The pupil is moderately enlarged, seldom fully dilated and less often normal. The subjective symptoms are those of contusion and dazzling except in complicated cases.

Other injuries, as lacerations of the ciliary body, dislocations of the lens, bleeding and formation of membranes in the vitreous and rupture of the choroid, frequently accompany this lesion. No inflammation follows, but the iris never heals, as the endothelium grows over the torn edges. Thus (objectively) the defect may be seen many years after, and histologic examination shows the want of union.

If not obscured by bleeding, or upon resorption of same, the solutions of continuity may very readily be seen by the naked eye or by the magnifier. In some cases dialysis is combined, and as a rule there are other injuries, before described, which are apparent to diaphanoscopy and the ophthalmoscope.

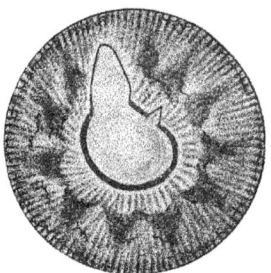

Sphincter Rhexis. Marginal Tears of the Iris.

The *prognosis* depends upon the complications, especially of the vitreous, retina and choroid. Single sphincter tears have no special significance as to vision.

Therapy. Theoretically, miotics should bring the torn pupillary margins together and cause healing, but such is not the case. Atropin, however, is contraindicated, as its action would only tend to deepen the tear.

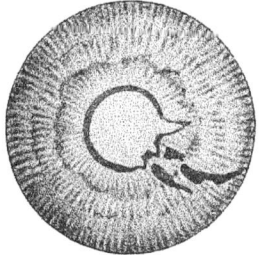

Marginal and Radial Tears of the Iris.

Rhexis iridis; tears through the entire width and extent of the iris. A continuation of the marginal tear through the entire thickness and extent of the iris forms a traumatic coloboma which may be so regular that it seems as if surgically accomplished. This may happen in the case of scleral rupture when a piece of the iris is nipped off. Without an opening of the globe, the condition must be both a sphincter tear and dialysis accompanied by a doubling over, or inversion, of the torn lips of the iris.

Dehiscences between the pupillary edge and the ciliary processes, or dialyses anterior to the root of the iris, and between it and the pupil, are rare and are usually the result of a spent shot or other

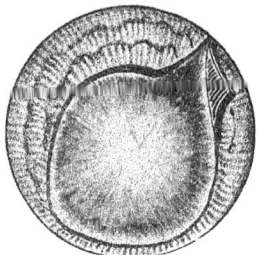

Iridorhexis with Inversion and Eversion of the Iris.

substance striking the globe between the ciliary region and the pupil, denting it in and rupturing the iris in a circular manner. Usually several such tears exist and are parallel to each other and to the root of the iris.

Traumatic pigment coloboma is seldom seen, but it is, however, very common after cataract operations, as may be readily shown by trans-

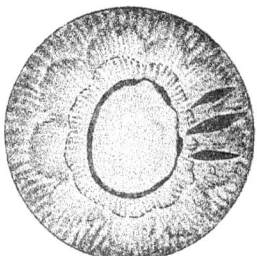

Radial Tears of Iris; Small Marginal Tear of the Sphincter.

illumination. In but few cases does the lens escape from the globe without removing some iris pigment. The writer has likewise noticed this condition in many cases of contusion which involved the iris. The trauma is not apparent by direct examination; if much of the posterior coat has been rubbed away the red reflex of the fundus may show through by the ophthalmoscope, but diaphanoscopy renders the diagnosis easy, showing the dehiscences which appear reddish through the thinned membrane, almost as red as the pupil.

A *cross-like adhesion of the iris to the posterior layer of the cornea* has been described as following an accident.

Mydriasis and miosis traumatica. Traumatic iridoplegia. This condition is very common after severe contusions, especially from blows upon the eye, spent shot, and injury from lightning. Injury to the sphincter is the usual cause and can, in the majority of cases, be elicited by transillumination. In other cases the nerve endings of the oculomotor may be directly bruised, or bleeding into the iris tissue may prevent contraction.

As a rule, irregular and moderate dilatation of the pupil is found with tears of the iris. More seldom is the pupil round. The reaction is absent or diminished. Hypotony usually exists. The pupil is usually oval or moderately and irregularly dilated, as in the cadaveric position. Maximal mydriasis or miosis rarely exists. Fuller dilatation may be effected by atropin but the pupil dilates more slowly than normally. If the pupil fully dilates to atropin there has been no lesion of the dilator muscle; if contracting fully to eserin, none of the constrictor. Enlargement and diminution of the pupil, in themselves, do not cause any special interference with vision, if not combined with paralysis of accommodation. Slight dazzling may exist.

One may add that the chief evidence of these changes in the pupil after injury is that there is generally a deep-seated trauma, combined with paralysis of accommodation; fine opacities of the cornea; bleeding into the anterior and vitreous chambers, followed by retinal, choroidal, and optic nerve hemorrhages and atrophy; disassociation of contiguity of the lens, choroid and retina, in some cases with Berlin's opacity of the retina and destruction of the macula. In a few cases, myopic astigmia follows from spasm of accommodation, or a myopic lens astigmia arises.

The pupil is moderately enlarged, maybe irregularly, and does not react to light or accommodation. Accommodative paralysis or spasm exists, frequently with myopia. If no bleeding obscures the view injury to the sphincter may be seen on transillumination. The patient should be questioned as to previous use of mydriatics and it should be remembered that paralytic mydriasis is seldom maximal. Diseased conditions must be excluded. Slight degrees may get well in the course of a few weeks, but many cases persist for the patient's life time.

Protective smoked, euphos, amethyst or amber glasses give relief to the slight dazzling. Strychnin internally, eserin locally, the high tension and high frequency electrical currents may all assist Nature in the return to normal.

Atrophy of the iris after contusion may occur, forming a simple membrane in which the pupil may persist, but within function; or holes in the iris may form. See, also, **Holes in the iris.**

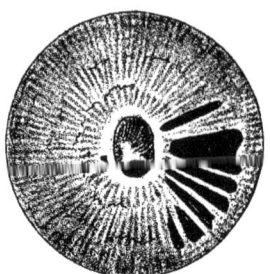

Radial Atrophy and Holes in the Iris, after Injury.

INJURIES OF THE LENS.

The effect of external force upon the lens is manifested either by solutions of continuity or contiguity, and by opacification of the lenticular capsule, cortex or body; commonly both participate in the injury and its results.

Traumatic cataract. Direct wounding of the lens occurs from pointed or cutting objects and flying foreign bodies, which as a rule pass through the thin capsule into the cortex or nucleus, or even through the structure into the vitreous.

All injuries which make an opening in the lens capsule result in opacity. This is usually complete, as the edges gape, the lens fibers absorb the aqueous humor, and swell, becoming opaque and finally separating from each other in layers through a process of cleavage. When the traumatism affects the posterior capsule, the vitreous acts in the same way. The operation of discission affects the lens in a like manner. In many cases of contusion it is likely that rupture of the capsule, probably in the equator, is likewise caused, but lenticular opacity may also result from simple concussion.

Of the traumatic opacities of the lens there appear some that are stellate and situated in the posterior cortical area. These are interesting, first, because in perforative traumatisms the foreign body need not reach the posterior zone to produce this form of cataract; second, because such a cataract may appear from injuries with blunt objects without tearing the capsule or causing a visible lesion of the zonule; and, third, because the opacity may remain stationary or clear up and disappear.

Fresh cases show the corneal or corneo-scleral wound, older ones the cicatrix. If the injury be in the pupillary area the wound in the capsule may be seen: if through the iris the wound may be so small in the latter that the first evidence thereof is the opacity of the lens, following hours, days, weeks, or months later. If the wound of the ocular coats be extensive there will likely be prolapse of the iris, and the lens may be even partially or completely extruded from the eye. If the lens capsule be greatly torn and the lenticular substance broken up pieces of the lens may be seen in the anterior chamber.

If the wound in the capsule be very small, as from a needle, none of the lens substance comes out and on first observation we note but a grayish spot on the capsule, with perhaps the line of penetration showing on oblique illumination as a grayish canal in the body of

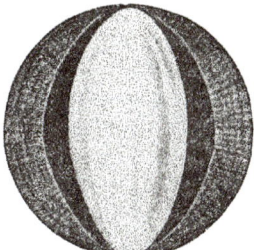

Veasey's Case of Traumatic Anterior Total Luxation and Version of the Lens.

the lens and proceeding from the latter in more or less radiating lines of opacity.

Linear wounds are caused by such instruments and objects as knives and glass splinters; contused and lacerated wounds by more blunt objects, as thorns, forks and perforating foreign bodies, etc.

In fresh cases the wound canal of perforating foreign bodies may be made out, and in many instances the resistance of the lens substance is sufficient to stop their passage so that they may be retained anterior to the posterior capsule of the lens.

The pupil does not respond readily to atropin, as the iris is often hyperemic, and the wounded iris adheres to the capsule of the lens. The tension is lowered so long as the wound of the ocular envelope is open, then as the lens swells it becomes increased, the tumefaction of the lens perhaps becoming so great as to occlude the angle of the anterior chamber, and the aqueous so heavy from lenticular débris that glaucoma arises.

In small wounds the process of tumefaction and opacification may

be watched from hour to hour, until in a few hours to days the whole
lens becomes opaque. As early as a few hours after injury the lens
substance is found cloudy in the region of the capsular wound. Some
swollen lens fibers protrude through, projecting in the form of gray
floccules into the anterior chamber until in some cases the entire
chamber is found filled with lenticular débris. As a rule these prolapsed masses dissolve in the aqueous, are absorbed and new floccules
keep protruding through the wound. At the same time the opacity
proceeds into the lens substance so that in a few days the whole
lens is opaque. In favorable cases the lens goes on to absorption, but
in most instances the absorption comes to a stop from healing and
closure of the capsular wound. Then opaque portions of the lens
remain in the capsule and discission is required to obtain a clear
pupil and vision.

Lenticular absorption varies from completeness in children from six
weeks, or so, to but partial absorption of the cortex in adults of over
forty years; the nucleus in adults not absorbing but remaining as an
obstacle to vision as a shriveled cataract. The anterior capsule does
not absorb. There is great tendency to closure and healing by proliferation of the epithelium if the wound edges are close together.
When not, the cut edges of the capsule retract and curl over, as they
do after cataract extraction.

The posterior capsule and the hyaloid membrane likewise have a
strong tendency to regeneration, so that wounds of these membranes
tend to close and heal quickly. Thus it is that the vitreous is held in
place and even forced back after free posterior discission. When
either or both anterior and posterior capsules remain, unless proliferation occurs, they are sufficiently transparent to offer but little obstacle
to vision after the lens body is absorbed.

The opacity may be mainly capsular and partial and exist in any
part of this membrane. If the cortex be involved the opacity may first
radiate from the nucleus in a star-shaped form.

After most of the lens nucleus and cortex has been absorbed or
removed, as after cataract extraction, the edges of the capsule curl
over, imprisoning some lenticular substance which may not become
entirely absorbed, but as it is locked up behind the iris out of the pupil,
offers no obstacle to a clear pupil and vision.

Complications of traumatic cataract. The irritation of the injury,
especially of the lens and iris, causes hyperemia and may lead to
iritis. The course of traumatic cataract is unfavorable if inflammation or tension occurs. The inflammation is probably always due to
some form of infection, although in some cases it is regarded as a

direct result of the mechanical injury, especially of the uveal tract. Slight inflammation of the iris may occur as the result of pressure or traction from the swelling of the traumatic cataract. This leads to proliferation of the capsule (cataracta accreta), or posterior synechia, seclusion and occlusion of the pupil, which render the relief of sight by operation more difficult. Other cases go on to loss of vision from irido-cyclitis, or of the globe from panophthalmitis.

As in the case of other wounds, the character of the injury to the lens should be ascertained; its length, width and depth; whether punctured, linear, bow- or sickle-shaped, lacerated, etc.; the direction from which it came and the character of the foreign body or object producing the injury; whether or not a foreign body may be retained in the globe; the wound of entrance to the eye, etc., all of which have a bearing upon the injury, its prognosis and treatment.

After some time has elapsed the wound of entrance through the cornea, and that in the lens capsule, may have so healed that they cannot be recognized, or are seen only on the closest examination. Such may not be recognized when in the sclera. If the wound be in the lens capsule behind the iris, the diagnosis is only made after opacification has proceeded so that it is seen in the pupil, the enlargement of which by atropin helps the diagnosis.

Traumatic iritis is signalized by discolored iris, slow dilatation of the pupil, presence of synechia, cyclitis, minus tension, as a rule, and precipitation on Descemet's membrane; irido-cyclitis, from plastic exudates in the pupil and vitreous. Secondary glaucoma manifests itself by increased tension, extreme pericorneal congestion, loss of vision, typical one-sided head pains, etc.

The *prognosis of traumatic cataract* as a general thing is unfavorable, as most cases are complicated by inflammation of the uvea. One must, however, strongly differentiate between simple, clean, uncomplicated traumatic cataract, as produced by small wounds, being practically a traumatic discission, and complicated cases in which at least one-half the eyes lose their vision, and a comparatively large percentage are lost through infection.

The prognosis is good in simple cases, particularly in children, where the lens substance may go on to absorption without operation, and a convex glass may later give good vision. It is likewise good where one or more discissions may remove the obstruction to vision. In old people, however, the lens does not absorb and even simple wounds of the lens are apt to result in irido-cyclitis and glaucoma, especially if the lens is well broken up and portions fall into the anterior chamber.

If inflammation develops the prognosis is bad, for the lens substance is excellent food for germs and the eye soon goes on to panophthalmitis.

The *treatment of traumatic cataract is both* medicinal and surgical.
In recent cases the first indication after antisepsis of the conjunctival
cul-de-sac is atropin to dilate the pupil and to paralyze the ciliary
muscle. One per cent. atropin solution should be dropped into the
eye 3 to 5 times a day, or even a 5 per cent. solution may be used at
first to insure dilatation of the pupil, care being taken not to poison
the patient, for this strong solution saturates the system, and may
cause a general intoxication.

In the case of non-penetrating wounds of the eyeball a bandage
should not be applied until mydriasis is obtained; but in open wounds
of the anterior chamber the mydriatic action of atropin is not secured
until the wound has closed. Atropin causes increase of intra-ocular
tension and thus the eye should be carefully watched and the tension
estimated daily during its use.

Dionin in 5 to 10 per cent. solutions, or the pure powder, is the
most effective local analgesic, and from its lymphagogue action leads
to absorption of the cataractous masses from within the lens capsule
and anterior chamber, and in some authoritative instances is known
to have caused clearing of a lenticular opacity. It gives an analgesia
of from 3 to 24 hours with each application. For the first few
instillations it produces great chemosis of the conjunctiva, and with
this much speedy absorption of intra-ocular exudates, but this reaction
is soon lost, so after a few applications but little lymphagogue action
is observed.

A protective bandage should always be put over the wounded eye,
and in large wounds over both, to protect from external infection,
from light and to keep it quiet. The 1:3000 sublimate salve and the
argyrol treatment are effective antiseptics.

Iced applications immediately after the injury for the first 24
hours, applied over compresses wet with 1:5000 sublimate solution,
reduce the immediate swelling of the tissues and the tendency to infection. The artificial leech may be applied on the temple for the same
purpose. If iritis or irido-cyclitis arises we endeavor to combat
this by hot compresses and mercurial subconjunctival injections. If
tension increases operative treatment must not be delayed beyond 24
hours.

Paracentesis of the anterior chamber may then be made, preferably
by a fine von Graefe knife—if there be no lens masses in the anterior
chamber. If, however, the anterior chamber becomes filled and tension

rises then linear extraction is indicated up to the age of 35 to 40 years, when nucleus formation begins, and then regular flap extraction may be preferable.

Operative discission. The danger of prolapse of the vitreous must ever be borne in mind on account of accompanying rupture of the suspensory ligament. Discission of the capsule should be small, to prevent escape of a large quantity of lens substance into the anterior chamber causing the development of glaucoma. The operation may have to be repeated in two weeks to two months, and perhaps several operations may be necessary. Although this method is slow, it is safe and sound. For details of the operation see p. 4022, Vol. VI. of this *Encyclopedia.* See, also, **Cataract, Traumatic.**

Foreign bodies in the lens. Flying missiles projected with suffi-cient force to pierce the cornea may also pass through the pupil or iris

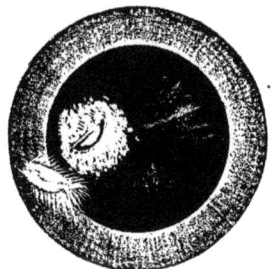

Steel Chip in the Lens Capsule.

Partial capsular cataract; scar in the cornea.

into the lens and be stopped therein by the anterior capsule, body of the lens or its posterior capsule. These are usually iron, steel or copper splinters and are frequently observed; more seldom wood, coal, glass and other particles; powder grains may lodge in the lens but shot pellets are rare.

According to the freedom of the body from infection, and its chemical qualities, foreign bodies may remain in the lens for a long time without causing reaction, and in a few instances produce but little opacity, but as a rule complete cataract ultimately occurs.

There are reported numerous instances where a foreign body has remained in the lens for a long time without causing full opacity. In these the wound of the lens capsule must have immediately coapted and healed, not allowing the aqueous to enter and cause swelling and disassociation of the lens fibers.

Most foreign bodies entering the lens do so through the pupil; those passing through the iris are noted elsewhere. The corneal wound will be noted in fresh cases, otherwise the cicatrix. After months or years the latter may with difficulty be observed. The aqueous has escaped and the anterior chamber is empty in recent cases, but if the corneal

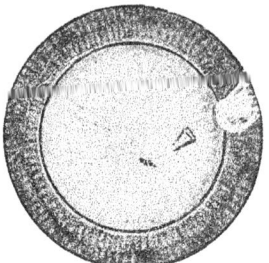

Steel Chip in the Lens.

Total lenticular opacity; scar in the cornea.

wound be small it soon closes and the chamber is restored. In these cases irritation is slight and iritis may not develop. The particle may usually be seen by the ophthalmoscope and diaphanoscope. Particles piercing the lens through the iris damage that structure and cause hyphema and iritis.

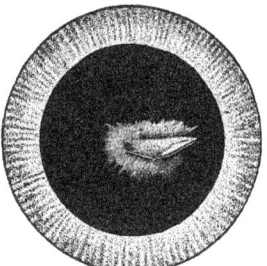

Steel Chip in the Lens.

Large foreign bodies break the lens up, cause immediate swelling of its fibers and falling of cortical masses into the anterior chamber. In this instance the foreign body may not be visible, except by the X-ray. If the entrance be by way of the ciliary body the damage to the eye is great and inflammation is apt to quickly occur with resultant danger of sympathetic ophthalmitis. The foreign body itself causes little irritation if enclosed in the lens and may be, as before noted, encapsulated and even cause but little opacity. Of course vision is immediately affected by the foreign body in the lens, becoming reduced to perception of light as the opacity progresses.

The main danger to the eye is from iritis and irido-cyclitis, aside from infection and chemical reaction of the intruding substance. From these sympathetic inflammation may occur.

Isolated infection of the capsular wound through pus cocci, carried in by the foreign body, may occur without the wound of entrance being infected.

The *diagnosis of foreign bodies in the lens* is made by the history; the wound of entrance through the cornea, or corneo-sclera; the lens opacity and resultant loss of vision; by seeing the object itself under direct or focal illumination assisted by magnification; by the ophthalmoscope and diaphanoscope. The parallactic displacement in ophthalmoscopy, the X-ray and the sideroscope give an idea of its localization; change in position of the foreign body in movement of the head and its movement under careful use of the magnet for diagnosis, and the sideroscope will explain its character if it is magnetizable.

Iron particles usually cause a change in the color of the lens, producing siderosis from rusting of the metal. Ocular inspection of the broken tool or material with which the patient was working may give some idea of the nature and size of the object.

When the lens masses have been extracted and no foreign body found, the Berlin blue reaction on the extracted material may show the presence of iron in solution, and that the foreign body has probably been left in the eye. Particles of iron in the interior of the eye may cause a central scotoma.

The *prognosis* is good if the foreign body be peripheral and become encapsulated without causing central opacity, which blinds the eye. This seldom occurs except in the case of particles of copper which, strange to say, are well tolerated by the lens, yet cases of steel and iron have been observed, as heretofore cited, which did not cause siderosis or progressive cataract. Siderosis from iron, however, usually occurs, and the opacity progresses.

If complicated by injury to the iris and ciliary body, the prognosis is not good, and at least one-third of these cases are lost from infection or irido-cyclitis.

Therapy. If a copper, stone, or other non-magnetizable body becomes imbedded in the lens and is well tolerated it may be allowed to remain until the lens has become opaque and then should be removed together with the cataract. But if the foreign body is of iron or steel it is better to extract it as soon as possible by the magnet, and then extract the cataract later.

If the steel splinter be loosely impacted in the lens capsule a peripheral corneal incision and the entrance of the tip of a Hirschberg or extended Victor magnet may be made into the anterior chamber upon withdrawal of which the chip will adhere and be removed thereby, or the Haab magnet may be used. If the wound of entrance be large it may be further enlarged, although where nature has already repaired the entrance wound by closure it is preferable to make a new clean incision, as this may usually be made nearer the foreign body than the wound of entrance. The magnetized lance may also be used with "safety, exactitude, and elegance." If the foreign body be more deeply impacted the large Haab, or the Victor, magnet may be used and the foreign body withdrawn with less danger of further rupture of the lenticular capsule.

If the lens be greatly swollen it may be removed, as previously described, at the same time; but as a rule the cataract is to be dealt with later. For fuller description of the magnet operation for non-magnetizable bodies see **Electromagnet**. Iridectomy usually has to be made in these cases, but should be avoided if the iris is not damaged and does not tend to prolapse.

Indirect traumatic cataract. Concussion cataract. Vossius' annular cataract. Besides cataract from wounds of the capsule, opacity of the lens may arise from actual contusion of its structure, both in the anterior and posterior lens capsule and in the lens structure itself.

Blows from projectiles, direct blows, falls and other injuries from blunt objects, more seldom spent shot or whip-lash injuries, may cause either rupture of the capsule, or failing in this, sufficient bruising of the lens structure as to disintegrate its cellular arrangement and thus produce opacity. These injuries are in some cases associated with penetration of the eyeball, while some show a brownish pigmentary deposit on the anterior surface of the lens.

In some cases the opacity may be attributed to direct crushing of the lens structure, where the lens comes in contact with the contusing object through a wound of the cornea or sclera; in others indentation of the ocular envelopes as a sort of forcible massage, and in others through disturbances of circulation.

In ring-shaped opacities (Vossius' annular opacity) on the anterior surface of the lens the consensus of opinion seems to be that these represent an impression of the pupillary margin on the lens. Some see the cause of them in the introversion of the cornea and the lens, others think that the iris is pressed against the lens by the suddenly increased pressure of the aqueous. See a full discussion of this lenticular opacity on p. 1769, Vol. III, of this *Encyclopedia*.

In indirect traumatic cataract the opacity may start in thirty-six hours, or not for days or weeks thereafter.

In direct bruising the opacity may commence in the posterior layers of the lens, the bruise starting with a tear in the equatorial region of the capsule; the neighboring zonule is also torn and this complication makes itself manifest by the appearance of a small portion of the vitreous in the pupil, which is often distorted and may be recognized under focal lateral illumination. The partial cataract forms a figure like a wreath at the posterior pole. The tear in the capsule usually enlarges and the lens masses then come forward into the anterior chamber.

In other cases the capsular tear closes and the opacity may remain stationary. Progressive loss of vision without pain or other symptoms, except that if the lens swells greatly or in complicated cases, is the only subjective symptom from contusions.

Rupture of the capsule is diagnosed from the solution of the continuity of the capsule, followed by opacity and swelling of the lens in an eyeball without external wound, seen by focal illumination, diaphanoscopy and ophthalmoscopy. Contusion cataract developing slowly after injury is apt to be a true contusion of the fibers. Complicated cases are attended by changes in the position of the lens, color of the iris and mobility of the pupil, and by lessened intraocular pressure.

Polar figures, either in the anterior or posterior cortex, are pathognomonic. Folds of the capsule may be seen. Equatorial capsule tears are apt to be connected with rupture of the zonule.

The *prognosis of indirect cataract* is apt to be better than in direct traumatic cataract; the opacity may progress to a certain extent and then remain stationary, as the broken capsule may close. Infection is excluded and if the lens does not swell greatly glaucoma is not apt to arise. Only complicated cases where the iris, ciliary body, choroid and retina are likewise affected by the injury, are apt to lose vision so completely that an operation cannot restore it, at least in part.

Therapy. Atropin to dilate the pupil and rest the accommodation is to be ordered in all cases. Dionin may be used for its lymphagogue absorbent action. If complicated, iced compresses at first, followed by hot compresses, may be used. Cataract discission, linear and flap extraction, after full opacity of the lens, are the operative procedures.

Cataract due to thermal and light injuries is discussed under

Electric ophthalmia; Cataract, Bottle finisher's; Dazzling; Cataract, Electric; Glass-blowers' cataract and similar captions. It may be added here that there is an etiologic connection between cataract formation and occupations entailing exposure to intense heat, as well as residence in hot climates. Of 30 men employed as glass-blowers, but 5 had reached the age of 40, and all them had developed glass-blowers' cataract. Cataract occurs in India at an average age of 40 years, while in western countries the average age is 66 years.

The frequency of cataract in glass blowers has been ascribed to the influence of extreme heat; to the bright light; to concentration of the aqueous by the constant evaporation on the surface of the cornea and the intense sweating; to changes of the aqueous in consequence of

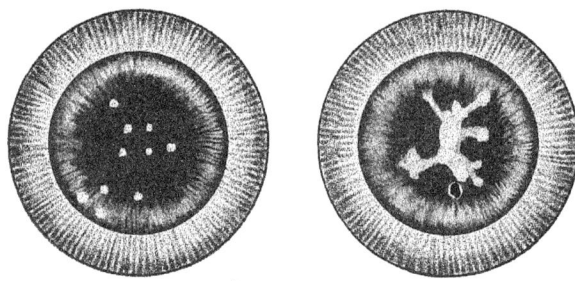

Electric Cataract.

congestion in the vortex veins, produced by the act of blowing. The latter view is not sustained by the fact that the glass-blowers' cataract is always unilateral and that nothing similar has been observed in trombone players.

Traumatic dislocation of the lens. Injury to the zonule of Zinn. Although this subject is also considered under the rubric, **Lens, Dislocation of the,** yet some special observations may be made here.

Wounds of the zonule are direct or indirect. Direct injuries are caused by the passing of a foreign body or the direct effect of a piercing or cutting instrument at the time of the accident. The foreign body may pass through the eye or remain therein. Direct wounds of the zonule are complicated by wounds of the cornea, sclerocornea and ciliary body through which the trauma is first applied. Through the tear in the suspensory ligament vitreous escapes into the anterior chamber and perhaps also through the external wound. There is an immediate effect upon the lens, for the tension of the zonule at this place of injury is lost and the lens at the site of injury regains its elasticity, contracts, and causes a lenticular astigmatism in the meridian. Correction by cylindric glasses cannot be made, for the refraction is only changed in a portion of the meridian, corresponding to the tear in the capsule, the other parts of the lens remaining normal. As a rule opacities of the vitreous or lens and other intraocular changes appear, having an unfavorable effect upon vision. Foreign bodies may remain in this location, but usually pass through; small ones without injury to the lens itself. The tear in the zonule heals, but the tension of the ligament is never so good, so some defect in vision remains. Such is seen after the Haab method of pulling a foreign body around the edge of the lens from the vitreous by magnetic attraction.

In a few cases the opening in the zonule may be visible.

Relaxation of the zonule. Myopia has been reported after contusion of the globe without other apparent injury. This has been referred to by many authors as due to a slackening of the zonular fibers.

Fuchs states that such a relaxation may take place from simple elongation and loosening, or from rupture or complete destruction, and that changes of this sort may affect either single portions or the entire circumference of the zonule.

Partial laceration of the zonule without displacement of the lens results if the zonule be completely torn. The tension of the ciliary muscle is then taken off and the lens becomes thicker antero-posteriorly and its circumference lessened, thus increasing the refraction, bringing in the far point to meet the near point, so only one focus is possible and myopia is produced. If only partially lacerated the tension is removed at the injured meridian and less astigmatism results.

The diagnosis may be made by tremor of the iris and of the lens on movement of the head, and by the subjective testing of the accommodation and refraction. The diagnosis is certain when the lens changes in position or when from an iridectomy the defect is actually visible. The lens may remain in position for a long time until some movement of the body, such as occurs from shivering, sneezing or a fall or blow, puts it out of position, causing dislocation or lens luxation.

Partial laceration of the zonule with subluxation of the lens, or subluxation, may consist in the lens being tilted a little so that one edge is somewhat forward, the opposite edge backward *(dislocatio ad axem)*; or it may be moved partially out of the fossa patellaris to the side where the ligament still holds *(dislocatio ad laterem)*.

This condition is recognized from the unequal depth of the anterior chamber, it being deeper than normal in one side and shallower in the opposite half. If the pupil be dilated, or if the displacement be marked even with the normal pupil, the edge of the lens will be seen by direct and focal illumination.

The portion of the pupil situated beyond the edge of the lens is a deep-black color, the lenticular portion shows dark-gray, the lens itself reflecting some light while the vitreous reflects so little that it appears black. By ophthalmoscopy or diaphanoscopy the edge of the lens appears dark, while the red of the fundus shows through its body and through the extra-lenticular point of the pupil. The part of the pupil not filled in by the lens is highly hyperopic (about 10 D. in emmetropia), while the lenticular part shows an astigmatic variance from the normal refraction. There is usually paralysis of accommodation and if the edge of the lens divides the pupil monocular double vision occurs. The lens may remain clear, but as a rule gets opaque, when the visual acuity is markedly lowered.

Subluxation generally goes into complete luxation. If the iris and vitreous remain normal the lens is apt to keep its position. Congenital disease and weakness, as myopia, fluid vitreous, etc., predispose to weakness of the zonula and dislocation of the lens. Glaucoma from pressure, interference in the iridic angle and the irido-cyclitis from injury to the ciliary body are the complications mostly to be found.

While tremulous iris and lens is not a positive sign yet this condition points strongly to laceration of the zonule. The movement of the lens is only to be directly seen when there is lenticular opacity; the pupil is usually enlarged from the trauma and hence these signs sometimes fail. If full mydriasis be produced, or when an iridectomy has been made, in some cases the torn zonular fibers can be seen.

Complete dislocation of the lens. If the zonule be completely torn the lens will come out of the patellar fossa and pass into the anterior chamber or into the vitreous. In partial luxations it remains attached to the suspensory ligament by a few strands of tissue.

Dislocation of the lens is usually caused directly by blows from stone-throwing, lumps of coal and large pieces of iron, falls and blows from blunt objects. The shrinking of a hypermature cataract may cause stretching of the zonule, with atrophy, and thus give rise to spontaneous dislocation; or a slight traumatism, or even sneezing, bending over, etc., might dislocate the cataract and restore the vision. Indirectly the lesion happens from severe shaking of the body, as from a fall upon the buttocks or a severe blow upon the head. Double-sided dislocation has been observed.

Foerster showed that a blow on the front of the eye pushes the aqueous humor with it, inverting the iris so that the zonule is pressed upon and burst. Another reason must be shown in lateral blows and

in severe concussion of the body. When the limbus is impinged upon
the lens springs back and tears away from its support. In concussion
of the head or body the lens may tend to tear away from the force
of the blow, suspended as it is by the delicate and easily torn ligament of Zinn.

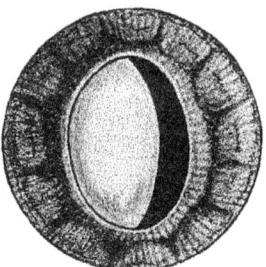

Partial Luxation of the Lens Laterally into the Vitreous.

The ligament is more fragile and the lens has less support in anomalous and diseased eyes, such as in high grades of myopia, staphyloma
of the cornea, fluid vitreous and congenital lenticular anomalies.

In *complete anterior luxation* the lens shows as a round, convex,
usually transparent body nearly filling the anterior chamber in front

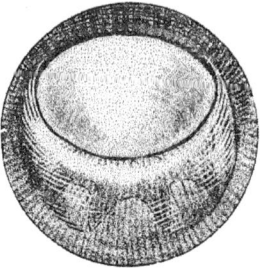

Partial Luxation of the Lens Forward and Upward into the Anterior Chamber.

of the iris. If the lens be clear the pupil may be seen through and
behind it. The rim of the lens appears like a curved line of golden
luster so that it looks like a great drop of oil in the anterior chamber.
The iris is pressed backwards by the posterior surface of the lens
which is more convex than when it is in the natural position, as it is
no longer kept flat by the tension of the zonule. The anterior chamber is deeper, especially below. The effect of gravity keeps the center

of the lens a little below the center of the pupil and the iris shows above its upper rim, but not below. If the patient lie on one side the lens may gravitate to that side, but upon regaining the erect posture again seeks the former position.

Every dislocation of the lens entails considerable disturbance of vision. If completely forwards the eye will become myopic from the

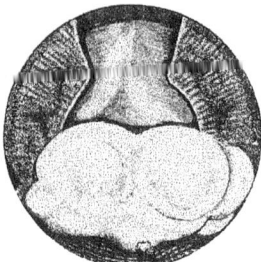

Complete Luxation of Lens Substance into the Anterior Chamber. Iridectomy.

increased refraction; if somewhat to one side there will also be astigmia, and if a portion of the pupil be unfilled by the lens diplopia will result. On examining with the ophthalmoscope when the visual line of the observer passes through the rim of the lens, thus looking through the stronger refracting lens and the unfilled area of pupil, the fundus details will be seen doubled.

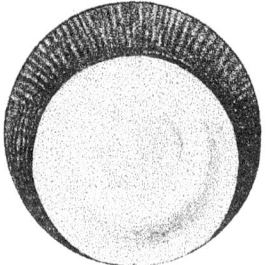

Complete Luxation of the Clear Lens in Capsule into the Anterior Chamber.

Irritation caused by the prolapsed lens on the iris produces spasm of the sphincter, the pupil contracts and the return of the lens to the posterior chamber is prevented. It may even happen that on account of this spasm the lens is held tight at the moment of passing through the pupil. It is then jammed in the pupil and irritation is at once set up. There are also cases where the lens may slip back and forth through the pupil (wandering lens).

The rule is that a lens luxated into the anterior châmber generally stays there, on account of the inflammation which it excites, becoming attached to the cornea and iris by exudates. As a rule such eyes become blind from glaucoma with formation of staphyloma of the sclera, or from irido-cyclitis. Sympathetic inflammation in the other eye has also been reported.

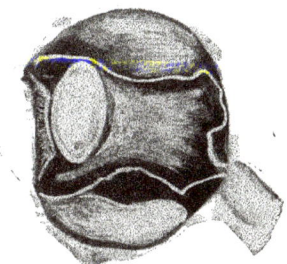

Chronic Irido-cyclitis following Dislocation of the Lens into the Vitreous from a Blow on the Eye.

Incomplete anterior luxation. If a cramp of the sphincter retains the lens part way in the passage a more or less transparent rounded object remains in the pupil, the edge of the lens partly in the anterior chamber, partly in the posterior or indenting the vitreous. If increase of tension and inflammation arise there is opacity of the cornea and

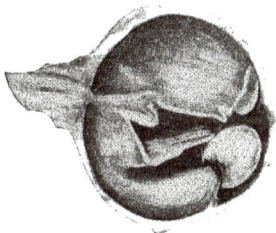

Detachment of the Retina, Inversion of the Iris, Dislocation of the Lens into the Anterior Chamber after Blunt Injury.

exudation into the anterior chamber. In a few cases the condition may be tolerated for a long time, but as a rule inflammation occurs.

. The lens may turn a somersault so that its posterior surface looks forwards. In the numerous other cases of partial dislocation, cataract has followed, which has ordinarily been dealt with by discission, as most of these are juvenile.

Posterior luxation of the lens into the vitreous is the commonest form of lens luxation. The anterior chamber is deep because of the recession of the iris, which is tremulous. The pupil is a pure black and the lenticular reflections of the anterior and posterior capsule are not elicited. If the lens be opaque it may sometimes be seen upon direct or focal illumination, but as a rule the ophthalmoscope is required to see it. It is usually in the lower part of the fundus, attached to some spot by masses of exudation, or it floats freely about in the vitreous *(cataracta natans)* and is seen to move as the head is moved. The lens becomes speedily opaque, and, in a few cases of young persons where the capsule has been torn, is absorbed.

Glaucoma and cyclitis, with the termination in atrophia bulbi, may here occur even after months or years of quiet, as was seen in many instances of the old method of cataract operation by depression of the lens into the vitreous.

Luxation of the lens into the vitreous is better tolerated than the forward form of dislocation.

In some cases a lens may pass back and forth through the pupil, even voluntarily, without causing irritation. The patient can bring the lens forward into the anterior chamber by bending his head and shaking it, while to carry it behind the iris he lies on his back. In such cases the lens is always small and thus passes through the pupil without difficulty. In some instances these movable lenses are still attached to the zonule, which is then greatly elongated.

Fuchs advises us, in the extraction of such lenses, to first bring them in position by an appropriate maneuver, then to imprison them behind the iris before making the corneal incision.

Cases where the lens shows capacity for making such extraordinary excursions are rare. Once the lens is luxated it tends to remain in the new location.

Complications of lens luxation. At the same time as the lens dislocation, mydriasis traumatica, dialysis, tears and inversion of the iris, rupture of the choroid, vitreous and retinal bleeding and dislocation, but seldom lens capsule laceration, may occur.

Berger saw retinal detachment with dislocation of the lens in a 35-year-old needle-woman who 19 years before had been hit in the eye with a fork. A cataractous lens was seen in the fundus, and also a retinal detachment.

The *diagnosis* of lens luxation is made by the deep anterior chamber, tremulous iris, viewing of the whole or the edge of the lens, which, in the anterior chamber, looks like a large drop of oil if clear, or a cataract if opaque. It is readily seen in the vitreous if the latter is

clear and the lens is opaque. The absence of the intraocular reflections from the anterior and posterior capsule of the lens, and the
hyperopia of about 10 D., will show the aphakia. In other cases opacities of the media and the blindness will obscure the diagnosis. Contact
of the lens with the cornea causes corneal opacity and perhaps
ulceration.

The *prognosis* is doubtful, but practically all cases of anterior dislocation lead to inflammation and blindness if the lens be not extracted.
The lens in the vitreous tends to get smaller or to be encapsulated; the
sight may be restored by the dislocation of the cataractous lens, but as
a rule after a few years the eye is lost by chronic irido-cyclitis.

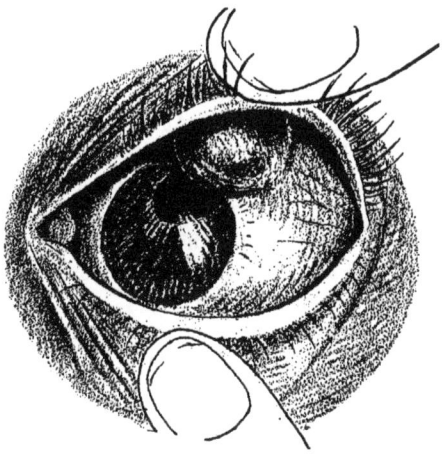

Dislocation of the Lens under the Conjunctiva through Wound of the Cornco-
scleral Margin, with Prolapse of the Iris.

Therapy. All injuries causing rupture of the zonula of Zinn, producing partial or complete displacement of the lens from the fossa
patellaris, are attended with commotio bulbi. They are generally complicated, particularly with rupture of the iris, ciliary body, vitreous
and hyphemia; in fact, they are seldom recognized until the case has
been under observation sufficiently long to permit of the exudated
blood being resorbed, therefore the treatment is usually that of a
non-penetrating injury to the eye; rest in bed, atropin to dilate the
pupil and get the edge of the iris out of harm's way before the setting
up of an iritis; cold compresses to hinder bleeding and, after 48 hours,
hot compresses to secure resorption of the blood clot and to relieve
pain; and the use of eserin and dionin. If hypertension occurs, the
atropin must be discontinued and paracentesis of the cornea may be

made to let out the blood clot. If the lens be partially luxated and remain clear, optical treatment to neutralize the resultant astigmia is needed. If it becomes cataractous, this may be dealt with by diseission or extraction, depending upon the age of the patient. If at the same time there is rupture of the capsule, complete or partial absorption may spontaneously occur; if the lens swells the pupils should be kept widely dilated by atropin and the lens extracted when its swelling causes reaction. If the lens be dislocated into the anterior chamber, it should, as a rule, be extracted, although when seen early an effort may be made to reduce it by gentle pressure or by massage of the cornea either with or without scleral incision behind the ciliary body to diminish the tension. Extraction of the lens dislocated into the anterior chamber is attended at times with much difficulty, as, on opening the cornea, it may slip back into the posterior chamber, hence, it should be transfixed by a knife-needle before the incision and supported thereby, or the bident of Agnew may be used to transfix it after the incision. The writer usually operates with a downward section, the patient being in a sitting position, or have allowed the head of the patient to hang over the edge of the table for the upward incision in order to facilitate the dropping out of the displaced lens.

The dressings and *after-treatment* of removal of dislocated lens are similar to ordinary cataract extraction.

Where the lens is dislocated under the conjunctiva, it may be left to disintegrate and absorb, but as a rule it is preferable to remove the foreign body by incision and extraction.

If the lens be in the vitreous chamber, it should not be disturbed unless it gives rise to irritation, when an attempt should be made to extract it through a scleral incision, but this may prove futile, especially with a freely movable or a floating lens. If inflammation takes place, it is advisable to enucleate the eyeball on account of possible sympathetic inflammation of the other eye.

It is a difficult operation to extract a dislocated lens, for the zonule is ruptured and allows the vitreous to present and some is always lost. Even complicated cases may, however, be dealt with successfully in skilled hands.

INJURIES OF THE CILIARY BODY.

Wounds of the ciliary body have already been discussed in connection with traumatisms of the sclerocorneal junction.

Foreign bodies in the ciliary body usually lodge there after explosions, as of gun-caps. Less often do we find chips of iron, glass, stone, wood or shot pellets, although the last furnish a large proportion of foreign bodies which penetrate and pass through the ciliary body into the interior of the eye. These may reach the ciliary body either directly through the sclera, or after penetrating the sclera or cornea at another point may traverse the ocular contents until the ciliary body is reached, wherein they may lodge. Frequently foreign bodies entering the eye and lodging first in the vitreous or retina may wander, later on, to the ciliary body and become impacted therein, to be found upon enucleation and section.

Gradle found spirillæ in the ciliary body in five cases of perforating injuries; whereas six cases, examined with the same methods, were negative. He is far from asserting that the spirillæ have any significance for irido-cyclitis, or even sympathetic ophthalmia, as long as experiments on animals have not yielded positive results, but wishes to call attention to these interesting findings.

The most intense irritation, pain, tearing and dread of light are produced by a foreign body in the ciliary body, through its extreme sensitiveness from the ciliary nerves and the constant contraction of the muscles.

A sector of the limbus corresponding to the site of the intruder may be injected and especially tender to the touch. Unless the foreign body is removed, and often even then, cyclitis begins and extends to the iris, the disease going on to irido-cyclitis and atrophia bulbi. After the acute symptoms subside the foreign body becomes encapsulated, and from time to time new attacks with subsidence of inflammation occur.

In a few cases, most often those where copper chips have been retained, the chemical reaction is intense, and spontaneous extrusion of the intruder follows, either through the port of entry, or another opening, generally downwards, to the corneal limbus. A foreign body does not stay long in this location without giving trouble.

The *diagnosis* of a foreign body in the ciliary body may only be positively made when it can be seen or felt by the probe. It may even extend out of the scleral wound or be seen upon atropinization, through the enlarged pupil, as a grayish object. Certainly diaphanoscopy or the X-ray helps if the object be large enough to cast a shadow; but exact localization cannot be made by either, and the foreign body may be in the vitreous clear of the ciliary body when the X-ray plates seem to show it there. The ciliary region may be tender and in some cases abscesses have been caused and have pointed at this location. The *prognosis* is generally most unfavorable, even when speedy extraction of the foreign body is made, especially if the eye does not soon become quiet. In previous years most such eyes were immediately enucleated by the conscientious surgeon. Now perhaps we are getting ultra-conservative, and are saving many eyes for the couse-quences of sympathetic disease.

When the foreign body can be seen the wound may be opened and the unwelcome visitor removed by forceps; in magnetizable cases aided by the magnet. If the foreign body cannot be removed the eye should be immediately enucleated, as dilatory and deficient methods lend a false security and may lead the patient to blindness of both eyes

Isolated traumatic cyclitis seldom occurs, as the ciliary body is part of the uvea and with it the iris and choroid are usually affected. Praun describes the disease as accompanied by severe pain, lachrymation, much photophobia, pericorneal injection, hyperemia of the iris without synechia, stationary contracted pupil, spasm of accommodation, exudate in the vitreous and sometimes into the aqueous. So long as the inflammation remains confined to the ciliary body, not proceeding anterior to the iris or back into the choroid, it may get well in a few weeks, but often it proceeds to irido-cyclitis with resultant atrophia bulbi.

Accommodation cramp and paralysis from blows. When associated with mydriasis there is usually paralysis of accommodation; when with miosis, spasm. Perhaps cases of brief duration may be accompanied by commotio retinæ, and those of longer duration by bleeding into the ciliary muscle or macular rupture. Of special interest is the accompanying accommodative myopia.

Rupture of the ciliary body. In severe cases of scleral rupture the ciliary body is usually implicated. There may be even pronounced laceration of the ciliary body at its attachment, or entire separation from the sclera. Fuchs remarks that this sort of injury is found quite often in anatomical specimens, while clinically it cannot be diagnosticated, because we cannot see the ciliary body in the living eye. By laceration of this sort the anterior chamber is placed in direct communication with the space between the sclera on one hand, and the ciliary body and choroid on the other (peri-choroidal space). It thus becomes possible for the aqueous to enter this space and detach the choroid from the sclera.

See, also, p. 3625, Vol. V, of this *Encyclopedia;* as well as **Cyclitis.**

INJURIES OF THE CHOROID.

Wounds of the choroid occur from all the causes of perforating traumatisms of the eyeball, especially from without, as those which pass through the sclera, such as cuts and foreign bodies. Penetrating wounds of the posterior portion of the eyeball involve the choroid; they are likewise accompanied by injuries to the retina and vitreous. If clean, they heal by cicatricial tissue, if septic, inflammatory changes result, producing irido-choroiditis and panophthalmitis.

Small foreign bodies may also pass through the vitreous and injure the fundus, passing through the retina to the choroid and lodging against the sclera. Double penetration may likewise occur, particularly in case of shot wounds, and occasionally chips of metal may be projected with such great force as to pass entirely through the globe. Sewing-needle, hatpin, and other piercing wounds of the sclera may pass into the interior of the globe by way of the choroid and retina, causing circumscribed hemorrhage into the vitreous at the point of passage. In larger wounds the hemorrhage into the vitreous is severe and leads to formation of membranous opacities with great loss of vision. Larger wounds of the choroid are so intimately connected with those of the sclera that they have already been discussed with the latter.

If the hemorrhage occurs under the choroid, detachment of this membrane results. If the cut in the sclera heals without inflammation, an atrophic spot remains in the choroid. In other cases retinal detachment ultimately results from cicatricial contraction, or the eye may go on to irido-cyclitis plastica and atrophy, or, if infected, to chorioretinitis suppurativa, formation of abscess in the vitreous and panophthalmitis.

Foreign bodies in the choroid. It is possible for very small copper or iron particles to become imbedded between the retina and sclera in the choroid. There it must have first penetrated the eye, passing through the vitreous and becoming imbedded in the posterior coats. The vitreous is readily penetrated, the choroid also, but the sclera offers great resistance and stops the flight of the particle, and it thus remains on the sclera imbedded in the choroid and is seen through the retina, as it does not become encapsulated in this location for a considerable period of time.

But foreign bodies within the posterior part of the globe, in the vitreous and retina, usually cause acute inflammation which leads to plastic shrinking of the bulb. A foreign body near the sensitive ciliary body is very dangerous.

The *diagnosis* is made when the foreign body is seen under and through the retina.

The *prognosis* is that of retained foreign bodies, generally poor unless speedily removed.

The *treatment* is that of intraocular foreign bodies generally; removal or enucleation.

Prolapse of the choroid and ciliary body should be replaced within the scleral capsule and retained by scleral and conjunctival sutures if these structures be not penetrated, otherwise the protrusion should be snipped away by the scissors placed flat to the globe and the wound toilet be completed before suturing.

Hemorrhage from the choroid may occur from the ruptured choroidal vessels following contusions of the eyeball.

In slight cases the hemorrhage may be circumscribed and appear in spots under the retina. In severe forms the blood does not remain in the parenchyma of the choroid but spreads between it and the sclera, causing detachment of the choroid, or between that membrane and the retina, causing retinal detachment. If the latter be also perforated the blood oozes into the vitreous. The blood may pass by way of a ruptured zonule into the anterior chamber.

Diagnosis is made by the ophthalmoscope. Irregular blotches of blood are seen under the retina. At times these may be rounded and bluish-red; their centers dark-red; their edges blurred. The retinal vessels pass undisturbed over these hemorrhages. When the retina is torn its edges appear apart and rolled up as whitish-gray membrane.

If the hemorrhage is not accompanied by other damage it may be absorbed after a month or more, leaving a whitish plaque which later becomes replaced by pigment, the function being little altered. If, however, the hemorrhage causes dislocation of the choroid or retina, or the retina be involved in the trauma through cicatricial shrinking, the function of vision is lost.

Therapy. Rest. Ergot and calcium chloride internally, followed by iodides; local treatment by galvanism and high frequency electric currents induce resorption.

Detachment of the choroid from hemorrhage under it is rare in eyes that have not been opened. It is often seen in scleral rupture, has occurred after cataract, iridectomy, and staphyloma operations, and is often found in anatomic examination of atrophic eyes.

The accident is due to rupture of a large vessel of the choroid near the posterior pole, most likely at the venæ vorticosæ. After operations it is due to the sudden relief of intra-ocular tension.

Immediate loss of vision follows bleeding under the choroid. If acute glaucoma, with diffuse opacity or bleeding into the media, does not prevent examination by the ophthalmoscope, then may be seen a reddish-brown or yellowish prominence in the vitreous behind the retina. The blood vessels of the choroid may be seen over the surface of the swelling. Retinal opacity and hemorrhage often obscure the view. This is direct from the retina, and from migration of blood from the choroid.

If the blood vessels of the choroid be seen by ophthalmoscopic examination over the reddish tumor a diagnosis may be made. Even here there is a distinction to be made between a hematoma and sarcoma. The history should help, as the loss of sight is sudden from bleeding, and slow from a true tumor. The hemorrhagic swelling may change in position, as the head is carried to one side, while a true tumor remains in the same place.

The *prognosis* is bad as regards sight, and even as to retention of the globe, for acute glaucoma sets in and in most cases these eyes have

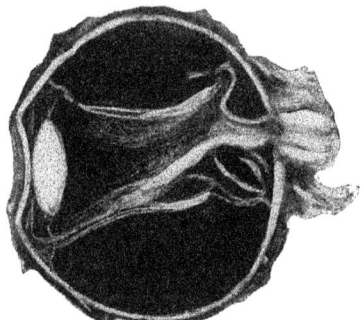

Detachment of the Choroid and Retina from Subchoroidal Hemorrhage.

to be enucleated. In cases where the globe has been opened, as after cataract, the bleeding may be extremely severe.

Therapy. Iced compresses, ergot, calcium chloride, and, when acute glaucoma with great pain sets in, enucleation. See, also, Choroid, **Detachment of the.**

Indirect rupture of the choroid. While ruptures of the choroid are looked at even now with some curiosity by ophthalmologists, yet since they were first pointed out by von Graefe, in 1854, there have been many cases reported.

Rupture of the choroid is caused by all contusions which affect the bulb in its surroundings, the most common of which are corks flying out of bottles, the impact of shot or blunt pieces of wood and iron, whiplash and pencil injuries, and industrial accidents. In a few cases the choroidal rupture may come, as noted, from an injury distant from the eye.

One choroidal rupture is found in about every thousand patients. In 289 cases 70 per cent. were single ruptures, some 16 per cent. double; while a radial rupture was found in some 10 per cent. Those combined with arc-like rupture happened only in 7 per cent. of the cases, that is, once in 15,000 eye patients.

Parsons says: "The early stages of rupture of the choroid have not been examined microscopically. In indirect wounds caused experimentally or by foreign bodies, other structures are invariably injured in addition. In experimental wounds in rabbits Tepljaschin found the changes to be essentially inflammatory and reparative. The tissues were separated by serous exudate and infiltrated by wandering cells, whilst karyokinetic figures formed a distinct feature in vertical sections. They were principally 'internal to the chorio-capillaris,' in the layer described as the musculus choriodæ in rabbits by Hällsten and Tigerstedt. Karyokinetic figures were also seen in the cells of the muscular layer of the walls of the large choroidal vessels. He found similar results in experimental injuries on monkeys, and it is to be noted that the choroid affords the chief means of repair in these cases, as might be expected from its highly vasular nature."

Temporal ruptures occur in 82 per cent., nasal ruptures in 14 per cent., horizontal ruptures in 4 per cent. of the reported cases. The tear is usually found in the posterior pole of the eye, concentric with the optic nerve, between the optic disc and the macula, forming a half circle about the papilla. In a recent case the eye is often so swollen and photophobic, and the injury is so obscured by obstructions in the anterior chamber, vitreous, and bleeding into the retina, that it is difficult to see; but it may be observed as a yellowish streak with its edges covered by blood, mixed with pigment. Upon resorption of the blood and clearing of the media, as a rule the injury appears to be about ⅓ to ½ the width of the disc, and two or three times its length, sharp at its ends, with its concavity directed toward the optic nerve, forming a concentric defect of a yellowish-red color, later becoming white, which is caused by the sclera showing through its edges, and still later becoming pigmented. In the neighborhood of the tear, the retina shows streaks of blood and the swelling of its blood vessels is seen over the defect when the tear does not also extend through the retina; but as a rule the pigmented epithelium of the latter membrane is likewise torn. The bleeding is confined to the tear and its neighborhood, and in some cases is very slight, so that the vitreous and the anterior chamber show effusion of blood in few cases. The tension of the eyeball remains about the same unless the bleeding is severe, except in the case where there is a perforating wound of the eyeball with loss of vitreous, when the tension is lowered and much blood may be observed in the interior of the eye.

The defect is white when the lamina fascia remains unbroken and in connection with the sclera, and not bluish, which is the case when the sclera itself is uncovered in the line of the rupture.

Atypical conditions are mainly confined to the form of the tear, which may be even three or four times the width of the optic nerve and very much longer. Enormous ruptures occupying the entire posterior portion of the fundus have been described. In another case the end of the crescent was in the form of a fork and directed towards one side. In a 14-year-old patient, who had a stick of wood fly against the eye, it was noted that the region of the macula was occupied by the choroidal defect which had two processes from above and two downwards.

The position of the tear in perhaps one-tenth of the cases occurs inward from the papilla, while a number have been described which occurred radially from the papilla to the periphery; in a few the tear was horizontal, more seldom vertical.

Accompanying the rupture of the choroid may be other injuries, such as traumatic mydriasis, paralysis of accommodation, rupture of the iris and sphincter, irideremia, dialysis, aniridia, tearing of the zonula and capsule of the lens and luxation of the lens. In many cases bleeding into the macula occurs.

The secondary degenerative changes are due to cicatrization of the choroid, atrophy and degeneration of the retina, especially at the macula, leading to atrophy of the optic nerve.

Immediately after the occurrence of this accident there is traumatic mydriasis, loss of accommodation, etc., the loss of vision depending upon the opacity of the media. Commonly the pigment layer of the retina is involved in the rupture, and a loss of function is shown which goes hand in hand with the loss of the visual field. By streakiness, opacity, and bleeding in the neighborhood of the retina the sight is interfered with. In many cases peripheral defects of the visual field are found, ascribed to tearing of the nerve fibers in the optic nerve itself. The loss of vision is later due to interference with the nutrition of the retina, and particularly of the macula, from connective tissue forming in the choroid. These occur without the sight being complained of. The retina, however, especially the macula, is affected in the formation of scar tissue. If the retinal tissue is not affected the vision may return entirely.

The blood in the neighborhood of the injury is absorbed and the opacities in the media disappear; the hemorrhage due to the rupture is also resorbed, and pigment is deposited at the edges. The region of the rupture is now made clear, and blood stripes are found in the retina here and there, especially at the macula. The tear in the choroid commences to cicatrize and may be observed from time to time to grow smaller. Large tears very seldom come together, smaller ones more commonly, with or without the healing up of pigment, and then will be found choroidal changes and pigment deposits and atrophic spots.

If increase of vision occurs and the choroidal tears come entirely together, and the retina is not affected, which is only occasionally observed, sight may fully return, but as a rule the retina becomes atrophic from changes and the sight declines. Detachment of the retina and atrophy of the optic nerve may likewise follow.

The most common *complication* of choroidal rupture is contemporaneous tearing of the retina, which renders the prognosis of the injury very unfavorable. Rupture of the retina may likewise occur primarily from the contusion of the eye, and secondarily from blood effusion from the torn blood vessels of the choroid. The pigment layer of the retina is commonly affected with the choroidal injury, but not so often does the injury extend through the entire membrane.

A *restitutio ad integrum* is of course impossible in such unpromising cases. The retina degenerates and sight diminishes.

Diagnosis. One can see how rupture of the choroid may happen more commonly than is shown by clinical research. At first it is obscured by bleeding and opacity. Later, it is often overlooked, or the patients do not return for further treatment. One should observe these patients for a long time and examine them from week to week, but many indolent patients allow their eyes to become blind without the cause of it being ascertained. The ophthalmoscopic picture of a rupture of the choroid is so typical that it cannot well be mistaken for any other condition.

In a very few cases complete healing occurs with resultant good sight, but as a rule the vision deteriorates from secondary changes in the retina and optic nerve. In extraordinary eases the vision remains good.

Therapy. At first atropin should be ordered so that the ciliary muscle remains quiet, followed by strychnia in full doses by injection; then high frequency and high tension electric applications. The patient should be quiet for a long time. Leeching, sweating, and the dark-cure are without any particular benefit. Atropinization does no harm and keeps the eye quiet during the course of changes following the injury to the choroid.

Direct rupture of the choroid. The tear of a direct rupture is sit-

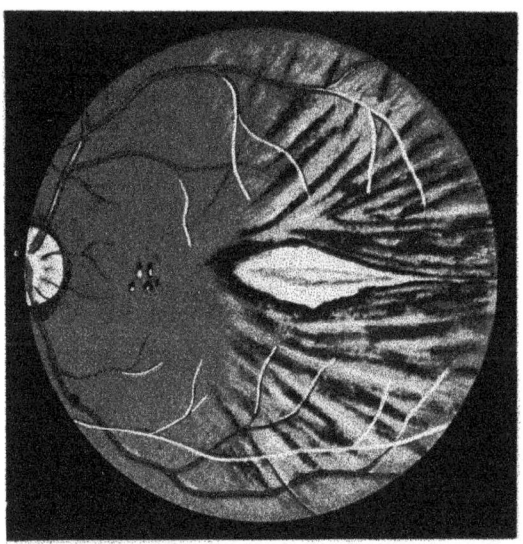

Instrumental Operative Wound Through the Capsule,
Resulting in Large Cicatrix of the Choroid and Retina,
atrophy of the optic nerve, retina, choroil and vessel
walls, pigmentary leposits in retina and striate retinal
changes.　(Würdemann.)

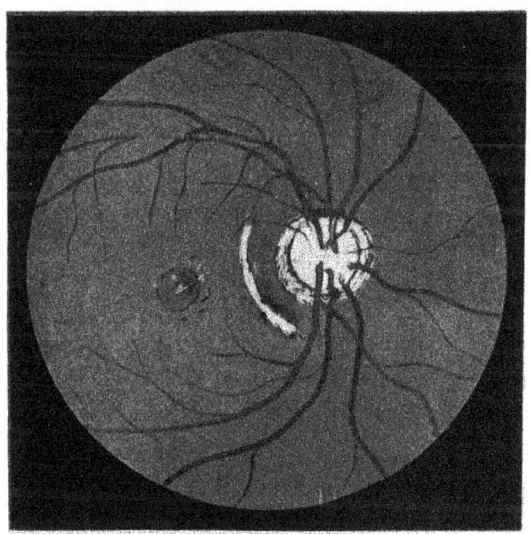

Rupture of the Choroil Two Months After Injury from
a Whip-lash.　(Würdemann.)

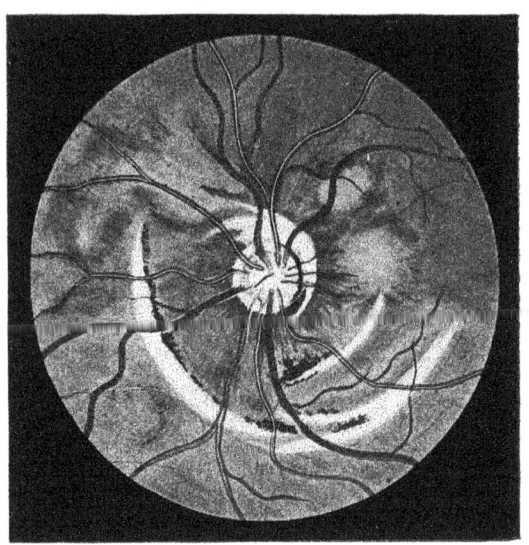

Old Multiple Ruptures of the Choroid.

Atrophy of optic nerve, atrophy and pigment degeneration of the retina, three months after injury from a cow-horn.

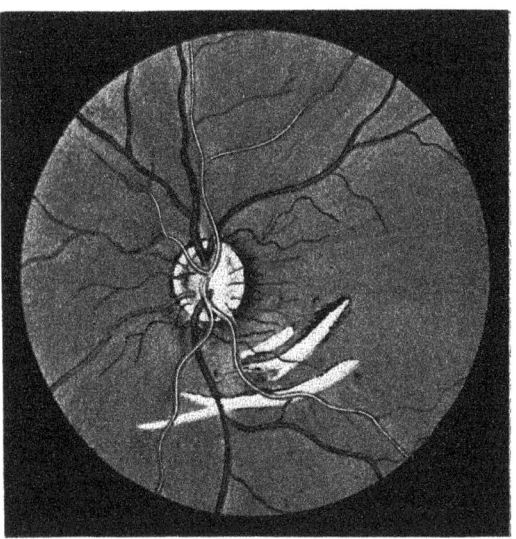

Recent Multiple Ruptures of the Choroid, One Month After Kick from a Horse on the Eyebrow. (Würdemann.)

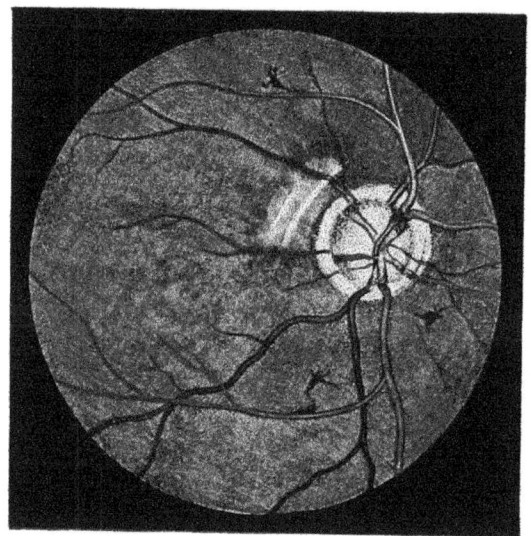

Recent Ruptures of the Choroid. Small Detachment
of the Retina. Two days after blow from a fist.
(Würdemann.)

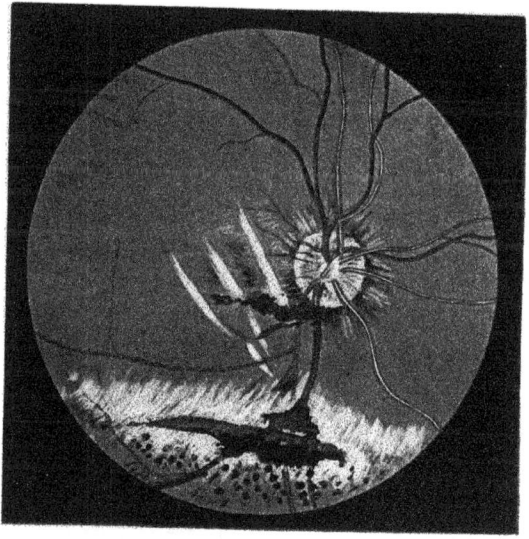

Recent Multiple Ruptures of the Choroid.

Recent vitreous hemorrhages, peculiar partial rupture
and detachment below with pigment migration. Two
weeks after a blow from whip-lash.

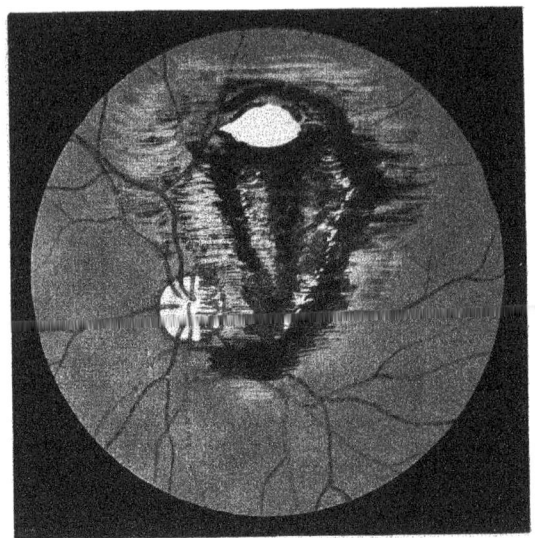

Point of Impact of a Foreign Body in the Fundus
with Resulting Blood Clot in the Vitreous. (Würdemann.)

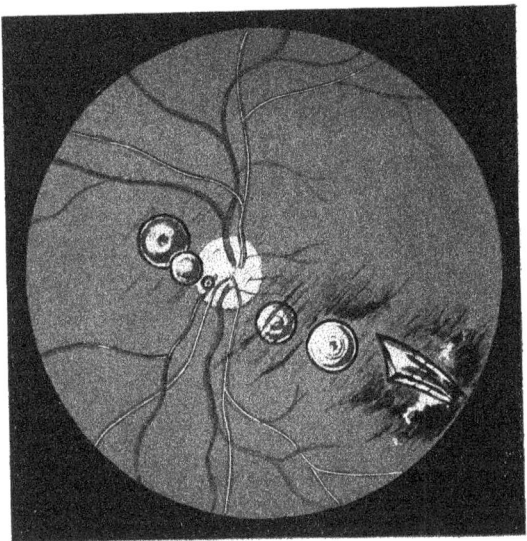

Glass Chip in the Vitreous with Air Bubbles in the
Course of the Wound through the Vitreous. (Würdemann.)

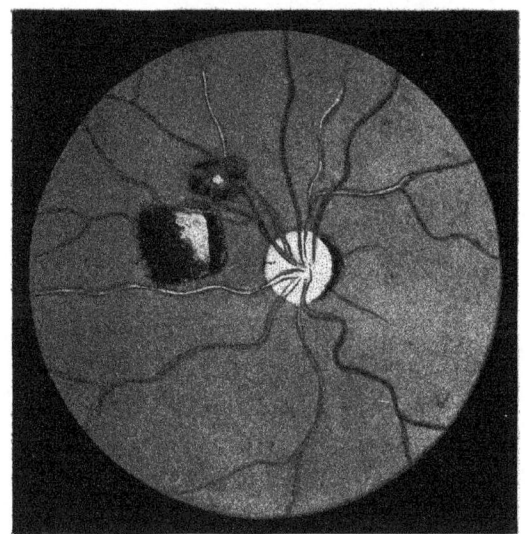

Steel Chip in the Vitreous. (Würdemann.)

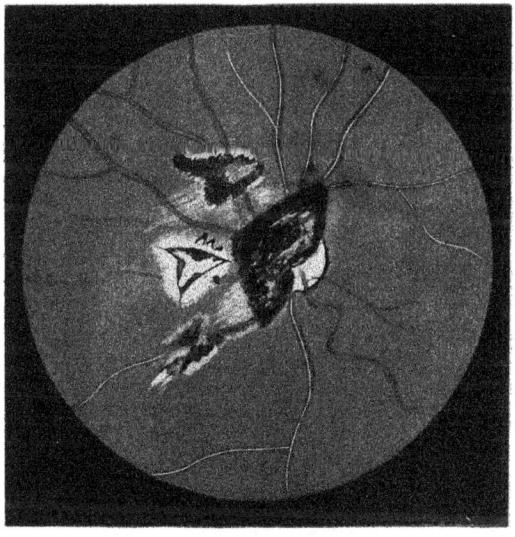

Double Perforation of Globe by Chip of Steel. Perforation to Nasal Side. (Würdemann.)

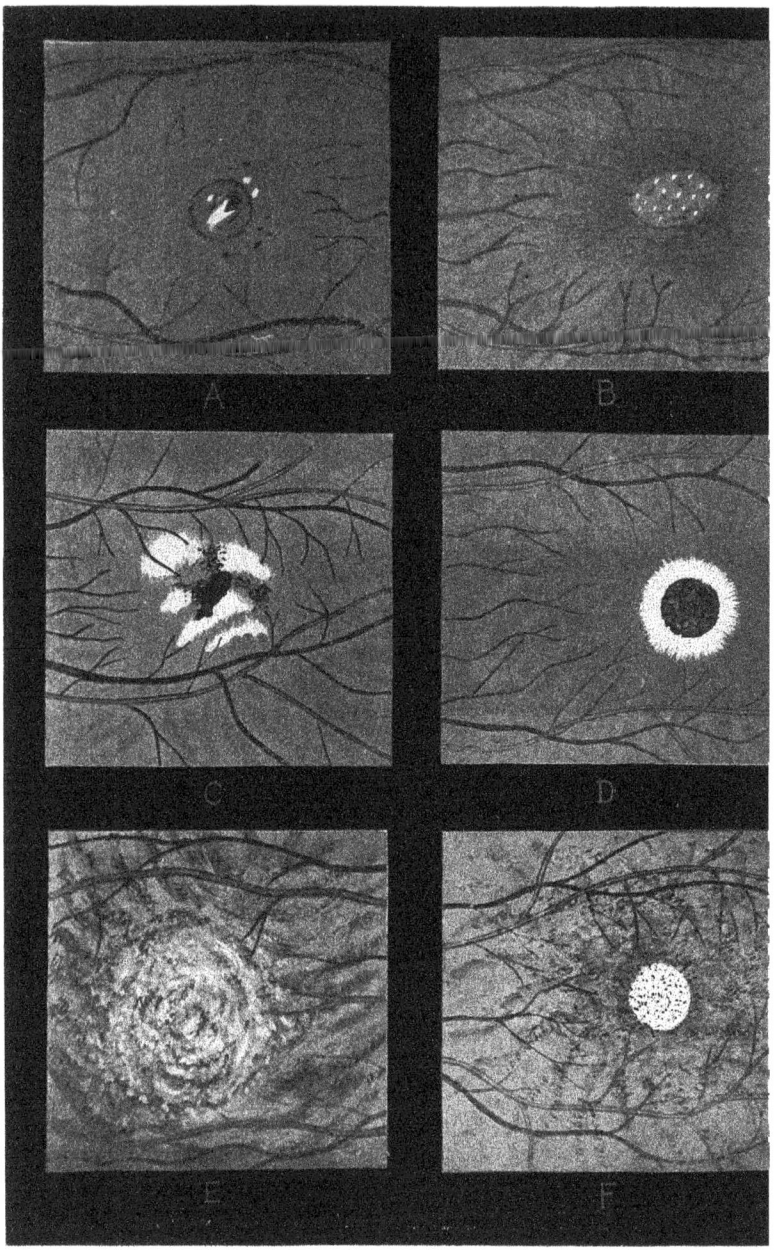

A. Macular Injury, Contusion of Globe from Rope End. B. Blow from Fis
Blow from Door. D. Hole at macula from snowball. E. Iron in vitreous, 6
changes at macula. F. Iron in vitreous, 6 days, changes and lisease of macula
contusions of globe and retained foreign boly in vitreous. (Würdemann.)

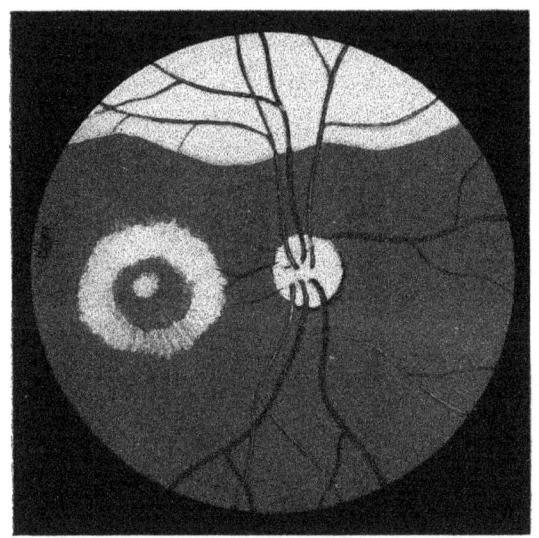

Opacity of the Retina Due to a Blow on the Eye
Berlin's Opacity. Taken a few hours after being hit in
the eye by a wedge. (Würdemann.)

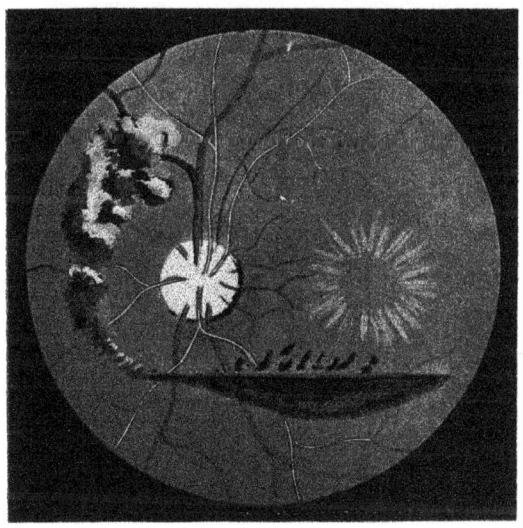

Rupture of Superior Nasal Branch of the Central
Retinal Vein. Pre-retinal Hemorrhage. (Würdemann.)

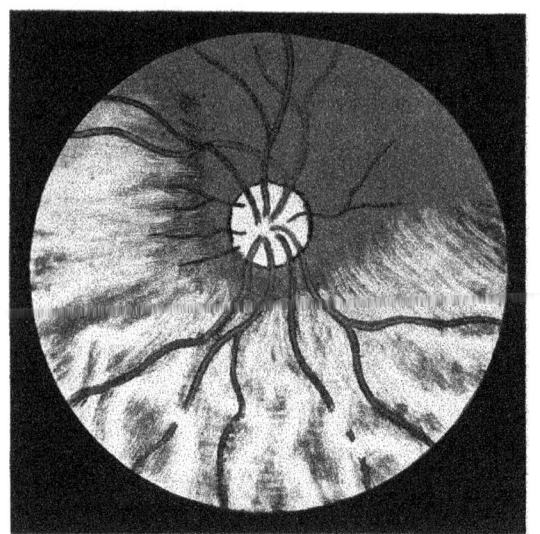

Dialysis of the Retina from Injury. (Würdemann.)

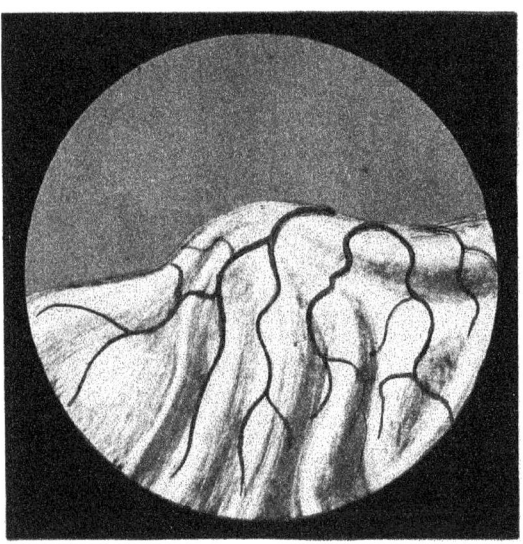

Total Detachment of the Retina Following Injury.
(Würdemann.)

uated, in contra-distinction to the indirect, at the periphery of the fundus at the ciliary region. An irregular, wide tear in the choroid is here seen, through which the sclera shows bluish-white. The retina may be ruptured, opaque, or detached. The sclera may be indented or opened. It is usually combined with laceration of the ciliary body and generally connected with contused wounds or rupture of the sclera. Choroidal tears parallel to the scleral opening may occur in rupture of the sclera. See, also, p. 2165, Vol. III, of this *Encyclopedia.*

DETACHMENT OF THE RETINA FROM INJURY.

This subject has been so fully discussed under **Detachment of the retina** that there remains little to be added here except to repeat that the *prognosis* in recent cases of traumatic separation of the retina is, generally speaking, good, in strict contrast with the ordinary form which does not readily yield to any therapeutic measure.

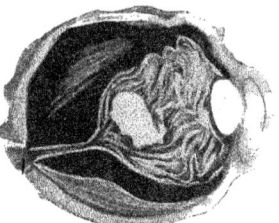

Total Traumatic Detachment of the Retina.

Purtscher (*Centralbl. f. prakt. Augenheilk.,* January, 1913) reports two cases of *angiopathia retinæ traumatica* with changes in the fundus, which he considered as typical of severe traumatisms of the head. They consisted of bright, white patches in the inner layers of the retina of varying size and number generally grouped around the disc and macula, mostly in the course of the large retinal veins. The discs were perfectly normal, but there were more or less numerous venous hemorrhages in the retina in the form of stripes or spots. In one case, the affection was bilateral, in the second case, unilateral, but the other eye was completely amaurotic from atrophy of the optic nerve, in consequence of fracture of the optic canal. The impairment of vision in the three eyes was only moderate. The white patches and hemorrhages disappeared entirely in the second case, which was under long observation. Similar cases have been described by Gonin and Liebrecht. The etiological element in all the cases seemed to be an increase of intracranial pressure and an entrance of cerebrospinal fluid into the retina. Purtscher attributes the white patches to a direct extravasation of lymph from the perivascular lymphatic spaces into the retina tissue.

Macular injury occurs occasionally. Kaz describes two cases seen immediately after an accident, and which were seen again two years later. In the first there was a flat detachment of the retina which left behind a hardly perceptible darkening of the fovea with vision 0.5. In the second, a boy of eight years old, the macula was torn across and this was followed by retinitis proliferans, with a vision of 0.2. In both these cases a light, arch like line was noticed in the retina, in the first case between the macula and the optic disc, and in the second to the outer side of the macula; the concavity being in both cases turned towards the macula and indicating the limits of the post retinal edema.

Souter's review of J. Gonin's (*Annales d'oculistique,* Jan., 1912) case of *partial rupture of the optic papilla* is well worth reading. The author believes that tears of the optic nerve at its entrance into the globe are not infrequent as a result of penetrating injuries of the orbit, and in such cases the disc usually disappears and is replaced by a mass of cicatricial connective tissue in no wise resembling the papilla, but partial ruptures may also be found from traumatism to the eyeball itself.- Such results, however, are very rare, and Gonin has found but two in the literature. He gives notes of two cases where he believes that the conditions are explainable by this lesion.

A young man of twenty while skiing on an ice slope accidentally struck his face with the end of his ski. Besides brow and lid wounds he showed, when seen two days after the accident, a rupture of choroid in the lower periphery of the fundus, and a hemorrhage about the lower outer border of the papilla. The corresponding sector of the optic disc showed more the appearance of a deep, glaucomatous excavation, involving about one-third of the disc surface, but with abrupt edges and a brilliant white coloration, without any trace of vessels in the depths. The macular area showed signs of a slight edema, but it did not have that retinal ischemia suggestive of one of the arteries having been torn. Yet the upper part of the visual field was entirely absent up to 10° from centre of fixation. Visual acuity was 2/10. The clean-cut nature of the crack at the lower border of the papilla and the abolition of the visual field above combined to make him conclude that there had been a rupture of the whole of a fasciculus of the optic nerve fibres. The absence of ophthalmoscopic opacity in the corresponding region of the retina does not by any means negative this diagnosis but supports the experimental finding that the porcelain tint which involves the retina as a result of resection of the optic nerve has for its determining cause retinal ischemia and not ascending degeneration of the nerve fibres. Five months later the vision had risen to ⅓, but the field was unchanged. The affected part of the optic papilla was now covered by a whitish, cotton-wool-like mass obscuring the excavation. A mass of pigment had collected beyond on a level with the papillary border. At the moment of the accident the young man had reflexly shut his eyes and the globes had therefore turned up. The lower part of the sclerotic thus received the impact of the point of the ski in the region where the ophthalmoscope showed the choroidal rupture, and this impact acting from below up had naturally produced a forcible retraction of the eyeball in such a way as to stretch sharply the inferior surface of the optic nerve at its entrance into the globe, and so rupture of the optic nerve fibres at that part.

An analogous mechanism had been in force in the second case. A student had fallen with a ruler in his hand and had received a violent shock on the left eye from below upwards. It caused hyphema and the vision was much reduced by a large absolute central scotoma. Six months later the ophthalmoscope showed on the disc a cicatricial mass as in the last case, occupying the temporal sector of the optic disc and covering partially the origin of the vessels. As he did not have any visible alteration of the retinal tissue there had been a lesion of the fasciculi of the macular fibres which had caused the central scotoma. In the two observations from the literature, the lesion produced was like a coloboma of the optic nerve. Lang's case showed a rupture of the lower third of the papilla and Casper's a rupture of the lower part with suppression of the upper part of the field as in Gonin's own case. Casper expected complete optic atrophy to follow but in Gonin's case this did not occur.

INJURIES OF THE OPTIC NERVE.

This important organ is rarely injured alone. Still, in gun-shot wounds of the orbit, a subject discussed under **Military surgery of the eye,** the optic tissues may be the chief parts involved. See, also, **Optic nerve, Injuries of the; Hemiopia; Evul**sion of the optic nerve; as well as **Automutilation, Ocular.**

Indirect or associated injuries of the optic nerve are not uncommon. *Wounds,* according to Adams, are either sagittal or transverse, and he says that the subsequent course differs in the two varieties; while retinitis proliferans is the rule in the latter, it is exceptional in the former, and only occurs where the nerve has been torn away from the globe. He supports his views by the findings in 4 cases—two of each variety.

Reis reports a case in which the upper margin of the orbit was comminuted by the kick of a horse, and the eyeball torn loose except for the sheath of the optic nerve and a strand of the internal rectus. The nerve sheath was quite empty, the nerve having been torn off just back of the lamina cribrosa. In Schmidt's case a crochet hook penetrated

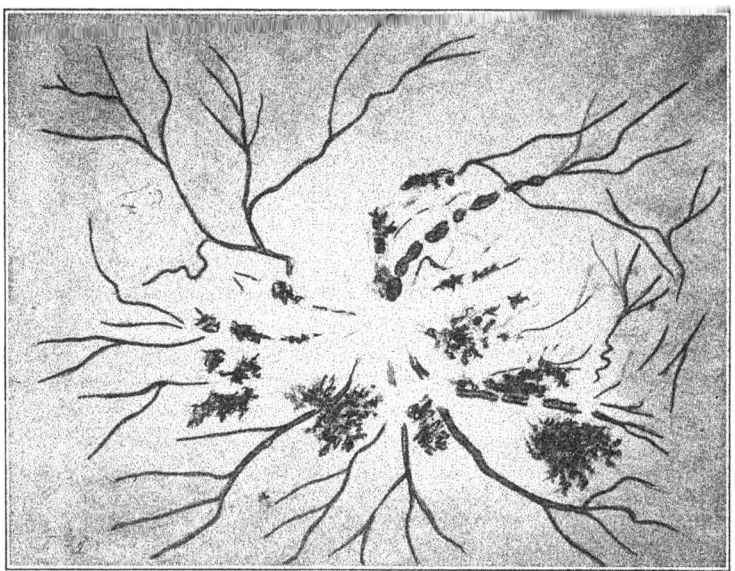

Traumatic Rupture of the Optic Nerve.

the orbit to the optic foramen, divided the nerve at that point and entered the cranium. The wound healed promptly after extraction of the hook; four weeks later the disk was atrophic.

Parker (*Oph. Year-Book*, p. 285, 1912) describes a case in which the patient was injured by an elevator falling upon him. The line of demarcation separating the darkened area from the normal ran around the neck above the clavicle. Immediately after the accident the right eye was almost blind. There was bilateral exophthalmos with great swelling of the conjunctiva from extravasation of blood. The optic nerve was white and there was great engorgement and tortuosity of the veins. In the other eye there was retinal edema with venous engorgement. The discoloration and most of the conjunctival blood rapidly disappeared.

Le Roux reports the occurrence of unilateral optic atrophy after compression of the thorax in a railway accident. Neither the head nor the extremities were injured. On regaining consciousness the man was blind. There was diffuse ecchymosis of the head, neck and later of the lids and conjunctiva of both eyes. The left eyeball remained normal throughout. The right pupil was moderately dilated and there was a papillitis which resulted in almost complete atrophy. The initial loss of vision was attributed to commotio retinæ and the permanent monocular blindness to a hemorrhage within the sheath of the nerve.

De Schweinitz and Holloway record a case of fracture of the skull extending from the posterior occipital protuberance near the parieto-temporal suture to the base of the zygoma, in which there were numerous large hemorrhages scattered over the fundus and more or less concealing the papilla in both eyes. Autopsy showed that the whole cerebrum was involved in a subdural hemorrhage and there were ampulliform enlargements of the sheath of both optic nerves. The sheaths of the nerves were distended with blood. Heed records an instance of optic nerve atrophy following a blow on the supra-orbital margin. The day after the injury the eye was blind. Not until six weeks later was the atrophy recognizable with the ophthalmoscope. Rupture of the optic nerve by fracture into the optic canal is assumed to have occurred.

INJURIES TO THE EYEBALL AS A WHOLE.

Traumatic enophthalmos is sufficiently discussed on p. 4318, Vol. VI, of this *Encyclopedia,* and the same may be said of *evulsion of the globe* under **Dislocation of the Eyeball; Automutilation;** and **Evulsion of the optic nerve.**

For an account of the various forms of *exophthalmos the result of injury,* see p. 4850, Vol. VII, of this *Encyclopedia.*

ORBITAL AND LID INJURIES.

Aside from the infections, the blood vessels and the orbital walls may acquire certain surgical affections following an injury. After some contusions gangrene of the lids may occur, after blows upon the bony parts, periostitis, osteitis, caries, and necrosis. After injuries to the blood vessels an aneurysm may develop in the orbit, causing pulsating exophthalmos. Aneurysms of the retina may likewise develop from blows upon the orbit. Emphysema of the orbit and lids may be seen after fracture of the ethmoids, causing air to enter the tissues.

The *development of tumors,* more particularly epithelioma, sarcoma, and carcinoma, after contusion of the part has been recognized for ages. Even yet, however, we do not know the reason therefor unless the attractive theory of Cohnheim is substantiated. By this theory a trauma releases and sets to growing slumbering embryonal elements and these grow into a mass which we call tumor. Laboratory and clinical experiments have not yet proven this theory. Be this as it may, many patients with tumors remember a previous accidental injury to which they ascribe the development of the disease.

Ciliary neuralgia may be due to the development of a small neuroma in the wounded ciliary nerves, or be reflex from an impacted iris. The irritation may cause clonic and tonic reflex spasms.

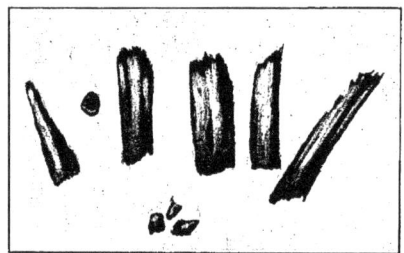

Nine Pieces of Sage Brush Wood Removed from the Orbit.   Exact Size.

INJURIES OF THE EYELIDS.

On p. 5012, Vol. VII, of this *Encyclopedia* will be found a short account of this subject, to which a few additional observations are in order.

Injuries of the lids are very common, not only from industrial accidents but even in family practice, and are to be noted for forensic purposes as they may be an important factor in evidence.

Incised wounds. All kinds of sharp objects used in work or play, accident or assault, cause these lid wounds, many of which are but the external signs of deeper injuries, and complicated by those of the frontal, nasal, or temporal regions and the face, as well as those of the eye and orbit. Injuries to the eyeball by broken lenses are extremely rare; injuries to the ocular appendages are more common; they occur more frequently among wearers of spectacles than nose glasses, and the injury is usually due to breaking of rimless glasses. The wound may be superficial, cutting only the skin or through the muscle, tarsus and conjunctiva, in some cases only penetrating, in others dividing, the lid, in which it may be followed by a permanent coloboma and great deformity. From the cicatrization ectropion, entropion, lagophthalmus and other deformities result. In many cases the patient appears with the lid-wound gaping and full of dust, but the blood supply is so rich that infection rarely results.

Horizontal wounds, parallel with the fibers of the orbicularis muscle, come together and often heal without suturing, leaving but little cicatrix unless the entire lid has been cut through, in which case a lengthy wound results. If the wound should be vertical the edges gape widely and do not tend to heal together unless rendered aseptic and properly stitched.

Ptosis occurs from cicatrization of the upper lid, while interference with the drainage of the tears through the lachrymo-nasal duct from injury to the lower canal, whereby chronic irritation with eczema of the lid and cheek is produced. From incomplete closure of the lids chronic conjunctivitis and ulceration of the cornea result. If the septum orbitale or fascia tarso-orbitalis be divided the lid is not well supported, and ectropion or entropion results.

Longitudinal wounds that do not gape tend to heal kindly unless they are deep or of some extent, otherwise stitches may not be needed, but if the deeper structures be injured, especially in the case of the levator tendon of the lid so that ptosis is produced, the divided ends should be sought and joined together with several interrupted catgut sutures and the skin wound sewed with silk. Where the lid is divided vertically, so that a coloboma is produced, the edges should be brought together not only by interrupted fine silk sutures, but as the skin is so delicate and thus easily torn, and swelling is apt to ensue, deep tension stitches should also be placed outside of the wound sutures. In old cases the edges of the coloboma are to be freshened and then sutured together. Where sloughing has caused loss of tissue, flap and whole-skin grafts may be made.

Punctured wounds. Small punctures from clean instruments are not at all dangerous, but those which perforate the lid through to the conjunctival surface, or to the lachrymal sac or gland, may leave a permanent fistulous opening through which the tears flow. Symblepharon may likewise occur.

The fascia tarso-orbicularis is easily torn by such wounds, the healing resulting in dislocation of the lid from the eye because of cicatricial contraction. The direction of these wounds is generally backwards.

At times cilia may be torn away or carried into the wound if it be at the ciliary margin of the lids.

. The complications of penetrating wounds of the lids are coincidental injury to the globe and the orbit, usually through foreign bodies of some size. But often smaller foreign bodies, as shot pellets, chips of metal, glass, sand and stone from explosives may pass through the lid. Recognition of the port of entry should be made by stretching the lids and by close examination. The probe may be sparingly and carefully used.

Stabs of the eyelids from sabres and knives were more common in former days than in this age, but are occasionally seen.

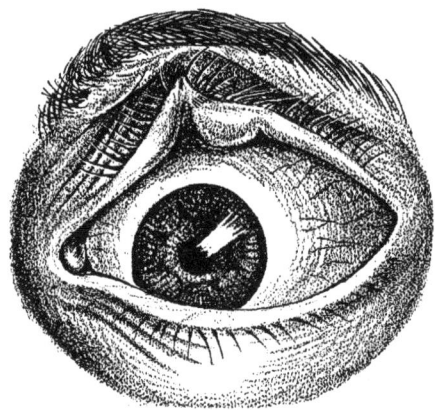

Ectropion and Deformity of the Upper Lid from Dog Bite.

Tears and bruised wounds of the lids are perhaps more common than cuts and punctures, as they obtain, in most cases, from foreign bodies entering the orbit, particularly in the case of broken timbers, handles of tools, bullets, explosives of powder and dynamite, cowhorns, tears from claws and lacerations from bites, and contused wounds from hoofs of animals. The butcher's meat hook has caused several such injuries. Bites from human beings and animals are usually complicated, involving other parts of the face, or at times, the eyeball.

Several cases of *cow-horn injury* in America have been seen, and this has generally involved the upper lid. These accidents are probably more common amongst the peasantry of Europe than in America, where milch cows are usually dehorned. One such case is illustrated herein. A number of cases of fracture of the bones of the face and orbit have been seen, resulting from kicks of animals, in one of which the lower lid was badly torn.

Lacerations and contused wounds vary in appearance according to their character and that of the object producing the injury. The edges of the wounds are turned in or out, lacerated, bruised, ragged and usually impregnated with dust. Where there is entrance to the orbit wounds of the globe and contents occur, and in deeper, direct injuries fracture of the walls or base of the brain. Care should be taken to determine the presence of foreign bodies. The course depends upon the amount of tissue lost, the quality of infection and

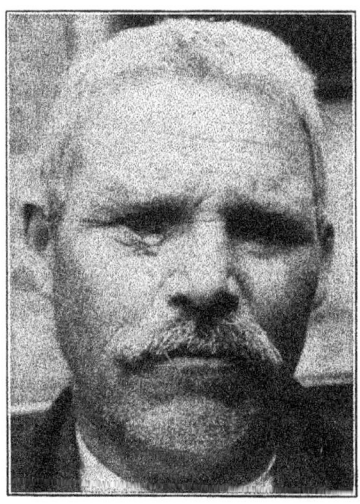

Cicatrical Ectropion from Cow-horn Injury.

the complications. Where a portion of the tissues is removed by the injury or by ulceration the function of the lid is affected and cicatricial contraction causes ugly deformities.

Infection leads to erysipelas and gangrene of the lid.

A number of instances of infection by syphilis of a scratch wound of the lid have been observed.

The *therapy of wounds of the eyelids* is asepsis and coaptation of the wound. Ragged and bruised edges must be cut away and in old cases the cicatricial tissue removed and the wound edges freshened and coapted by sutures, with or without undermining the adjacent skin to make sliding flaps. Wounds over 5 mm. in length should be sutured with fine silk and thin needles, always taking care to secure proper coaptation by entering the edges of the skin wounds by forceps after tying the stitches. As the swelling is usually great several tension stitches should be put in to insure the fine skin sutures remaining. When the lid has been completely torn through deep stitches of fine catgut may be laid in the depths of the wound and remain buried therein upon closure by superficial sutures.

When sloughing or trauma has caused loss of tissue, and when cicatricial contraction has ensued, various surgical procedures, for ptosis, entropion, ectropion, lagophthalmus, symplepharon and anklyoblepharon, as well as to replace large defects, must be used. These operations are described in detail elsewhere in this *Encyclopedia*.

As regards lid plastics a great variety of operations has been proposed and used in former days but are not now in such vogue, their places being better supplied by the Thiersch and Wolff grafts. In order to cover a defect of the skin caused by removal of tissue, either by accident or design, these flaps may be taken from the neighborhood, as the temple or cheek, according to the principles used in general surgery, shown under **Blepharoplasty.** See, also, **Ectropion**; as well as the caption **Entropion**.

Foreign bodies in the eyelids. With the exception of powder and sand grains impacted into the lids from explosions, other foreign bodies are rarely seen, as the lids are thin and objects projected with much force usually pass through into the eye and orbit. Glass splinters, chips of metal and sharp pieces of wood are occasionally seen in the skin of the lids.

Most foreign bodies cause a certain amount of inflammation and suppuration and are extruded thereby through the wound of entrance. Sterile stone, pellets of shot and powder grains, however, become impacted, and from the latter extensive tattooing and resultant deformity takes place, these cases being quite common in practice from careless handling of gunpowder and fireworks. In some instances the powder or other particles pass entirely through the lids into the globe, causing ulceration and granuloma of the conjunctiva, and various injuries to the eyeball, previously described in these pages.

Abscess of the lid is uncommon from retained foreign bodies but does occur at times.

The diagnosis is not difficult, but it should be remembered that in explosions many foreign bodies may be impacted in all parts of the face and eyes. The finger tip is useful for feeling the foreign body, which may be brought to view by small incisions.

Injuries of the lids from blunt objects. Where hemorrhage into the lids results from a blow upon the ocular region and no other complications ensue the case is one of ordinary "black eye" so common from fisticuffs and striking the face against a door in the dark, and such a patient generally ascribes the event to some such cause as the latter. See p. 1006, Vol. II, of this *Encyclopedia.*

But we should ever be on our guard in examining such cases to search thoroughly for a deeper and more important lesion, as the discoloration of the lids by extravasation of blood under the skin is in some cases but one of the symptoms of a grave injury to the cranium, as previously described.

Of particular importance in diagnosis are those suggulations coming from direct and radiating fractures of the bones of the face, orbit,

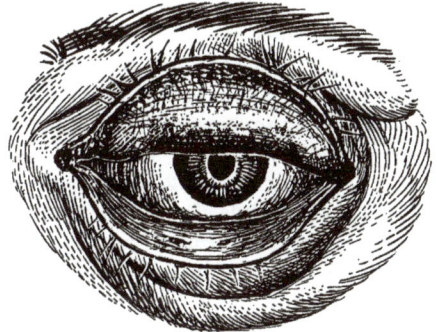

Ectropion of Both Lids from Cicatricial Contraction following Burn.

and skull. The bleeding occurs immediately in the two former and in orbital injuries is often accompanied by an immediate and extensive hematoma. The bleeding from fracture of the base of the skull appears 12 to 24 hours after the accident, at first in the lower lid near the orbital margin; then it extravasates slowly through the cellular tissue under the nose to the other eye.

This form of extravasation coming on after an injury to the head, with or without unconsciousness, is pathognomonic of basal fracture and not favorable as regards vision, so the acuity and field should be carefully noted from time to time.

Emphysema of the lids is a symptom of fracture of the floor or inner wall of the orbit and laceration of the mucous membrane, periosteum, and orbital tissues, with communication with the nasal accessory sinuses. Dentists sometimes cause emphysema of the face and lids after drilling a tooth through and blowing out the cavity by compressed air. See p. 4301, Vol. VI, of this *Encyclopedia.*

The chief symptoms of emphysema of the orbit and lids are proptosis, limited movement, diplopia, swelling, gaseous crepitation supervening after blowing the nose, violent sneezing, or forced expiration. Usually emphysema of the orbit and lids is confined to these structures by the strong anterior lamina of fascia between the lids and orbital margins. The usual causes are traumatism, disease or necrosis of the bones, surgical operations, or because of the presence of erosion of the buccal mucous membrane. A break in the continuity of the mucous membrane lining the accessory cavities and a fracture of the bony walls of the orbit, with a rupture of the periosteum, are common causes. Fuchs explains the mechanism of many fractures by the giving way of the lamina papyracea due to the increase of pressure in the orbit by the ball being forced backward. This theory throws no light on those cases in which the injury involves the back of the skull. Extensive hemorrhage is not likely to occur because of the tortuosity of the larger vessels, and their protection by the soft tissues.

Severe *contusions,* and prolonged pressure, as from hematoma and emphysema, are usually combined with wounds which are readily infected and in a few cases become gangrenous.

Burns of the skin of the lids show the several degrees of burns, the symptoms of redness, vesicularization and gangrene. These injuries are part of burns of the face and eyes, the cornea and conjunctiva being generally involved.

Continuous iced compressing in weak individuals has given rise to gangrene of the lids.

The prognosis depends upon the extent and character of the burn. The complications are not only those of the eye, but also from contraction of the lids, lagophthalmus, entropion, ectropion, trichiasis, narrowing of the lid aperture, cauterization and closure of the lachrymal puncta and canals.

The therapy of burns of the lids is placed upon general surgical principles. See the general sub-section on BURNS.

Wound infection in injuries of the lids and soft parts of the orbit. Infection of the skin of the lids is not common, and considering the large number of palpebral injuries and infections they all do well, the circulation being free and the nutrition plentiful. Penetrating wounds of the orbital tissues, however, are apt to become infected, causing orbital cellulitis and phlegmon, and if so give rise to serious disturbances, septicemia and pyemia, anthrax, glanders, and lyssa.

Erysipelas is common, and phlegmon occurs from infected lesions of the lids and orbital margins. Deeply penetrating wounds of the orbit may give rise to phlegmon, followed by meningitis, sinus thrombosis, encephalitis and, perhaps, death. Abscess of the orbit or retrobulbar phlegmon also comes from entrance of foreign bodies, or secondary infection of the wound by the streptococcus or staphylococcus; or periostitis, caries or necrosis may occur, followed by infection of the orbit or surrounding nasal sinuses; and yet aseptic bodies have been retained therein for many years.

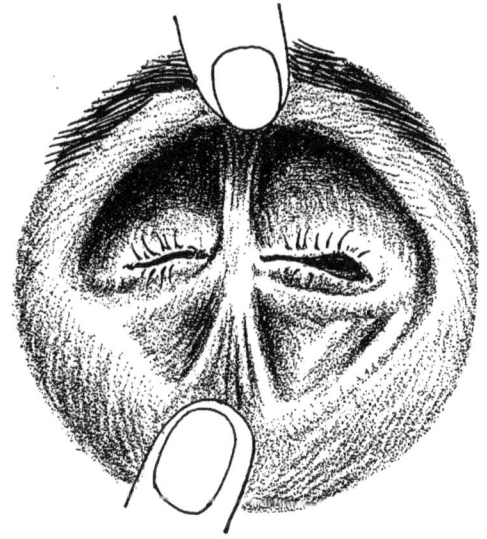

Cicatricial Contraction of Lids and Orbit after Burn by Lime.

The clinical course begins with symptoms of septicemia, fever, pain; followed by marked local symptoms, exophthalmos and immovability of the globe, which differentiates it from a panophthalmitis beginning within the eye. The exophthalmos is caused by many smaller collections of pus situated in the cellular fatty tissues and the ocular muscles, which accounts for the loss of ocular nutrition. This also accounts for those cases where deep incisions may not evacuate pus, yet the relief of the tension by the free bleeding thus produced gives much relief to the symptoms. When a large pus cavity forms it may push the globe to the opposite side and fluctuation be felt.

The principal danger of orbital cellulitis and phlegmon is from passage of the inflammation to the brain, causing meningitis and encephalitis, or a septic thrombus beginning in the ophthalmic vein and continuing to the carotid sinus. Such cases may likewise cause an optic neuritis with resultant optic nerve atrophy.

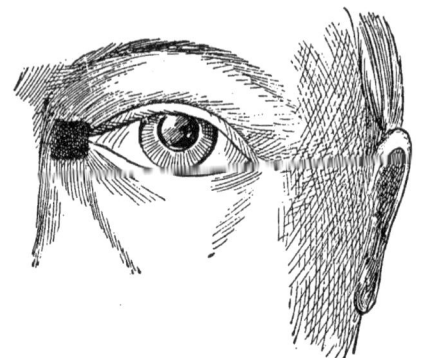

Breech Block in the Orbit.
Sketch of Patient before operation.   (Wright.)

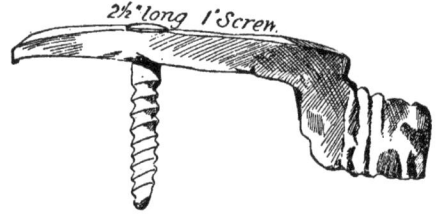

Breech Block after Removal (reduced to one-third).

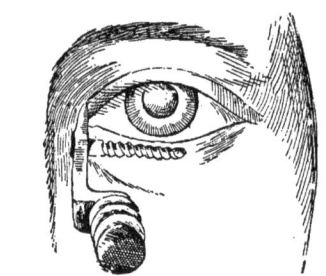

Sketch Showing how the Breech Block Entered.

The *therapy* consists in general antiphlogistic treatment, especially by quinin, antistreptococcic serum injections, retrobulbar injections of 1:5000 mercurial sublimate or oxycyanide, free and early incisions to relieve the chemosis and aid the pointing of the pus cavities, hot compresses, 5 per cent. phenol injections at the margins of inflamed areas in erysipelas. Where fluctuation is felt, deep incisions and gauze or tube drainage may be established. In only exceptional instances may it be advisable to enucleate a panophthalmitic eye attended by orbital cellulitis.

Tetanus may develop from injuries to the orbit, especially with retention of foreign bodies, from contused and lacerated wounds of the lids or even from retention of a foreign body in the conjunctival sac. The therapy is antitetanic serum and chloral.

Injuries to the walls and contents of the orbit are included mainly under **Orbit, Injuries of the.**

Foreign bodies in the orbit are of a variety and size that pass belief. See, for example, the figure depicting the breech-pin described by Gifford. Lead-pencils, shot, bullets, broken glass, pieces of stone,

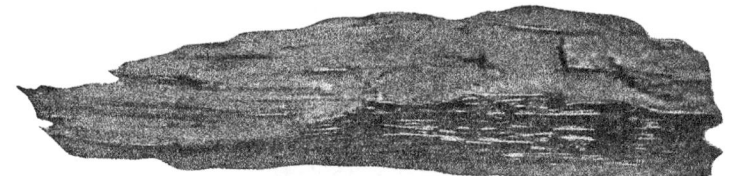

Actual Size of Piece of Wood Penetrating the Orbit.

splinters of wood, etc., have been not only found but have lain hidden within the orbit for months and even years, without exciting even a suspicion of their presence. Of course, the use of the X-ray and careful probing will generally clear the diagnosis. Removal of the foreign body and subsequent cleansing generally ends in a cure, but the prognosis always depends chiefly upon the extent and character of the injury to the orbital contents.

Injuries of the extraocular muscles are almost invariably part of a more extensive trauma of the orbit and orbital contents, such as occur in cow-horn accidents. Wertheim describes a case of traumatic laceration of the belly of the superior rectus, and the tendon of the superior oblique posterior to the trochlea. The tendon had to be abscised. The muscle was sutured. The reporter ascribes the perfect cure which resulted (no diplopia) to the fact that the power of the rectus as an elevator was weakened to the same degree as the function of the oblique as a depressor was interfered with. See, also, the major heading **Muscles, Injuries of the ocular.**

Injuries to the eyes occurring during or as the sequelæ of ocular and other operations. It quite frequently happens that the *cornea is abraded by the anesthetist* in testing the lid closure reflex by the finger during the giving of an anesthetic, or a drop of ether or chloroform may enter the eye and give rise to irritation. The lethargy induced by the anesthetic, lasting for twenty-four hours afterwards, as a rule does not permit of much complaint from this source from

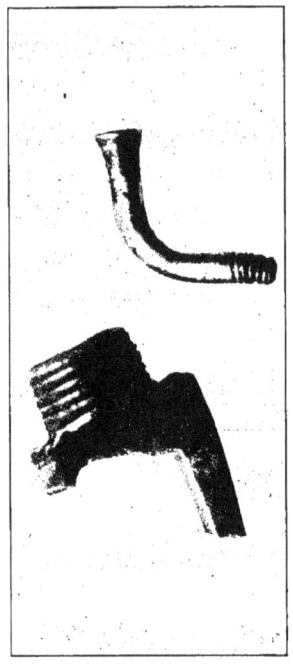

Gifford's Case of Breech-pin in the Orbit.

Breech-pin, 1½ inches long, weighed 11 drams.

patients, and by that time restoration of epithelium has usually occurred. Occasionally, however, the oculist is called to see such a patient.

In old patients the conjunctiva may be very friable and tear on fixation by forceps. This event, however, is of little moment as repair always and speedily ensues. Occasionally also instrumental injury of the cornea occurs.

For accidents in *cataract operations,* see **Cataract, Senile;** and **After-treatment of operations.**

Portions of instruments, as ends of knives and needles or buried threads, may inadvertently be left in the ocular tissues. Sooner or later these give rise to irritation, as would any other foreign body, and have to be removed. The breaking of knife or needle points in tissues during operation is generally due to their becoming brittle through sterilization.

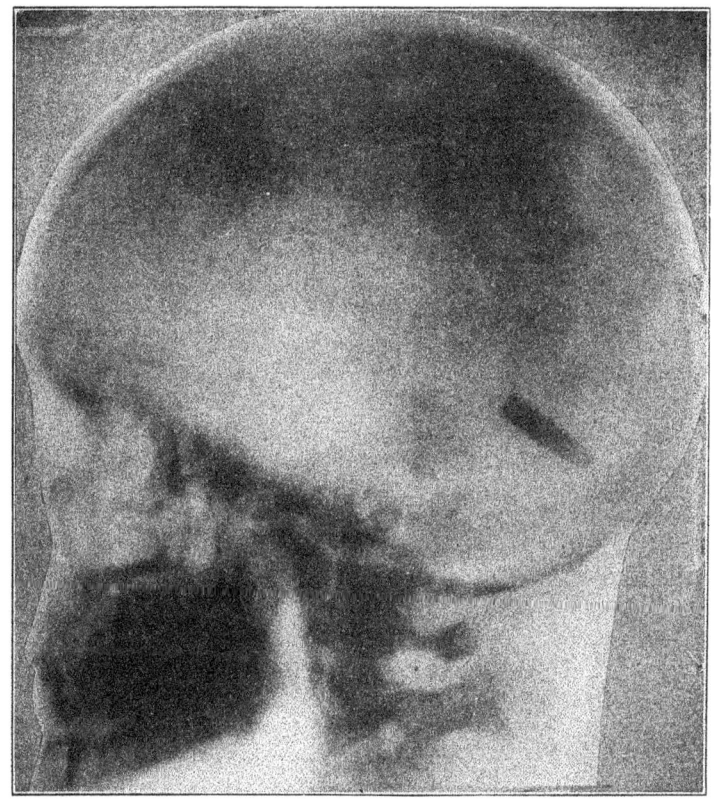

Bullet Wound of the Orbit. Skiagram Shows Bullet Impacted in the Posterior Chamber of the Cranium. (Girard.)

Injuries during childbirth, with the exception of ophthalmia neonatorum produced by infection during or after labor, occur during spontaneous or instrumental delivery from mechanical causes, mostly coming under the head of injuries from blunt force, being due to compression, contusion, and rupture. Here we differentiate: 1,

Fractures of the skull, especially of the orbital walls; 2, Injuries to the soft parts of the orbit, and particularly the lids; 3, Evulsion of the eyeball; 4, Paralysis of the ocular muscles; 5, Injuries to the eyeball. See **Birth injuries.**

Drugs used for medicinal purposes may cause injury to the eyes locally or internally. Accidental or purposeful instillation of certain remedies into the eyes may, if wrongfully or too freely used, produce not only unpleasant symptoms but in some cases permanent injury. The quantity used; the appropriateness of the place chosen for its use; the absorption; the power of resistance of the individual, sometimes make a drug poisonous, whereas in others it is a remedial agent.

It is a common complaint of the dissatisfied patient that the last doctor he went to used too strong a remedy for the eye, and thereby aggravated the previous existing disease or ignorantly damaged the eye. In the vast majority of cases there is no cause for such complaint, therefore the physician should ever be careful to disabuse the patient's mind of such a delusion, and in no case to give rise to further criticism of the previous consultant.

Occasionally, however, either from accident, idiosyncrasy or actual ignorance, damage is done to the eyes from such applications. Both idiosyncrasy of the patient and toxicity of the medicament may cause untoward symptoms in, or damage to, the eyes from drugs administered internally in therapeutic or toxic doses. Inhalation also claims its victims, as in the optic nerve atrophy following the fumes of wood alcohol.

Of local applications the most common complaint is from the use of mydriatics and cycloplegics for measuring the refraction, to which even yet in this enlightened age some persons ascribe damage, needless to say without cause. The effects of cocain and homatropin usually pass away within 24 hours; rarely exceeding 48 hours. Full cycloplegia by atropin may last as long as 14 days, but usually disappears within 10 days. Instillations of eserin or pilocarpin relieve the mydriasis and cycloplegia. Systemic toxic symptoms are often produced, but are not to be discussed in this connection. Continuous use of atropin for a long time locally may produce a chronic conjunctivitis. The same may be said of many other applications.

The instillation of even the feebler mydriatics may, however, precipitate an attack of glaucoma, or cause it in eyes predisposed to the affection, and hence should be used with caution in patients after middle life. The mistaken application of atropin in glaucoma may produce fulminating symptoms and cause permanent blindness. The miotics, eserin, pilocarpin and morphin used locally, however, have no evil effects, although used internally to toxicity they may produce amblyopia. Iodoform used locally in the form of powder or ointment may produce irritation of the conjunctiva and a dermatitis of the lids, and orthoform is very apt so to do.

When iodoform is used locally, as in dressing wounds of other parts of the body, by injection of emulsions, as well as internally by pills, untoward symptoms may be caused in the eyes, a form of descending atrophy of the optic nerve from the toxemia developing. There is failing sight, central color scotoma and normal outer boundaries of the visual field, the temporal side of the pupil is often paler in these cases—symptoms we group under the title of retrobulbar neuritis. Retinal hemorrhages, with or without a neuroretinitis, are occasionally observed. The poisonous effect of iodoform depends chiefly upon the free iodin. See **Argyrosis.**

The ingestion, inhalation, epidermic, hypodermic, endermic, intramuscular, or any other method by which certain toxic substances may get into, or be developed within, the system, may induce changes in the tissues of the eye by which diverse effects are produced, denominated, commonly, **Toxic amblyopia.**

Traumatic glaucoma. Typical glaucoma may be produced by trauma. Eyes with glaucoma and arterio-sclerosis are predisposed to hemorrhage from the brittleness of their vessels. The affection is rare and it is not peculiar to old age. The ages of the patient vary from 6 to 66, and there have been more instances in young subjects than in old.

In all the cases reported, traumatic glaucoma had been a primary affection, occurring suddenly in subjects who before the accidents had never presented any symptoms of glaucoma. The time after the traumatism at which it appears varies from a few hours to several days. In one case it appeared nine days, and in another nineteen days, after the injury. It may be preceded by intraocular hemorrhage, but this is often absent. Rather frequently it has been accompanied by a subluxation of the lens.

Where atropin is not used in traumatic cataract the swollen lens presses upon the iris, and with the increase in the sp. gr. of the aqueous closes the communication between the anterior and posterior chamber and causes increased tension. In young people the eye capsule yields, which it does not do in older persons with hard sclera and secondary glaucoma, when excavation of the papilla arises. Traumatic glaucoma occurs from inflammation, swelling and edema of the ciliary body by closing the space between it and the lens.

Luxation of the lens into the vitreous, resulting from accident or reclination, produces increased tension, as it surely does in forward dislocation. Some authors think that glaucoma is consecutive to a slight subluxation of the lens which, pressing at a point on the ciliary zone, provokes a reflex hyperemia of the whole uveal tract and a mechanical obstruction of the paths of excretion, but this explanation is not applicable to all cases, since in some there was an entire absence of luxation.

Rupture of the pectinate ligament allows the ciliary body to slip backward, at the same time drawing upon the iris, then causing pupillary distortion and a deepening of the anterior chamber in the region of the pectinate rupture. The lesion is usually caused by a blow on the eye from a blunt instrument without rupture of the globe. A hyphema usually follows at once, which, after absorption, presents the above picture. The canal of Schlemm usually becomes obliterated and increased tension is a symptom which finally develops and ultimately demands excision of the eye.

Finally, some claim that traumatic glaucoma is to be explained, not by an obstruction of the paths of excretion, but rather by an obstruction of the suprachoroidal lymphatic spaces following a hyperemia and serous exudation of the choroid.

The *prognosis* is very variable. In a large proportion of the cases a complete and lasting cure has been obtained, while in many a loss of vision has been reported.

The medical *treatment* includes strong miotics, hot compresses, local bleeding and dionin, and generally bromids, chloral, antipyrin, quinin, etc., may be given.

In the surgical treatment, iridectomy is the operation of choice, though it appears from reported cases that sclerotomy, or even simple paracentesis, acts more decidedly in traumatic glaucoma than in the spontaneous form.

INJURIES OF THE LACHRYMAL APPARATUS.

Wounds and dislocations. In a few cases of wounds of the lids and intraorbital tissues, especially those from broken bottles, sharp stones, or pieces of wood, the orbit may be entered and the lachrymal gland be cut, evulsed or prolapsed through the wound, especially in the case of children.

In 13 cases of *dislocation of the lachrymal gland* collected by Jackson, ten occurred in children of 11 to 14 years of age. The slight development of the upper margin of the orbit in childhood leaves the gland unprotected, just as in adults this accident is most likely to occur in those having undeveloped orbital margins.

In children the accident usually results from falling and cutting the lid; in adults, from wounds penetrating beneath the brow.

The symptoms and course are those of wounds of the orbit; the signs of dislocation of the gland are the presence of a tumor and diplopia. The eyeball is forced forwards, downwards and inwards, and its movements are limited.

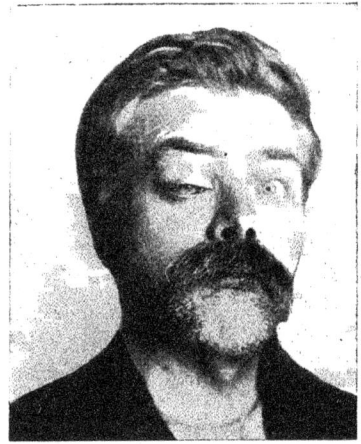

Pseudo-ptosis and Suppuration of the Lachrymal Gland, due to Penetrating Splinter of Wood. Operation; recovery. (Würdemann.)

Injury to the *canaliculi, sac* and *nasolachrymal duct* occurs from lid and nasal wounds, especially from shot and pointed sticks. Horizontal wounds are less common than vertical.

Inflammation of the lachrymal gland may occur from blows on the brow or gland. It is seldom of moment and not often recognized. The writer has seen a number of cases in connection with ordinary black eye. Several cases of *dislocation of the gland* without an external wound, as well as of spontaneous prolapse, have been reported.

Coughing, epilepsy and "moral emotions" have been suggested as etiologic factors in lachrymal gland luxations; sudden hyperemia of the gland following vaso-dilatation causes its displacement and subsequent prolapse. Congenital dislocation is also known to occur as a result of defects in the conformation of the orbit.

Symptoms. There is a rather hard tumor of oval form at the outer angle of the orbit, contained in a fold of skin in which it rests as in a sac or hammock. It may hang down over the commissure of the lids. It is freely movable between the skin and the tarsus in the horizontal and upward directions, but not downward, and unless too large can be replaced in its proper position in the orbit, but falls out by its own weight or as the result of lowering the head, or straining.

Spontaneous reduction of the dislocated lachrymal gland has been observed; attempts have also been made to keep it in place by various devices, and it has been extirpated.

The replacement of the gland is rather difficult, and if not successful, it continues to be a disfigurement of the patient.

The *diagnosis* of wounds and dislocations is not difficult. Where both are combined the gland may be seen protruding from the wound, and in other cases may be felt as a tumor about the size of a shelled almond.

The abuse of probes in the treatment of lachrymal obstruction may cause false passages and infections.

The *prognosis* in lachrymal injuries depends upon the incidence of infection and whether foreign bodies are, or are not, retained in the orbit.

Therapy. In most cases proper antiseptic treatment and restoration of the parts to their normal position by suturing will be followed by complete restoration, except that a cicatrix remains. It may be necessary, in the surgical treatment of these cases, to excise all or a portion of the protruding gland. Secondary operations for relief of lachrymal stricture may be required in some wounds of the lachrymal passages.

Rupture of the lachrymal sac or canal sometimes occurs in fractures of the nasal and lachrymal bones. It is hardly recognizable except when emphysema of the orbit, or obliteration of the passage, after wounds, occurs. The writer has seen such a case following a forceps delivery.

In connection with *burning* of the lids and conjunctiva, partienlarly by glowing metals, acids, alkalies and lime, the lachrymal passages may be involved. They usually close up and may in favorable cases be again opened by surgical methods.

The writer has observed this sequel in lime burns, as well as from molten lead, and carbolic acid.

The *lachrymal gland* is seldom the seat of a foreign body, but all kinds of foreign bodies may be found sticking in the *lachrymal canaliculi*, especially cilia, portions of insects, grains of chaff, wood, fingernail clippings; infrequently iron, stone or sand particles. These generally lodge first in the conjunctival sac and are then carried by the tears and movements of the lids into a canaliculus. They may cause considerable irritation and are often overlooked.

Naturally, as the *sac* has such a small entrance through the canaliculi, foreign bodies seldom gain entrance to it save where the canaliculus has been previously divided.

Canalicular concretions may also form in dacryocystitis, and foreign bodies may wander into the sac from the nose.

Styles have been retained for many years in the lachrymal canal.

The evident therapy is removal of the foreign body. See **Canaliculus, Foreign bodies in.**

Traumatic neuroses are observed after injuries to the eyes, as after other bodily injuries, but, with the exception of so-called hysterical blindness and changes in the visual field, are less often seen. It is difficult to distinguish between hypochondria, hysteria and actual malingering in patients who claim damages at law following alleged accident.

See **Blindness, Simulation of,** and **Legal relations of ophthalmology.**

Following erosions and small wounds of the cornea severe hysterical pain, lasting for weeks or months, may be complained of in the seat of the scar. This symptom may also be due to bacteria remaining in the depths of the tissues, in which case it is relieved by excision of the scar or by the local use of the galvano-cautery.

Of special importance is *traumatic hysteric blindness.* In all cases there is a local exciting defect or trauma which cause accommodative cramp and pain, the impression being so vivid that patients forcibly close their eyes, and finally fail to recognize objects by sight, although in no case is there an actual, permanent lesion. These cases are cured by suggestive therapeutics, combined with visual training, even though the blindness has lasted for days or years.

This subject is partly discussed under **Hysteria, Ocular manifestations of.** ·Here it may be added that the "ocular symptoms of *traumatic neurasthenia and hysteria* do not differ particularly from those of the nontraumatic varieties. The cornea and conjunctiva may be anesthetic or hyperesthetic; the eye muscles relaxed from fatigue, or be in a state of spasmodic contracture; the visual perceptive apparatus may show fatigue, while there may be also psychical perversions of visual perceptions.

In *traumatic hysteria* the subjective complaints are mostly of pain and paresthesia in various parts of the head after using the eyes, of spots before the eyes, of apparent increase or decrease in size of objects seen, blurred vision after close work dependent upon fatigue of the muscles of accommodation, doubling of print due to inability to maintain convergence, and of fluttering and confusion of print, on account of abnormal duration of after-images in the fatigued retinas. In other words, hysterical amblyopia from injury exhibits much the same symptomatology as from other causes.

A fine tremor of the lids is always noticeable when they are gently closed. There may be lachrymation without inflammation, and photophobia causing drooping of the upper lids; this droop occurs also as a symptom of fatigue as the examination proceeds. The patient not only may fail to raise the lid when directed to do so, but may also forcibly resist the examiner's effort to elevate the lid with his finger.

Reflex closure of the lids when the cornea or conjunctiva is touched is frequently slow or wanting, indicating anesthesia of these parts; and this anesthesia is likely to be more pronounced in the eye having the more marked disturbances of vision, or on the side corresponding to a general hemianesthesia. The pupil is usually normal in size and in reaction, although in cases of hysterical blindness it may be large and unresponsive.

The extraocular muscles often exhibit a lack of balance and particularly a varying latent divergence of exophoria, which may be regarded as a sign of fatigue from convergence. Again, a spasm of any of these muscles may give rise to diplopia, which might suggest an actual paralysis, but the anomalous behavior of the double images in different directions of the gaze, and the presence of corroborative symptoms, lead us to the diagnosis of a purely functional disturbance.

Diplopia of another sort and of a purely physical nature is absolutely characteristic of hysteria, and is a very valuable diagnostic sign when it exists. This is uniocular diplopia. With one eye closed the patient sees a light double, when it is carried a certain distance away from the eye, and when asked to count fingers he sees double the number presented.

The acuteness of vision is usually normal, but the patient often reads the distant letters slowly, and with an effort, and only after considerable urging. There may be even more difficulty in reading print near by, and the patient will hold the test-card close to his face, or far away or to one side, assuming cramped positions, and even repeated urging may not make him read the smallest print. But if an indifferent glass, plain, smoked, or weakly refracting, is held before the eye the psychical effect is such that both distant and near vision at once become normal, or as nearly normal as the patient's refractive condition will permit.

In rarer cases vision in one eye is very poor or the patient may be unable to see at all. But if we employ any of the tests for detecting simulated blindness, which consist in arranging lenses, prisms or colored glasses in such a manner that the patient uses the eye with supposed poor vision while believing that he is using only the eye with good vision—we find that the sight of the poor eye is in fact normal.

For the still rarer cases in which there is apparent blindness in both eyes we have no test to reveal the actual amount of vision, but the diagnosis can usually be made from the presence of other hysterical symptoms, the previous history of aphonia and the like, and the lack of organic changes in the eyes. The patient, however, finds it too difficult to maintain this fiction long, and usually the vision which was lost suddenly, after a few days as suddenly returns.

Anomalies of the visual fields are the most frequent and the most characteristic eye disturbances in neurasthenia and hysteria. The typical condition, if the examination is made deftly without overfatiguing the patient, is a normal field for the usual white test object, a concentric contraction of the color fields in their regular order, and a diminution of central color perception in that a small area of color is not recognized as far away as by the normal eye. These anomalies of color perception are to be regarded as evidences of fatigue of the retina or of the psychical centers, or of both. If the examination is tediously made or purposely long-continued, evidence of increased fatigue is manifest in further narrowing of the fields, giving them the watch-spring or spiral type. That is, if the limits of the fields are plotted a number of times continuously, the boundary line recorded will be a diminishing spiral.

Besides the typical concentric contraction of the color fields in their regular sequence, there is occasionally a reversal of their sequence, the field for red being larger than that for blue, and occasionally a contraction of the field for white. But rarely is there a central defect in the field or a defect of an hemianopic type. The contraction of the field is often more pronounced in the eye of the side which is more anesthetic. Size of fields varies from day to day; forms of color fields are bizarre. These functional eye disturbances are not only common in young women, but most marked and persistent disturbances are found in strong men with hysteria following injury or nervous shock.

Traumatic neurosis consists in an abnormal fatigue not only of the retina but of the neuroptic apparatus, including its cerebral centers. The fatigue found in the field as a whole also exists for the macula and is shown by the condition of quantitative perception of color.

There are two forms, one simulated amaurosis, and the other true amaurosis, hysterical in origin. In the former the patient sees and knows that he sees; in the latter the patient does not see, or if he does, he is not conscious of it.

Amblyopia is comparatively frequent, while total bilateral amaurosis is extremely rare. It is liable to occur in persons debilitated from any cause, and even in previously robust subjects.

A valuable contribution to the study of *nervous symptoms from contusion of the eye* is that of E. R. Williams (*Trans. Am. Oph. Soc.*, p. 40, 1915). He discusses these traumas and divides their consequences into: (1) surgical shock at the time of the accident, its relation to cerebral concussion, its exaggeration by psychic influences, as, for instance, the emotions of fear, anxiety, etc.; (2) psychic shock of the eyeball, sub-divided into two classes; (a) shock causing reduced vision without permanent damage of the retina, (b) shock effecting serious retinal damage, with permanently reduced vision; (3) traumatic delirium, often a complication of head injuries, eye operations, etc.; (4) traumatic neuroses, tending to incapacitate the individual from quickly resuming work, and necessitating special after-treatment; (5) permanent damage to different internal parts of the eye.

In *characteristic shock symptoms* the patient, upon being hit on the eye, usually staggers and sinks to the ground, where he remains dazed, but conscious. In some instances the patient may lose consciousness several minutes. He groans or cries out in anguish. Severe pain in the globe may come instantly, but sometimes is delayed an hour or more; with severe blows it persists one or several days. The individual feels faint or chilly, looks pale and haggard, is nauseated, and often vomits. Being much weakened, he staggers if he attempts to walk. The pulse is weak and rapid, due to the decrease of blood-pressure. These shock symptoms are usually gone after the first night's sleep. Disturbing dreams occurred in two of these cases. The prostration, both mental and physical, often will last several days.

Psychic shock of the eyeball was studied by von Merz (*Klin. Monatsblätter für Augenheilk.*, Beilageheft, 1907), who had many opportunities to treat eye patients during the Russo-Japanese war. The most interesting contusion injuries of the eyes were caused by air concussion following the bursting of shells. He divided his cases into two classes: (A) psychic shock; (B) a paralytic dilatation of the vessels between the retina and the choroid (Beck's theory).

If shock alone is present, there occurs a molecular change in the structure of the retina, but one which is neither macroscopic nor microscopic.

If transudation of fluid from the choroidal vessels occurs (even in small amounts), the delicate retinal elements will be more or less destroyed. Ordinarily, there is no ophthalmoscopic change seen. Vision may never be regained, and, later, an atrophy of the optic nerve will be seen.

Williams further says that in the *traumatic neuroses of globar contusions,* if the injury is severe enough to have the patient admitted to hospital, it seems best to him that he shall be kept quietly in bed, at least one day—just as cerebral concussion cases are handled. Worry over the condition of his eye and the doubt in his mind about the final outcome will often be enough to start true traumatic neuroses. An excellent plea for careful watching of all such accident cases during convalescence has been made by **J.** J. Thomas (*Modern Treatment of Nervous and Mental Diseases,* p. 439). He believes that those who treat contusions of the eye should realize that a great deal can be done to prevent the development of neuroses by the proper care of the patient during the late convalescence. After the healing of his wounds, or after the first shock symptoms have subsided, it is not good practice to discharge the patient and tell him he is fit to resume work. The individual does not always feel cured; he is still nervously weakened, and consequently timid of serious complications which may affect the restoration of his full eyesight. The effect of attempting to resume his duties, especially if they are intellectual, is to increase the remaining symptoms. It frequently confirms the fear he has, perhaps unacknowledged to himself, that he never will be able to use his eye and do good mental work again. This fear sets in motion very frequently the chain of symptoms known as traumatic neuroses. The patient should be kept away from too solicitous friends, who, by frequent allusions to his recent accident, tend to keep active a chain of thought which might lead easily to further neuroses. The patient needs repeated assurances that his injured eye is regaining its normal functions. This will do more than any other one thing to restore his confidence.

TRAUMATIC PSYCHOSES.

Outbreaks of mania and the onset of insanity are occasionally observed after surgical operations, especially those upon the head and eyes. These psychoses usually take the form of hallucinations, are seen in chronic alcoholics, or are due to somatic diseases, or perhaps in some cases to the systemic effects of atropin.

Post-operative mania after cataract extraction is not so uncommon.

While but few cases of psychoses due to ocular accidents have been reported, yet the etiology is similar, and occurs from the fretting and worry of the patient over the pain, or other symptoms, and especially as to the ultimate outcome of the injury, the loss of time and money and the necessary confinement. The long waiting for a cataract to ripen, with the gradual loss of vision and the doubts as to the favorable outcome (in the patient's mind), together with the introspection common to the aged are wanting in the usual run of ocular injuries which generally occur in younger and non-neuropathic individuals.

ERRORS OF REFRACTION PRODUCED BY TRAUMA.

Pressure behind the globe, in the case of traumatic exophthalmos and alterations in the orbital walls from fracture, may produce shortening of the optic axis and hyperopia or irregular pressure astigmia.

Myopic eyes are predisposed to detachment of the retina and intraocular hemorrhages from the weakness of their walls, a slight, direct blow, or the effects of contre coup, being more apt to cause injury than in the case of emmetropic or hyperopic eyes. Temporary myopia from spasm of the accommodation and miosis traumatica may occur. Myopia likewise occurs in commotio retinæ, the cause in each case being perhaps the complete filling of the bloodvessels or bleeding into the ciliary muscle which causes the cramp. These cases are usually acute and disappear after a few days' use of atropin.

The beginnings of traumatic cataract from contusion are characterized by swelling of the lens and temporary increase or production of myopia. See Index myopia.

The effects of wounds of the cornea in the healing by scar tissue may leave regular astigmatism if the wound be clean cut, as in the astigmatism after cataract and glaucoma operations, or if the healing be attended by much loss of tissue, as following ulcerations, irregular astigmatism is produced.

Sympathetic ophthalmitis. Certain forms of traumatism in one eye may induce a disease in the other. Sympathetic ophthalmitis, **or**

ophthalmia, has been long classified as either irritative or inflammatory, and it is of the greatest importance that the clinical difference between the two should be early properly diagnosed in a given case.
Simple irritation quite frequently produces alarming, although
slight, loss of function; while the other is a true inflammation with
exudation, which almost invariably results in blindness, which may
be more complete than that in the originally injured or exciting eye.
See **Sympathetic ophthalmia.**

INJURIES TO THE INTRACRANIAL ORGANS OF VISION.

This subject belongs mostly to the general surgeon although it is
largely treated under **Optic centres, Injuries of the,** and such captions
as **Hemiopia; Brain abscess** and various **Orbit** headings; also under

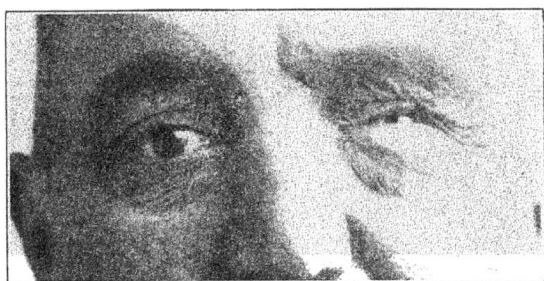

Traumatic Euophthalmos.

Military surgery of the eye. A few instances of the relation between
both direct and indirect injuries of the cerebral optic centres and
vision will suffice here.

A case of revolver bullet lodged in the chiasm is reported by Roy
(*Canadian Med. Assocn. Jour.,* August, 1912). The disturbance of
vision included complete loss of sight of the right·eye, with optic
atrophy. In the left eye there was atrophy of the nasal half of the
disk. The patient could count fingers at 8 inches, and later at 12
inches; and retained a contracted nasal field. Both oculomotor nerves
were paralyzed for a time, but later recovered. X-ray pictures
showed the bullet lodged in the chiasm.

Sulzer and Chappé report the case of a man who fell 15 meters,
causing a fracture of the frontal bone,. and typical bitemporal
hemianopsia, with preservation of good central vision, and without
paralysis of either cranial nerve. The pupillary reaction to light was
lost for the blind half of each retina, but preserved for the nasal

field. The reflex contraction with convergence was lost. They believe that there was fracture of the optic foramen and division of the chiasm.

Meyer saw a man three months after a severe fall, striking on the forehead. In the left eye only a small portion of the peripheral field remained. In the right there was narrowing of the temporal fields for colors, and subsequent contraction of the field with concentric narrowing of the nasal portion, and vision reduced to 1/20. The ophthalmoscope showed in the left eye a complete whitening of the nerve and in the right whitening of the temporal portion. Muskens saw a boy who ten days previously had fallen from a window; and on recovery from coma was found blind and without reaction of the pupils to light.

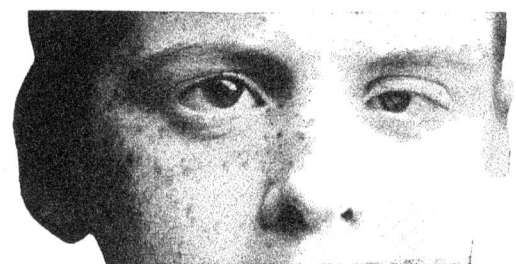

Traumatic Enophthalmos.   Paralysis of the External Rectus.

At the end of a month there was some recovery of vision, but left hemianopsia. A month after that it was stated that he saw as well as other boys. Hemorrhage pressing upon the chiasm was supposed to be the cause of the blindness.—(H. V. W.)

Inné. (F.) Innate; congenital.

Innenglied. (G.) Internal or inner membrane.

Inner canthus.. INTERNAL CANTHUS. The inner commissure of the lids. See **Anatomy of the eye.**

Inner capsule of the eye. In certain *Cephalopoda,* a layer of cartilage between the tapetum and the retina.

Innere Augenentzündung. (G.) An intraocular inflammation. ·

Innere granulirte Sehschicht. (G.) Inner granular layer (of the retina).

Innere Kornerschicht. (G.) Inner nuclear layer.

Innerer Augenwinkel. (G.) The internal canthus.

Innerer gerade Augenmuskel. (G.) The internal rectus muscle.

Inneres Augenlid. (G.) Nictitating membrane.

Inneres Augenlidband. INNERES AUGENWINKELBAND. (G.) The internal tarsal ligament.

Inner-pole magnet. See **Electromagnet.**

Innesto di pezzi di cute. (It.) A skin graft.

Inocular. Inserted in the eyes (said of antennæ).

Inoculation. The insertion of a virus into an abrasion of the skin or other similar wound in order to communicate a disease. Weeks (*Diseases of the Eye*, p. 909), gives directions for inoculating various ocular tissues.

To inoculate the *conjunctival sac* drop an emulsion of the growth to be tested into the conjunctival sac and rub the emulsion into the mucous membrane by means of a sterile glass rod, or small sterile cotton probang, or employ friction through the lid.

To inoculate the *cornea* make a wound in the cornea by means of an infected knife or make a small pocket in the corneal tissue by means of a knife and rub in some of the emulsion of the germ from a platinum loop or needle.

In piercing the fibrous coat of the eye with a needle or knife for the purpose of *inoculating the interior of the eye,* the puncture should be made diagonally so that it will close after the instrument is withdrawn.

To inoculate the anterior chamber. If solid tissue is to be introduced, the eye is cocainized, a small incision is made through the cornea near the scleral margin in the upper-outer quadrant and a drop of cocain is again instilled. The piece of tissue is now pushed through the opening by means of a spatula and carried well into or below the pupillary area. If this is not done the mass is liable to be extruded by the flow of aqueous through the wound. Emulsion or fluids are introduced through the needle of a hypodermic syringe, a portion of the aqueous having first been permitted to escape in order to reduce the intra-ocular tension.

In introducing solids or liquids into the *vitreous chamber for inoculation purposes* the tension of the globe should be reduced after the puncture is made by tapping the anterior chamber (if the puncture were made after the aqueous had escaped the eye would be flaccid). Inoculation is then performed with relative ease.

Inouye, Tatsuya. The most famous of Japanese ophthalmologists. Born in the Province of Awa, Japan, in 1848, the son of a family physician of the feudal lord, and of a family which had been physicians by occupation for eight generations, Tatsuya Inouye was known as an extremely earnest and studious person even in his early boyhood. His medical degree was received at the Tokio University in 1871, when he was only 23 years of age. Five years later he was made ophthalmic assistant at the Tokio University. In 1878 he became a docent, and in 1880 a professor extraordinarius.

Two years later he resigned his professorship and established a private hospital for eye diseases at Surgadai of Tokio, an institution which is still flourishing. In his capacity as surgeon in this institution he acquired an international reputation.

In 1885 he went to Germany, where, for four years, he studied under all the famous masters of the time.

Returning to his native land, he continued to practise until his untimely death, July 10, 1895, when he was only 48 years of age. He left three sons, however, who are still living, and all of whom are noted ophthalmologists practising in Japan.

Regarding the personality of Inouye, we quote the following words of Professor M. Takayasu, of Kanazawa Medical College, Kanazawa, Japan: * ''He was a rather small and thin man, always enthusiastic and nervous, but quite calm at the time of operation. He was generally recognized as rather eccentric, being of very strong will and disinclined to yield even to the noble and rich. He paid but little attention to the etiquette of society in general, and to all such minor matters. He was very kind, but strict, to patients and assistants. He visited the wards of the hospitals every day and even every night, when serious cases were on hand. Of a morning he would begin his work at five o'clock in the summer and at six in the winter, and, after two hours' work, he rode for an hour and then again took up his work. He never accepted any assistance in the examination and treatment of patients. Every evening at seven o'clock he met and asked his assistants what they had learned and studied in the day. There were no holidays in his hospital at any time of the whole year, and he often asked, 'Is there any holiday in disease?' Inasmuch as he was extremely earnest and diligent, he often became angry and scolded patients, when they were not obedient.

''He taught and warned many disciples in his house day and night, and everybody was allowed to ask him at any time about any matter. Several hundred pupils succeeded in their studies, and are attending now their service in Japan. A clinic was held in his hospital, where several thousand people attended. Simplicity was the guiding principle throughout his whole life, but he never hesitated to give away a great deal of money for his beloved science. All the rest of his money

---

* I have given this passage but little editing, because of the excellent English written by Professor Takayasu. For the facts of all this article, furthermore, I am chiefly indebted to Professor Takayasu—though these I was obliged to condense.—(T. II. S.)

he spent for books and instruments, or else for the support of pupils, of whom he always kept a great many living in his house.

"His only interest was reading, and nothing concerning art, exercise and animals interested him, excepting only horses. He believed in Buddhism, and was accustomed to invite the priest to his house for conversation once or twice each month. Even on the street he was always thinking about his special science and nothing else, and sometimes he mixed up the street with house. In Japan it is the well-known custom to take off shoes in buildings and houses. One day Inouye visited a patient, and was found in shoes and with umbrella in hand in the patient's room.

"Absolutely he never regarded the distinctions between different classes of people, and noble and mean were treated quite alike in his house and hospital. A daughter of the prime minister of that time was admitted, and it was the custom of the hospital that every patient to be operated on was obliged to take a bath in the same tub, which was also used for other patients without changing the hot water, just as is the case in the public baths of Japanese towns. But she never had had a bath in such a common tub before, and so she proposed not to bathe in the tub of the hospital, but in another tub. The ophthalmologist soon refused to treat her and commanded her to leave the hospital. An accommodating assistant, however, set secretly a new tub in a room for her, and then told the ophthalmologist that she had finally bathed in the common tub, just as she had been commanded to do. Matters then were satisfactory."

Inouye was an excellent writer, an ingenious inventor of instruments, and a man of much executive ability. The record of his work in all these three capacities is as follows:

A. Books: 1. *Handbook of Ophthalmology.* 2. *Handbook of Ophthalmoscopy.* 3. *Atlas of Background of Eye.* 4. *Hygiene of Eye Diseases.* 5. *Operation for Cataract.* 6. *Operation for Strabismus.*

B. Articles: 1. On Cases in which the Fundus Presents Dark Spots, Caused by Embolism of the Central Retinal Artery. 2. On the Douching Method of the Anterior Chamber. 3. On the Methods for the Incision of the Deformed Sclera Resulting from Staphyloma. 4. Treatment of the Cornea and Conjunctiva after Injuries by Particles of Explosive Powder.

C. Instruments: 1. Cataract knife. 2. Forceps and knife for making the very small pseudo-pupil. 3. Needle for tattooing. 4. Irrigator for the anterior chamber. 5. Knife for corelysis. 6. Keratoscope. 7. Cup for eye bath. 8. Glass chamber for eye operations. 9. Sterilising apparatus.

D. Foundations: In 1889 Inouye founded the first ophthalmologic periodical and also organized the first special ophthalmologic society in Japan.—(T. H. S.)

Insane, General paralysis of the, Ocular signs of. General paresis is rarely accompanied by optic-nerve atrophy; when present it is apt to occur early in the disease. The most important pupillary sign is the absence of the light-reflex. Miosis may be extreme in the early stage, followed in the late stage by mydriasis. There is variable inequality in the size of the pupils. Simple constant inequality is met with in ordinary insanity —(J M R)

Insane root. HEMLOCK. It was once supposed that those who ate hemlock became possessed of remarkable powers of vision. Thus, Greene *(Never Too Late),* ''You have eaten of the roots of hemlock, that makes men's eyes conceit unseen objects.'' The idea was that the drug in question both produced hallucinations and at the same time conferred the power of beholding actual objects which were unseen by others.— (T. H. S.)

Insanity, Ocular relations of. Alterations in the normal fundus picture and other ocular disturbances are so rare as generally to be considered coincident. Visual hallucinations may annoy the patient, while miosis, mydriasis, Argyll Robertson pupils, paradoxic pupils, hippus, deformities of and inequality in the size of the pupils have also been observed.

Insects, Eyes of. The eyes of insects are considered in detail under **Comparative ophthalmology**; it will be sufficient to say at this juncture that they are mostly bilateral, compound eyes, i. e., are composed of a large number of minute eyelets, each, as a rule, exhibiting hexagonal facets set in the surface of the head. These facets number from 20 to several thousand in each composite eye. In some insects these eyes make up almost the entire mass of the head. Their outline is generally spherical, but sometimes kidney-shaped. Rarely, these faceted eyes are composed of a group of ocelli *(Punctaugen),* or of single, bilateral eyes as in Fleas and Lice.

In Crabs, one finds not infrequently punctuated eyes, one to three in number, placed in the median line of the head.

Insexé. (F.) Having no sex or no sexual organs.

Insitio ciliorum. (L.) An old term for an operation for the restoration of the eyelashes to their normal position, and indirectly of the eyelid to its proper shape.

Insolation. Subjection to the influence of the sun's rays; also, exposure of a susceptible substance to sunlight in order to render it phosphorescent.

Inspection, Ocular. See **Examination of the eye.**
Inspection of the eye. See **Examination of the eye.**
Inspection, School, Laws of various lands relating to. See **Legal relations of ophthalmology,** in last third of the section; as well **Conservation of vision.**

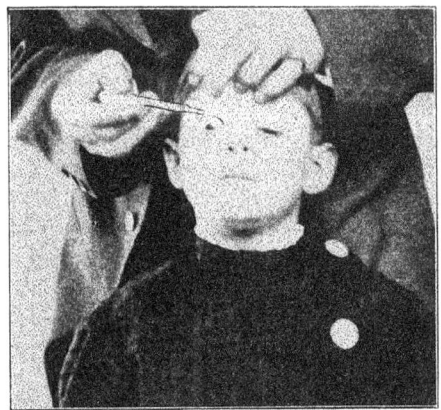

Instilling Drops into the Upper Cul-de-sac.

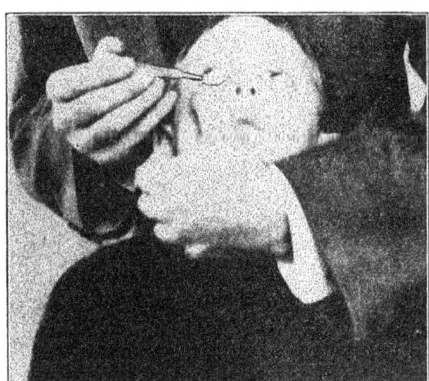

Instilling Drops into the Lower Cul-de-sac.

Inspergation. The application of a fine powder or spray to a surface, as of the eye, by sprinkling or dusting.
In-sphere. An inscribed sphere.
In-square. An inscribed square.

Instantaneous lens. Any lens which, when used with a large aperture, gives a sharply-defined image.

Instantaneous photography. The reproduction, by photographic means, of scenes, etc., too rapid to be distinguished by the eye.

Instantaneous shutter. A mechanical device for rapidly uncovering and covering photographic lenses.

Instilling eye-drops. Dropping various collyria into the conjunctival sac is best accomplished—apart from irrigation—by forming single drops at the end of the dropper and then touching the up-raised edge of the lid with the latter. The pendant drop is then "sucked" beneath the (upper) lid, runs over the upper palpebral conjunctiva, thence into the upper cul-de-sac, over the eyeball and, finally, reaches the lower sulcus and spreads over the conjunctiva of the lower lid. In this way the medicated fluid spreads most effectually over the largest surface of the external eye and is most likely to become absorbed.

The usual method of instillation of drops into the lower sulcus is shown in the figure.

Institutions for the blind. OCCUPATIONS, SCHOOLS AND OTHER FORMS OF INSTRUCTION FOR THE BLIND.

These important subjects will be considered by several writers under the following captions: (A) *European institutions and schools for the blind;* (B) *Institutions and schools for the blind outside of Europe and America;* (C) *American institutions and schools for the blind.*

A. EUROPEAN SCHOOLS, HOSPITALS AND OTHER INSTITUTIONS FOR THE
BLIND.

During ancient and mediæval periods the handicap of the blind was considered as practically insurmountable, and the majority of the sightless remained in an almost imbecile condition. From time to time, there were, of course, exceptional blind persons who emerged from the obscurity of their fellows—but they were few in number. The discovery that the blind can be satisfactorily educated, and can learn to read and write by means of embossed lettering, is of comparatively recent date.

In times past the only occupation open to the blind was that of a beggar, and the sightless appear frequently in that rôle in art and literature.

While there were some asylums for the blind founded prior to modern times, as one in Cappadocia in the fourth century and one in Syria in the fifth century, they were refuges only and contemplated no plan of constructive education. A government hospital for the blind was founded in Paris in 1260 and is still in existence today. From this time on there is record of sporadic efforts to educate blind individuals, but there seem to have been devised no methods of particular merit.

Touch system of reading. The education and training of the blind is so inseparably bound up with the development of the touch system of reading that it is desirable to consider this matter in some detail.

One of the first to conceive the idea of the touch system of reading and education was an Italian physician, Girolamo Cardan (*c.* 1500),

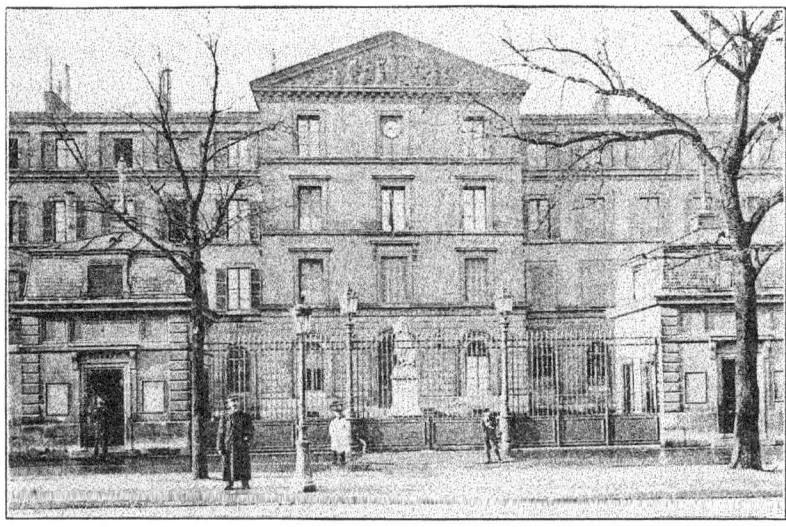

L'Institution.Nationale des Jeunes Aveugles, Paris, France.

who had become interested in the handicapped through his work for the deaf. During the early part of the sixteenth century **F**rancesco Lucas, a Spaniard, devised a plan of engraving letters on blocks of wood for the use of the blind, dedicating the invention to Philip II of Spain. Rampazetto did similar work in Italy. In 1640 Pierre Moreau, a writing master in Paris, cast a movable lead type for the blind, but was forced to abandon the plan being without means to develop it. Pins inserted in cushions were next tried, and large wooden letters. After these came a contrivance of Du Puiseaux, a blind man, who had cast metal letters set in a small frame with a handle.

While these experiments were going on in **France**, R. Weissem-
bourg, a resident of Mannheim, Germany, who lost his sight at the
age of seven, made use of letters cut in cardboard, and later pricked
maps in the same 'medium. By these means he instructed a blind
Austrian lady, Thérèse von Paradis, a talented musician and the
friend of Valentin Haüy.

The subsequent development of types for the blind is well described
by Sir **Francis** Campbell.

''To Haüy belongs the honor of being the first to emboss paper as a
means of reading for the blind; his books were embossed in large

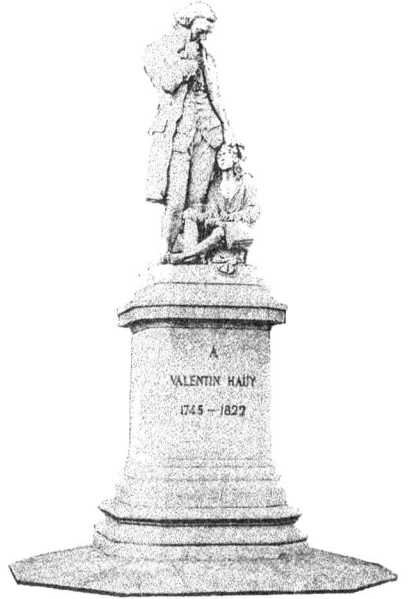

Statue of Valentin Haüy Outside the Institution Nationale des Jeunes Aveugles,
Paris, France.

and small italics, from movable type set by his pupils. The following
is an account of the origin of his discovery. Haüy's first pupil was
François Lesueur, a blind boy whom he found begging at the porch
door of St. Germain de Prés. While Lesueur was sorting the papers
on his teacher's desk, he came across a card strongly indented by the
types in the press. The blind lad showed his master he could decipher
several letters on the card. Immediately Haüy traced with the handle
of his pen some signs on paper. The boy read them, and the result

was printing in relief, the greatest of Haüy's discoveries. In 1821 Lady Elizabeth Lowther brought [to England] embossed books and types from Paris, and with the types her son, Sir Charles Lowther, Bart., printed for his own use the Gospel of St. Matthew.''

Various other efforts in the development of printing for the blind were made in Europe and work was begun in the United States. James Gall of Edinburgh, made great claims for a system which involved the use of regular capital letters with curves eliminated and angles thrown to the outside substituted in their stead; his theory was that the outside contours of the letters were more distinguishable to the touch than the outlines of the inside. His plan, however, seems to have met with little favor though several schools for the blind gave it determined trials. In 1827 Gall did the first printing under his system and in 1834 issued the *Gospel of St. John* in his embossed text. The Society of Arts of Edinburgh in 1832 offered a prize for the best system of embossed printing for the blind. After considerable deliberation Gall's plan was rejected and the award made to Edmond Fry who submitted an alphabet which consisted of capital letters with the smaller strokes omitted. John Alston of Glasgow became the most prominent user of this new system, raising a fund of contributions and securing a government grant to aid the work. In 1838 he issued the New Testament in Fry's type and in 1840 the complete Bible. A little later two stenographic systems of printing were proposed by Lucas and Frere.

The next system which was devised has proven of great value. Its originator was William Moon, himself blind, who promulgated it in 1847. The Moon type as it has since been called, bears a general resemblance to regular capital letters. All unnecessary parts were omitted and some radical changes were made to make the embossed letters easily distinguishable to the touch.

Up to this juncture all the systems proposed had been based on an adherence, more or less close, to existing characters in ink printing or writing. They are all known as line types. An epochal advance was made by the introduction of a point system—that is an alphabet formed by different combinations of embossed points. Charles Barbier, a French army officer, devised a system of speech sounds represented by units embracing twelve positions in which varying numbers of raised dots could occur. The particular sound was determined by the number and location of the dots in the possible positions. Each unit was made up of two vertical rows of six points or positions each. The objection to this system was that the number of dots used was too great to be easily sensed by touch and thus read. But it was reserved for a blind man to create the first alphabet destined to come into general use.

A teacher in the Institution Nationale des Jeunes Aveugles, Louis Braille, in 1834 brought forth an alphabet similar in general principle to that of Barbier but with the number of point positions reduced to six. These positions are arranged in two vertical rows of three points each. This system is now known as European Braille, and with several modifications is the one now used in most of· the institutions on the continent and in England. **See** also **Alphabets and literature for the blind.**

Institutions for the blind. Meanwhile there had been manifested interest in other aspects of the subject. As early as 1646 there appeared a book by an Italian on the condition of the blind, published in Italian and French, the title in the latter language being *L'Aveugle affligé et consolé.* In 1670 a book was written on the instruction of the blind by Lana Terzi, the Jesuit. In 1749 Denis Diderot, the French litterateur, wrote an essay [1] on the lot of the blind which attracted considerable attention and to which frequent reference has since been made. This purported to show how far the intellectual and moral nature of man is modified by blindness, but the heterodox speculations therein contained caused Diderot to be imprisoned for three months in the Bastile. While thus incarcerated he was visited by Rousseau who is reported to have suggested a system of embossed printing.

J. Locke, G. W. Liebnitz, Molineau, and others have discussed the effect of blindness on the human mind.

The development of provision for the blind being a natural concomitant of a higher type of civilization, came first in Europe, the two most important advances being the inauguration of the institutions at Paris and Vienna.

The inception of modern provision for the blind in **France** is effectively described by Sir **Francis** Campbell as follows:

"The degraded state of the masses of the blind in **France** attracted the attention of Valentin Haüy. In 1771, at the annual fair of St. Ovid, in Paris, an innkeeper had a group of blind men attired in a ridiculous manner, decorated with peacock tails, asses' ears, and pasteboard spectacles without glasses, in which condition they gave a burlesque concert, for the profit of their employer. This sad scene was repeated day after day, and greeted with loud laughter by the gaping crowds. Among those who gazed at this outrage to humanity was the

---

[1] *Lettre sur les aveugles à l'usage de ceux qui voient.*

philanthropist Valentin Haüy, who left the disgraceful scene full of sorrow. 'Yes,' he said to himself, 'I will substitute truth for this mocking parody. I will make the blind to read, and they shall be enabled to execute harmonious music.' Haüy collected all the information he could gain respecting the blind, and began teaching a blind boy who had gained his living by begging at a church door. Encouraged by the success of his pupil, Haüy collected other blind persons, and in 1785 founded in Paris the first school for the blind (Institution Nationale des Jennes Avengles), and commenced the first printing in raised characters. In 1786, before Louis XVI and his court at Versailles, he exhibited the attainments of his pupils in reading, writing, arithmetic, geography and music, and in the same year published an account of his methods, entitled *Essai sur l'éducation des aveugles*. As the novelty wore off, contributions almost came to an end, and the Blind School must have ceased to exist had it not been taken, in 1791, under the protection of the state.

"The emperor of Russia, and later the dowager empress, having learned of Haüy's work, invited him to visit St. Petersburg for the purpose of establishing a similar institution in the Russian capital. On his journey Haüy was invited by the king of Prussia to Charlottenburg. He took part in the deliberations of the Academy of Sciences in Berlin, and as a result a school was founded there."

With this introduction we may pass to a description of the situation in individual countries.

AUSTRIA.

The blind Thérèse von Paradis, an Austrian lady whose accomplishments impressed Valentin Haüy, also influenced her compatriot Johann Wilhelm von Klein to make positive efforts to ameliorate the lot of the blind. It is said that Klein was not acquainted with Haüy's work and methods, but acted solely upon his own initiative and plan. An institution was founded in 1816, the state taking it under public auspices, and placing Klein at its head.

Under Klein's influence there were also founded other European institutions, particularly those at Munich, Breslau, and Zürich.

The institutions for the blind in Austria in chronological order of their foundation are as follows: Vienna, Imperial Institution for the Education of the Blind, 1804; Prague, private institution, 1808; Linz, private institution, 1824; Vienna, asylum and occupational institution for adults, 1828; Prague, Klar's institution for the blind, 1832; Brünn, 1845; Lemberg, Galician institute for the education of the blind, 1851; Vienna-Hohe-Warte, Jewish institution for the blind, 1872; Purkersdorf near Vienna, 1873; Graz, school and asylum, 1881; Linz, work-shop and asylum for women, 1883; Vienna-Neulerchenfeld, school, 1884; Vienna-Hernals, asylum for blind children before school-age, 1885; Prague, "Francisco-Jerefinum," an asylum for the blind who are able to support themselves and for mental defectives, 1893; Linz, work-shop and asylum for men, 1893; Brünn, home for girls, 1895; Wien-Hütteldorf, for girls, 1895; Wien-Breitensee, home for men, 1896; Kla-genfurt (Kärnten), 1898. There has also been projected a new plant in the country outside of Prague, for the Klar School for the Blind and its kindergarten.

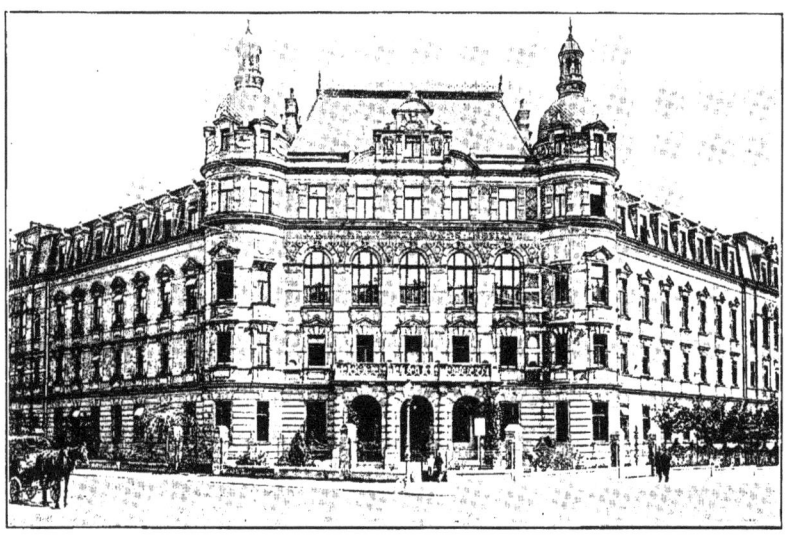

Imperial Institution for the Blind, Vienna, Austria.

According to a description by Dr. Alexander Mell, director of the Imperial Institution at Vienna, some of these institutions devote their efforts more particularly to the instruction of the blind, others rather to the care of the blind after graduation, although all institutions share to some extent in the latter work. Especial attention is paid to the fate of women after graduation. The Imperial institution in Vienna has a library of 2,500 volumes partly written and partly printed in Braille. Throughout Austria, music takes second place as a subject of instruction, the major emphasis being placed on manual arts. Of these the most widely taught are broom and basket making and the manu-facture of wicker furniture.

The Imperial Institution in Vienna had its press completely re-fitted for the Braille printing in 1890. It is said that 80 p. c. of the books it produces go abroad.

The institutions follow in general the same tendencies as the German ones, which are described further on in some detail (*vide infra*). They are covered also by the critical remarks cited with reference to the German institutions. Taken in connection with these it may be said that a little more attention is paid to the esthetic and individual factors. The following reply of a director of an Austrian institution

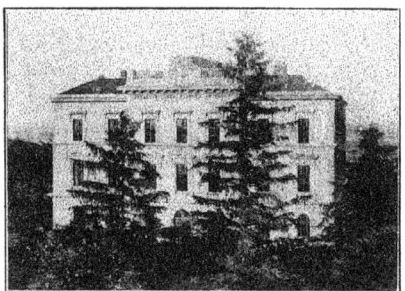

Jewish Institute for the Blind, Vienna, Austria.

to a comment upon the greater care he bestowed on the personal appearance of his pupils is illuminating:

"Yes, some of my fellow-directors, especially from Germany, have often blamed me for this, and called it an unwise and unwarranted luxury. We in Austria, in spite of the fact that money is less plenty here, do not commonly carry expediency so far; for example, we do not generally centralize our local efforts for the blind under one management and within one enclosure, preferring to classify and scatter them even in the same city. Perhaps this is less businesslike, and there is doubtless less harmony among our institution heads; but the blind benefit."

Regarding other features reference should be made to the section dealing with conditions in Germany.

BELGIUM.

In Belgium according to the census of 1906 there were 3,076 persons totally blind, or 434 blind persons per million of population.

Most institutions for the blind in Belgium are combined with institutions for deaf mutes and are conducted by religious organizations.

The institutions are: Bruges, founded in 1836 by Canonicus Carlton; the number of inmates in 1896 was 31 boys and 26 girls. Brussels, founded in 1819 and another institution in 1839 by Canonicus Triest; the first took care in 1897 of 56 boys, the second of 56 girls. Ghlin-les-Mous, an institute for blind children founded by B. Limonou (blind) in Namur in 1876, from where it was moved to Ghlin-les-Mous in 1884; this is the only institution for the blind in Belgium which is not connected with one for deaf mutes. Liège, founded in 1819 as an institution for the deaf; a section for the blind was opened in 1837; in 1896 the number of inmates was 29, 15 boys and 14 girls. Maeseyk, founded in 1840 by Abbé Y. A. Polus. All institutions for the blind in Belgium are recognized by the state, and poor pupils are provided for by the state or the provincial authorities. Braille is used and a variant of it introduced by Abbé Carlton which is probably restricted in its use to Bruges, the home of the inventor. A peculiar flat script is also used which is based on Latin *italics*. Hockman's script, in which Latin capitals are represented by a series of points and which has the advantage of being intelligible to the blind writer, is hard to produce, and therefore it is little known outside of Belgium. The Fédération des Aveugles Belges is an organization founded in 1886 by the blind graduates of the Woluwe Institute. They offer assistance to the blind in cases of disease and unemployment.

DENMARK.

In 1901 there were in Denmark, 1,047 blind, 427 to the million of population.

The most prominent organization in Denmark for the care of the blind is the one called "Die Kette" (the Chain), a society which founded an institution for the blind on June 1, 1811, and opened it in Copenhagen on June 10, 1811, with 12 inmates. In 1881 the number of inmates had risen to 100. When in 1862 a society for the promotion of self-support by the blind was founded, the Copenhagen institution closed its doors to all but women (1865). In 1861 "Die Kette" founded a home and preparatory school for blind children, and the first graduate of the new school became a teacher in it. The society also assists the blind (especially women) outside the institution as well as persons who have to undergo ophthalmic operations.

The society founded in 1862 assists graduates of the institution, takes care of cases of late blindness, sickness and old age, sells the products of blind workshops and supplies them with raw materials, and attempts to secure employment for the blind in public workshops.

According to the census of 1901 France had among her population 27,174 blind, or 698 per million. To make provision for some of these, there are about thirty institutions.

In Paris there are four institutions for the blind; the National Institute for the Young Blind (founded 1874); the Braille School (founded 1883); the Home of the Blind Sisters of St. Paul (1852); and the Institute of the Brothers of St. Jean de Dieu (1875). The National Institute is controlled by the Ministry of the Interior, and pro-

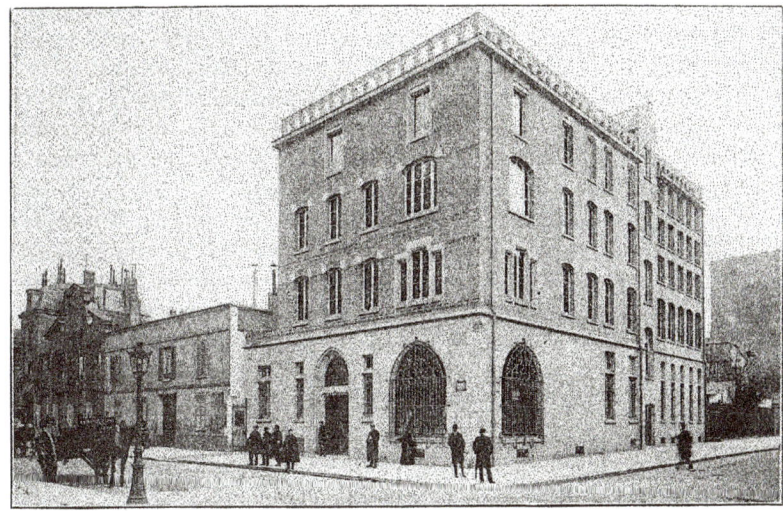

The Association Valentin Haüy, Paris, France. An organization to promote the general interests and welfare of the blind.

vides for 150 boys and 80 girls. It has achieved signal successes in musical training, many of its pupils having won medals in conservatory competitions, while others have become piano merchants in the provinces. The Institute runs its own printing press and boasts a library of 100,000 volumes. The Braille School devotes itself mainly to training in the manual arts. The St. Paul Home devotes itself to the education of young girls along intellectual, musical and industrial lines. Since 1879 two public schools of Paris have been offering special courses by two blind teachers in music and piano tuning.

In addition to these institutions France has over twenty schools in the provinces. Of these three are for boys only (Ronchin-Lille, Bordeaux and Nantes); six are for girls only (Lille, Larmay, Alençon, two at Lyon and Laon); and ten are for both sexes (Amiens, Angers, Arras, Bison, Clermont-Ferrand, Limoges, Marseilles, Montpellier, Nancy and Toulouse.) We also find six associations for the welfare of the blind; three industrial schools; seven workshops, of which four are independent and three combined with schools; one asylum and eight organizations for the assistance to the blind. Of the seven institutions for the welfare of the blind founded in the Middle Ages only one survives, the so-called Quinze-Vingts, which since 1779 has become a general hospital. It is self-supporting but co-operates with the Ministry of the Interior. In it reside three hundred blind of both sexes, married and single. They must be at least forty years old. About 1,800 blind outside of the institution receive yearly subsidies of from 100 to 200 francs from the funds of the institution.

There are in French over 600 works printed in Braille, which are read by more than 800 school children, by more than 600 self-supporting adults, and by some 1,000 blind cared for in homes and asylums. In all, some 3,000 blind read Braille.

The main organization for the care of the blind in France is the "Valentin Haüy" Society, founded in 1889 by Maurice de la Sizeranne. The society publishes three journals devoted to the interests of the blind in France; it maintains a museum of articles and appliances relating to the care of the blind; a large library; a school of broom-making; a workshop in which paper-bags are made; a dressmaking shop; and a savings-bank.

In the history of the education of the blind in France may be observed a gradual decline of the manual arts and the ascendency of music. The Braille school alone persists in its devotion to the manual arts. It keeps its workers for life and provides them with work. They must all be former pupils of the school, must be residents of the Department of the Seine and at entrance be less than thirteen years old. They live in houses belonging to the school and receive salaries proportionate to the amount and quality of the work done. All the work is done under the direct supervision of foremen (not blind). Moreover while the more mechanical and simple tasks are performed by the blind, the finishing stages of the work are in the hands of workmen who are not blind.

GERMANY.

The first institution for the relief of the blind in Germany was founded in Berlin in 1806 at the instance of Frederick William III, who had become impressed with the achievements of Haüy with his pupil, Fournier. At the present time there are about 35 educational institutions and 26 workshops and homes. According to Frederick Rose, the annual income of these organizations is derived approximately as follows: From states, provinces, and communes, $350,000; From private sources, $300,000. Of the 35 educational institutions, 24 are public in character (state, province, or municipality) and 11 private (religious, endowed, etc.). Eight of the public institutions are conducted by the states; namely those at Steglitz, Dresden, Munich, Ilvesheim, Weimar, Neukloster, Friedberg, and Braunschweig. And of these only those at Steglitz and Neukloster were originally founded by the states. The institutions in question provide in all for about 13,000 blind pupils.

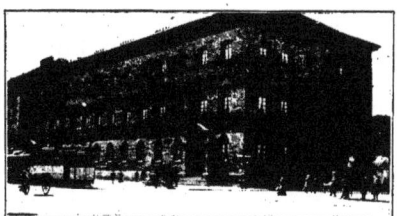

Institution for the Blind, Munich, Germany.

Children ordinarily leave the school division to enter the workshops between the ages of twelve and sixteen. Some trade instruction is given during the school period and some continuation work in ordinary school subjects is given during the trade instruction period.

In addition to instruction in the ordinary elementary and industrial subjects, much attention is devoted to physical exercises and music, especially singing, the latter less for purposes of self-support than for recreation and pleasure.

In Saxony a special follow-up system to care for the blind after they leave the institution, and to provide for industrial activity and sales of goods has been in operation for some time. It is known as the Saxony system, and is described as follows by Director Büttner, of the Dresden institution:

"When twenty years of age, the blind are usually discharged from the institution. Long experience has taught us that the care and supervision of the blind after their discharge from the institution are quite as important as their education and training in the institution. It would, in our opinion, be unjust to remove them from their sad surroundings, educate and accustom them to higher wants, and then allow them to sink backward into their former miserable way of life. After much deliberation it was decided to remain in connection with the discharged blind, to visit them in their places of abode, to learn their wants, to study the difficulties which they experienced in supporting themselves independently, and, as far as possible, to remove their grievances. Director Georgi began this work in 1843. Director Reinhard continued it from 1867 to 1879, and the present director has followed the same path. With the knowledge of these difficulties the *Fürsorge* (care) for discharged blind has steadily advanced, and has won the confidence of the Saxon people. It was decided that, on the discharge of the blind person, the director should select a trustworthy person, residing in his future place of abode, to give him advice and practical help, to protect him from imposition; and to keep up communication with the director. If this guardian is unable to advise or help, he then writes to the director, who, if necessary, comes to the place, and this is all the easier as he travels free on all railways in Saxony. The result of these visits, as well as all communication from the guardian, the letters from the blind person, and every document relating to him, are entered in a register kept at the institution. These guardians are respectable, benevolent, practical men, capable of procuring work for their wards. But there was no doubt that, in spite of these arrangements, the discharged blind were unable to support themselves without the assistance of capital, whether in money or outfit. The blind man can do as good work as the man who can see; but as a rule he does not work so quickly and if the man who is not blind has to use every exertion to support himself and his family, the blind man to do the same requires some special help, without which he will either not be able to compete, or will have to lead a life of great privation.

"The first difficulty when a blind pupil is starting in life is to provide himself with the necessary tools and material. These the institution supplies to him, and continues through life to afford him moral and material help; and by this means the greater part, of the blind are enabled to save money for sickness and old age. Those who cannot return to their relations cannot at once meet all their expenses, and the weak and old need special help. A part of the money for their board and lodging is paid for those who have to be settled in other places on account of the death or untrustworthiness of their relatives.

"The fund for the discharged blind is administered by the director of the institution. The number of those assisted amounts at present to about 400, who live respectably in all parts of Saxony, are almost self-supporting, and feel themselves free men. For, just as a son does not feel galled by a gift from his father, so they are not ashamed to receive assistance from their second paternal home, the institution.''

With regard to the results of the ''Saxony System'' as regards industrial features, it seems that the utility is most apparent in districts densely populated. It is not so successful in the country, owing to the distance to which the goods have to be conveyed and the difficulty of finding customers.

From the benefits of the fund for the assistance of the blind in Saxony, the following are specifically excluded: blind beggars, blind organ players, blind girls who marry, and blind men who marry blind women. The fund was founded in 1843 with a small gift and now amounts to over $400,000.

In Prussia the instruction and care of the blind are not undertaken directly by the state but by the provincial governments. The provincial administrative districts either possess their own institutes or enter into contract with private institutes for the boarding, lodging, training and employment of blind persons at so much per capita per annum. For example, the private institution at Königsberg receives from the provincial authorities $150 annually for blind persons over 15 years of age and $100 for those under 15. In the Rhine provinces, the instruction is divided into preparatory, ordinary, and continuation classes. The trade instruction includes rope-making, brush and basket making, cane-plaiting, mat, cord, shoe, and bee-hive making, piano tuning, typewriting, piano, and organ playing. Brush and basket making are the most remunerative. The annual expenditure per blind person amounts to $140. Of this sum $100 is estimated for board and lodging, $25 for instruction, and $15 for clothes. In the majority of cases the blind are boarded, lodged, and instructed free of cost, or partially so. The annual income of the Düren institution (185 boys and girls) is $28,000, that of the Neuwied institution (85 boys and girls) is $17,200.

The majority of pupils in the institutions are able to maintain themselves after they complete the course or leave the institution. Many are able to pass the journeyman's examination and test, and this has been instrumental in dissipating much of the prejudice attaching to work performed by the blind. Some of those who have been trained in music pass the examination for organist and obtain positions in churches.

All institutions for the blind in Germany, whether provincial, municipal, or private, Protestant or Catholic, are subject to state

inspection. All entrance and graduation regulations, the appointment of principals, plans of instruction, and details of internal organization must be sanctioned by the state authorities. In Prussia
these duties have been delegated to the provincial educational authorities with the right of appeal to the State Minister of Education.
In Saxony the functions are performed by the Ministry of the Interior.

As has been mentioned, the majority of German institutions for
the blind owe their foundation to private persons or societies. A
few, notably those at Breslau, Halle, and Stettin, were founded by
blind persons. But a very large number are now managed by the
public authorities or receive subsidies from these sources. This has
been instrumental in improving the methods and extent of the instruction and the quality of the equipment. It also increased the number
of blind children under instruction from 744 in 1878 to 1,340 in
1893. But in spite of all the efforts undertaken on behalf of the
blind, it was calculated that in 1900 there were still about 1,000 blind
persons between the ages of 5 and 20 lacking suitable instruction.

There has thus grown up a movement in favor of compulsory
attendance of blind children at educational institutions until they
become proficient in some occupation. The congress for the blind
held in Munich in 1895 passed a resolution calling upon all the
German states to introduce compulsory trade instruction for the blind
and to furnish suitable buildings supported by public funds. The
states of Saxony, Brunswick and Baden have already enacted such
laws. A similar bill was introduced in Prussia in 1892 but was later
withdrawn. It appears, however, that paragraph 1666 of the new
German civil code provides sufficient powers for the purpose in question. As far as Prussia is concerned, this paragraph is supported
by a clause in the Act of 1900 relating to the welfare of children
under 18 years of age. The movement for compulsory and adequate
training of the blind is furthered by the fact that 97 p. c. of the
youthful blind in Germany belong to very poor families. The existing
compulsory educational requirements, however, seem rather ineffective
because compulsory *institutional* attendance is a different matter, and
the latter is but little enforced.

The industrial features of provision for the blind in Germany have
been described first because greater importance is attached to that
branch of the work. With regard to primary education along standard lines, progress in modern methods dates from 1870. Up to that
time even reading and writing were almost completely neglected.
Now all German institutions use an eight-volume reader, and many of
them maintain extensive libraries. Almost all printing is done in

Braille (Voll und Kurz-Schrift). To diminish the size of the volumes, at first, both sides of the pages were printed upon; later the *Zwischendruck* was introduced. In their communication with the seeing the blind use the *Blauschrift* of Nebold as well as Klein's *Stacheltypenapparat* improved by Mell. Typewriters are in common use.

In 1870 the entrance age of all state institutions was 9-10 years, but this has since been reduced to 5-6 years.

In addition to the regular elementary instruction, which varies from two to seven grades, some institutions provide advanced courses for especially able pupils. There are also special classes for backward children.

Tactile instruction with various objects has reached a high degree of efficiency and most of the institutions are well provided with material. According to Edward E. Allen: "In every school there is a profusion of objects for instruction. No American school can show anything like such an array. These are not so much the expensive, stuffed specimens we are apt to think of as belonging to a school museum as they are common, every-day articles which children with sight see at one time or another and understand. There are the manifold objects for nature study, minerals, nuts and seeds, and native birds, not those of foreign countries; and the somewhat elaborate school productions, partly of former pupils, partly of teachers, representing in miniature (nearly all of them dissectible) such things as a coal or a salt mine, a church and steeple, a tannery, a mole's nest, an electric street car, and, floor by floor, the institution itself."

Practically all the schools are resident ones, continental conviction being that the blind require institutional life and schooling. In Berlin, however, there is a non-resident school for blind children, much like the classes in such wide operation in England and the United States. It is operated in conjunction with a school for orphan girls and these latter pupils conduct the blind children, either on street cars or otherwise, to and from the school.

Throughout the article critical comment has, in general, been refrained from. There is available, however, on the German and Austrian work, such a valuable *kritik* by a competent authority, Edward E. Allen, that it may be of value to quote from it certain passages. He points out that European institutions for the blind will be found to be "little school and big workshop; often to embrace also a boarding home for blind men, either learners or regular workers in the shop, a living home for blind women ditto, and occasionally even a retreat for the aged and infirm—a *Blindenfeierabendheim*, as the Germans very beautifully call the latter. Now the gathering together in one inclosure of all these departments, excellent though each is by itself, is what astonishes and perhaps shocks the American whose conviction is that children are children, adults adults, invalids invalids, and that neither blindness nor deafness nor any other physical defect should throw them into one community, even though they are more or less isolated from one another, school children, adult workers, and the invalid aged.''

With regard to the character of training with reference to the later career of the blind, ''In Germany,'' Mr. Allen says, ''the whole matter has been thought over, worked over, and settled once for all, and this conclusion reached: that blindness incapacitates one for earning his living; that it is folly as well as cruelty to expect the

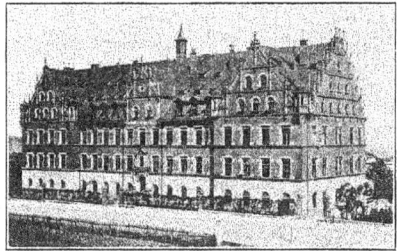

Institution for the Blind at Nuremburg, Germany.

blind to get on in the world of competition without special aid; hence they must be spared the effort and the mortification of attempting it. The blind are therefore no problem, as are the insane, and any excess of expenditure must go to the latter. One director told me that the blind should certainly not receive pure charity for nothing, but should be trained to receive it for something. This man, who is an extremist, not only believes but carries out his belief that all blind children of his community should be gathered into the institution, schooled and trained to the maximum efficiency in some trade, and be given regular employment at it within the institution throughout their whole working life, and thereafter be kept on there in comfort until they die—a living illustration, this, of the completed system of caring for the blind from the cradle to the grave. Perhaps as they grow older they enjoy seeing ahead of them increased doles of tobacco, snuff, and beer. Most Germans, however, go on the principle that the blind should be trained to leave the institution in early adult life, but because they cannot take care of themselves, even though skilled, industrious, and businesslike, the institution must keep in touch with them always, and aid them as a parent would its children. It is settled that a few stock trades supply the best and most nearly self-sustaining occupations for the blind. Hence it is that the institutions seem to be mainly workshops—shops for beginners, for adult apprentices, and for skilled workmen. But such shops, with such industry, such results, we American school-men, with our industrial departments, never see at home. Our product is usually but incidental to instruction; the European is the real thing, and will stand competition. The instructors themselves are skilled artisans, real masters of handicraft, and are always men with sight. They are conscious of teaching the only practical subject of the school, and of being the chief agents of the effectiveness of the institution. To be sure, the girls are taught sewing and other women's handiwork, but only as a useful side issue.''

In a general summary, Mr. Allen states that methods are not as yet wholly settled and that the various directors were of different

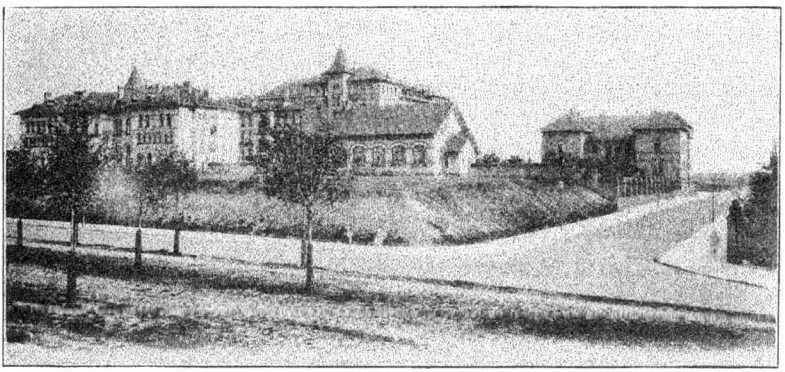

Provincial Institute for the Blind, Halle, a. S., Germany.

minds on many questions. ''I found the general tendency was towards either small institutions or the division of large ones into small groups for living and working; the building or rebuilding, according to the pavilion plan, of small, separate houses; and the expenditure of a good deal of money for beautiful structures and grounds, not omitting attention to decorations and to modern sanitary and hygienic conditions. I was surprised to find compulsory school attendance generally inapplicable to the blind—surprised to see expediency in dress and personal appearance so strongly and barely economical, and this part of the pupil's care so often left to servants, and morning prayers so perfunctorily carried out in Protestant communities; surprised to perceive the institutions so much more workshops than schools, even the school life from the beginning being directed to a studied end; and the potent subject of music relegated to the province of mere pleasurable resource and publicity. I was not prepared to find co-education everywhere; nearly all the teachers men; no official, not even the director, receiving his living at the institution. I was profoundly impressed with the thoroughness of the teaching and the abundance of the equipment for object teaching and sense perception lessons, but disappointed at discovering no enterprise in sports and athletics. The whole tendency seemed to be more quieting than stimulating a schooling of the blind for contentment with their lowly lot.''

The principal institutions for the blind in Germany, together with the dates of their foundation are located as follows: *Baden:* Freiburg, 1837 (started as a private institution in 1826), workshop and school; Ilvesheim, 1868, school. *Bavaria:* Augsburg, 1889, school and workshop; Munich, 1826, school and workshop; Neuhausen, 1893, home for girls; Nuremberg, 1854, school, asylum, and workshop; 1884, society for the support of the blind; Würzburg, 1854, school and workshop; 1866, asylum; Ursberg-Pfaffenhausen, 1894, school and workshop. *Braunschweig:* Braunschweig, 1829 (revived in 1894 as state institution), workshop and school; 1884, asylum. *Bremen:* 1855 (institution not fully organized before 1896). *Alsace-Lorraine:* Illzach, 1857, school and workshop; Still, 1895, workshop, school and asylum. *Hamburg:* 1830, school and workshop, from which a special school of music and languages branched off in 1835. *Hesse:* Friedberg, 1850, school, workshop, and asylum. *Mecklenburg-Schwerin:* Neukloster, 1864, workshop, asylum, and school. *Prussia:* Berlin, 1806, later transferred to Steglitz; 1878, school; 1852, school for adults; 1860, Moon's Society for the Blind; 1877, society for the promotion of self-support among the blind; 1874, general society for the blind; 1883, society for promoting the interests of the blind. Hanover, 1843, school and workshop; 1891, society for the blind; Frankfort, 1837, school and workshop; Wiesbaden, 1861, school and workshop; 1846, school and workshop; New-Torney, 1850, school for boys; 1857, division for girls. *Rhine Provinces:* The Society for the Blind of the Rhine Province has branches and institutions in Aachen, Barmen, Birkesdorf, Crefeld, Düren (2), Ehrenfeld, and Elberfeld. There are also institutions at Neuwied and Rheydt. Cologne, 1887, workshop; Barby, 1896, workshop and school; Halle, 1833, workshop and school; 1853, society for the support of adult blind. There are minor organizations for the blind at Apenrade, Eiderstede, Kellinghusen, Kiel (2), Paderborn, Soest, and Königsthal. *Saxony:*

Dresden, 1809, school and workshop; Konigswartha; Leipzig, 1865, school and workshop; 1895, society for the blind; Moritzburg, two preparatory schools. *Saxe-Coburg-Gotha:* 2 institutions at Gotha. *Saxe-Weimar:* Weimar, 1858, school and workshop. *Württemberg:* Schwäbisch-Gmund, 1832, school and workshop; Heiligenbronn, 1860, workshop; Lustnau, 1865, workshop; Stuttgart, 1830, school and workshop.

GREAT BRITAIN.

The relative number of the blind in Great Britain is decreasing, according to official data. In England and Wales the number of persons enumerated as afflicted with blindness in 1901 was 25,317. The decrease from one census period to another is set forth as follows:

Year	Number of Blind	Blind per Million of Population	Persons Living to One Blind Person
1851	18,306	1,021	979
1861	19,352	964	1,037
1871	21,590	951	1,052
1881	22,832	879	1,138
1891	23,467	809	1,236
1901	25,317	778	1,285

The first institution for the blind in Great Britain was founded in 1791 through the efforts of Edward Rushton, himself blind. This was the Liverpool School for the Indigent Blind. In 1790 Rushton suggested to the literary and philosophical society of which he was a member, the establishment of a benefit club for the indigent blind. Bringing the matter to the attention of his friend, J. Christie, a blind musician, the latter thought the plan should also provide for the education of young blind persons. Through circulating letters and enlisting the assistance of others interested, the proposal was brought to fruition. Thomas Blacklock of Edinburgh, a blind scholar and poet, then translated Haüy's work on the *Education of the Blind.* He succeeded in interesting others in the subject and after his death there was established the Edinburgh Asylum for the Relief of the Indigent and Industrious Blind (1793). The order of establishment of institutions in Great Britain was as follows:

School for the Indigent Blind, Liverpool....................1791
Royal Blind Asylum, Edinburgh...........................1793
Bristol Asylum...1793

School for the Indigent Blind, Southwark (now removed to
  Leatherhead) 1799
Norwich Asylum and School................................1805
Richmond Asylum, Dublin..................................1810
Aberdeen Asylum..1812
Molyneux Asylum, Dublin..................................1815
Glasgow Asylum and School................................1827
Belfast School...1831
Wilberforce School, York.................................1833
Limerick Asylum..1004
London Society for Teaching the Blind to Read, St. John's
  Wood N 1838
Royal Victoria School for the Blind, Newcastle-on-Tyne........1838
West of England Institute for the Blind, Exeter..............1838
Henshaw's Blind Asylum, Manchester.......................1839
County and City of Cork Asylum...........................1840
Catholic Asylum, Liverpool...............................1841
Brighton Asylum..1842
Midland Institute for the Blind, Nottingham................1843
General Institute for the Blind, Birmingham................1848
Macan Asylum, Armagh 1854
St. Joseph's Asylum, Dublin..............................1858
St. Mary's Asylum, Dublin................................1858
Institute for the Blind, Devonport.......................1860
South Devon and Cornwall Institute for the Blind, Plymouth...1860
School for the Blind, Southsea............................1864
Institute for the Blind, Dundee..........................1865
South Wales Institute for the Blind, Swansea................1865
School for the Blind, Leeds..............................1866
College for the Sons of Gentlemen, Worcester...............1866
Northern Counties Institute for the Blind, Inverness..........1866
Royal Normal College and Academy of Music for the Blind, Upper
  Norwood 1872
School for the Blind, Sheffield..........................1879
Barclay Home and School for Blind Girls, Brighton............1893
Homes for Blind Children, Preston........................1895
North Stafford School, Stoke-on-Trent....................1897

Many of the early institutions were asylums. With nearly all
the present day schools for the blind workshops have been connected.
In 1856 Miss Gilbert, the blind daughter of the Bishop of Chichester,
established a workshop in Berners Street, London, and since that
date workshops have been started in many of the provincial towns.

A great advance in provision for the blind followed upon the appointment in 1886 of a royal commission on the blind and deaf, which, after taking much authoritative evidence, issued a valuable and instructive report. Following the practical recommendations of the commission there was enacted the Elementary Education (Blind and Deaf Children) Act, 1893, under which the education of the blind became for the first time compulsory. The local school authorities were made responsible for the provision of suitable elementary education for blind children below the age of sixteen, and annual grants of £3, 3s. for elementary subjects, and of £2, 2s. for industrial training, were contributed by the National Education Department to the local school boards towards the cost of educating such children. As a result of this Act there are day-classes for blind children in the public schools of almost every city of reasonable size.

England and Wales. The statistics for this division of the United Kingdom have already been given. In 1907 according to Sir Francis Campbell there were twenty-four resident schools and forty-three workshops for the blind in addition to the day classes for blind children maintained by the public school authorities in almost every city of reasonable size. At the same time there were forty-six home teaching societies. All of these societies lend books in tactile print and a good many public libraries make similar provision.

The British and Foreign Blind Association is one of the largest organizations for promoting the interests of the blind, through education, employment, and the distribution of books. The International Lending Library in London sends embossed books to all parts of the Kingdom. There are also fourteen magazines published in embossed type. There are thirty-six pension societies. The Gardner Trust is a large foundation with a purpose of instructing the blind in music, trades, and professions; it also makes grants for special purposes.

Scotland. According to the census of 1901 Scotland had 3,253 (or 727 per million) blind persons. A unique feature of work for the blind in Scotland is the Outdoor Mission. Twenty-four missionaries or teachers are employed in addition to a large number of volunteers and the blind are visited throughout all of Scotland. There are several societies with a view of providing work for the blind. There are five schools for blind children and connected with these are workshops for adults.

Ireland. By the census of 1901 there were in Ireland 4,253 totally blind persons, a proportion of 954 per million. Of these 2,430 were over 60 years of age and 11 over 100. These figures do not include the partially blind who numbered 1,217. The large number of aged blind persons is probably to be explained by an ophthalmic epidemic which occurred during the Irish Famine. The following table sets forth the number of blind in age-groups in 1901:

Age-Period	Number	Age-Period	Number
Under 5 years	10	50-55	392
5-10	38	55-60	314
10-15	64	60-65	617
15-20	73	65-70	000
20-25	95	70-75	540
25-30	116	75-80	306
30-35	146	80-85	372
35-40	146	85-90	118
40-45	205	95 and upwards	95
45-50	224		

There are twelve institutions and a home mission and home teaching society. Nine of the institutions are, unfortunately, asylums, that form of provision having been largely adopted in Ireland. The scarcity of manufacturing industries entails a scarcity of work adapted to the abilities of the blind.

HOLLAND.

In 1907 there were 2,710 blind in the Netherlands, or 462 per million of population. The care of the blind in Holland dates from 1806 when four men resident in Amsterdam approached Daniel Fürst of Copenhagen, a teacher with Valentin Haüy, and asked him for information on the present status of instruction of the blind. William Holtrop, a Freemason, took especial interest in the matter and persuaded a number of masonic lodges to co-operate. Thus it came about that on November 13, 1808, a school was opened in Amsterdam with three pupils. In 1810 ten pupils were admitted to the examinations. In 1823 the institution erected its own house, which in time proved too small for its various activities, and in 1883 a large structure was erected for its use. Since then nearly a thousand boys and girls have been educated in the institution. The entrance age is six or more, and the pupils leave at nineteen. Braille and other systems are used, as well as typewriting machines. Music is taught, this including tuning, harmony and composition. The manual arts suitable for the blind are taught, also sewing by sewing machines. The present number of inmates is seventy.

In 1843 an institution was founded in Amsterdam for adult blind. It was used at first as an asylum, but later opened its doors to unemployed young men until they succeed in securing positions. There is also a workshop for adult blind, married or single, of both sexes; about 150 blind are brought to the shop daily for the working hours from 8 A. M. to 4 P. M.

Other similar institutions were established in Rotterdam, the Hague, Utrecht and Middelburg. Among them is an institution supported by the ''St. Heinrich's'' Fund. The Prince Alexander Fund is devoted to training the blind for the main Amsterdam institution. A kindergarten is organized, and parents are advised as to the proper way of handling their blind children. The age of admission is from 3 to 9 years. The 'Verein zur Verbesserung des Loses der Blinden' has 430 members. It provides that the children of indigent blind are taken care of in institutions, furnishes them with clothing and so forth. Branches of the 'Verein' have been opened in other towns in Holland and in the colonies. The Union of the Blind of Holland is an organization for mutual assistance with a membership of about one hundred. Since 1893 the Amsterdam institution has published a bimonthly, *The Friend of the Blind,* in Braille, which is sent free to all the blind in Holland. The Braille-Library of the Netherlands was founded in 1901 at the initiative of G. T. Kolff and his sister. It contains over 2,000 volumes. There is also another smaller library at the educational institution in Amsterdam.

ITALY.

According to the census of 1901 there were in Italy 38,160 blind, or 1,175 per million of population.

The first institution for the blind in Italy was established at Naples in 1818 at the initiative of King Ferdinand I. It was in the form of a hospital, 'St. Giuseppe e Lucia,' which formed part of the King's poor-house. The next one to open was in Padua (1838), then one in Milan (1840). The next after that was not opened until 1859.

A list of institutions for the blind in Italy is given herewith. The statements of capacity are not exactly accurate and up-to-date but they are approximate, and will help to give an idea of the extent of provision in Italy. The dates of foundation are also given.

Assisi (1871), capacity 10; Bologna (1881), capacity 50, another (1877), capacity 12, and an institution for blind and near blind (1885), capacity 10; Cagliari (1897), capacity 9; Como, an asylum 1875, capacity 15; Florence (1870), capacity 50; Genoa (1868), capacity 60; Milan (1840), capacity 120, Mondolfio asylum (1873), capacity 30, and Zirotti workshop (1881), capacity, 38; Naples, Hospital 'St. Giuseppe e Lucia' (1818), capacity 150, the 'Principe' Institute (1873), capacity 80, and the 'Strachan Rodino' school (1869), capacity 15; Padua, central institution (1838), capacity 32, and a home (1895), capacity 14; Palermo (1892), capacity 40; Pavia (1896), capacity 4, and 1870, capacity 12; Reggio-Emilia (1883), capacity 20; Rome, Institute of 'St. Alessio' (1868), capacity 80, and the 'Margherita' Hospital (1873), capacity 25; Turin (1897), capacity 70.

There are two societies for rendering assistance to the blind in Florence, the 'Tommaseo' and the 'Margherita.' They have three branches located in Padua, Rome, and Naples. These societies owe their success to the work of Dante Barbi-Adrieni of Florence. He was also the editor of the *Mentore dei Ciechi* (Braille) and the *Amico dei Ciechi.*

From the point of view of frequency of blindness Italy may be divided into three districts. The frequency is lowest on the Alps and in the valley of the Po; then comes the region of the Apennines and their water-sheds; and it is highest in Sicily and Sardinia. The main cause of non-congenital blindness in Italy is the conjunctivitis of infants resulting from the ignorance and neglect of parents in the lower strata of society. Congenital blindness constitutes only 15 p. c. of the total, but from the point of view of instruction most cases of non-congenital blindness must be classed with congenital, since occurring in the first two years of life, no memory of visual impressions is retained.

Practically nothing is done for the blind in Italy by the government. There is a law making instruction obligatory, but as the law does not specifically refer to the blind, it is interpreted as not applying to them. The schools for the blind, all supported by private contributions, provide four classes of two years duration each. Pupils are taught the Roman alphabet to familiarize them with the script used by their seeing fellows. Braille and other methods are also employed. In Milan the so-called Vitali ink is used, which is applied thick, and, when dried, leaves an elevated ridge which is perceptible to the touch. In many institutions didactic museums have been established, in which are displayed geometrical forms, models of animals, plants, and so forth. The teaching of music includes theoretical instruction. Attempts to teach the writing of notes have not proved successful.

The music students are subjected at the end of each year to an examination by professors of the conservatory in the presence of the teachers of the particular institution. The more talented ones are admitted to the examinations of the Royal Conservatory and receive diplomas which open to them the doors of the teaching profession. The manual arts are, on the whole, neglected in Italy. The situation, in general, is far from satisfactory, only about 1,000 or 20 p. c. of these of school age (8 to 20) receiving instruction. Of the graduates of the various institutions about two-thirds are said to become self-supporting.

Much valuable information on the blind in Italy is contained in the proceedings of the National Congress of Teachers of the Blind, held in various years at Florence, Padua, Naples, and Milan.

NORWAY.

The census of 1910 gave the number of blind in Norway as 2,097 or 889 per million of population.

The first society for the care of the blind in Norway was organized in 1858 by F. Johansen. In 1859 he applied to the government for a grant with which to erect a building for the proposed institution, but was refused. At the initiative of the King, however, means were provided for a study of the instruction of the blind in other countries and a subsidy was also assured the society for the erection and maintenance of an institution to be housed in a structure built according to plans approved by the King.

The institution was opened on August 1, 1861. The school provided six classes and 70 pupils matriculated. There was also a special class for backward children. The subjects taught were: religion, language, writing (using the Danish Guldberg apparatus for pencil-writing), arithmetic, geography, history, natural science, Froebel exercises, modelling, gymnastics, singing, and playing of the organ, piano, and other instruments. All the manual arts suited to the blind are taught. Embossed school books are imported from Copenhagen. The entrance age is 9-20.

In 1886 another institution was established in Glöshaugen near Trondhjem. It was supported partly by the state, and partly by various organizations, but failed and its place was taken by a public school for the blind opened in Klaebu. In Christiania there is a school of manual arts founded by Lönwig (blind). Blind missions publish religious writings in embossed script. According to the law of June 8, 1881, elementary education is obligatory in Norway, and it is made to extend to the blind as well as other abnormal children. The age of admission to the institutions of Norway varies from 9 to 21 years; the average period of residence is eight years. In June, 1898, the institution in Christiania was taken over by the state and is now supported by it together with the school at Klaebu.

PORTUGAL.

There were in Portugal 5,650 blind about the year 1900, this being in proportion of 1,040 per million inhabitants. The proportion is rather high for a European country, yet almost nothing is done for their care.

The state has taken no steps for the assistance of the blind. The Lisbon institution is antiquated and insufficient. In 1895 Dr. Mascaro published a pamphlet, which received wide circulation, and in which he discusses the various aspects of the blind problem. Its contents show with great clearness how little is done for the care of the blind in Portugal. In 1894 a commission was organized to study the question, but it achieved nothing. There is one other institution at Castilo-del-bide.

RUSSIA.

There are a large number of blind persons in Russia, the last census returns showing a total of 215,413, or 2,097 to the million. The prevalence of blindness is said to increase from the western to the eastern provinces. Thus, in Poland there are 600 blind persons to the million of population, while in the states of Ufa, Viatka and Kazan, there are 6,000 in the same proportion.

The first interest in the welfare of the blind was manifested in 1806 when Tsar Alexander I invited Valentin Haüy to visit Russia and establish in Petrograd (St. Petersburg) a school for the blind. Haüy remained ten years, but the seed sown by the French philanthropist fell in unprofitable ground. After his departure nothing further was done for many years. Most of the present institutions for the blind have been founded and are maintained by the Maria Alexandrovna Association for Promoting the Interests of the Blind. There are, however, fourteen other societies.

The Maria Alexandrovna Association was founded in 1881. The Tsarina Maria Alexandovna, wife of Alexander II, took an interest in blind and partially blind soldiers who were survivors of the Turkish war. Those with eye diseases received proper treatment, while the totally blind were placed in a workshop in Petrograd, where they were taught basket-making in order to make them self-supporting. The experiment proved successful, received wide publicity and was repeated in many other cities. The member of this association most instrumental in advancing the interests of the blind was Constantin Grot. The association has representatives in all the provinces, who work without compensation. The membership is nearly 6,000. The original fund amounted to 217,000 roubles, but large sums are collected annually in churches, synagogues, and Mohammedan prayer-houses throughout the country during the so-called "Blind Week" beginning with the Sunday on which is read the scriptural account of the healing of the blind. The general activities of the association may be enumerated as follows: the education of blind children; the care and instruction of adults who become blind in later life; the provision for aged and infirm blind persons in asylums and so forth; the establishment of a sound public opinion with reference to blindness; the prevention of blindness.

For incurable blind children the association has founded 23 non-sectarian schools, in which are received pupils between the ages of seven and eleven. The curriculum covers fully the course of regular preparatory schools and lasts from eight to ten years, according to the capacity of the pupils. After the kindergarten and primary courses the pupils are taught trades such as brush and basket making, and in the provincial schools, shoemaking, weaving, music, singing, piano-tuning, and massage. Schools are in operation at Vladimir, Vologda, Yelabuga, Irkutsk, Kamenetz-Podolsk, Kiev, Kostroma, Minsk, Moscow, Odessa, Perm, Poltava, Reval, Samara, Petrograd, Saratov, Smolensk, Tver, Tiflis, Tula, Charkov, and Tchernigov. The present number of pupils in these schools is about 950. Up to 1910 there had been over 850 graduates.

For the instruction of the adult blind the association maintains two establishments: an industrial home for blind women at Viatka, exclusively for local needs; and the Grot workshops at Petrograd. In the Viatka home 20 blind young women learn brush-making, weaving, and shoe-making. The Petrograd workshops, which are much larger, are housed in a three-story structure built at his own expense by Constantin Grot. The school department trains over 20 pupils, the instruction (in brush and basket-making) lasting three years. The pupils live not far from the shops in the Nicholas Alexander Home for the Blind. In addition to the educational function, the shops provide daily employment for over sixty adult blind men, who live in various parts of the city.

The workshops also provide work for blind men working at home as well as for blind girls, living at the Elisabeth Coudurat Home. All the blind persons working either in or outside the shops, bring their products to the salesroom, where orders are taken and goods sold. Many of the workers are self-supporting and others need only slight assistance from a special fund.

For the blind who have to leave the Maria Alexandrovna institution or the industrial classes at the Grot workshops to return to the provinces, however, the situation is not as favorable. For such persons the delegates of the association endeavor to find locally persons who will act as protectors and friends to assist the blind man in every possible way.

In 1907, the association made an inquiry regarding the status of graduates of schools for the blind in order to ascertain whether the training provided was adequate to assure subsequent self-support. The result showed 440 or 55 p. c. of the total to be self-sustaining; 178 were practising brush making, 69 basket making, 110 music and singing, and 25 were teachers or masters in schools for the blind.

For the old and unemployable blind, the association maintains in Petrograd two asylums for women: the Elisabeth Coudurat Home for 47 blind women fifty years of age and over; and the Princess Volkonsky Home for 120 blind women, twenty years of age and over. Both institutions are maintained by their endowments. For men there are available 20 beds in the Nicholas-Alexander Home and 11 beds in the Municipal Asylum, the latter paid for out of the funds of the association.

It should also be stated that there have recently been opened in the Elisabeth Coudurat Home departments for feeble-minded girls and for orphan girls.

Five other homes for the incapable blind are maintained by the association in Vladimir, Voroney, Kazan, Orel and Tula. The latest statistics show that the association was caring for 300 incapable blind. Pecuniary assistance is also given to the destitute blind, though monetary grants are regarded as the least desirable form of aid.

The association maintains its own printing office for the production of books and music in embossed characters. Three blind printers are constantly employed. This press has provided the schools with all the books required in their instruction. In addition the school libraries are augmented by books produced by societies of lady copyists. The press also issues one monthly magazine in embossed type and another in ink print, the latter being designed to spread among the sighted knowledge regarding work for and needs of the blind.

Since 1893 one of the most important features of the Association's work is the prevention of blindness. In this campaign 21 ophthalmic hospitals have been established, and in localities where the means did not permit of a hospital ophthalmic stations were founded. Securing the gratuitous services of local surgeons, the association provides instruments and medicines, salaries for nurses, and lodging for poor dispensary patients. At the total of 148 hospitals and stations, in 1909 there were received 198,487 patients who made 800,000 visits. There were performed 44,725 operations.

The association also sends out traveling staffs consisting of one ophthalmologist with one or two assistants who make tours in the distant or sparsely settled provinces. Known to the people as "royal staffs" they have gained complete popular confidence, and they attract a considerable number of patients. During the year 1910 there were received by 32 traveling staffs, 74,415 patients who made 184,701 visits, and profited by 18,232 operations.

The total number of patients received during the years 1893-1910 by hospitals, stations, and staffs was 2,300,965, and that of operations was 600,000.

In addition to these extensive activities of the Maria Alexandrovna Association there are in Petrograd under the care of the Royal Philanthropic Society the institution founded by Haüy with about 40 inmates; the Maria Home for girls, founded 1871, with about 15 inmates; and another asylum for girls founded in 1882.

In Moscow there are the following institutions: an educational institution for both sexes, founded 1882, with 60 inmates, and having its own press; an asylum for 140 men and women between the ages of 20 and 80; the Prince Oldenburg Home, for 20 boys; an asylum for 15 men; and an institution founded by a merchant, Nemirov-Koldkin, for 40 men and women. In Riga there is a private institution for 22 children. In Warsaw there is an institution for the deaf and dumb and the blind with 30 inmates of both sexes; and an asylum for 58 inmates. In Finland there are two institutions, one in Helsingfors for 15 boys, and one in Kuopio for 30.

It should be observed that of all the institutions in Russia but three are supported by government funds, one in Warsaw and the two in Finland. All the rest are provided for by private philanthropic endeavor.

SWEDEN.

The number of the blind in Sweden, according to the census taken about 1900, was 3,413, or 664 per million.

The father of care for the blind in Switzerland is Per Aaron Borg, who educated a blind girl at his house and examined her in the presence of several persons (1808). All were greatly impressed. This led to the establishment in 1809 of an institution for the deaf and blind. In 1810 the institution extended its activities to the feebleminded as well, and began to receive a yearly subsidy from the government. In 1816 the institution was supposed to educate 13 deaf or blind free, but at this time the acceptance of blind pupils was discontinued. Nothing was done until 1845 when instruction of blind was begun in a section of the institution. The number of pupils was 60 out of 324 in the country between the ages of 10 and 20. In 1879 a special institution for the blind was founded. At first it was located in temporary quarters in Stockholm, later a house was built by the state for the institution at Tomteboda near Stockholm, with a capacity of one hundred (1889). The age of admission was fixed at 9-14. The period of instruction was 6 years for those who came from the preparatory school, and 8 years for others. The Moon alphabet is in use, also Braille. Small square Latin letters prepared by a special Swedish apparatus are also employed. A workshop was established in 1884 in Christinehumn. In 1885 the Society for the Welfare of the Blind founded a home for women and a shop for selling the products of the blind. In addition to these there are also: in Stockholm, a workshop for men; in Upsala a workshop for adult girls; in Norrbacka, a workshop for women. The law of May 29, 1896, makes the instruction of the blind obligatory.

SWITZERLAND.

In 1895 the census returns recorded 2,107 blind persons, or 722 per million of inhabitants. In Bern only does the compulsory education law extend to the blind. There are three institutions in Bern, one in Lausanne, and one in Zürich; all private. An asylum was founded in 1884 in the Bern canton. The Vaud canton has an organization which extends its activities over all western Switzerland and the neighboring districts of France. In the Zürich canton there is an institution for the blind and a fund (established 1865) which supports 35 blind persons. Another organization is located in Schaffhausen.

SPAIN.

The last available figures place the number of blind in Spain in 1877 at 24,608, or 1,006 per million of population. Work for the blind is not active. There are fourteen institutions, the first of which was established at Barcelona in 1820, the second in Madrid in 1842, then following in order: Alisante, 1861; Santiago, 1864; Burgos, 1868; Saragossa, 1871; Seville, 1873; Valencia, 1887. There are also institutions at Salamanca, Taragona, and later two more were founded at Barcelona and Madrid. Most of these institutions also provide for deaf-mutes. In accordance with the law of obligatory instruction (1857) one school for the blind and deaf must be located in each university district.

The latest available statistics regarding the blind in European countries is appended in the following table:

STATISTICS OF THE BLIND IN EUROPE.

Country.	Date.	Number of blind. Individuals.	Per million inhabitants.	Authority.
Ireland	1901	4,253	954	British Empire Census, 1901.
Scotland	1901	3,253	727	British Empire Census, 1901.
England and Wales	1901	25,317	778	British Empire Census, 1901
Belgium*	1906	3,076	434	Annuaire Statistique, 1908, Page 27.
Netherlands*	1909	2,710	462	Jaarcijfers voor het IConinkrijk, 1910, page 27.
Denmark	1901	1,047	427	Statistisk Aarbog, 1911, page 15.
Norway	1910	2,097	889	Statistisk Aarbog, 1911, page 15.
Sweden	(about 1900)	3,413	664	Statistisk Tidskrift, 1910, page 11.
Germany*	1900	34,334	609	Statistisches Jahrbuch für das Reich, 1908.
Switzerland	1895	2,107	722	Enc Brit., 11th Edition, iv., page 60.
France	1901	27,174	698	Annuaire Statistique, 190, page 8.
Portugal *	(about 1900)	505	1,040	Enc. Brit., 11th Edition, iv., page 60.
Spain	1877	24,608	1,006	Enc. Brit., 11th Edition, iv., page 60.
Gibraltar	1901	33	1,200	British Empire Census, 1911.
Malta	1901	418	2,011	British Empire Census, 1911
Italy	1901	38,160	1,175	Censo della Popolazione, 10 Febbraio, 1901, ii., page 344.
Austria*	1905	14,052	515	Statistisches Handbuch, 1907 pages 52 53.
Hungary	(about 1900)	19,377	1,006	Official Publicati (No).
Servia	1900	2,345	941	Annuaire Statistique, 1906, page 96.
Bulgaria	1905	5,319	1,318	Annuaire Statistique, 1910, page 114.
Roumania	1899	4,967	834	Date de Dec., 1899, Résultats Défi-nitifs.
Poland (Russian)	1897	7,005	745	Census, 28 Jan., 1897; St. Petersburg, 1905, ii., page 186.
Finland	1900	3,229	1,191	Befolkningsstatistik No 37; Aperçu de la pop-ulati de la Finlande au., Dec, 190
Russia (in Europe)	1897	215,413	2,097	Census, 28 Jan., 1897; St. Petersburg, 1905, ii., page 196.
Cyprus	1901	1,732	7,300	British Empire Census, 1901.

* Relates specifically to the *totally* blind.

Authorities. In the preparation of this necessarily synthetic article extensive use has been made of suitable material in the literature of the subjects. Especial indebtedness is acknowledged to Alexander Mell's *Handbuch,* to Sir Francis Campbell, Edward E. Allen, and Frederick Rose.

Literature. The literature on the provision for the blind is not plentiful and there is but little of general value apart from the contributions just cited. There is no good history of the care and education of the blind. The most useful sources are periodical files: the *American Outlook for the Blind;* the English *Braille Review;* the French *Valentin Haüy;* and the German *Blindenfreund.*— (D. C. McM.) See, also **Blind, The,** and **Blindness,** in Vol. II of this *Encyclopedia,* as well as the article on BLINDNESS in the eleventh edition of the *Encyclôpedia Britannica.*

(B.) SCHOOLS, HOSPITALS AND OTHER INSTITUTIONS FOR THE BLIND
IN ASIA, AFRICA AND AUSTRALASIA.

With the exception of Australasian, Egyptian and Japanese institutions, there is comparatively little organized aid for the unfortunate blind to be found outside of Europe and America. Yet one finds on other continents that much progress is reported towards an effective alleviation of the sufferings of those who have lost their useful vision.

EGYPT.

This is the country in which partial or complete blindness in either one or both eyes is almost the rule rather than the exception. Kenneth Scott, whose account of the care of the blind in this country is given in the following paragraphs, says it is computed that there is in Egypt at least one totally blind person to every fifty of the population. This is principally the result of acute ophthalmia occurring in infancy, and it is fostered by the superstitious observance which prevents the mothers from washing their children from the time of birth until they are two years old, at which late date they are weaned. There is also a great deal of infection carelessly and ignorantly conveyed direct from eye to eye, by means of unwashed fingers, and this is accountable for the occurrence of much more eye-disease than any that may be caused by the proverbial flies.

The only employment followed by the blind, both Mohammedan and Coptic (or native Christian), and that only to a limited extent, is recitation aloud—the former repeating portions of the Koran at funerals, and the latter chanting the church ritual in their services; blind girls and women are without occupation. Practically, no education is given to the blind as a class, and anything which they learn has to be acquired orally and by frequent repetition. The blind were not always so completely neglected, as the native ecclesiastical authorities *(Wakf)* gave an annual grant of £2,000 for the continued maintenance of a school for the blind, the deaf and dumb in Cairo, which taught about 80 day-pupils; the latter years of the school were passed under the Ministry of Education, and it was ultimately discontinued. Such a condition of affairs appealed to Dr. T. R. Armitage, and explains his motive in trying to establish some proper means for affording the blind in Egypt the necessary scholastic instruction and other training. In

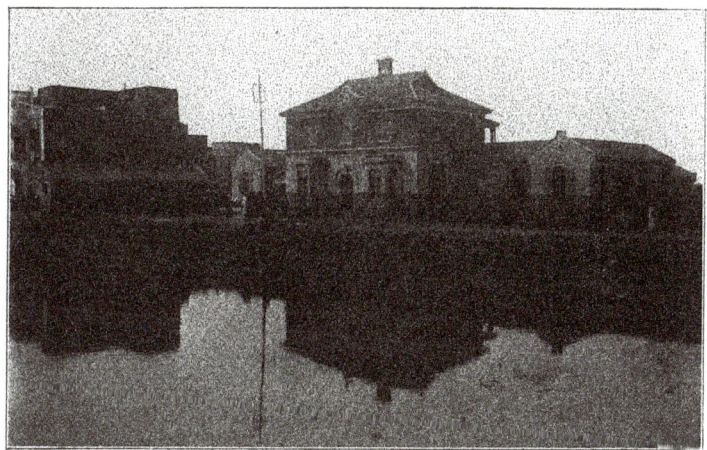

Permanent Ophthalmic Hospital, Tanta, Egypt.

Egypt, as in other countries, it is occasionally very difficult, and takes some time, to start any enterprise such as this on a satisfactory and practical footing, and it was left for Mrs. T. R. Armitage to be the means of successfully carrying out her husband's wishes in this particular. In 1900 Mrs. Armitage asked Dr. Kenneth Scott to prepare a scheme for the education and welfare of the blind in Egypt, on lines suggested to her. This, through the British and Foreign Blind Association, was submitted to Queen Victoria, who graciously commanded it to be sent, through the foreign office to the khedive, who in mark of approbation and encouragement generously gave a handsome donation towards its realization. The Institution for the Blind was established at Zeitoun, Cairo, early in the year 1901, through funds provided by Mrs. T. R. Armitage. The object of the institution, which is wholly unsectarian in character, is to educate and train the blind mentally and physically and in industrial occupations, and at the same time to improve their moral standards, so that eventually they may become in great measure, or even completely, self-supporting.

However, the most effective work for the blind of this stricken country has been more recently done under the supervision of A. F. MacCallan (*Ophthalmic Record*, Dec., 1910), now Director of Egyptian Ophthalmic Hospitals, under the Ministry of Public Health.

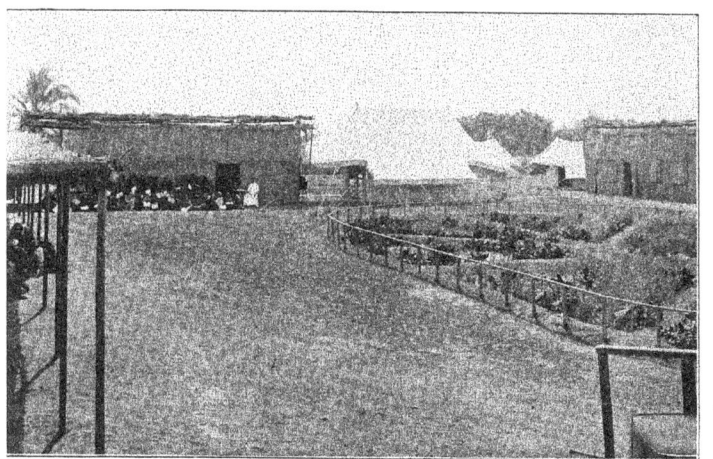

Traveling Tent Hospital, Luxor, Egypt. (MacCallan.)

He says that trachoma is ubiquitous and affects more than 90 per cent. of the population. This dictum is based on regular examinations of the pupils of some of the large government primary schools and of thirty-seven *kuttabs* or preparatory schools, where during last year it was found that more than 90 per cent. of the pupils showed unmistakable evidence of active or quiescent trachoma. As the result of experience and local knowledge now extending from one end of Egypt to the other, it may be said that the incidence of trachoma in different places among the middle and lower classes varies very little. The extraordinary density of population naturally favors the spread of the disease. This is 939 per square mile and is greater than that of any European country, of which the most densely populated is Belgium with 588 per square mile.

The mode in which the disease is spread is mainly by the fingers; clothing also is a fruitful source of contagion, used as it is indifferently as a mosquito net, a towel and a protection from the heat or cold. Acute ophthalmias occur at all times during the year but are more prevalent in the hotter months during the period of increased microbic activity, when the contagion may be fly-borne, although it is probable that it is more commonly digital. The uncleanly habits of the lower classes, habits in some cases consecrated by custom, and in others aggravated by the difficulty in obtaining water; the crowded huts with crumbling mud walls in which the poorer fellahin sleep together with their cattle; the dust of the streets, unpaved and unwatered except in a few of the

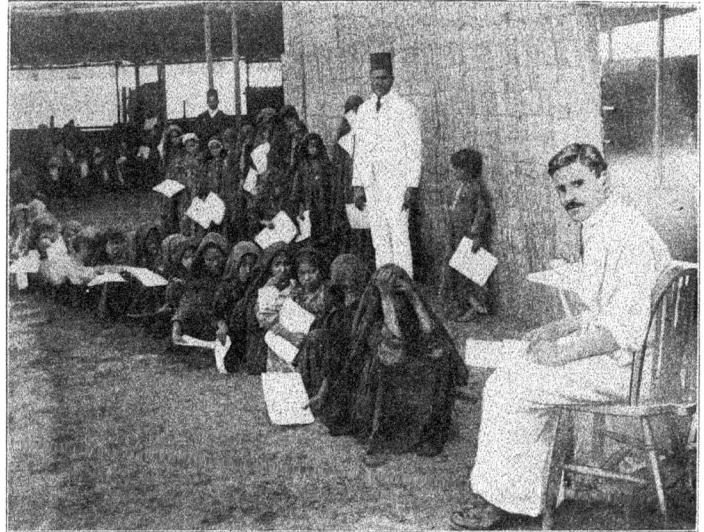

Luxor Traveling Trachoma Hospital in Egypt. Patients awaiting
treatment. (MacCallan.)

larger streets, and continually ground to powder by the tramping of the cattle, which are daily driven from the huts to the fields; the gales of daily occurrence during some periods of the year, which drive the dust about until it permeates the whole atmosphere, both without and within the most hermetically sealed house; all these are fertile causes of acute ophthalmias.

The occurrence of acute ophthalmias materially assists the spread of trachoma. A non-secreting case of trachoma is only slightly infective, but as soon as the secretion caused by the addition of an acute ophthalmia to the chronic trachoma is transferred to unaffected persons, it may be by the fingers, by towels, or by clothes, trachomatous contagion rapidly spreads.

Trachoma may have various sequelæ, but the most important are trichiasis and entropion, of which ten thousand cases were seen at the ophthalmic hospitals in 1909; the time at MacCallan's disposal enabled him to operate on only three thousand of these cases. Trachoma alone rarely causes blindness; this is the effect of the acute ophthalmias. Six per cent. of all cases seen by the ophthalmic staff in 1909 were blind in both eyes (1,385 in all), and 15.64 per cent. were blind in one or both eyes (3,501 cases).

The 1907 official census showed that Egypt was nine times as much affected with blindness as the colored population of the most affected state (Idaho) and fifty-five times as much as the average in the United States (1900 census).

Between the beginning of the year 1904 and the end of 1914 sixteen ophthalmic hospitals have been opened in various parts of Egypt. The cost of maintenance of all, except two, of these hospitals, is assured; two were endowed by Sir Ernest Cassel, with a capital sum of £40,000; four are maintained by local self taxation (Provincial Councils); eight are maintained by the Government, while two are closed for lack of funds.

Of the total cost of provision of these hospitals, which amounted to rather more than £68,000, £49,000 was obtained by gift (apart from the Cassel Fund), public subscription, or local taxation, while £17,000 only was contributed by the Government.

Different types of *permanent hospitals* have been erected in various places, but it has been found, as the result of experience, that a satisfactory hospital can be built for £4,000. Such a hospital contains a commodious out-patient department and beds for sixteen patients. This number of beds is quite sufficient for a daily clinic of 200 to 300 patients, when the majority of operations such as those for trichiasis-entropion are performed on out-patients.

The permanent hospitals at Tanta, Assiût, Mansûra, Beni Suef, and Zagazig, have, during 1914, been carrying on satisfactory work. At Mansûra and Zagazig a considerable lull in the number of patients treated was noticed during the colder part of the year, but measures were taken which resulted in a return to the normal number. New hospitals were opened at Damanhûr (provided by the Provincial Council of Beheira) and at Shibin el Kôm and Sohâg (provided by subscription). Hospitals are under construction at Minia and Fayûm.

The permanent hospitals erected and maintained by the Provincial Council of Gharbia at Mahalla el Kubra and Kafr el Zayât continue to do satisfactory work. A hospital is also being built at Santa by the same Council.

The usefulness of *traveling hospitals* and their popularity among the *fellahîn* is very great. The type of traveling hospital which has been found most satisfactory consists of a commodious tent with a double roof for operations, and accommodation for a British Inspector, an Egyptian doctor, eight or ten in-patients, with the necessary attendants and servants.

During 1914 two large traveling hospitals known as the Cassel Fund Hospitals have worked at Maghâgha, Shibîn el Qanâter, Damietta, Minia el Qamh, Delta Barrage. The period spent in each locality is about six months. The places previously visited are Damietta, Mansûra, Menûf, Shibin el Kôm, Qaliûb, Benha, Shibin el Qanâter, Zagazig, Damanhûr, Abu Hommos, Rosetta, Zifta, Giza, Fayûm, Beni Suef, Minia, Maghâgha, Assiût, Sohâg, Luxor, Aswân.

The cost of each of these hospitals is about £1,350 a year; each hospital has two surgeons who can get 200 operations done per month, together with the daily treatment of 250 patients.

The Provincial Councils of Daqahlîa and Assiût maintain traveling hospitals which are managed on behalf of the Councils by the Director of Ophthalmic Hospitals. The activities of each of these hospitals is naturally confined to the limits of the province to which it belongs. The cost of each of these hospitals is £750 a year, each has one surgeon who can get 150 operations done per month, together with the daily treatment of 150 patients. It is to be regretted that the Provincial Council of Assiût has felt obliged to reduce the expenses of the hospital to £500 a year, which will make it impossible to retain the accommodation for in-patients, thereby diminishing the utility of the hospital.

The two traveling hospitals belonging to the Provincial Council of Gharbia were not opened during the year, their places having been taken by two permanent hospitals erected and maintained by the Council. It is to be hoped that when the financial situation improves these hospitals may be reopened.

The traveling hospital was, in 1910, encamped close to the American Mission School at Luxor on the road to the temple of Karnak. An acre of land is dotted over with large tents of Indian make, the little garden forming a restful patch of green on the brown soil. The large mat-shelters shield the patients from the glare of the sun. Under the shelters are three or four hundred natives of all sorts, conditions and ages, but all poor. The majority of them are children. Most are animated and interested, pleased to wait as long as is required; for them every hospital day is a fête where they meet their friends and indulge in

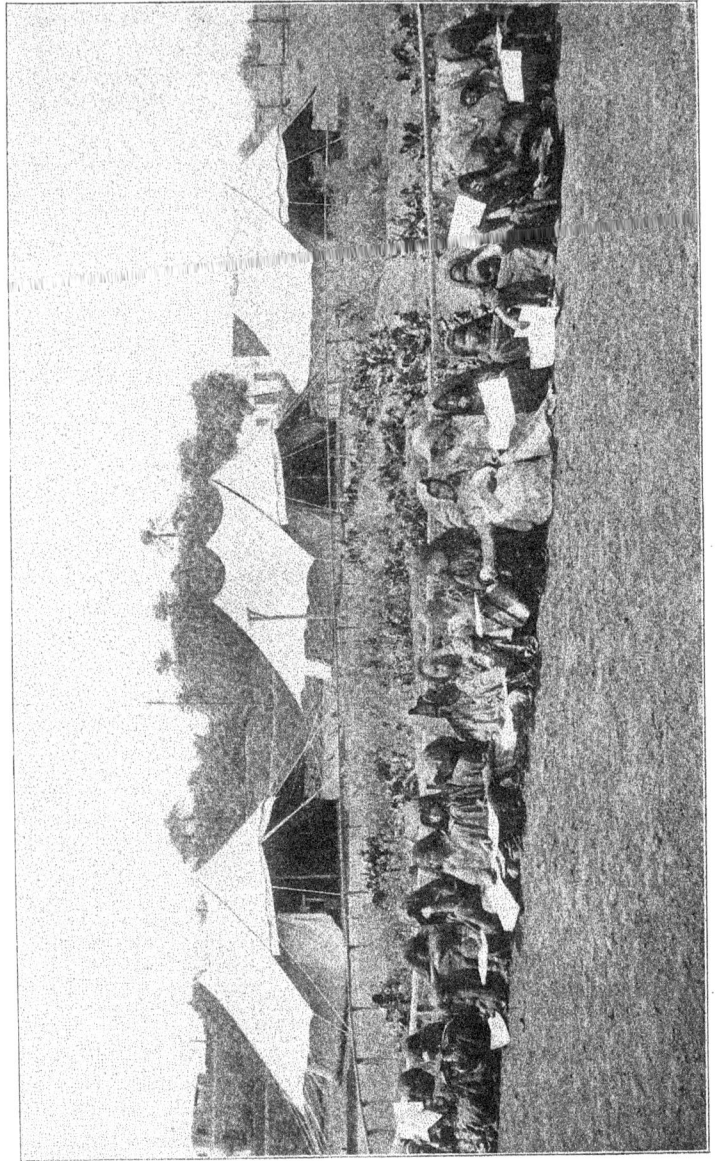

Luxor Treatment of Trachoma in Egypt. Children at the Camp. (MacCallan.)

agreeable converse. There are pretty little girls in gaily striped gowns, filthy babies in the arms of filthy mothers, who will be refused treatment inexorably until the baby's face has been washed by the mother; boys of all ages; a row of old men squatting on the ground, each of whom is blind or nearly blind with cataract, but all will be operated on for this condition sooner or later.

A sad and silent little group is squatting on the ground in front of bowls of sublimate solution, each patient with two little platters, one containing clean pledgets of cotton-wool to dip in the solution, and another to contain them when they have been used for swabbing their eyes. These are the cases of acute ophthalmia of every degree of severity. There is a sheyal or porter in a short blue gown, in the prime of life, magnificently built, with ulceration of both corneæ and prolapse of the irides, stoically mopping his eyes, miserable but unimaginative and not thinking of his future. There is an undersized little man in European clothes, a katib at the Mudiria, who, accompanied by his father, has arrived with a profuse conjunctival discharge; the father beats his breast and scratches his face in grief, for if his son becomes blind and can no longer be an honored servant of the Hukuma or government, who will give his poor father the luxuries he has learned to require, the cigarette and the frequent cup of coffee?

A good-looking girl of fifteen with one of her corneæ almost entirely destroyed is swabbing away for dear life. Poor thing, she hopes that her beauty may be preserved, for if not she will no longer be talked of as a prize in the marriage market; so, careless of exposing her features, she carries out her treatment.

The large group of black-robed figures sitting together are women with trichiasis; there are twenty or thirty such cases every day, easily cured by operation, but the operation for each one takes about half an hour. So that if all the operations were done for this condition alone, without touching all the other cases, the surgeons would operate for twelve hours a day; most of them must therefore be inevitably postponed.

The two traveling hospitals carried on work at Mansourah, Beni Suef, Gizeh, and Luxor. The only permanent hospital at present opened is that of Tanta, which was at work during the whole year. The traveling hospitals naturally are closed for purposes of transfer from one locality to the other, and one of the hospitals was closed during the summer in order that leave might be given to the overworked surgeons and employes.

The average number of patients seen per day was 221. The number of new patients treated was 12,092, each of whom attended the hospital about 14 times; 4,071 of the total number were under the age of fifteen years. The number of operations performed was 9,930, of which 2,783 were done under the influence of chloroform. The number of patients seen with ingrowing eyelashs, trichiasis or entropion, was 10,060, but the time at our disposal enabled us to do only 3,128 operations for the relief of this condition, which is not merely painful, but frequently leads to blindness. The disability caused is such that the fellahin, unable to obtain advice or operation from a skilled surgeon, for there are none available for the prices they can afford to pay, frequently resort to charlatans to cure them. The operation usually performed by

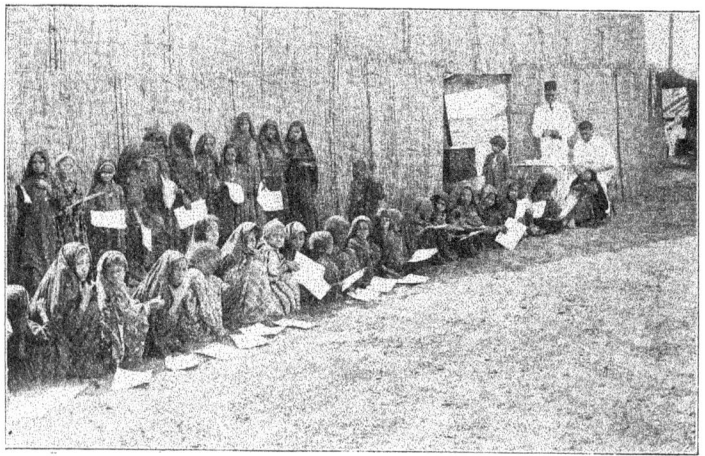

Luxor, Egypt. Children being Treated in the Traveling Hospital.

these "fakirs" is this: A fold of skin of the upper lid is included between two pieces of reed, the ends of which are tied tightly together to such a degree as to cause eversion of the ingrowing eyelashes. The included skin naturally necroses and falls away, the raw area granulates up, and in a certain number of cases in which the operation was done for the relief of entropion the condition is cured. But trichiasis is much more common than entropion in Egypt; and the majority of people who resort to these quacks, not only are not cured, but with a large piece of the skin of their upper lid removed, they are unable ever to close their eyelids again (lagophthalmos), causing great disability in all cases and frequently resulting in complete opacity of the corneæ with dire results to vision. One thousand four hundred eighty-one such cases were seen last year.

The regular staff at one of the permanent or complete camp hospitals consists of two Egyptian surgeons, one of whom has spent at least two years learning ophthalmic surgery on the Ophthalmic Hospital Staff after taking his medical diploma at the Government Medical School in Cairo; and two senior ophthalmic surgeons or inspectors, of whom one is English and the other Egyptian, are always in residence at the various hospitals in turn. Frequent visits are also made by the chief inspector to the hospitals for the general management of which he is responsible.

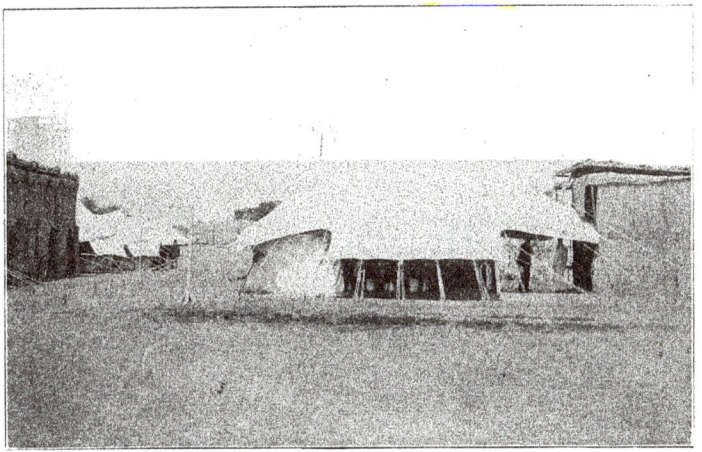

Luxor, Egypt. Operation Tent.

The clerical staff consists of a clerk, a headman of the camp, two trained male hospital attendants and seven servants, including a woman who looks after the comfort of the women in-patients, and a cook to prepare food for all the patients in the hospital, all of which is provided for them gratis.

The regulation period for each traveling hospital to stay in one place is six months, after which it is moved to another place. This is not because the need for the hospital's services is apparently less after six months, but because it is only just to give different places the advantage of the hospital's presence. It is impossible in most places in Upper Egypt to carry on traveling hospitals in the summer. The heat, dust and flies make surgical work unsatisfactory. Therein lies the advantage of permanent hospitals, in which surgical work can be carried on all the year round.

In 1903, Sir Ernest Cassel placed a sum of £40,000 at the disposal of

Lord Cromer for ophthalmic relief in Egypt. The form that the relief took was the establishment of Traveling Ophthalmic Hospitals. These hospitals became a definite branch of the Egyptian Government service in 1906, in which year the first permanent hospital was built at Tanta. In the next year a hospital was built at Assiout to which the inhabitants of the province contributed a sum of £5,000 and last year a similar sum was given by an Egyptian gentleman for the erection of a permanent hospital at Mansura. The Ministry of Finance has undertaken to maintain ophthalmic hospitals, built by private effort, on approved plans in the capital provincial towns, if they are handed over to the control of the ophthalmic section of the Public Health Department. This very valuable undertaking was obtained by Mr. Graham, the present Director General of the Department of Public Health.

"It is too much to expect that an immediate provision could be made for the maintenance of a complete system, but we have the active sympathy of Sir Eldon Gorst, the British agent, and of Mr. Paul Harvey, the financial adviser to the Khedive, and we hope in the course of time to give effect to a complete scheme. The laisser-aller attitude of the majority of the Egyptians as regards the suffering from eye diseases, which they are so accustomed to, makes it improbable that any comprehensive effort will be made by the Egyptians themselves. Some financial assistance has been received from a few American and English visitors to Egypt, though not in sufficient amounts to produce any great result."

A complete scheme of ophthalmic relief in Egypt means the provision in each of the fourteen provinces [several have been founded since this article was written] of a permanent hospital in the capital town and of a complete traveling hospital to tour the districts of each province. There should be in addition a complete hospital of flying columns in every province, each consisting of two or three tents in charge of a single surgeon; these would visit the more remote districts and smaller villages. Each of these elements would have a well-defined function. The flying columns would only treat trachoma and conjunctival affections and should preach a propaganda of ophthalmic hygiene. No operation, except scraping or expression of the lids for trachoma would be performed. The two flying columns could be located an hour's journey by road from one another and could be worked by a single surgeon, who would do clinical work at one hospital in the morning, say from eight o'clock until ten or eleven o'clock, and at the other from three o'clock till five or six o'clock, riding from one to the other. The flying columns should remain not more than three months at each camping ground.

The traveling hospital should work at a considerable distance from the permanent hospital of the same province, staying in each place at least six months. All kinds of ophthalmic surgical work might be carried on, except the more serious cataract and orbital tumor operations, which should be sent to the permanent hospital. ·

The permanent hospital should act as a base for the traveling hospital and for the flying columns. It should receive all the more important operative cases and any cases of exceptional clinical interest met with in the province; these would form clinical material for teaching purposes, and one of the most important functions of the permanent hospital should be that of a center of ophthalmic instruction for postgraduate students.

The cost of building each permanent hospital would be, at the lowest possible estimate, £5,000, and the cost of equipment £1,500. Three permanent hospitals having been already provided, the cost of these items for the remaining eleven provinces only remains. The cost of equipment and installation of each complete camp hospital is £1,000. Two being already in existence, the cost of the remaining twelve hospitals would be £12,000. Twenty-eight flying columns at £500 each, would cost £14,000, giving a grand total of about £100,000 or half a million dollars.

The upkeep of this organization at the rate of £2,000 a year for each permanent or complete camp hospital and £1,000 a year for each flying column would be about £75,000, or less than four hundred thousand dollars, in addition to the present yearly expenditure which is about fifty thousand dollars.

SOUTH AFRICA.

The proportion of blind persons to the total population is not large in the Union as a whole. In 1904 there were 68 blind in Natal, but there were 2,802 in Cape Colony. The large percentage and number in the latter province was due to an abnormal increase between 1875 and 1891, but between 1891 and 1904 the rate per 10,000 had decreased to 23.78.

Governmental provision is made for the instruction of the South African blind, especially for the education of children, and in some cases adults are trained in various handicrafts. There is an institution in Worcester (founded in 1881) for both blind and deafmutes. It is supported by fees and public subscriptions supplemented by a government grant.

AUSTRALASIA.

The number of blind in the Australian Commonwealth and New Zealand was, according to the census of 1901, as follows:

New South Wales 884
Queensland 209
Victoria 1,082
West Australia 121
South Australia 315
New Zealand (1901)............................. 274
Tasmania 173

The Commonwealth provides instruction for her blind, especially for the young, and generally trains adults in one or more handicrafts. Embossed literature is carried free of expense, while in Victoria no charge is made for the rail transportation of a guide who accompanies a blind person. In Australia proper there are institutions for the blind at Sydney, Maylands, Brisbane, Brighton, Adelaide and Melbourne. New Zealand supports a similar institution at Auckland.

INDIA.

As in most oriental countries India has a large proportion of inhabitants blind chiefly from trachoma—most of them beggars. In some Provinces the proportion is as high as 600 to the million; in others, it falls as low as 400. In all there must be at least half a million blind native Indians. Very little had been done to educate these unfortunates until quite recently, although many missionaries have assisted individuals. At Amritsur in the Punjab well organized work for the blind has been carried on for years. The school founded there has since been removed to Rajpur and is attended by nearly 100 blind women and children. In 1913, a government hospital and school were established at Bombay in memory of Queen Victoria. In this establishment carpet weaving, tailoring, lathe-work, typewriting, carpentering, as well as reading, writing, and arithmetic are taught the blind students. In addition to this useful institution there are small blind schools at Chota-Nagpur, Coorg, Calicut, Palancottah, Calcutta, and Parantij; there is, in addition to these a school at Moulmein in Burma.

PALESTINE.

As in Egypt and India, blindness, particularly from trachoma, is exceedingly common in both Syria and Palestine. There is a large ophthalmic hospital with effective medical attendance in Jerusalem.

Similar opportunities for treatment are now available in the other larger towns, while the missionary schools are doing much to teach habits of cleanliness to the natives, thus reducing the chances for infection and its consequent blindness. A home and school for blind girls in Jerusalem is really an extension of a day school opened in 1896 by an American missionary. A small school, also under American auspices, has been established at Urfa.

CHINA.

In addition to the ever-prevalent trachoma, smallpox, and leprosy are common in China and are among the most potent causes of blindness. Begging, the immemorial occupation of the blind both in the near and far East, prevails in this country. The first effective work to relieve the condition of these unfortunates was done by missionaries. W. H. Murray, a Scottish missionary of Pekin, made a simple and ingenious adaptation of the Braille symbols to the complicated system of Chinese printing, in which over 4,000 characters are required. It was necessary to represent at least 408 sounds, and each one was given a corresponding Braille number. When a pupil reads the number he knows instantly the sound for which it stands. A school for the blind was established at Pekin, and the version of the Scriptures printed there can be read in all the provinces where the Northern Mandarin dialect is spoken.

A complete account of this interesting publication is given by Miss Gordon Cumming in *The Inventor of the Numerical Type for China.* A Braille code has also been arranged for Mandarin. At Fukien, Canton, Amoy, Ningpo and Foochow there are schools—some of them large—for the blind, carried on by missionaries.

JAPAN.

Recent statistics show that there are 70,506 blind men and women in Japan. Blind adults have long been trained in massage, acupuncture and music; indeed, until lately the Japanese blind had almost a monopoly of these occupations. From three to five years is spent in perfecting himself in the study of massage, after which the blind student is able to support himself. In Yokohoma, a city of half a million inhabitants a thousand men and women are engaged in massage, nine-tenths of whom are blind. It has been estimated that today in Japan the occupations of the blind are as follows: masseurs and acupunctors, 4,587; moxa practicers (cauterizing by burning the leaves of *Artemisia moxa* on the skin), 618; musicians, 4,706; story tellers, 246; teachers, 386; other occupations, 9,159; no occupation, 3,253.

There is, also, in Japan a blind caste, with its important special privileges. This is an association of blind monks, the legal provisions requiring the education of blind sons, along their appropriate lines, and the giving over of certain occupations to the blind. The most important and profitable of these occupations is massage. There are also three newspapers devoted to their entertainment and instruction.

In 1878 a school for the blind—including deaf-mutes—was established in Kioto, and, shortly afterwards, one in Tokio. Japan has now at least four large schools exclusively devoted to instruction of the blind, as well as seven other combined schools for both blind and deaf-mute pupils.

Lightning Source UK Ltd.
Milton Keynes UK
UKHW010632010219
336547UK00009B/741/P